THE OPHTHALMIC ASSISTANT

ELEVENTH EDITION

THE OPHTHALMIC ASSISTANT

A TEXT FOR ALLIED AND ASSOCIATED OPHTHALMIC PERSONNEL

Harold A. Stein, MD, MSc(Ophth), FRCSC, DOMS(London)
Professor of Ophthalmology and Visual Sciences, University of Toronto, Toronto, Ontario, Canada; Emeritus and Past Chairman, Department of Ophthalmology, Scarborough General Hospital, Scarborough, Ontario, Canada; Emeritus, Mount Sinai Hospital, Toronto, Ontario, Canada; Past Secretary General, International Contact Lens Society of Ophthalmologists, Denver, Colorado; Past President, International Joint Commission on Allied Health Personnel in Ophthalmology, St Paul, Minnesota; Past President, Contact Lens Association of Ophthalmologists, New Orleans, Louisiana; Past President, Canadian Ophthalmological Society, Ottawa, Canada; Co-Director, Bochner Eye Institute, Toronto, Ontario, Canada

Raymond M. Stein, MD, FRCSC
Medical Director, Bochner Eye Institute, Toronto, Ontario, Canada; Professor of Ophthalmology and Visual Sciences, University of Toronto, Ontario, Canada; Board of Directors, Foundation Fighting Blindness, Toronto, Ontario, Canada; Attending Ophthalmologist, Scarborough Hospital, Scarborough, Ontario, Canada; Attending Ophthalmologist, Mount Sinai Hospital, Toronto, Ontario, Canada; Editor, Past President, Canadian Society of Cataract and Refractive Surgery, Montreal, Quebec, Canada; Past Commissioner, International Joint Commission on Allied Health Personnel in Ophthalmology, St Paul, Minnesota

Melvin I. Freeman, MD, FACS, FACEHP
Clinical Professor of Ophthalmology, Emeritus, University of Washington School of Medicine, Seattle, Washington; Affiliate Clinical Investigator, Benaroya Research Institute at Virginia Mason, Seattle, Washington; Past Head, Section of Ophthalmology, Virginia Mason Clinic and Medical Center, Seattle, Washington; Medical Director, Emeritus, Department of Continuing Medical Education, Virginia Mason Medical Center, Seattle, Washington; Past President, Alliance for Continuing Medical Education, Birmingham, Alabama; Past President, Contact Lens Association of Ophthalmologists, New Orleans, Louisiana; Past President, International Joint Commission on Allied Health Personnel in Ophthalmology, St Paul, Minnesota; Chair, Joint Commission on Allied Health Personnel in Ophthalmology Education and Research Foundation, St Paul, Minnesota

Rebecca L. Stein, MD, FRCSC
Medical Degree from University of St Andrews, Scotland, and University of Manchester, England; Ophthalmology Residency, University of Toronto, Ontario, Canada; Fellowship in Cornea, External Disease, Cataract, and Refractive Surgery, Ophthalmic Consultants of Long Island, New York; Staff Ophthalmologist, Bochner Eye Institute, Toronto, Ontario, Canada

ELSEVIER

Contents

Preface

Many ophthalmic assistants and technicians have no opportunity for formal training and learn their duties on the job. Experience and repetition alone may become excellent teachers. To paraphrase Sir William Osler, experience without knowledge is to sail an uncharted course, but knowledge without experience is never to go to sea at all. *The Ophthalmic Assistant* was written expressly for ancillary ophthalmic workers who assist eye doctors in the day-to-day care of eye patients. This book was designed to fill a vacuum in our community by providing a training basis for eye care personnel and meeting their needs for a reference source. The textbook has become a textbook of practical ophthalmology.

Originally published over 55 years ago in 1968, *The Ophthalmic Assistant* has grown in size by over 300%. It became necessary to continually expand the textbook to reflect the explosive growth of ophthalmic knowledge and ophthalmic technology. Over the years, we broadened the scope of the textbook to provide not only practical technical information but also background information on ophthalmic disease processes and surgical procedures. In this 11th edition, we attempted to keep pace with the ever-expanding new developments in the field of eye care by updating each chapter. At the same time, we have tried to retain the original concept: to provide a concise, up-to-date review of the field of eye care that is easily readable, interesting, and illustrated.

The Ophthalmic Assistant provides reliable and competent information on eye care procedures, including visits to offices, clinics, and hospitals. Ophthalmic assistants must be familiar with sterile procedures, types of emergencies, and many technical aspects of eye care. This knowledge can increase the ophthalmic assistant's efficiency, ensuring that all details of diagnostic workup and regimen are understood and carried out. Although *The Ophthalmic Assistant* emphasizes the paramedical functions of the ophthalmic assistant and not the secretarial duties, we recognize that both positions in a small office may have to be carried out by the same individual.

We purposely avoided controversial subjects and highly specialized technical areas because of the varying degrees of training of eye care assistants throughout the world. Rather, the emphasis is placed on illustrations and photographs that illuminate and clarify ophthalmic technology and foster interest wherever possible.

Although the main thrust of this book is toward the ophthalmic assistant, we hope the clarity, organization, and readability of the book will attract others in the ophthalmic community. To accommodate these readers, we included sections for the hospital ophthalmic assistant who aids in surgery, for the nurse who aids in the surgical and postoperative care of patients after surgery, and for the optometrist and their assistants to provide information in recognizing diseases and disorders, particularly glaucoma and retinal disorders. We also include material of interest to those individuals working for optical and associated pharmaceutical companies. We have added and updated material for contact lens technicians, with a more detailed review to be found in our companion book, *Fitting Guide for Hard and Soft Contact Lenses*, 4th edition, published by Mosby. A companion book, *Ophthalmic Terminology*, 3rd edition, published by Mosby, serves to expand the glossary and is designed for learning vocabulary and the origins of words. An additional publication, *Ophthalmic Dictionary and Vocabulary Builder for Eye Care Professionals*, 4th edition, authored by H.A. Stein, R.M. Stein, M.I. Freeman, and J.S. Massare and published by Jaypee-Highlights Medical Publishers, is also available for learning vocabulary and original words.

Refractive surgery and computerized corneal topography are two areas of eye care delivery that generate great clinical interest. The 11th edition expands on the chapter on refractive surgery with new emphasis on corneal and intraocular techniques, as well as the section on computerized corneal topography.

We miss the influence and contributions of our previous coauthor, Dr. Bernard Slatt, whose passing came shortly after the seventh edition was published. His memory gave us input, motivation, and direction in continuing this work.

We are also deeply saddened by the passing, just after the 11th edition manuscript was submitted to the publisher, of our dear colleague, Harold A. Stein, MD, FRCSC. Dr. Stein was a true scholar, a visionary, a gentleman, a leader, and a true friend and mentor. He took his coauthors under his wing and offered us opportunities to participate with him in his many lectures, programs, books, and papers. He will truly be missed by all of us, but his accomplishments will live on in those he mentored and in his vast contributions to medicine, ophthalmology, and the education of allied ophthalmic personnel.

We are delighted that Rebecca L. Stein, MD, FRCSC has joined us as a coauthor and editor of the text. She represents the fourth generation of the Bochner/Stein's in their dedication to optimal patient eye care and the education of allied and associate ophthalmic personnel.

We gratefully acknowledge our newly invited 23 chapter authors and coauthors whose names appear in the List of Contributors with our continuing chapter authors. Our deep appreciation is extended to our nine retiring chapter authors and coauthors whose names join our Acknowledgments list of past contributors and reviewers of previous editions.

New chapters have been added for the 11th edition on refractive surgery, eye banking, and an updated, atlas of common ocular conditions.

Harold A. Stein
Raymond M. Stein
Melvin I. Freeman
Rebecca L. Stein

Acknowledgments

For aid and support for the eleventh edition, we thank Kayla Wolfe, Nicole Congleton, Manikandan Chandrasekaran, and the contributors and reviewers.

Acknowledgments for aid as reviewers or contributors in previous editions:

Bud Appleton	Therese Fredette	Laurette LaRocque	Penny Cook Pilliar
Richard Augustine	Ivan Gareau	Les Landecker	Christine Quach
Howard S. Barneby	Alice Gelinas	Daniella	Karen Quam
Joseph T. Barr	Paul Graczyk	Lent-Schochet	Paula Quigley
Tony Benson	Desmond Grant	John Lloyd	Robert Rosen
Bernard R. Blais	Mark Grieve	Sze Kong Luke	Barnet Sakler
Maxwell K. Bochner	Darrell Guthmiller	Bernice Mandelcorn	Abraham Schlossman
Arielle Brickman	David L. Guyton	Theodore Martens	Ernest R. Simpson
Zijie Cai	G. Peter Halberg	Lynn D. Maund	Anne Skryzpnik
Albert Cheskes	Barbara T. Harris	Gerald E. Meltzer	Bruce E. Spivey
Jordan Cheskes	Keith Harrison	Richard P. Mills	Laurie Stein
John Crawford	William Hunter	Edyie G. Miller-Ellis	Kenneth Swanson
Norman Deer	John Hymers	Donald Morin	Spencer Thornton
Katherine Delmer	Anne Jackson	Korosh Nikeghbal	Alyssa Tipple
William H. Ehlers	Mo Jalie	Sherrine Nunes	Russell N. Van Gelder
Saul Fainstein	Jerome Kazdan	Kenneth Ogle	Perry Yan
Tina Felfeli	Edna Kelly	Thomas D Padrick	Len Waldbaum
Zoraida Fiol-Silva	D'Arcy Kingsmill	John Parker	Becky Walsh
Desmond Fonn	Jill Klintworth	Thomas Pashby	E. Edward Wilson, Jr.
John Fowler	Steven Kraft	Charles J. Pavlin	Sheffield Wo
		Scot M Peterson	Kenneth Woodward

List of Contributors

The editors would like to acknowledge and offer grateful thanks for the input of all previous editions' contributors without whom the new edition would not have been possible.

Sara M. AlShaker, MD, FRCSC
Cornea, External Ocular Diseases and Refractive Surgery
Department of Ophthalmology and Vision Sciences
University of Toronto
Toronto, ON, Canada;
Department of Ophthalmology, College of Medicine
King Saud University
Riyadh, Saudi Arabia
(Chapters 8 and 21)

Lynn D. Anderson, PhD
CEO, Executive
International Joint Commission on Allied Health Personnel in
    Ophthalmology
St. Paul, MN, USA
(Chapters 50, 51, 52, and 53)

Parnian Arjmand, MD, MSc, FRCSC
Vitreoretinal Surgery Fellow
Department of Ophthalmology and Vision Sciences
University of Toronto
Toronto, ON, Canada
(Chapter 24)

William F. Astle, MD, FRCSC
Pediatric Ophthalmology Vision Clinic
Alberta Children's Hospital;
Professor, Surgery
University of Calgary
Calgary, AB, Canada
(Chapters 50, 51, and 52)

M. Bernadette Ayres, MD
Kellogg Eye Center
Department of Ophthalmology and Visual Sciences
University of Michigan
Ann Arbor, MI, USA
(Chapter 43)

Michael S. Berlin, MD, MSc, FAAO
Founder and Director
Departments of Clinical Care and Laser Research
Glaucoma Institute of Beverly Hills
Beverly Hills, CA, USA;
Professor of Clinical Ophthalmology
Department of Glaucoma
UCLA Stein Eye Institute
Los Angeles, CA, USA
(Chapter 25)

Bernard R. Blais, MD
Clinical Professor
Albany Medical College
Albany, NY, USA
(Chapter 9)

Lisa Buckland
Manager
EyeBank
Lions Eye Institute
Perth, Australia;
Chair, Member
Eye Bank Association of Australia and New Zealand
Melbourne VIC, Australia
(Chapter 54)

Masako Chen, MD
Assistant Professor of Ophthalmology
New York Eye and Ear Infirmary of Mount Sinai
New York, NY, USA
(Chapter 27)

Daniel Epstein, MD, PhD, FARVO
Professor Emeritus
University of Uppsala, Sweden
Bern, Switzerland
(Chapter 38)

Peter Y. Evans, MD
Professor Emeritus
Department of Ophthalmology
Georgetown University
Washington, DC, USA
(Chapter 53)

Eleanor E. Faye, MD
Formerly Ophthalmic Surgeon
Manhattan Eye, Ear and Throat
    Hospital, New York
Ophthalmic Consultant, Lighthouse
    Internationale Continuing Education
New York, NY, USA
(Chapter 44)

Joseph D. Freeman, MD, FACEP
Emergency Medicine
Cottage Health
Santa Barbara, CA, USA
(Chapter 45)

Fatimah Gilani, MD, FRCSC, FACS
Ophthalmologist
Ophthalmology
Bochner Eye Institute
Toronto, ON, Canada
(Chapter 40)

Michael J. Gilbert, MD
Comprehensive Ophthalmologist & Medical Retina Specialist
Ophthalmology
Northwest Vision Institute
Bellevue, WA, USA
(Chapter 20)

Michael L. Gilbert, MD
Medical & Surgical Director
Northwest Vision Institute;
Comprehensive Ophthalmologist & Cornea Refractive Specialist
Ophthalmology
Northwest Vision Institute
Bellevue, WA, USA
(Chapter 20)

Richard E. Hackel, MA, CRA, FOPS
Retired, Instructor
Director of Ophthalmic Photography
WK Kellogg Eye Center
Department of Ophthalmology
University of Michigan
Ann Arbor, MI, USA
(Chapter 39)

Melissa A. Jones, MEd, BA
Assistant Administrator
Practice Management
Florida Health Care Plans
Ormond Beach, FL, USA
(Chapter 6)

Susan B. Larson, MBA
Chief Standards\Credentialing Director
International Joint Commission on Allied Health Personnel in
    Ophthalmology
St. Paul, MN, USA
(Chapter 51)

Daniel Lavinsky, MD, PhD
Professor
Ophthalmology
Universidade Federal do Rio Grande do Sul
Porto Alegre, Brazil
(Chapter 35)

Andrea K. Leung, MD, FRCSC
Lecturer
Department of Ophthalmology and Vision Sciences
The Hospital for Sick Children
University of Toronto;
Division of Ophthalmology
Scarborough Health Network
Toronto, ON, Canada
(Chapter 29)

Thellea K. Leveque, MD, MPH
Clinical Professor
Department of Ophthalmology
University of Washington Medicine
Seattle, WA, USA
(Chapter 26)

Alex V. Levin, MD, MHSc, FRCSC
Chief, Pediatric Ophthalmology and Ocular Genetic
Ophthalmology
Flaum Eye Institute;
Chief, Pediatric Genetics
Golisano Children's Hospital
Professor
Ophthalmology and Pediatrics
University of Rochester
Rochester, NY, USA
(Chapters 28 and 49)

Shoshana (Sue) M. Levine, LDO
Optical Manager, Visual Effects (Retired)
Virginia Mason Medical Center
Seattle, WA, USA
(Chapter 13)

Efrem D. Mandelcorn, MD, FRCSC
Associate Professor
University of Toronto
Department of Ophthalmology and Vision Sciences
Toronto Western Hospital
Toronto, ON, Canada
(Chapter 24)

Csaba L. Mártonyi, CRA, FOPS
Emeritus Associate Professor
University of Michigan Medical School
Ann Arbor, MI, USA
(Chapter 39)

Lynn D. Maund, BA, SC, CLS
Director
Contact Lens Services
Scarborough Eye Associates
Laser Surgery Consultant
Refractive Eye Surgery
Bochner Eye Institute
Past Director
Ontario Contact Lens Association
Toronto, ON, Canada
(Chapter 17)

John S. Massare, BA, MS, PhD
Former Executive Director (Retired), Contact Lens Association
  of Ophthalmologists
The Villages, FL, USA
(Chapter 9)

Chryssa McAlister, MD, MHSc, FRCSC
Ophthalmology Division
Saint Mary's General Hospital
Kitchener, ON, Canada
(Chapter 49)

Gerald E. Meltzer, MD, MSHA
Emeritus Assistant Clinical Professor
Ophthalmology
University of Colorado
Denver, CO, USA
(Chapter 20)

Richard P. Mills, MD, MPH
Clinical Professor
Department of Ophthalmology
University of Washington
Past President, American Academy of Ophthalmology
Seattle, WA, USA
(Chapter 19)

Hayley Monson, Bsc
Student
Department of Ophthalmology and Vision Sciences
University Health Network
McMaster University
Hamilton, ON, Canada
(Chapter 24)

Rod A. Morgan, MD, FRCSC, Dipl ABO, FAAO, LMCC
Clinical Professor
Ophthalmology & Visual Sciences
University of Alberta
Edmonton, AB, Canada
(Chapter 48)

Eduardo V. Navajas, MD, PhD
Clinical Assistant Professor
Ophthalmology
University of British Columbia
Vancouver, BC, Canada
(Chapter 35)

Anne K. Nguyen, MS, BS
Research Study Coordinator
Ophthalmology
Glaucoma Institute of Beverly Hills
Beverly Hills, CA, USA
(Chapter 25)

Korosh Nikeghbal
Refracting Optician
Contact lens
Bochner eye institute
Toronto, ON, Canada
(Chapter 17)

Neel D. Pasricha, MD
Assistant Professor
Department of Ophthalmology
University of California San Francisco
San Francisco, CA, USA
(Chapter 27)

Carol J. Pollack-Rundle, BS, COMT
Past President
ATPO, Association of Technical Personnel in Ophthalmology
Louisville, KY, USA;
Retired, Director of Clinic Compliance and Technician
  Education
Department of Ophthalmology and Visual Sciences
Michigan Medicine
Ann Arbor, MI, USA
(Chapter 7)

Phyllis L. Rakow, COMT, NCLEM, FCLSA(H)
Director
Contact Lens Services
Princeton Eye Group
Princeton, NJ, USA
(Chapter 47)

Hans-Walter Roth, MD
Visiting Professor
Eye Clinic
Contact Lens Department
The Institute of Contact Lens Optics
Ulm, Germany
(Chapter 46)

A. Ghani Salim, MD
Clinical and Research Director
Ophthalmology
Bochner Eye Institute
Toronto, ON, Canada
(Chapter 41)

Jonathan Shakibkhou, BA, MD Candidate
Research Manager
Ophthalmology
Glaucoma Institute of Beverly Hills
West Hollywood, CA, USA
(Chapter 25)

Victoria M. Sheffield, COMT
Consultant Senior Technical Advisor
USAID's Child Blindness Program at International Eye
    Foundation
Vice Chair
Advisory Board, International Pediatric Ophthalmology and
    Strabismus Council
Board Member, VISION2020/USA
Alexandria, VA, USA
(Chapter 53)

Jeremy Shuman, MPH, CEBT
International Business Development Manager
Lions Eye Institute for Transplant and Research
Tampa, FL, USA
(Chapter 54)

Craig N. Simms, COMT
Chief Learning Officer
Education Department
International Joint Commission of Allied Health Personnel in
    Ophthalmology
St. Paul, MN, USA
(Chapter 50)

Omar Sirsy, MD
Royal College of Surgeons in Ireland
Dublin, Ireland
(Chapter 25)

Tim Steffens, MS, CRA, OCT-C, FOPS
Director
Imaging and Information Systems
University of Michigan Ophthalmology
Kellogg Eye Center
Ann Arbor, MI, USA
(Chapter 39)

Gwen K. Sterns
Chief
Department of Ophthalmology
Rochester General Hospital;
Medical Director
Association for the Blind and Visually Impaired-Goodwill;
Clinical Professor of Ophthalmology
University of Rochester School of Medicine and Dentistry
Rochester, NY, USA
(Chapter 44)

Rahul Singh Tonk, MD
Assistant Professor of Clinical Ophthalmology
Bascom Palmer Eye Institute
University of Miami Miller School of Medicine
Miami, FL, USA
(Chapter 27)

James C. Tsai, MD, MBA
President
Ophthalmology
New York Eye and Ear Infirmary of Mount Sinai
New York, NY, USA
(Chapter 50)

Michael A. Ward, MMSc, FAAO
Instructor (Retired)
Ophthalmology
Emory University School of Medicine
Atlanta, GA, USA
(Chapter 5)

Joanne C. Wen, MD
Associate Professor
Ophthalmology
Duke Eye Center
Durham, NC, USA
(Chapter 19)

List of Reviewers

Lynn D. Anderson, PhD (Overall Review)

Barbara T. Harris, PA, MBA, OSC (Overall Review)

Korosh Nikeghbal, Refracting Optician (Chapters 14, 15, and 16)

Carol J. Pollack-Rundle, BS, COMT (Overall Review)

Craig Simms, BSc, COMT, ROUB, CDOS (Overall Review)

Dedication

Dr. Maxwell K. Bochner

A master ophthalmic clinician whose skillful guidance and use of ancillary personnel in ophthalmology permitted the delivery of quality eye care to a large number of visually disabled individuals. A caring and concerned physician who developed a strong bond with each and every patient.

Dr. Bernard J. Slatt

A gifted ophthalmologist whose untimely passing was a great loss to ophthalmology. He was a major contributor to previous editions of this textbook. An accomplished ophthalmologist, writer, father, and grandfather who contributed greatly in advancing the role of allied health personnel in ophthalmology.

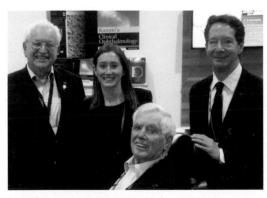

(L to R) Drs. Melvin I. Freeman, Rebecca L. Stein, Harold A. Stein, Raymond M. Stein

Dr. Harold A. Stein

A brilliant, kind, warm, and generous ophthalmic physician and surgeon with a great sense of humor. He was larger than life, a talented surgeon and teacher, an innovative and creative thinker, a renaissance man with a wide range of interests, and a storyteller with a twinkle in his eye. He loved to recount his adventures of working in developing countries, discovering new surgical techniques and to share his many observations and ideas for academic studies. He was a beloved father, grandfather, and great grandfather.

Chapter | **1** |

Anatomy of the eye

Although the eye is commonly referred to as the *globe*, it is not really a true sphere. It is composed of two spheres with different radii, one set into the other (Figs. 1.1 and 1.2). The front, or anterior, sphere, which is the smaller and more curved of the two, is called the *cornea*. The cornea is the window of the eye because it is a completely transparent structure. It is the more curved of the two spheres and sets into the other as a watch glass sets into the frame of a watch. The posterior sphere is a white opaque fibrous shell called the *sclera*. The cornea and the sclera are relatively nondistensible structures that encase the eye and form a protective covering for all the delicate structures within.

In terms of size, the eye measures approximately 24 mm in all its main diameters in the normal adult.

Surface anatomy

The eye itself is covered externally by the *eyelids*, which are movable folds protecting the eye from injury and excessive light. The lids serve to swab the eye and spread a film of tears over the cornea, thereby preventing evaporation from the surface of the eye. The upper eyelid extends to the *eyebrow*, which separates it from the forehead, whereas the lower eyelid usually passes without any line of demarcation into the skin of the cheek. The upper eyelid is the more mobile of the two and when it is open it covers about 1 mm of the cornea. A muscle that elevates the lid, the *levator palpebrae superioris*, is always active, contracting to keep the eyelid open. During sleep the eyelid closes by relaxation of this muscle. The lower lid lies at the lower border of the cornea when the eye is open and rises slightly when it shuts.

Normally, when the eyes are open, a triangular space is visible on either side of the cornea. These triangular spaces, formed by the junction of the upper and lower lids, are called the *canthi* (Fig. 1.3). These canthi are denoted by the terms *medial* and *lateral*, the former being closer to the nasal bridge. Most eyes are practically the same size; therefore when we speak of the eyes appearing large or small, we usually refer not to the actual size but to the portion of the eyeball visible on external examination, which in turn depends on the size of the *palpebral fissure*. The shape of the fissure also determines its appearance. In Asian persons, a fold of skin extends from the upper lid to the lower lid and covers the medial fissure, giving the eye its characteristic obliquity. In the medial fissure there are two fleshy mounds: the deeper one, called the *plica semilunaris*, and the superficial one, called the

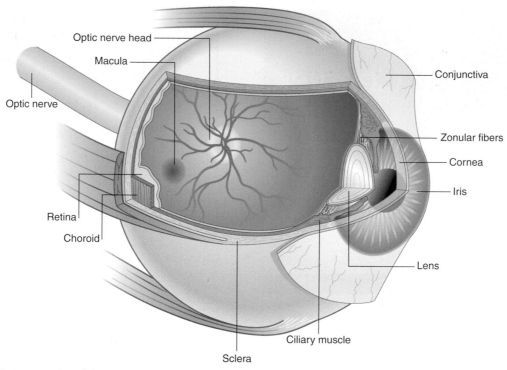

Fig. 1.1 Cutaway section of the eye.

Optic nerve head

Macula

Optic nerve

Conjunctiva

Zonular fibers

Cornea

Iris

Retina

Choroid

Lens

Ciliary muscle

Sclera

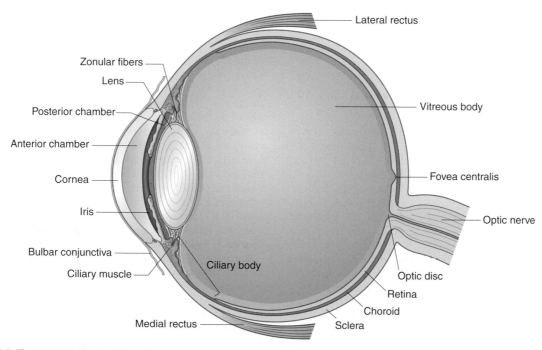

Fig. 1.2 The eye cut in horizontal section.

Lateral rectus

Zonular fibers

Lens

Posterior chamber

Anterior chamber

Cornea

Iris

Bulbar conjunctiva

Ciliary muscle

Ciliary body

Medial rectus

Vitreous body

Fovea centralis

Optic nerve

Optic disc

Retina

Choroid

Sclera

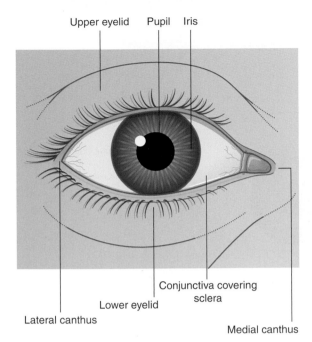

Fig. 1.3 Surface anatomy of the eye.

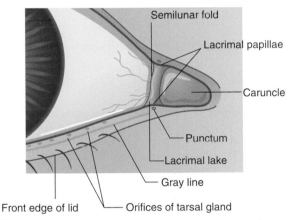

Fig. 1.4 Inner canthus, showing the semilunar fold and the caruncle. Normally, the punctum is not visible unless the lower lid is depressed.

caruncle (Fig. 1.4). The caruncle is modified skin that contains sweat and oil glands. Occasionally, it also contains fine cilia or hairs. When the eyes are open, the palpebral fissures measure about 30 mm in width and 15 mm in height.

The free margin of each lid is about 2 mm thick and has an anterior and a posterior border. From the anterior, or front, border rises the *eyelashes*, which are hairs arranged in two or three rows. The upper eyelid lashes are longer

and more numerous than the lower ones and they tend to curl upward. The lashes are longest and most curled in childhood. The posterior border of the lid margin is sharp and tightly abuts against the front surface of the globe. By depressing the lower lid, one can see the thin *gray line* that separates the two borders of the lid. This gray line is used in many surgical procedures to split the upper and lower lids into two portions. Also visible on both lids are the tiny openings that are the orifices of the sweat- and oil-secreting glands.

The largest oil-secreting glands, which are embedded in the posterior connective tissue substance of the lids (called the *tarsus*), are called the *meibomian glands*. The *lacrimal gland* is located above and lateral to the globe. Tears are produced by the lacrimal gland and travel through fine channels, referred to as *ducts*, to empty onto the conjunctival surface.

On the medial aspect of the lower lid where the lashes cease is a small *papilla*. At the apex of this papilla is a tiny opening called the *punctum* (see Fig. 1.4). The punctum leads, by means of a small canal, through the lower lid to the *lacrimal sac* (Fig. 1.5), which eventually drains into the nose. Tears are carried to the punctum by the pumping action of the lids and there they are drained effectively from the eye by means of tiny channels. A similar but smaller opening is found in the upper lid almost directly above it. The punctum normally cannot be seen by looking directly at the eye. It can be seen only by depressing the lower lid or everting the upper lid. The muscle underlying the eyelid skin is the *orbicularis oculi*, which is roughly circular. When it contracts, it closes the eye.

The portions of the eye that are normally visible in the palpebral fissures are the *cornea* and *sclera*. Because the cornea is transparent, what is seen on looking at the cornea is the underlying *iris* and the black opening in the center of the iris is called the *pupil*. The sclera forms the white of the eye and is covered by a mucous membrane called the *conjunctiva*. The conjunctiva extends from the junction of the cornea and sclera and terminates at the inner portion of the lid margin (Fig. 1.6). The conjunctiva that covers the eye itself is referred to as the *bulbar conjunctiva*, whereas the portion that lines the inner surface of the upper and lower lids is called the *palpebral conjunctiva*. The junctional bay created when the two portions of the conjunctiva meet is referred to as the *fornix*. The lower fornix easily can be viewed by depressing the lower lid.

The role of the conjunctiva is to defend and repair the cornea in the event of scratches, wounds, or infections. The almost invisible blood vessels that are present dilate and leak nutrients, antibodies, and leukocytes into the tears that then wash over the avascular corneal surface. The conjunctiva also secretes mucus and oil, both of which help to keep the cornea moist and clean and to reduce friction when the lids blink over the cornea. The conjunctival mucous

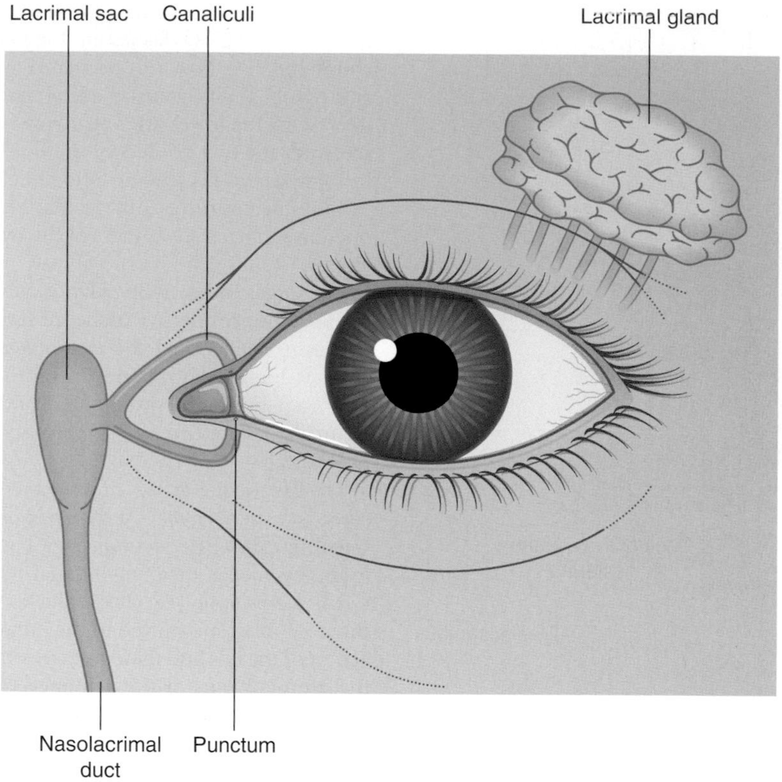

Fig. 1.5 Lacrimal apparatus. Tears produced by the lacrimal gland are drained through the punctum, lacrimal sac, and nasolacrimal duct into the nose.

film over the ocular surface catches microorganisms. This mucous net then condenses into a ball and is carried to the nasal canthus where it dries and rolls onto the skin. The conjunctiva also helps to resurface the cornea with epithelial cells if the entire corneal surface is scraped or burned.

Under the conjunctiva is a fibrous layer that overlies the sclera and rectus muscles. This is *Tenon's capsule,* a common surgical landmark.

Tear film

The tear film is composed of three layers (Fig. 1.7). The outermost layer consists of a lipid or fatty layer, mostly cholesterol esters, and is extremely thin. This layer is secreted by the meibomian glands and acts to prevent evaporation of the underlying aqueous layer. The central layer is chiefly aqueous, with some dissolved salts, as well as glucose, urea, proteins, and lysozyme. This layer is secreted by the lacrimal glands. The third layer is a very thin mucous layer lying over the surface of the conjunctiva and cornea. This layer is secreted by specific cells of the conjunctiva referred to as *goblet cells* and is important in the stability of the tear film. Tear film abnormalities may arise in association with a number of clinical problems in older adults and in particular problems related to contact lenses.

1. The precorneal tear film layer serves several functions. It forms a smooth refractive surface on the epithelium. It maintains a moist environment for the epithelium. It carries oxygen to the eye.

Cornea

The cornea is a clear, transparent structure with a brilliant, shiny surface. It has a convex surface that acts as a powerful lens. Most of the refraction of the eye takes place not through the crystalline lens of the eye but through the cornea.

The cornea is relatively large at birth and almost attains its adult size during the first and second years. Although

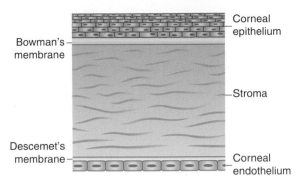
Fig. 1.8 The cornea in cross-section showing the position and sequence of the layers (illustration not to scale).

Labels in Fig. 1.8: Corneal epithelium, Bowman's membrane, Stroma, Descemet's membrane, Corneal endothelium

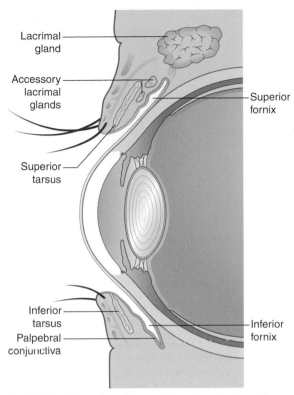
Fig. 1.6 Vertical section of the eyelids and conjunctiva. The lids act as a protective curtain for the eye. Only a small portion of the eye is actually exposed.

Labels in Fig. 1.6: Lacrimal gland, Accessory lacrimal glands, Superior tarsus, Superior fornix, Inferior fornix, Inferior tarsus, Palpebral conjunctiva

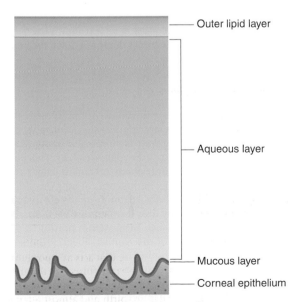
Fig. 1.7 Three-layer structure of the tear film.

Labels in Fig. 1.7: Outer lipid layer, Aqueous layer, Mucous layer, Corneal epithelium

the eyeball as a whole increases a little less than 3 times in volume from birth to maturity, the corneal segment plays a small role in this part, being fully developed by 2 years of age.

The cornea is thicker at its periphery (1 mm) than at the center (0.5 mm). It can be divided into five distinct portions (Fig. 1.8): the epithelium, Bowman's membrane, the stroma, Descemet's membrane, and the endothelium.

The *epithelium* is the part of the cornea usually injured by superficial abrasions or small foreign bodies. It is 5 to 7 cells thick (50 μm) and is composed of nonkeratinized stratified squamous cells. The epithelium functions as a barrier and as an important refractive optical surface. It regenerates rapidly and heals without leaving a scar. Injury to the deeper structures usually results in formation of an opacity in the cornea.

Bowman's membrane consists of randomly oriented collagen fibrils of greater periodicity than the underlying stroma. This acellular layer, which is 10 μm thick, has no regenerative capabilities. Its function is unclear.

The layer just under Bowman's membrane is the *stroma*. This structure is 950 μm at the periphery and about 450 μm centrally; it accounts for 90% of the corneal thickness. The stroma consists of 200 to 250 evenly spaced type I collagen lamellae, which are oriented at right angles to their adjacent lamellae. It is composed of 78% water.

Descemet's membrane is 3 μm thick at birth, and 10 to 12 μm thick in older adults. It is composed of type III collagen. This very elastic layer retracts if cut. It forms the basement membrane of the epithelial cells.

The *endothelium* is a 4 to 6 μm monolayer of 500,000 cells. There is a gradual decrease in endothelial cells with age. There is no known mechanism of attachment between the endothelium and Descemet's membrane. The endothelium is responsible for maintaining deturgescence of the cornea. No regeneration of this layer has been shown in humans. Corneal edema (swelling) can occur when contact lens materials, overwear, improper cleaning, or improper fit does not allow sufficient oxygen to reach the cornea.

The junction of the cornea and sclera is demarcated by a gray, semitransparent area referred to as the *limbus*. This transitional zone is only 1 mm wide and marks the point of insertion of the conjunctiva. The cornea, which contains no blood vessels, is completely nourished by three sources: a plexus of fine capillaries at the limbus, the tear film, and the aqueous humor.

In a paper published in *Ophthalmology* in 2013, by Dua et al, the existence of a newly described pre-Descemet's layer, hypothetically 15 μm thick, was suggested. Time will be needed to see if others can confirm the existence of this new layer and its potential significance.

Sclera

The opaque sclera forms the posterior five-sixths of the eye's protective coat. Its anterior portion is visible and constitutes the white of the eye. In children, the sclera is thin and therefore it appears bluish because the underlying pigmented structures are visible through it. In old age, it may become yellowish because of the deposition of fat. Attached to the sclera are all the extraocular muscles. Through the sclera pass the nerves and the blood vessels that penetrate the interior of the eye. At its most posterior portion, the site of attachment of the *optic nerve*, the sclera becomes a thin, sieve-like structure called the *lamina cribrosa*, through which the retinal fibers leave the eye to form the optic nerve. The episcleral tissue is a loose connective and elastic tissue that covers the sclera and unites it with the conjunctiva above. Unlike the sclera, the episcleral tissue is highly vascular.

Uvea

The *uveal* tract consists of three structures: the *iris, ciliary body*, and *choroid*.

Iris

The *iris* is the most anterior structure of the uveal tract. It is perforated at its center by a circular aperture called the *pupil*. The iris has many ridges and furrows on its anterior surface. Contraction of the iris, which occurs in response to bright light, is accomplished by the activity of a flat, washer-like muscle called the *sphincter pupillae*, buried in its substance just surrounding the pupillary opening. Expansion or dilation of the pupil is facilitated by relaxation of the sphincter muscle and by activation of the radially oriented dilator muscle of the iris found at its peripheral circumference.

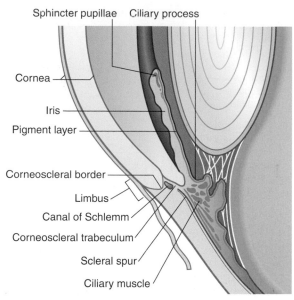

Fig. 1.9 Ciliary body and angle structures of the eye. The angle is formed between the iris and the back surface of the cornea, with the aqueous humor of the anterior chamber interposed. The angle structures include the corneoscleral trabeculum, Schlemm's canal, scleral spur, a small extension of the ciliary muscle, and the root of the iris.

Expansion and contraction of the iris, like an accordion, form circular pleat lines or furrows visible on its surface. In addition to these ridges and furrows, numerous white zigzag lines are formed by the blood vessels of the iris. Between the iris and the cornea is a clear fluid called the *aqueous humor*. This fluid occupies the space called the *anterior chamber* of the eye.

Ciliary body

The *ciliary body* (Fig. 1.9) is in direct continuity with the iris and is adherent to the underlying sclera. Directly posterior to the iris, the ciliary body is plump and thrown into numerous folds referred to as the *ciliary processes*. This portion of the ciliary body is only about 2.5 mm in length and is responsible for the major production of aqueous fluid. The equator of the lens is only 0.5 mm from the ciliary processes and is suspended by fine, ligamentous fibers known as the *zonular fibers* of the lens. The posterior portion of the ciliary body is flat. Most of the zonular fibers of the lens originate from the ciliary body. The ciliary body in general is triangular, with its shortest side anterior. The anterior side of the triangle in its inner part enters the formation of the angle of the anterior chamber. The iris takes root from its middle portion.

On the outer side of the triangle is the ciliary muscle, which lies against the sclera. Contraction of the ciliary muscle releases the tension of the zonular fibers, controlling the size and shape of the lens. This in turn allows the anterior surface of the lens to bulge forward and increase its power. Therefore the ciliary muscle directly controls the focusing ability of the eye. In children, this muscle is extremely active and the lens is easily deformed, which accounts for its powerful range of accommodation, or focusing abilities. The ciliary muscle declines with age; after the age of 40 years, its power becomes weaker and the lens is less able to change shape, so that focusing at near point, or accommodating, becomes difficult. This condition is commonly referred to as *presbyopia*.

Choroid

The choroid is in direct continuity with the iris and ciliary body and lies between the retina and sclera (see Fig. 1.2). The choroid is primarily a vascular structure. Its primary function is to provide nourishment for the outer layers of the retina.

Angle structures

The angle structures are formed by the tissues posterior to the cornea and anterior to the iris, with the aqueous humor intervening (see Fig. 1.9). Included in the angle structures are: (1) the root of the iris, (2) a portion of the anterior surface of the ciliary body, (3) a *spur* from the sclera, (4) the *canal of Schlemm*, and (5) the *corneoscleral trabeculum*.

Aqueous humor leaves the eye by filtering through the crevices of the *trabecular meshwork*. The trabecular meshwork consists of tiny pores through which aqueous humor travels until it reaches *Schlemm's canal*. From Schlemm's canal, the aqueous humor leaves the eye through the aqueous veins that penetrate the sclera. Obstruction within the trabecular meshwork or the angle structures, by iris or scar tissue, results in raised intraocular pressure and glaucoma.

Lens

The lens of the eye is a transparent biconvex structure situated between the iris and the vitreous (Fig. 1.10). Only that portion of the lens not covered by iris tissue (i.e., only that portion directly behind the pupillary space) is visible. The center of the anterior surface of the lens, known as its anterior pole, is only about 3 mm from the back surface of the cornea. The diameter of the lens is about 9 to 10 mm. Its peripheral margin, called the *equator*, lies about 0.5 mm

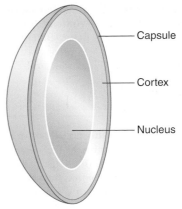

Fig. 1.10 Crystalline lens.

Capsule

Cortex

Nucleus

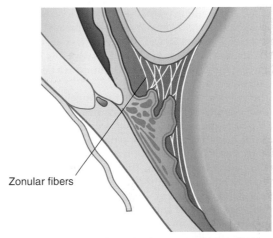

Zonular fibers

Fig. 1.11 Distribution of zonular fibers. Zonular lamella forms the external layer of the lens capsule, consisting of the anterior insertion 1 mm from the equator and the posterior insertion 1.5 mm from the equator. (Modified from Jaffe NS. *The Vitreous in Clinical Ophthalmology*. St Louis: Mosby, 1969.)

from the ciliary processes. It is attached to the ciliary processes and to the posterior portion of the ciliary body by means of fine suspensory ligaments referred to as the *zonular fibers* (Fig. 1.11).

The lens is surrounded by a capsule, which is a transparent, highly elastic envelope. The lens material within this elastic bag is rather soft and putty-like in infants. With age it tends to grow harder, especially toward the center of the lens. The harder central portion of the lens found in adults 30 years of age or older is called the *nucleus* of the lens, and the outer lens fibers form the lens *cortex*. The harder nucleus is a product of the normal developmental growth of the lens. As new lens fibers are produced, the older fibers are pushed more toward the center and are compressed in a concentric fashion. It is this constant lamination of lens fibers over a period of years that eventually produces the nucleus.

Vitreous

The vitreous is a jelly-like structure, thick and viscous, that occupies the vitreous chamber in the posterior concavity of the globe. Actually, it fills the largest cavity of the eye, occupying two-thirds of its volume. It is surrounded mainly by retina. Anteriorly, it forms a slight depression behind the lens and is attached to it around the circumference of this depression. Normally the vitreous is quite transparent.

The vitreous is not simply an inert jelly. Within the body of the vitreous, fine collagen fibers crisscross in a scaffolding manner. The resulting matrix is filled with a viscous mucopolysaccharide, called *hyaluronic acid*. Vitreous is almost 99% water. Hyaluronic acid is a great shock absorber and can compress slowly and rebound slowly. This is important in injuries to the eye from such things as a fast-moving squash ball.

The envelope that surrounds the vitreous is primarily a condensate of the gel and is anchored to the more forward part of the retina, the *ora serrata*, and at the head of the optic nerve along the major retinal blood vessels. If the vitreous shrinks, the resulting tension on its anchors can produce a tear in the retina. This may permit the adjacent vitreous to enter between the choroid and retina and produce a retinal detachment.

With age, some of the collagen fibers of the vitreous often break away from the main structure. These may condense into strands and float freely in the watery sections of the vitreous. Patients often see floating specks or webs that move as their eyes move and that are mildly annoying but usually harmless. These often disappear in time.

Retina

The retina, which contains all the sensory receptors for the transmission of light, is really part of the brain. The retinal receptors are divided into two main populations: the *rods* and the *cones*. The rods function best in dim light; the cones function best under daylight conditions. The cones number only about 6 million, whereas the rods number 125 million. Cones enable us to see small visual angles with great acuity. Vision with rods is relatively poor. Color vision is totally dependent on the integrity of the cones. The cones form a concentrated area in the retina known as the *fovea*, which lies in the center of the *macula lutea*. Damage to this area can severely reduce the ability to see directly ahead. The rods are distributed in the periphery of the retina (not in the macula). Damage to these structures results in night blindness but with retention of good visual acuity for objects straight ahead.

The junction of the periphery of the retina and the ciliary body is called the *ora serrata*. In the extreme periphery of the retina there are no cones and only a few rods. The retina is firmly attached to the choroid at the ora serrata. This is the reason that retinal detachments never extend beyond the ora serrata. The other site of firm attachment of the retina is at the circumference of the optic nerve. The posterior layer of the retina, called the *pigment epithelium*, is firmly secured to the choroid. Retinal detachment occurs as a result of cleavage between its anterior layers and the posterior pigment layer.

Optic nerve

The optic nerve is located at the posterior portion of the globe and transmits visual impulses from the retina to the brain itself. Only the head of the optic nerve, called the *optic disc*, can be seen by ophthalmoscopic examination (Fig. 1.12).

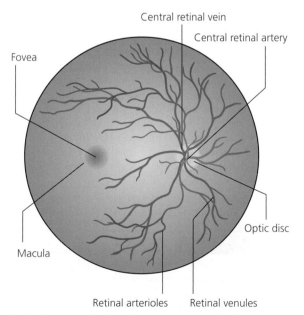

Fig. 1.12 Normal fundus. Note that the central retinal vein emerges from the optic disc lateral to the central retinal artery.

The optic nerve contains no sensory receptors itself and therefore its position corresponds to the normal blind spot of the eye. Branching out from the surface of the optic disc are the *retinal arterioles* and *veins*, which divide soon after leaving the optic disc and extend out on the surface of the retina to supply the inner one-third with nutrients.

As the optic disc enters the globe, it goes through a fibrous, sieve-like structure, visible on ophthalmoscopic examination, called the *lamina cribrosa*. When the lamina cribrosa is prominent, it forms the base of a depression in the disc called the *physiologic cup*.

The optic nerve consists of 1 million axons arising from the ganglion cells of the retina. The nerve emerges from the back of the eye through a small circular opening. It extends for 25 to 30 mm and travels within the muscle cone to enter the bony optic foramen. From there it travels another 4 to 9 mm to pass into the intracranial cavity and joins its fellow optic nerve to form the optic chiasm.

Visual pathway

As the retinal fibers leave the optic nerves, half of them cross to the opposite side (Fig. 1.13). The fibers that cross are derived from the retinal receptors nasal to the macula. The structure so formed by the mutual crossing of nasal fibers by both optic nerves is the *optic chiasm*. From the optic chiasm, the nasal fibers emanating from the nasal half of the retina of one eye intermingle with the fibers derived from the temporal sector of the retina of the opposite eye, forming a band called the *optic tract*.

Fibers in the optic tract continue toward a cell station in the brain called the *lateral geniculate body*, so named because it is shaped like a knee (Latin *genu*). The geniculate body is a relay station from which fibers spread out in a fan-shaped manner and extend to the parietal and temporal lobes of the brain. They continue to their final destination, the posterior portion of the brain called the *"occipital" lobe* in an area denoted as the *visual striate area*. It is in this area of the brain that conscious recognition of visual impulses takes place.

Ocular muscles

Six ocular muscles move the globe: the *medial, lateral, superior,* and *inferior rectus muscles* and the *superior* and *inferior oblique muscles* (Fig. 1.14). The medial rectus muscle moves the eye toward the nose or *adducts* the eye. The lateral rectus muscle moves the eye horizontally to the outer side or

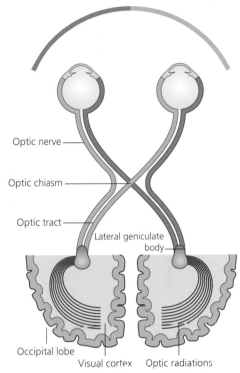

Optic nerve

Optic chiasm

Optic tract

Lateral geniculate body

Occipital lobe

Visual cortex   Optic radiations

Fig. 1.13 Visual pathway. One-half of the visual field from each eye is projected to one side of the brain. Thus visual impulses from the right visual field of each eye will be transmitted to the left occipital lobe.

abducts the eye. The superior rectus muscle elevates the eye primarily, whereas the inferior rectus muscle depresses the eye. The rectus muscles are inserted very close to the limbus, the medial rectus lying approximately 5.5 mm and the lateral rectus approximately 7 mm from the limbus. The rectus muscles are not normally visible because they are covered with conjunctiva and subconjunctival tissue. Because they lie on the surface of the globe, they are readily accessible for muscle surgery.

The superior oblique muscle functions primarily as an intorter by rotating the vertical and horizontal axis of the eye toward the nose; it also functions to depress the eye. The inferior oblique muscle acts to extort and elevate the eye. The oblique muscles are inserted behind the equator of the globe.

In the lid, the *levator palpebrae superioris* muscle serves to elevate the lid, whereas the *orbicularis oculi* muscle closes the eye during winking, blinking, or forced lid closure. If the levator muscle is weak or absent, the lid droops and *ptosis* results.

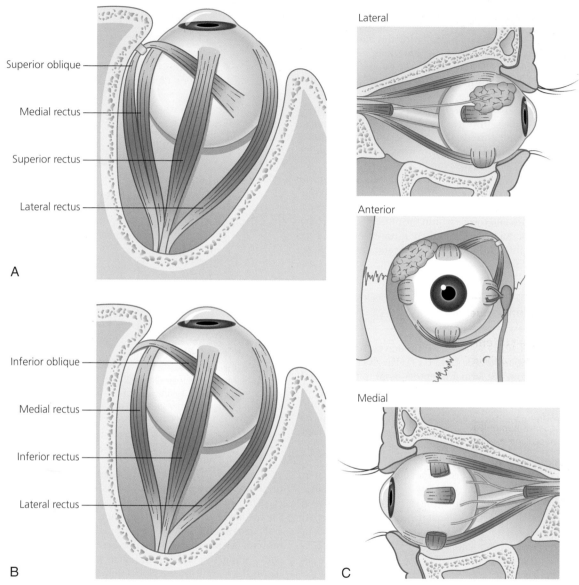

Lateral

Anterior

Medial

Superior oblique

Medial rectus

Superior rectus

Lateral rectus

A

Inferior oblique

Medial rectus

Inferior rectus

Lateral rectus

B

C

Fig. 1.14 (A) Ocular muscles of the right eye viewed from above. Only the oblique muscles are inserted behind the center of rotation of the eye. All the rectus muscles are inserted in front of the center of rotation of the eye near the limbus, where they are easily accessible for muscle surgery. (B) Ocular muscles of the right eye viewed from below. (C) The right eye viewed laterally, anteriorly, and medially.

Summary

A brief sketch of the anatomy of the eye and its surrounding structures has been presented. Each of these structures, when diseased, can give rise to problems, depending on its anatomic location and function. Because many diagnoses made in ophthalmology are formulated from anatomic terminology, familiarity with these structures is essential before any understanding of patients' problems can be realized. The foundation of any course in medicine is based on anatomy. The ophthalmic assistant is advised to learn this section well and use it as a foundation for further reading.

Questions for review and thought

The questions that follow, as well as those following the chapters in the rest of this book, are designed for review of the material. They are intended to sharpen your understanding by testing your knowledge of the material and stimulating you to think. Answers to some of the questions at the end of each chapter may be found in other parts of this book or, in some cases, only in other sources.

1. Draw a horizontal section of the eye with attached muscles and label as many parts as you can without referring to the text.
2. Outline the production and flow of tears.
3. Name the five layers of the cornea.
4. How does the iris contract and expand?
5. Discuss the functions of the rods and cones.
6. Draw the pathway of fibers from the optic nerve to the visual cortex.
7. What is the limbus?
8. How many ocular muscles are attached to the eye? Name them.
9. Describe the muscles that open and close the eye.
10. Describe the macula.
11. What is the ora serrata?
12. At what age is the cornea fully formed? At what age is the rest of the eyeball fully formed?
13. Describe the vitreous.

Self-evaluation questions
Q

True–false statements

Directions: Indicate whether the statement is true (T) or false (F).
1. The main function of the sclera is to keep out light. **T** or **F**
2. If the epithelium of the cornea is damaged, a fine scar will appear. **T** or **F**
3. Aqueous humor leaves the eye by filtering through the trabecular meshwork. **T** or **F**

Missing words

Directions: Write in the missing word(s) in the following sentences.
4. The transparent lens of the eye is attached to the ciliary body by fine suspensory ligaments called _____.
5. The retina consists of rods and cones. The _____ function best in daylight.
6. The head of the optic nerve is called the _____.

Choice-completion questions

Directions: Select the one best answer in each case.
7. The meibomian glands are:
   a. in the ciliary body.
   b. in the tarsus.
   c. in the hair follicles.
   d. associated with the lacrimal glands.
   e. in the conjunctiva.
8. The vitreous body comprises:
   a. the pigment structure of the eye.
   b. the aqueous-forming part of the eye.
   c. the sensory structure of the eye.
   d. two-thirds of the volume of the eye.
   e. the heat-absorbing portion of the eye.
9. The orbicularis oculi is the muscle that:
   a. dilates the pupil.
   b. affects accommodation.
   c. closes the eyelids.
   d. opens the lids.
   e. constricts the pupil.

Answers, notes, and explanations
A

1. **False**. The main function of the sclera is protective. The sclera is a firm fibrous coat that prevents injury from outside the eye and prevents rupture when there is increased intraocular pressure to the globe. The sclera has an opaque white appearance, in contrast to the transparent cornea, because of the greater water content of the sclera and the fact that the collagen fibers are not as uniformly oriented. In some situations, however, the sclera may become exposed and dehydrated and it can become transparent.

2. **False**. The epithelium may be removed partially or completely from the cornea and it has an amazing ability to regenerate completely and cover the other layers of the cornea without leaving a scar. Only if the injury involves the deeper layers of the cornea, such as Bowman's membrane, stroma, or through-and-through lacerations of the cornea, will an opacity form because of scar formation.

3. **True**. Water, electrolytes, and nonelectrolytes enter and leave the eye by diffusion from the ciliary body and by secretion from the epithelium of the ciliary process. From the posterior chamber, the fluid then passes through the pupil into the anterior chamber and out through the filtering trabecular meshwork. From here it passes into Schlemm's canal where about 30 collector channels conduct the fluid to about 12 aqueous veins out into the venous system.

4. **Zonular fibers**. These fine suspensory ligaments are composed of numerous fibrils arising from the surface of the ciliary body and inserting into the lens equator. Normally, the ciliary muscle is relaxed and consequently the zonular fibers are taut, which reduces the anteroposterior diameter of the lens to its minimal dimension. However, when the ciliary muscle contracts to focus light from a near object, the tension is released on the zonular fibers and the lens of the eye assumes a thicker shape, with a correspondingly greater refractive power. This is what occurs during accommodation.

5. **Cones**. The cones are used during daylight to allow detailed vision and color perception. They predominate in the macular area and receive visual images, partially analyze them, and submit this modified information to the brain. If these cones are damaged, the central vision is affected and the patient will have difficulty in reading and discerning small objects in the distance.

6. **Optic disc**. The optic disc is seen with an ophthalmoscope and represents the head of the optic nerve as the nerve bundle fibers pass from the eye back toward the brain. The optic disc corresponds to the normal blind spot of the eye and represents about 1 million axons, which arise from the ganglion cells of the retina. The optic nerve then travels about 25 to 30 mm in the orbit within the muscle cone to enter the bony optic foramen and then the cranial cavity.

7. **b. In the tarsus**. The meibomian glands lie in the tarsus and secrete sebaceous material, which creates an oily layer on the surface of the tear film. This oily layer helps prevent evaporation of the normal tear layer. When these glands become obstructed, they give rise to a condition known as *meibomianitis* and produce internal hordeolum or chalazion.

8. **d. Two-thirds of the volume of the eye**. The vitreous is a structure that occupies the largest cavity of the eye, over two-thirds of its volume. Normally the vitreous is transparent and jelly-like. However, it changes with age and becomes more fluid-like and less jelly-like in high degrees of myopia.

9. **c. Closes the eyelids**. The main function of the orbicularis oculi muscle is to close the eyelid. An accessory function is to evacuate the tear sac so as to continue the pumping action and removal of tears from the conjunctival sac. This muscle is innervated by the seventh cranial nerve so that when this nerve is paralyzed, the eye will fail to close. During intraocular surgery a facial block is often given to paralyze this nerve.

Chapter | 2 |

Physiology of the eye

Physiology of the eye deals with the function of the eye, its capacities, and its limitations. The actual perception of light takes place in a well-delineated area called the *field of vision*. What is not seen beyond these boundaries is cataloged and stored in our visual memory center, so that we are not uncomfortable or handicapped by this imposition. Most eyes cannot form a sharp image on the retina without an internal adjustment made by focusing or by some external appliance, such as lenses placed before them. There is a limit to how much detail the eye can resolve, its magnifying abilities being only 15×, considerably less than most microscopes. The spectrum of light to which our retinal receptors are sensitive is confined to specific wavelengths of light; the world of ultraviolet and infrared is invisible to ordinary perception.

Despite these limitations, the human eye is an extremely versatile instrument capable of seeing both in daylight and in dim light, registering colors, appreciating depth, and exercising rapid focusing adjustments. This chapter deals with the mechanisms that enable the eye to carry out these tasks.

Alignment of the eyes

In human beings the two eyes work as though they were one, both projecting to the same point in space and fusing their images so that a single mental impression is obtained by this collaboration. Without this delicate balance we would "see double" because two images would be formed by the independent action of each eye. In other words, stereopsis would be lost because this faculty is totally dependent on the eyes seeing in unison. The ability of the eyes to fuse two images into a single one is called *binocular vision*.

Binocular vision depends on an exquisite balance of motor and sensory function. The eyes must be parallel when looking straight ahead and they must be able to maintain this alignment when gazing in other positions. Each impulse that directs an eye to move in one direction must be equally received by the other eye. Further, the contraction of an eye muscle pulling the eye in one direction must be accompanied by an equivalent amount of relaxation of its opponent muscle. Without perfectly harmonious eye movement, binocular vision would be impossible because eyes that do not move together do not see together.

Each eye must have good vision because a clear image and a fuzzy image cannot be fused. The brain usually ignores the fuzzy image (suppression). Each macula must have its projection straight ahead, so that the line of vision from each eye intersects at one point in space. Also, the field of vision from each eye must overlap (Fig. 2.1). Although we can see more with two eyes than with one, this difference is not great (~35 degrees) because most of the field of vision from one eye overlaps the field from the other eye. Overlapping visual fields act as a locking device, forging our peripheral vision in place and thereby ensuring central fusion.

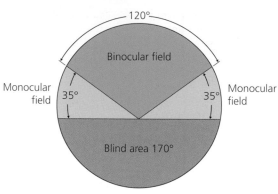

Fig. 2.1 Field of vision. Binocular field of vision (120 degrees) represents the overlapping field of vision from each eye.

Looking straight ahead (fixation)

Fixation involves the simple task of looking straight ahead toward an object in space. Fixation requires stability of the eyes and good monocular function. If the eyes are constantly moving, such as occurs with congenital nystagmus (shaking of the eyes), the eyes can make only scanning motions around an object and never adequately see it in detail. Needless to say, if the ability to fixate becomes compromised by constant eye movements, then the visual acuity of the affected eyes is reduced. If the macula is damaged, then fixation is difficult because anything viewed directly ahead becomes enshrouded in relative darkness.

Fixation can be reduced without organic changes in the eye. Children with strabismus often are found to have poor vision in the turned eye. If a child has crossed eyes, we would think that double vision would occur because the two eyes would not be directed to the same point in space (Fig. 2.2). Children, however, have a wonderful faculty for completely ignoring the image in the turned eye to avoid confusion. It is this constant habit of actively suppressing the image in the turned eye that eventually leads to loss of vision or amblyopia. In some of these children, in whom the suppression mechanism has become profound and the resultant vision very poor, foveal function becomes so depressed that a new point just outside the fovea is used. Such an eye can no longer see straight ahead and the fixation pattern is described as *eccentric*.

Locking images (fusion)

Fusion is the power exerted by both eyes to keep the position of the eyes aligned so that both foveae project to the same point in space. Because fusion is a binocular act, it is

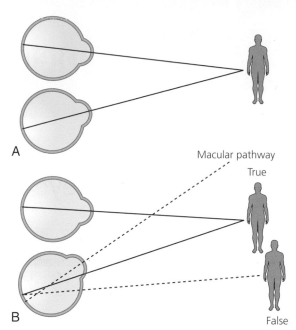

Fig. 2.2 (A) Binocular vision (both eyes looking at the same figure). (B) One eye is turned in, resulting in double vision. In this case the figure is received by the macula of one eye and a point nasal to the macula of the turned eye. The projection of this nasal point results in the person seeing two images instead of one of the same figure. This is an example of uncrossed diplopia, as seen in esodeviations.

easily disrupted by covering one eye. The eye under cover drifts to its fusion-free position. The amount of movement that the eye makes is a measure of the latent muscular imbalance kept in check by fusion, or the amount of heterophoria. *Heterophoria*, then, may be defined as the position the eyes assume when fusion is disrupted. The eye under cover may drift in, called *esophoria*, or drift out, called *exophoria*. The eye also may drift up and down; this position is called *hyperphoria*. Fusion also may be disrupted by placing a Maddox rod before one eye. The Maddox rod changes the size and shape of the image presented to the eye under cover so that fusion becomes impossible.

The power of fusion is measurable by prisms (see Ch. 3). For example, a four-diopter prism is placed with the base toward the nose of an observer looking at a small letter placed 16 inches (40 cm) from the eye. The prism will displace the image before that eye in a direction toward its apex and the eye moves outward to follow it because of the power exerted by the fusional reflex (Fig. 2.3A). Now the prism is removed and the uncovered eye returns to its original position in response to the fusional reflex (Fig. 2.3B). Normally, 20- to 40-prism diopters can be exercised by fusional convergence. The amount of fusion exercised with

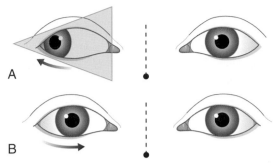

Fig. 2.3 (A) The prism displaces the image toward its apex and the eye moves outward because of the fusional reflex. (B) When the prism is removed, the eye returns to its original position because of the fusional reflex.

respect to divergence is less, being only 10- to 20-prism diopters. This is measured by using base-out prisms. Vertical imbalances are difficult to overcome because our eyes can overcome only about 2- to 4-prism diopters.

Eye movements

The *primary* position of the eyes is the straight-ahead position as they look at a point just below the horizon with the head held erect. Movement of the eye from the primary position to a secondary position occurs when the eyes are moved either horizontally or vertically. If the eyes are directed in an oblique position (up and in or down and in), they are said to be in a tertiary position.

- The movement of one eye from one position to another in one direction is called *duction*. In duction, the fellow

eye is either covered or patched. The movement of two eyes in the same direction is called a *version* (dextro-, levo-, sursum-, and deorsumversion) (Fig. 2.4).

- Eyes right: dextroversion
- Eyes left: levoversion
- Eyes up: sursumversion
- Eyes down: deorsumversion

An outline of the functions of the extraocular muscles is given in Table 2.1. The medial and lateral rectus muscles have only one action: to move the eye horizontally. The other four muscles of the eye have auxiliary functions.

Table 2.1 Actions of extraocular muscles

Muscle	Prime action	Secondary action
Medial rectus	Turns eye inward toward nose or adducts eye	None
Lateral rectus	Turns eye outward toward temples or abducts eye	None
Superior rectus	Elevates eye	Intorsion Adduction
Inferior rectus	Depresses eye	Extorsion Adduction
Superior oblique	Intorts eye	Depression Abduction
Inferior oblique	Extorts eye	Elevation Abduction

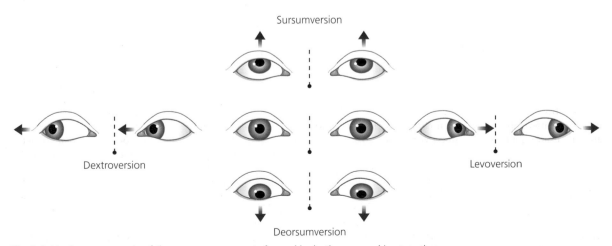

Fig. 2.4 Version movements of the eyes or movements formed by both eyes working together.

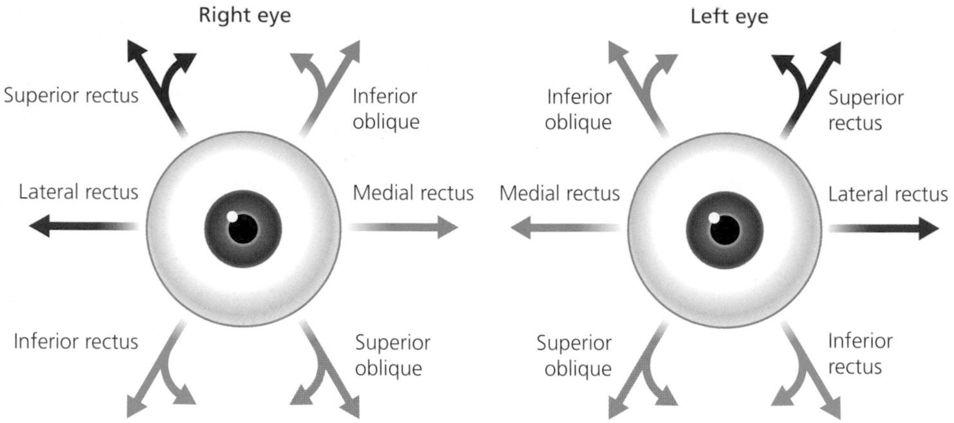

Fig. 2.5 Action of the extraocular muscles. The *arrows* reveal that the superior and inferior rectus muscles function best as an elevator and a depressor, respectively, when the eye is abducted. The inferior and superior oblique muscles function best as an elevator and depressor, respectively, when the eye is adducted.

When these secondary roles are used, assisting the lateral or medial rectus muscles to abduct or adduct, these muscles are called *synergists* (Fig. 2.5).

The main function of the oblique muscles is to rotate the globe either inward *(intorsion)* or outward *(extorsion)*. Intorsion occurs when the eye rotates on its long axis so that the 12 o'clock position on the cornea moves toward the nose. For example, if a point on the cornea of the right eye moves inward from 12 to 1 o'clock, then intorsion is said to occur because of the primary action of the right superior oblique muscle or secondary action of the right superior rectus muscle. Similarly, if the point on the right cornea moves outward from 12 to 11 o'clock, then extorsion is said to occur because of the primary action of the right inferior oblique muscle or secondary action of the right inferior rectus muscle.

Control centers for eye movements

The eyes move in response to our own volition or in a passive manner, such as in following a slow-moving target. Volitional eye movements usually are rapid, starting at high speeds and ending just as abruptly. Such movements occur with reading, when words or phrases are quickly scanned, with an abrupt halt coming at the end of a section or a line. These voluntary eye movements are controlled from centers in the frontal lobe of the brain.

Whereas voluntary eye movements tend to be short and choppy, following or pursuit eye movements are rather slow, smooth, and gliding. The velocity of a following movement depends entirely on the speed of the object the eye is tracking. If the fovea is fixed on a moving target with an angular velocity (<30 degrees per second), the eye follows the target almost

exactly. With greater speeds, following movement becomes difficult and the smooth, gliding movement is replaced with an irregular, jerky movement. Pursuit movements are controlled from centers in the occipital lobe of the brain.

Looking toward a close object

Vergence is the term applied to simultaneous ocular movements in which the eyes are directed to an object in the midline in front of the face. The term is usually applied to *convergence*, in which the eyes rotate inward toward each other, or to *divergence*, in which they rotate outward simultaneously (Fig. 2.6).

Convergence is invariably accompanied by narrowing, or constriction, of the pupils and by accommodation. The triad of convergence, pupillary constriction, and accommodation is often called the *accommodative reflex*, although in the true sense these movements are merely associated reactions (synkinesis) rather than a true reflex. Each component of the triad facilitates fixation at near. The constriction of the pupil is the attempt by the eye to form a pinhole camera device so that a clearer image is seen. Accommodation enables the object to be focused on the retina; convergence brings the eye inward toward the object of regard.

Seeing in depth

The ability to see in depth enables us to travel comfortably in space. Without it, we could not judge distances,

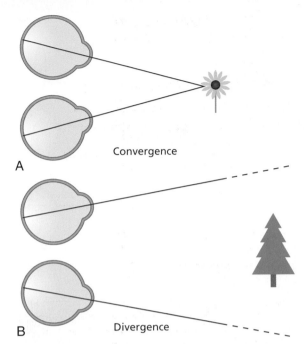

Fig. 2.6 (A) Convergence. The eye is turned in toward the midline plane. (B) Divergence. The eye is turned out, away from the midline plane.

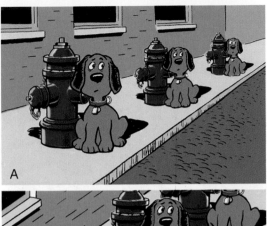

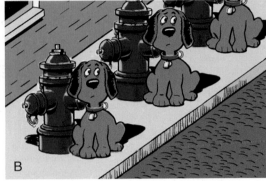

Fig. 2.7 (A) Artist has drawn the picture with proper depth perspective. Monocular clues include decrease in size of dogs and confluence of lines toward a point. (B) Artist has ignored the usual monocular clues so that our appreciation of depth and size is erroneous. The second dog appears larger than the first, although both are the same size.

estimate the size of objects beyond us, or avoid bumping into things. Without depth perception, even the simplest of tasks would be difficult. We would be unable to reach accurately for our morning coffee, and passing a car on the highway would be tantamount to suicide. Fortunately, everyone has some depth perception, whether the person has one eye or two. Those with only one eye learn to estimate depth with monocular clues (Figs. 2.7 and 2.8). They know that the speck in the distance that becomes a huge train standing beside them in the station has not grown larger but has merely come closer. There are other clues in addition to changes in object size. The train tracks spread from a point and become parallel, the color of the train changes from a misty blue-gray to dark green, the sound increases, and when the train is alongside, one can feel the heat.

- There are many monocular clues that facilitate depth perception, including the following: magnification: well-recognized objects, if they become larger, are deemed to be nearer
- Confluence of parallel lines to a point (e.g., railway tracks)
- Interposition of shadows
- Blue-gray mistiness of objects at a great distance
- Parallax: if two objects situated at different points in space are aligned and the head of the observer is moved in one direction, the nearer object will appear to move in the opposite direction

A monocular person, however, if removed from familiar surroundings, would have great difficulty in judging distances because of a lack of any intrinsic depth-perception mechanism. For example, a one-eyed pilot would create a hazard because of the difficulty he or she would experience in maneuvering in space without the normal monocular clues.

Stereopsis is a higher quality of binocular vision. Each eye views an object at a slightly different angle, so that fusion of images occurs by combining slightly dissimilar images. It is the combination of these angular views that yields stereopsis. The same method is used in photography in making three-dimensional pictures. The stereoscopic picture is taken at slightly different angles and later viewed that way.

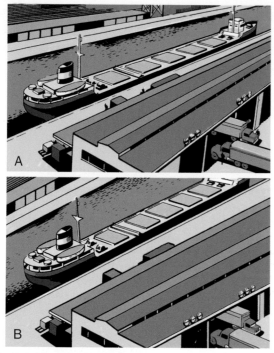

Fig. 2.8 (A) The scene is drawn using normal monocular clues of distance, thereby giving it perspective. (B) The same scene is drawn without regard to the normal impressions of distance. Therefore the scene loses its perspective.

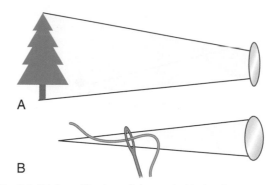

Fig. 2.9 (A) Crystalline lens of the eye is thin for distant objects. (B) Crystalline lens accommodates for near objects by becoming thicker. This increases its effective power.

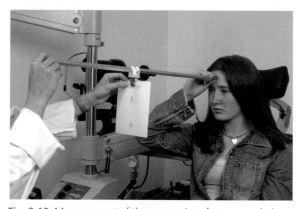

Fig. 2.10 Measurement of the near point of accommodation.

Focusing at near (accommodation)

Any object can be moved from a distance to about 20 feet in front of an observer and still be seen clearly without accommodation. This distance is called the *range of focus*. As the object is brought closer than 20 feet, however, the eye must continuously readjust to keep the image of the object clearly focused on the retina. This readjustment requires an increase in the power of the eye and is brought about by an automatic change in the shape of the lens in response to a blurred image (Fig. 2.9). This zoom-lens mechanism in the eye is very active in children; they are able to see a small letter in clear focus only 7 cm from the eye, whereas an adult of 55 years can focus no closer than 55 cm. The *range of accommodation* is the distance in which an object can be carried toward an eye and be kept in focus. The power of accommodation of an eye is the dioptric equivalent of this distance. By age 75 years, this power is zero.

Both the range and the power of accommodation are measured quite easily (Fig. 2.10). When the full spectacle correction is worn, it is merely the closest point at which an

accommodative target (such as a small letter) can be seen clearly. It usually is equal in both eyes. The range of accommodation is measured in centimeters, whereas the power is converted to diopters (Table 2.2).

This stimulus for accommodation is a blurred image on the retina. As an object is moved closer to the eye, the rays of light entering the pupil must be continuously converged. This change in focusing power of the eyes is brought about by active contraction of the ciliary muscle. The contraction of this muscle causes the zonular fibers of the lens to relax, which in turn allows the lens of the eye to change its shape (Fig. 2.11). In the child and the young adult, the lens can be molded, and it increases its power by becoming thicker and increasing the curvature of its anterior space. In an adult, the ability of the ciliary muscle to effectively contract declines with age and the lens becomes harder and less malleable with advancing years.

The decline in accommodation with age, called *presbyopia*, is remedied with reading glasses or bifocals. It usually becomes apparent by the age of 45 years.

Table 2.2 Accommodation and near point of the normal eye

Age (years)	Near point in centimeters	Available accommodation in diopters
10	7	14
20	9	11
30	12	8
40	22	4.5
45	28	3.5
50	40	2.5
55	55	1.75
60	100	1
65	133	0.75
70	400	0.25
75	Infinity	0

Transparent pathway for light

For light to effectively stimulate retinal receptors, clear media for transmission are necessary. One of the prime functions of the eye is maintenance of the transparent pathway for light (Fig. 2.12).

The *cornea* is the window through which light rays pass on their way to the retina. It is a five-layered transparent structure whose cells and collagen fibers are arranged so that light can pass through it with a minimum of diffraction and internal reflection. The cornea is transparent because its fibrils are arranged in a parallel manner and are tightly packed and separated by less than a wavelength of light. When the cornea is swollen, this arrangement is distorted and the cornea becomes hazy. The cornea contains no opaque substances, such as blood vessels, that would mar its clarity. It receives its nourishment from perilimbal vessels, the tear film, and the aqueous humor. The cornea is kept shiny and lubricated by tears that keep its surface moist and fill out any irregularities in its superficial epithelium.

The *tears* are composed of three main layers. The outermost *oily*, or *lipid*, layer comes from the meibomian gland

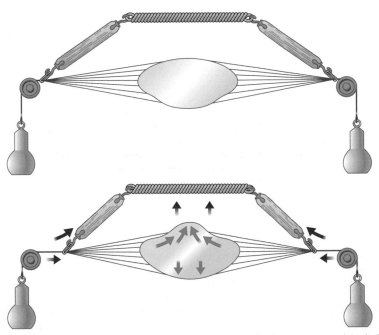

Fig. 2.11 Adjustment of the crystalline lens by accommodation. When the zonular ligaments are relaxed, the inherent elasticity of the lens causes it to increase in thickness and therefore increase in power. (Redrawn from Krug WFS. *Functional Neuro-Anatomy.* New York: The Blakiston Co.; 1953.)

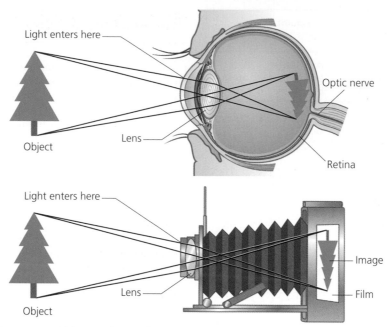

Fig. 2.12 The eye is like a camera. Light must have a clear pathway to be clearly focused on the sensory receptors of the retina or the film of a camera.

and retards evaporation of the aqueous or watery layer. *Aqueous water* makes up the middle layer and arises from the main lacrimal and the accessory lacrimal glands in the conjunctiva. It is filled with inorganic matter, salts, and varying amounts of mucin. This functions to keep the cornea moist. The innermost layer of the tears is *mucin*, which arises from the goblet cells of the conjunctiva and fills in the tiny irregularities of the corneal epithelium, thereby producing a mirror-like finish to the cornea.

The most important factor in maintaining corneal transparency is the ability of the cornea to keep itself relatively dehydrated. If a section of cornea is placed in isotonic saline solution, it becomes hydrated, opaque, and edematous. However, if the sclera is dehydrated, it becomes transparent.

The cornea has an active, pump-like mechanism located in the corneal epithelium and endothelium that enables it to keep itself relatively dehydrated. Damage to the corneal epithelium or endothelium results in the cornea's becoming hydrated and swollen. Swelling of the cornea, be it localized or diffuse, always results in a loss of transparency. If the swelling (i.e., corneal edema) is located centrally, then vision will be blurred. In acute angle-closure glaucoma (see Ch. 25), the sudden rise in intraocular pressure causes epithelial edema. The individual droplets in the epithelium break up white light to its colored spectral components and the patient complains of seeing colored halos around lights. The rainbow we see after a storm is similarly

explained. It is merely the effect of suspended water droplets in air breaking up white light.

Transparency is also aided by the ability of the corneal epithelium to rapidly regenerate. The corneal epithelium, by sliding over defects and regenerating its cells, can cover a large abrasion within 24 hours and without leaving a scar. If Bowman's membrane or the corneal stroma is damaged, however, repair takes much longer and a permanent scar forms.

The *aqueous humor* found between the lens and the cornea is a clear, colorless, watery fluid. It is formed by active secretion from the ciliary processes and to a lesser extent by diffusion from the vessels of the iris. The aqueous humor is in constant circulation, flowing from the posterior chamber through the pupil to the anterior chamber, where it leaves the inner eye proper through the trabecular meshwork, Schlemm's canal, and the aqueous veins (Fig. 2.13). If the exit of aqueous humor from the eye is blocked, the volume of fluid within the eye increases; because the coats of the eye are relatively nondistensible, the pressure within the eye also increases.

As light travels through the eye, the next structure it encounters is the *iris*, with its central round opening called the *pupil*. The iris is the shutter mechanism of the eye, controlling the amount of light entering the eye in the interest of clear vision. If the amount of available light is excessive, the pupil constricts by the action of the sphincter muscle of the iris to reduce excessive light or glare. If the illumination

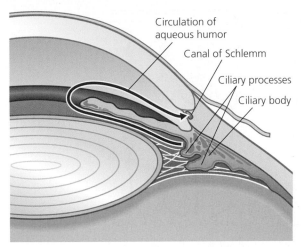

Circulation of
aqueous humor

Canal of Schlemm

Ciliary processes

Ciliary body

Fig. 2.13 Flow of aqueous humor. Aqueous humor is produced largely by the ciliary processes in the posterior chamber; it flows into the anterior chamber and leaves the eye through Schlemm's canal.

is poor, then the pupil dilates to increase the amount of light entering the eye. Other factors also control the size of the pupil. Emotional arousal (e.g., fear, anxiety, or erotic stimulation) tends to dilate the pupils. Pain in the body dilates the pupil. The pupils generally are large in the young, the blue-eyed, and the myopic and they tend to be smaller in the brown-eyed and in older adults. The pupils are normally round and equal in size. If a light is directed to one eye, both pupils constrict. The constriction of the pupil on the side toward which light is directed is called the *direct light reflex*, whereas the pupillary response in the fellow eye is called the *consensual light reflex*.

As light passes through the pupil, the next structure it encounters is the *lens*. The lens of the eye is a biconvex structure, completely surrounded by a capsule. It has only a single layer of epithelial cells under its anterior capsule, which does not significantly interfere with its transparency. Like the cornea, it contains no opaque tissue, such as blood vessels, nerve fibers, or connective tissue. It is nourished solely by the aqueous humor that bathes it.

Lens material in a child is very soft and putty-like in consistency. With age, however, the lens becomes harder, especially centrally. As new lens fibers form, they envelop the previously existing fibers, compressing them and pushing them into a compact unit toward the center. Thus growth of the lens is not accompanied by an increase in size after puberty but by compression and tight lamination of the older fibers. The central hard portion, called the *nucleus*, usually becomes well formed by the age of 30 years.

There are two main parts of the lens: the dense center, or nucleus, and the surrounding cortex. This arrangement

offers an optical advantage in making the total refractive power of the lens greater than if the index of refraction were uniform throughout.

The *vitreous body* is located directly behind the lens and occupies two-thirds of the entire volume of the eye. It is a transparent gel; that is, a viscous fluid midway in composition between a solid and a liquid. Functionally and metabolically, the vitreous is relatively inactive. If the lens and cornea are compared with the lenses of a camera, the vitreous body is the space before the film. Frequently with age, the gel breaks down in part, becoming liquid. This degeneration of the vitreous gives rise to the often-heard complaint of seeing spots before the eyes.

Once light has left the vitreous, the last great transparent structure of the eye, it finally strikes the retina, which contains all the receptors sensitive to light.

The *retinal receptors* are divided into two different populations of cells: the *rods* and the *cones* (Fig. 2.14). The rods are far more numerous (~125 million) than the cones (approximately 6 million) and function best in dim illumination *(scotopic vision)*. Without rods, night blindness occurs. Individuals affected by a disorder involving a selective loss of rod cells can see very well during the day as long as the illumination is high, however, under conditions of poor illumination, as in movie theaters or darkrooms, they are totally unable to adapt and behave as though blind. The cones function best in daylight *(photopic vision)* and mediate straight-ahead vision and color vision. A selective loss of cone cells results in a loss of visual acuity and an inability to perceive colors.

This difference of function among the retinal receptors is easily demonstrated by entering a darkroom illuminated only by a red light. The rods are relatively insensitive to red and therefore do not lose their function with this type of lighting. At first, everything appears quite dark, then hazy, and finally the definite shapes of objects at the sides come into view as the rods begin to function. The total duration for dark adaptation to be completed is about 30 minutes. Darkrooms (e.g., photography darkrooms and x-ray rooms) are usually equipped with a red light because it allows the cones to function and straight-ahead vision to be preserved while enabling the rods to become adapted to the dark.

The process of dark adaptation requires a rapid neural change in the rod cells and a slow (at least 30 minutes) chemical change in the outer segments of the rod cells. The chemical change is a complex process that requires the synthesis of the rod pigment called *rhodopsin*. Rhodopsin, or visual purple, forms under conditions of dark adaptation and is destroyed by light. Therefore it is continuously being used and restored. One of the main components of rhodopsin is vitamin A, found in carrots and other vegetables. Vitamin A deficiency causes night blindness, but the corollary that an excess of vitamin A will help the eyes is not true. The cones also contain a pigment called *iodopsin*.

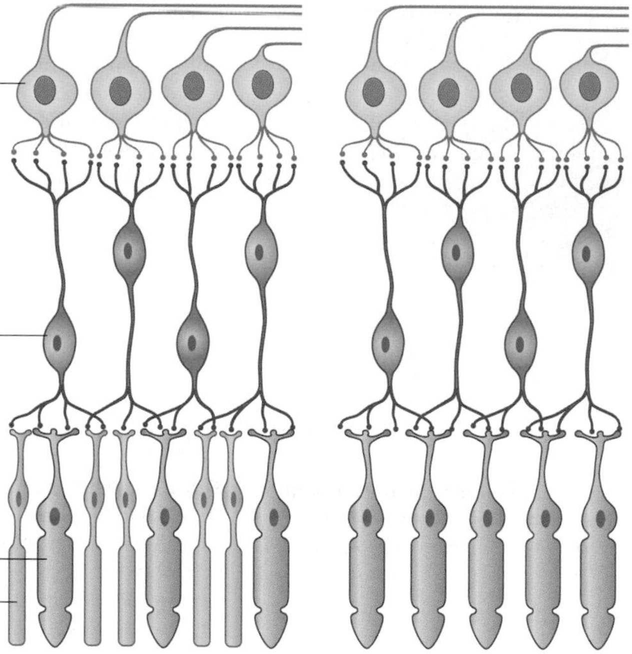

Fig. 2.14 Rods and cones of the retina.

Because the fovea contains no rods but only a concentration of specialized cones, it is found that when the eye is fully dark adapted there is a central loss of vision. Although visual acuity is not as good in this state, the perception of light is enhanced because the rods have a lower threshold for light sensitivity than do the cones. Visual information in the form of light strikes the photoreceptors and this sets off a chain of events that leads to the process of seeing. Impulses from the photoreceptors are carried to the bipolar cells and then in turn to the ganglion cells. The site of connections between cells is called the *synaptic zone*. The information from the ganglion cells then travels via axons through the optic nerves, the chiasm, and the optic tract to synapse with cells in the lateral geniculate body. Impulses are then carried by axons to the occipital cortex for the processing of the information.

Retinal images

Retinal images, once formed, persist for a very short time. They are called *positive afterimages*. Normally one is not aware of this persistence of retinal images because the eyes take up a new gaze that obliterates the former afterimage. In making movies, sensation of motion or flow is produced only when the film speed of the camera is sufficiently fast to enable fusion of the images produced by the moving frames on the film. If the camera is slowed, flickering occurs because there is a time gap between the afterimage of the first sequence and that of the next.

Negative afterimages also occur. This is commonly witnessed as a dark spot appearing before the eyes after one has been photographed with the use of a flashbulb. The high-intensity light exhausts the retinal receptors and they become unresponsive to further light stimulation for seconds after. Negative afterimages are used in a test for strabismus to determine the direction of fixation. High-intensity flashes placed in a vertical or horizontal position will produce a dark line of the same dimension as a flash. This line can be drawn by the patient. If fixation is central and straight ahead, the reproduction is exact. If the fixation pattern is eccentric, then the picture drawn will be off-centered by an amount equal to the degree of eccentric fixation.

Intraocular pressure

Normal intraocular pressure is between 13 and 20 mm Hg. These numbers are derived from measurements obtained with a tonometer and indicate the pressure in the eye that will not normally cause damage to the intraocular contents. Individual eyes respond to intraocular pressures differently. Some can tolerate pressures in the high 20s (ocular hypertension) and some will have damage to the optic nerve with lower pressures (low-tension glaucoma).

Transient and physiologic variations occur in the intraocular pressure. With respiration, these variations in intraocular pressure can amount to 4 mm Hg, whereas changes of 1 to 2 mm Hg occur with each pulsation of the central retinal artery. The changes with pulse beat are nicely demonstrated on tonographic recordings, which always show a sawtooth type of graph in rhythm with the beats of the pulse. Throughout the day the intraocular pressure can vary by as much as 2 to 3 mm Hg, with the maximum pressure being found around 6 a.m. In a glaucomatous eye, the fluctuations in diurnal pressures can be 6 to 8 mm Hg per day or even greater.

The pressure in the eye depends largely on the amount of aqueous humor secreted into the eye ($1–3 mm^3$ per minute) and the ease by which it leaves. The flow of aqueous into the eye varies with the general hydration of the body. In dehydrated states, the amount of aqueous produced decreases and so does the pressure within the eye. However, if large quantities of fluid are quickly ingested, the amount of aqueous secreted increases. Forced hydration is used in the water-drinking test: a rise of 8 mm Hg or more 45 minutes after drinking 1 L of water is suggestive of glaucoma. The drug acetazolamide (Diamox), used in the treatment of glaucoma, acts by reducing the volume of aqueous produced.

The rate of fluid exit from the eye, or its facility of outflow, is the most important single factor regulating the intraocular pressure. Glaucoma rarely or never results from an increase in aqueous production but invariably is linked to a decrease in the facility of outflow.

There are three primary methods of occluding the outflow channels of the eye. In *open-angle glaucoma* (the most common type), the diameter of the openings of the trabecular meshwork becomes narrowed, thereby increasing the resistance to fluid flow (Fig. 2.15). This situation is analogous to a drainage system in which the final common drain tube is suddenly reduced to only half its diameter at the very end. The amount of water leaving the system would be very small and the pressure in the tube in front of the narrowing would be very high.

In *secondary glaucoma* the trabecular meshwork becomes blocked. The obstructing matter can be in the meshwork and may consist of red blood cells with hyphemas, tumor cells, pigment, and debris. In addition, the obstructing matter may cover the meshwork itself in the form of scar tissue or anterior synechiae between the iris and the angle structures. These adhesions, which are commonly formed after a severe iritis, an episode of angle-closure glaucoma, or a central retinal vein occlusion, produce a severe and intractable glaucomatous state.

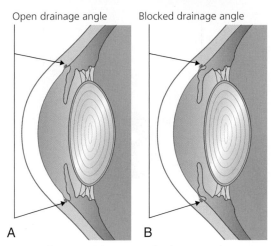

Open drainage angle   Blocked drainage angle

A   B

Fig. 2.15 Glaucoma. (A) Open-angle glaucoma. The obstruction to aqueous flow lies in the trabecular meshwork. (B) Closed-angle glaucoma. The trabecular meshwork is covered by the root of the iris.

Another method of occluding the outflow channels occurs with *pupillary block*, as typified in *primary angle-closure glaucoma*. In eyes predisposed to this condition, the angle formed by the root of the iris and the angle structures is narrow. If the pupil in such an eye is dilated, the iris tissue, which folds up like an accordion on dilation, abuts against the angle structures and partially blocks them. In addition, the aqueous humor in the posterior chamber has difficulty circulating through the anterior chamber. Therefore the pressure in the posterior chamber increases and bows the iris to a more forward position, obstructing even further the already compromised exit channels of the eye. This process occurs suddenly and the eye does not have the chance to accommodate itself to the high intraocular pressures reached. As a result, the eye becomes red, the cornea edematous, and the pupil fixed and dilated and the patient complains of considerable pain. Angle-closure glaucoma constitutes an ocular emergency. It is relieved by a peripheral iridectomy, where a small portion of the peripheral iris is removed to facilitate transfer of fluid between chambers. This procedure can be performed in the operating room; it is more commonly performed in the office with the use of argon or neodymium-yttrium aluminum garnet (YAG) lasers.

Tears

The surface of the eye is kept moist by tears formed by the lacrimal gland and the accessory lacrimal glands located in

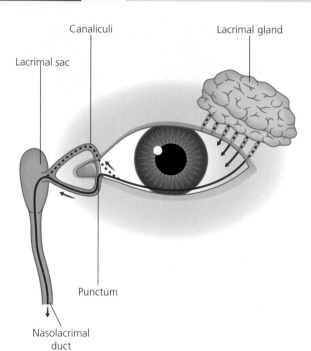

Lacrimal sac

Canaliculi

Lacrimal gland

Punctum

Nasolacrimal
duct

Fig. 2.16 Flow of tears. Note that most of the tears flow out through the lower punctum. Tears produced by the lacrimal gland are drained through the punctum, lacrimal sac, and nasolacrimal duct into the nose.

the superior and inferior fornices. Evaporation is minimized by a thin film of oil secreted by the meibomian glands over the layer of tears. Tears function to keep the globes moist and to fill in the interstices between the corneal epithelial cells, thus providing a smooth, regular corneal refractive surface.

Only 0.5 to 1 mL of tears is produced during the day; minimal tears are produced at night. About 50% of the tears are lost through evaporation; the rest are carried to the superior and inferior meatus of the nose located under the inferior turbinate (Fig. 2.16).

Tears contain an antibacterial enzyme called *lysozyme*, which is mainly effective against nonpathogenic bacteria by dissolving their outer coating.

Tear formation occurs as a result of psychic stimuli and reflex stimuli. Reflex stimuli involve uncomfortable retinal stimulation by bright lights or irritation of the cornea, conjunctiva, and nasal mucosa. The amount of tear production is measured by the *Schirmer test*. This test is performed by simply placing a strip of filter paper 5 mm wide into the lower fornix for 5 minutes; more than 10 mm of wetting indicates normal function.

Color vision

The cones of the human eye are believed to contain three different photosensitive pigments in their outer segments. These pigments act by absorbing light of certain definite wavelengths according to their period of vibration. The pigments of the cones are sensitive to red, green, and blue, the three primary colors of light. (This is not to be confused with the three primary colors of red, blue, and yellow, as found in the paint-mixing field and used by artists.) Other colors are formed by mixtures of these pigments.

Color depends on *hue, saturation,* and *brightness*. An object will have a particular hue because it reflects or transmits light of a certain wavelength. The addition of black to a given hue produces the various *shades*. Saturation is an index of the purity of a hue. The brightness of an object depends on the light intensity. Today we can experiment with all these aspects of color by altering the settings on a color television set to achieve the variations of hue, saturation, and brightness.

Color vision defects are believed to arise from a deficiency or absence of one or more visual pigments. Clinically, people with abnormal color vision fall into three major categories. The *trichromat* possesses all three cone pigments and has normal color vision. Those of us who have been tested and found to be normal belong to this category. The *anomalous trichromat* has a partial deficiency of one of the three cone pigments. This person may have (1) *protanomaly*, which is deficiency in sensitivity to the first color (red), as well as poor red–green and blue–green discrimination; (2) *deuteranomaly*, which is deficiency of one pigment mediating green, as well as poor green–purple and red–purple discrimination; or (3) *tritanomaly*, which is deficiency of the cone pigment for blue, as well as blue–green and yellow–green insensitivity. The *dichromat* has a complete deficiency in one cone pigment but preserves the remaining two cone pigments. This person may have: (1) *protanopia*, in which red is absent; (2) *deuteranopia*, in which green is absent; or (3) *tritanopia*, in which blue is absent. The *monochromat* has only one cone pigment.

The degree of color deficiency is determined by a series of plates or charts. The most common test used is the *Ishihara color plate test*, in which the ability to trace patterns on a multicolored chart is measured.

The milder deficiencies *(anomalous trichromacy)* are by far the most common, with red and green deficiency predominating. This type of color deficiency has a sex-linked recessive mode of inheritance and affects approximately 8% to 10% of all males and less than 1% of females.

Questions for review and thought

1. What keeps the cornea transparent?
2. What are the fixation and following reflexes?
3. What is amblyopia? What are the causes of amblyopia?
4. What muscles are involved in torsions? In the case of paralysis of the muscles that pull the eye horizontally and vertically, how do you test the function of the superior oblique muscle?
5. What is the accommodation reflex?
6. What are the clues that give a one-eyed person some appreciation of depth?
7. What structures in the human eye have no blood supply?
8. Describe the composition of the aqueous humor.
9. What would the visual acuity be in a person (a) with rods only, and (b) with cones only?
10. What are positive and negative afterimages? Why are surgical sheets in operating rooms green?
11. Why is the intraocular pressure higher than the pressure in the surrounding orbital tissue? What happens to the ocular structures when the pressure is too high and when it is too low?
12. What are the functions of tears?
13. What is the composition of the tear film?
14. What happens to an eye in which tear production is absent?
15. What are the primary colors?
16. Can a person who is totally color blind see?
17. The intraocular pressure varies during the day. What are the usual high and low periods in the normal person?
18. What visual functions are necessary to have binocular depth perception?
19. What happens to vision when the pupil is artificially dilated? Why?
20. What is the purpose of a normal pupillary response that involves constriction?
21. What is the function of blinking?

Self-evaluation questions   Q

True–false statements
Directions: Indicate whether the statement is true (**T**) or false (**F**).
1. Color vision should be tested binocularly. **T** or **F**
2. Loss of accommodation is caused by failure of the ciliary muscle. **T** or **F**
3. Tear production is increased during the night. **T** or **F**

Missing words
Directions: Write in the missing word(s) in the following sentences.
4. When an object is viewed up close, three reactions occur. The eyes converge, the eye accommodates, and the pupils _____.
5. The muscle that moves the eye up and in is called the _____.
6. The rod pigment _____, or visual purple, has vitamin A as its main component.

Choice-completion questions
Directions: Select the one best answer in each case.
7. The pupil is not affected by:
   a. Pain
   b. Light
   c. Accommodation
   d. Mydriatics
   e. Congenital color blindness
8. Night vision originates in the:
   a. rods.
   b. cones.
   c. choroid.
   d. macula.
   e. fovea.
9. The most powerful refracting surface of the eye is the:
   a. front surface of the cornea.
   b. back surface of the cornea.
   c. front surface of the lens.
   d. back surface of the lens.
   e. combined refractive index of the aqueous and vitreous.

Answers, notes, and explanations

1. **False**. Color vision should be tested separately with each eye. Although sex-linked color defects are present binocularly, certain acquired defects can occur with color vision that will produce color deficiencies in one eye only. Such conditions as optic neuritis may be responsible for a monocular type of acquired color defect and this would be missed if the examiner were testing binocular color vision.

2. **False**. Loss of accommodation is caused by a gradual hardening of the lens substance, beginning with the nucleus, so that it is more resistant to changes in shape. Stimulus for accommodation is caused by a blurred image, which causes the individual to contract the ciliary muscle and so relax the tension of the zonular fibers. This in turn allows the normal lens to assume a more spherical shape and increase its dioptric power. As the lens nucleus hardens with age, however, the lens is no longer as moldable and consequently is not able to bring the rays of light from a near object to focus onto the retina.

3. **False**. Tear production is decreased during the night and becomes almost nonexistent. There is, however, a compensatory lack of evaporation of tears during the sleep mechanism when the eyelids are closed. This provides adequate moisture for the cornea. The absence of tear production at night has important physiologic consequences in the development of an extended-wear contact lens of the soft variety, which is dependent on hydration.

4. **Constrict**. The pupils constrict during this triad in an effort to form a pinhole camera device so that a clear image is seen. This triad of pupillary constriction, convergence, and accommodation is often called the *accommodative reflex*.

5. **Inferior oblique**. The inferior oblique muscle moves the eye up and in. The other action is a torsional action in turning the eye outward, or extorsion.

6. **Rhodopsin**. Rhodopsin, or visual purple, forms with dark adaptation and is destroyed by light. It is continually being used and restored. Its main component is vitamin A, found in carrots and other vegetables.

7. **e. Congenital color blindness**. Pain causes dilation of the pupil. Light produces a constriction of the pupil. Accommodation produces synkinesis of convergence and pupillary constriction along with accommodation. Mydriatics are drops that produce dilation of the pupil. Color blindness, however, does not result in pupillary abnormalities.

8. **a. Rods**. There are approximately 125 million rods present in the extramacular area of the retina. These rods function best in dim light and are responsible for what is called *scotopic vision*. It is the adjustment after we enter a dark movie theater that permits us to walk up the aisles with some degree of accuracy. Pilots during World War II soon learned they had to become dark adapted for bombing missions at night. Rods are relatively insensitive to red and therefore do not lose their function with this type of lighting. Thus red goggles were the chosen method for airline pilots and those in a number of other occupations that require rod adaptation for night vision. About 30 minutes are required for dark adaptation to occur. The use of red glasses, darkrooms, and x-ray rooms permits individuals to maintain full cone function while the rods become dark adapted.

9. **a. Front surface of the cornea**. This surface contributes about two-thirds of the refracting power to bend the rays of light coming from a distant object. The lens of the eye contributes to the remaining one-third of the refracting power of the eye. The refracting power of the cornea is equivalent to a 43.00 diopter lens.

Optics

The study of optics can be divided into three parts: *physical*, *geometric*, and *physiologic*. Physical optics is primarily concerned with the nature and properties of light itself. Geometric optics is that branch of optics in which the laws of geometry can be used to design lenses that include spectacles, optical instruments, telescopes, microscopes, cameras, and so forth. Physiologic optics deals with the mechanism of vision and the physiology and psychology of seeing. We deal here primarily with physical and geometric optics.

Physical optics

What is light?

Our ancestors pondered and theorized about the nature of light. One theory proposed that light was wavelike and spread like ripples across a still pond (Fig. 3.1). Another theory held that light was a flight of particles similar to the shooting out of droplets of water from the nozzle of a hose (Fig. 3.2). In more recent times scientists have believed that there is truth in both theories: that light can be transmitted both as particles and as waves.

How does light travel?

Light, which is basically that aspect of radiant energy to which the eye responds as a visual experience, is called *luminous radiation*. The light waves travel in a specific direction. The movement of these waves is in an up-and-down motion perpendicular to the direction in which they travel (Fig. 3.3). These same light waves are capable of producing vision in human beings and lower animals by stimulating the very sensitive photoreceptors in the retina.

Nature of the world visible to humans

Human beings are continuously bombarded by electromagnetic energy, including waves from radio transmitters, infrared rays from heat lamps, and ultraviolet rays from the sun and quartz lamps, without receiving any visual sensation as a result of being in contact with these sources. It is only a portion of this *electromagnetic spectrum* that determines the visible world. The wavelengths of some of the waves of the electromagnetic spectrum are extremely short; for example, cosmic rays are only about 4 trillionths of a centimeter in length. Other wavelengths, such as those of radio waves, may be as long as 2 to 3 miles (3–5 km). The rays of wavelengths to which the eye responds lie in about the middle of this spectrum, namely, from 400 to 800 nm. Fig. 3.4, an illustration of the electromagnetic spectrum, indicates the range of wavelengths for various parts of the spectrum.

Speed of light

Light travels at a speed of 186,000 miles per second (300,000 km/s). It is many times faster than sound, as is evident by the fact that we see a lightning flash much sooner than we hear the thunder that follows. Each *wavelength* is

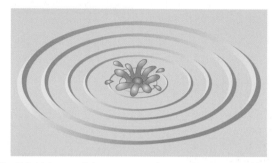

Fig. 3.1 Light travels in a wave motion, as demonstrated by ripples in a still pond when a stone is thrown.

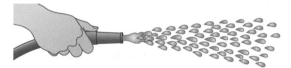

Fig. 3.2 One theory is that light behaves as water droplets shooting out of a hose.

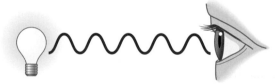

Fig. 3.3 Light travels not in a straight line but in a wave motion.

the distance from the crest of one wave to that of the next, whereas the *frequency* is the number of wavelengths passing a given point in 1 second. The product of these two quantities is equal to the *speed* of the electromagnetic radiation (*velocity* is the speed in a particular direction).

The speed of light in air is greater than that in other transparent media. For example, the speed of light in ordinary glass is only about two-thirds of the speed in air. However, we designate the wavelength of light in terms of its speed in air.

How do we measure intensity of a light source?

Light intensity is traditionally measured in terms of *footcandles*, a standard dating from preelectricity times. The light from a single candle falling on a surface at a distance of 1 foot illuminates the surface with an intensity of 1 candle per square foot. This is the premetric unit of measurement of light. If we hold a candle near a book to read, we soon find that as we move the candle away from the book, there is a distance at which the illumination is insufficient to permit us to read. The illumination of light on a surface is inversely proportional to its distance from the light source (Fig. 3.5). The luminance of an object depends on the light reflected, and the equivalent visual sensation is one of brightness. An illumination of 10 footcandles is sufficient for ordinary indoor tasks; 30 footcandles is adequate for sewing and reading, although we often choose a reading lamp that will give us as much as 50 footcandles (Table 3.1).

Because the original standard candle cannot be easily reproduced, it has been replaced by a group of carbon filament lamps operated at a carefully prescribed voltage and maintained in the vaults of the U.S. Bureau of Standards. In modern usage, the amount of illumination, or illuminance, is referred to in terms of *lumens* (the International System

1,000,000th of a millimicron   Kilometer

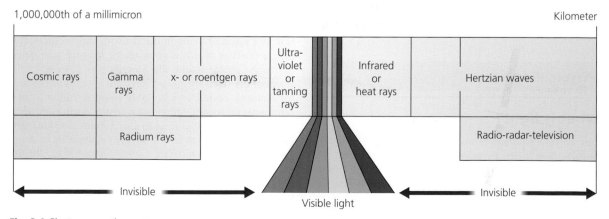

Fig. 3.4 Electromagnetic spectrum.

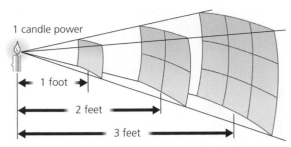

Fig. 3.5 Illumination is inversely proportional to the distance of the surface from the light source. (Modified from Adler FH. *Physiology of the Eye*. 4th ed. St Louis: Mosby; 1965.)

Table 3.1 Recommended minimum footcandles

Venues and tasks	Minimum footcandle level
Auditoriums	15
Waiting rooms	15
Building corridors and stairways	20
Libraries	70
Art galleries	30
Reading rooms	30
Study desks	70
Store interiors	30
School chalkboards	150
Kitchen work surfaces	50
Prolonged sewing	100

of Units [SI], commonly known as the *metric system*) *per foot* rather than candles per foot.

Color

The dispersion of white light into its many component colors was first demonstrated by Sir Isaac Newton, who allowed a narrow beam of light to pass obliquely through a prism and then intercepted the transmitted light, which appeared as colored bands or as a spectrum on a screen. The colors he found were spread into definite bands that the normal eye identified as red, orange, yellow, green, blue, and violet. The sequence of hues was always found to be in the same order. Newton called these bands of color the *spectrum* and he called the spreading effect caused by the prism *dispersion*. He was the first to show that white light is really a mixture of all colors. We enjoy everyday examples of this phenomenon of light breaking up into its constituent colors. Rainbows, for example, are produced by the dispersion of light into its spectral parts by droplets of rain or mist in the air.

Each wavelength range has a particular color hue. Red, having the longest wavelength, is deviated least by a water droplet or a prism and therefore appears at one end of the spectrum. Violet, which has the shortest wavelength, appears at the other end of the spectrum (Fig. 3.6).

Rays of light and the spectrum

A single *ray of light* is the path of a single corpuscle of light traveling through a tiny aperture through two successive screens.

A *pencil of light* is a group of rays that diverges from its point source. It might pass through the aperture of one screen but would not make it through the aperture of the other.

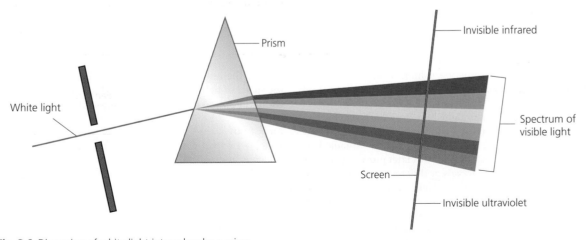

Fig. 3.6 Dispersion of white light into colors by a prism.

A *beam of light* is a group of pencils of light. A relatively large aperture is required to admit a beam.

Each filament in an electric bulb has a number of beams and pencils of light. These beams diverge and overlap one another. At close range, they strike an object and create overlapping shadows that are poorly defined. The further the light source, the more parallel are the beams of light. That is why shadows framed from the sun are sharper and more finely etched than those coming from an artificial light source.

Where rays of white light pass through cut glass, they frequently are broken down into lights of varying wavelengths. The longest wavelength is red, followed by orange, yellow, green, blue, and violet.

Red	650–750 nm
Orange	592–650 nm
Yellow	560–592 nm
Green	500–560 nm
Blue	446–500 nm
Violet	400–446 nm

The fragmentation of white light yields the visible spectrum. There are other wavelengths not visible to the eye, including ultraviolet, infrared, x-ray, radio, and electromagnetic waves.

White light is not regularly broken up unless it travels into and through a different medium, such as water droplets or glass. It is important to realize that the various wavelengths travel forward or outward at the same speed. Only their vertical vibrations differ in frequency. Thus the speed of violet light in air is the same as yellow, red, or green (i.e., 186,000 miles per second).

When white light enters the eye, all these light waves are moving at the same speed but with a different vibration. These waves fuse, giving the sensation of white even though they travel through the eye, which has a different index of refraction than air.

Bending of light

Most people will have observed that a straight pole placed in a clear pond no longer looks straight but appears to be bent at the surface of the water. Fish under the surface of the water appear to someone fishing to be at a different place from where they actually are (Fig. 3.7). This phenomenon is caused by *refraction* of light.

If light travels in a straight line, how does one explain this apparent bending of light? Snell discovered the law behind this everyday phenomenon: it was explained by assuming (and this assumption was later proved correct by experiment) that light travels at different speeds in different media. We have stated that light travels in a vacuum at 186,000 miles per second. However, as it travels through other media, such as water or glass, it travels at a slower velocity. The rate at which light travels through water is 140,000 miles per second (~225,800 km/s).

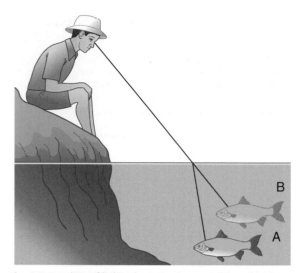

Fig. 3.7 Bending of light when entering a medium of higher index of refraction. The real fish is at A, although the boy sees it at B.

Other media, such as glass and the chambers of the eye, also retard the velocity and alter the direction of light. The ratio of the speed of light in a vacuum to that in a given medium is called the *index of refraction* of that medium. This index, which is a comparison of the speed of light through a particular medium to its speed through air, can be expressed as follows:

$$\text{Index of refraction} = \frac{\text{Speed of light in air}}{\text{Speed of light in substance}}$$

For water this index is:

$$\frac{186000}{140000} = 1.33$$

Thus the index of refraction of a substance determines the speed of light through it. The index of refraction of the common optical media can be expressed as follows:

Air = 1.00
Water = 1.33
Aqueous humor = 1.336
Cornea = 1.37
Lens cortex = 1.38
Lens nucleus = 1.40
Crown glass = 1.49
Polymethylmethacrylate (PMMA) plastic = 1.52
Flint glass = 1.65

How light can alter its direction

If rays of light pass from the air through another medium, such as a plate of glass, and pass perpendicularly to the glass, they will be slowed down somewhat but will emerge along the same line on which they entered the medium (Fig. 3.8A). If, however, these rays pass obliquely at any angle to the plate of glass, they will be bent a little at the surface. The oblique rays closest to the glass will enter the glass first, and these rays will be slowed down first on their pathway through the slower medium (Fig. 3.8B).

This is similar to the slowing-down effect when a line of soldiers marches at an angle toward a deep sandbar (Fig. 3.9). The soldiers who first enter the sandbar will be slowed down first, whereas those at the extreme end will continue at their original speed until they reach the sandbar. This will result in a bend in the straight-line formation. This same effect occurs when a beam of light strikes a glass surface at an oblique angle.

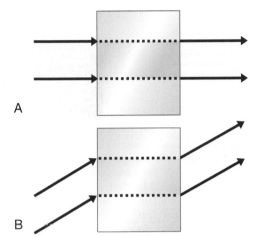

Fig. 3.8 (A) Light passing perpendicularly through a plate of glass remains unchanged in direction. (B) Light passing obliquely through a plate of glass is displaced laterally but continues in the same direction.

Geometric optics

Terminology

- **Divergence**. Rays of light from any luminous point of light will spread out or diverge (Fig. 3.10A).
- **Convergence**. When a bundle of rays is brought together, the rays are said to converge (Fig. 3.10B).
- **Parallel rays**. Light rays are assumed to be parallel if they emanate from a distant light source, such as the sun (Fig. 3.10C).

A ray of light entering a medium is called the *incident ray* and the same ray emerging from the medium is called the *emergent ray*. The angle that the incident ray makes with the perpendicular surface of the medium is called the *angle of*

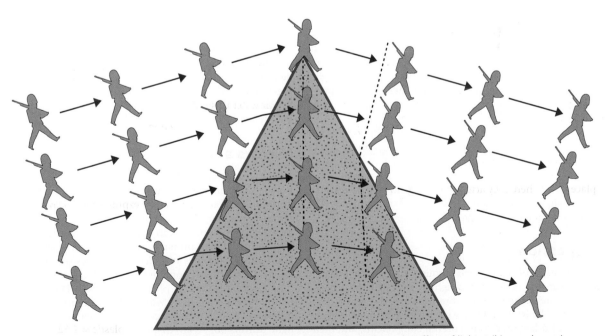

Fig. 3.9 The pathway of the soldiers' march is changed by a sandbar. This is similar to the effect of light striking a glass prism.

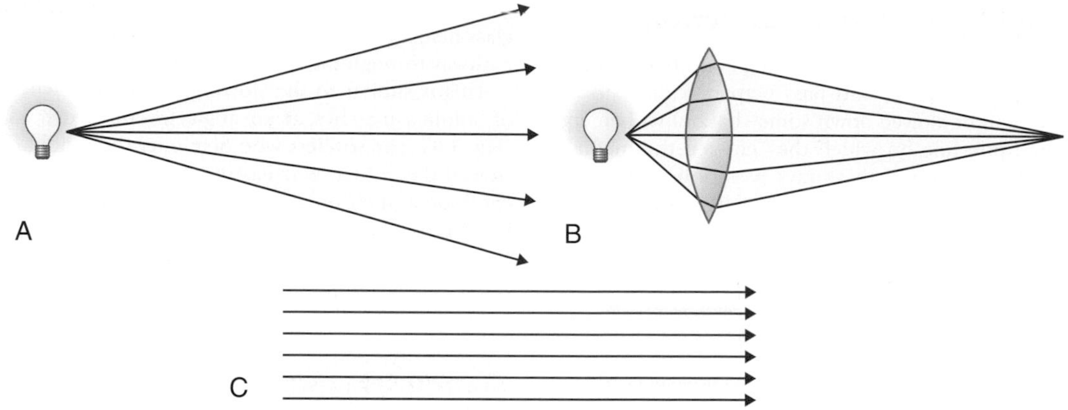

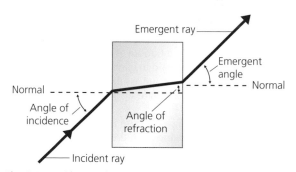

Fig. 3.10 (A) Divergence. (B) Convergence. (C) Parallel rays.

Fig. 3.11 Incident and emergent rays of light through glass.

incidence. The angle the ray makes within the medium by its change of direction is called the *angle of refraction* (Fig. 3.11).

The relationship between these two angles and the index of refraction of the medium through which the ray of light passes is the basis of *Snell's law*, a fundamental law in optics that governs the refraction of light by a transparent substance. Snell's law states:

$$\frac{\text{Sine of angle of incidence } (i)}{\text{Sine of angle of refraction } (h)} = \text{Index of refraction}$$

It is on this constant relationship of the angle of incidence, angle of refraction, and index of refraction of the medium that all lens design depends.

Dispersion

If a spectrum of light travels through a glass with parallel sides, then the deflection of light is such that the emerging rays are parallel to the direction of the original incident rays. The white light may enter a new medium, such as glass, be broken up into its spectral components, and then fuse on the way out into a white bundle of rays.

If a ray of light goes through a glass whose sides are not parallel, the white light will be broken up into its spectral components with the various wavelengths emerging in different directions. This effect, called *dispersion*, results in colored fringes found around anything viewed through prisms or unevenly cut glass. The dispersion value of different types of glass varies, depending on its index of refraction (Fig. 3.12).

Color

White light is made up of beautiful colors. This easily can be seen when a narrow beam of white light is passed through clear plastic, which bends the white light at different angles. Sir Isaac Newton, a famous English scientist, made this discovery in 1666. When mist disperses white light it gives rise to the rainbow. Red, green, and blue are the primary colors. In dim light, more sensitive cells in the rods of the retina take over, which explains why we see mainly black and white as it gets darker.

Mirrors and reflection

One way of changing the direction of light is to allow light to rebound from a surface and thus be thrown in another direction. This rebounding of light is called *reflection* and certain laws govern its behavior. Any reflecting surface, such as glass, water, or metal, can reflect light. Because glass and water transmit light primarily, their reflection is secondary. Many other examples of reflecting surfaces are found in nature, such as a still pond or lake (Fig. 3.13).

Mirrors illustrate this phenomenon best. They are primarily silver-coated glass, which allows a minimum transmission of light while reflecting the greater portion of the light. Mirrors obey a law that *the angle of incidence equals the angle of reflection* (Fig. 3.14). An analogous situation occurs

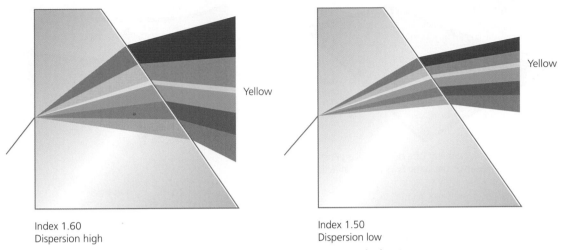

Index 1.60
Dispersion high

Index 1.50
Dispersion low

Fig. 3.12 Dispersion factor of light through oblique glass with different indexes of refraction.

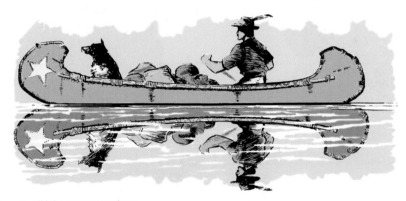

Fig. 3.13 Reflection. A still lake acts as a mirror.

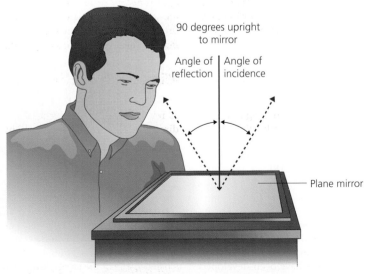

90 degrees upright
to mirror

Angle of
reflection

Angle of
incidence

Plane mirror

Fig. 3.14 Reflection from a plane mirror.

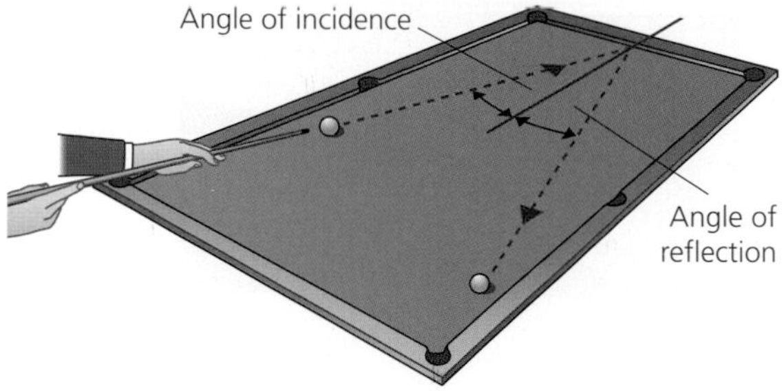

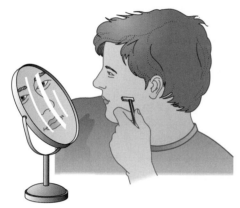

Fig. 3.15 Billiard table. Movement of a billiard ball against the cushion of the table observes the same laws as the reflection of light from mirrors.

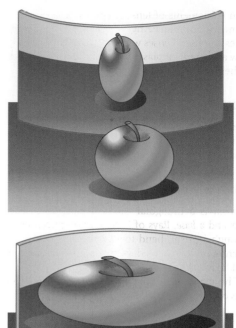

A

Fig. 3.16 Concave shaving mirror. The image is magnified.

B

Fig. 3.17 (A) Reflection from a convex mirror; the image is minified. (B) Reflection from a concave mirror; the reflection is magnified.

when a billiard ball strikes the rubber cushion of a billiard table. The angle at which the ball strikes the edge of the table is equal to the angle of the caroming ball (Fig. 3.15).

Mirrors may be *curved* or *planar*. Curved mirrors are of two types: *concave* or *convex*. *Concave mirrors* reflect light in front of them, so that if an object is placed before the focal point of a mirror, its image is magnified. This property is used to great advantage in the production of mirrors for shaving (Fig. 3.16). *Convex mirrors* reflect light away from their principal axes, so that if objects are placed before them the images will appear behind the mirrors in smaller size (Fig. 3.17). One application of this second type of mirror is used in retail stores, in which store managers can observe large areas through small mirrors (Fig. 3.18).

Lenses

Spectacle lenses were invented in about the 13th century and telescopes in the 17th century. In the past 100 years binoculars, cameras, projectors, periscopes, spectroscopes, and many other optical instruments have been developed

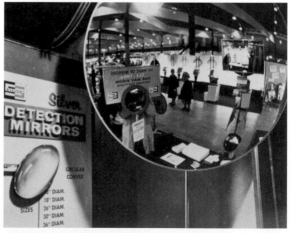

Fig. 3.18 Convex mirrors used to prevent shoplifting. The minified image of the store allows easy scrutiny of a large area.

with refinements of lens design; all have depended on the knowledge human beings have gained concerning the properties of lenses. Lenses were originally made of glass but are now also made of plastic. The main feature of curved lenses is their ability to bend rays of light.

How do lenses bend rays of light?

The basic principle of all lenses may be considered best by a discussion of prisms. One may consider a lens as being made up of prisms.

What is a prism?

A *prism* is a triangular piece of glass or plastic with an *apex* and a *base*. Rays of light, entering from air and going through a prism, bend toward the base of the prism. This phenomenon is related to the oblique surface of the prism and its medium (Fig. 3.19A).

The magnitude of the prismatic effect depends on the size of the angle at the apex of the prism. Light always is bent in the direction of the base of a prism. When one looks through a prism, however, the object of regard appears displaced toward its apex (Fig. 3.19B).

How are prisms measured?

Prisms used in ophthalmology are calibrated in diopters. By definition, *1 prism diopter* (D) is that prism which appears to displace an object 1 cm at a distance of 1 m from the eye (Fig. 3.20). At 0.5 m, if the object is displaced 1 cm, then the dioptric power of the prism is 2.00 diopters. At 2 m, if the object is displaced 1 cm, then the dioptric power is 0.50 diopter. This is expressed by the formula:

$$P = C/D$$

where:
  P = Prism power
  C = Displacement of object in centimeters
  D = Distance from prism in meters

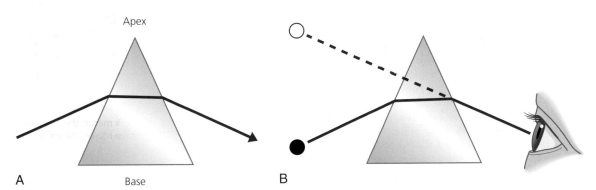

Fig. 3.19 (A) Light is deviated by the prism toward its base. (B) The observer views an object through the prism and the object appears to be displaced toward its apex.

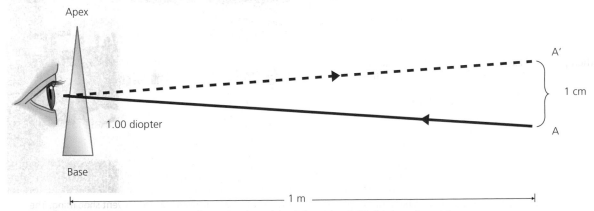

Fig. 3.20 An object at point A appears to be at A' when viewed through a 1.00 diopter prism at 1 m.

The use of prisms

Prisms are used in ophthalmology in the following devices and procedures:

1. Ophthalmic instruments, such as gonioscopes and ophthalmoscopes
2. Measurements of muscle balance of the eye in cases of strabismus: A prism can alter the direction of light so that the projection of the deviating eye is the same as its fellow eye, and, in effect, it corrects the sensory alignment of the eye without disturbing the motor alignment
3. Spectacles to correct muscle imbalance, especially those of a vertical nature
4. Eye exercises for muscular imbalance, such as convergence insufficiency

Prisms may be used as reflectors or mirrors. A ray of light usually travels through a piece of glass but there is a *critical angle* in which light is reflected rather than refracted. Any light rays striking a glass surface at an angle smaller than the critical angle will be refracted through the glass. When light hits the glass at an angle greater than the critical angle, the rays of light will be reflected as though the glass were a silvered mirror.

Convex lenses

A *convex lens* is a piece of glass in which one or both surfaces of the lens are curved outward. If two prisms are placed base to base (Fig. 3.21A) and the middle corners of the prism are smoothed off, a convex lens is created (Fig. 3.21B).

Alteration in the radius, or curvature, of the lens alters its point of convergence or focal point. A more curved lens will bend rays of light to a shorter focus than will a less curved lens. Lenses are considered as positive lenses, or *plus lenses*, if they converge rays of light to a focus behind the lens (Fig. 3.22).

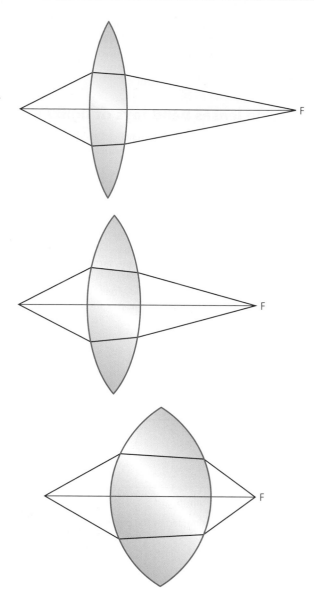

Fig. 3.22 Convex lenses. As the curvature of the lens increases, the focal point moves closer to the lens. Also the more curved the lens, the greater is its power.

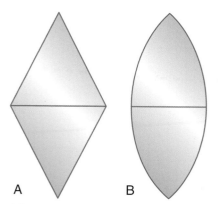

Fig. 3.21 (A) Two prisms placed base to base. (B) A convex lens derived from (A) by smoothing off the middle corners.

Concave lenses

A *concave lens* is a piece of glass in which one or both surfaces of the lens are curved inward. If two prisms are placed apex to apex (Fig. 3.23A) and the straight surfaces of the prisms are then curved, a concave lens is created (Fig. 3.23B).

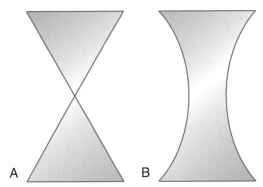

Fig. 3.23 (A) Two prisms placed apex to apex. (B) A concave lens derived from (A).

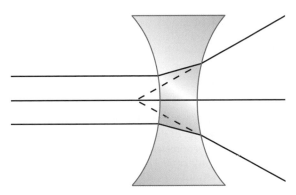

Fig. 3.24 Concave lens demonstrating an imaginary or virtual point of focus in front of the lens.

With a concave lens, the emergent rays of light diverge after refraction and thus cannot be focused behind the lens. If, however, we extend the direction of the rays of light backward, we can draw an imaginary focus in front of the lens. Thus this lens is called a *negative lens* or *minus lens* (Fig. 3.24).

Up to this point the lenses under discussion have all been spheres. The convex lenses are *converging lenses* and the concave lenses are *diverging lenses*. Converging means bringing together and diverging means spreading apart and that is what these lenses do to rays of light. Variations of the spherical lens occur when the curvatures of the anterior and the posterior surfaces are not the same (Fig. 3.25).

Focal length

In any lens, the ray penetrating through the center of the lens is undeviated, but all the rays on either side will converge to or from a point. This central ray, or *axial ray*, travels along a line called the *principal axis* of the lens. The rays on either side, or *paraxial rays*, converge to a point on this principal axis, which is called the *focal point*; the distance of this point from the center of the lens is called the *focal length* (Fig. 3.26).

A lens must be considered in terms of its focal length. The power of a lens is equal to the reciprocal of its focal distance measured in meters. The power is expressed in units called *diopters*.

The formula for conversion of focal length into diopters of lens power is:

$$D = 1/f$$

where:

D = Power of lens in diopters
f = Focal length in meters

For example:

Lens with focal length of 1 m = 1/1 = 1.00 D
Lens with focal length of 2 m = 1/2 = 0.50 D
Lens with focal length of 4 m = 1/4 = 0.25 D
Lens with focal length of 1/4 (0.25) m = 1/0.25 = 4.00 D

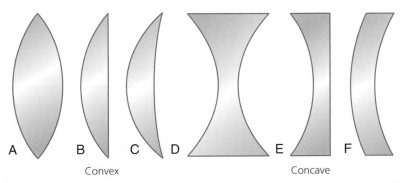

Convex   Concave

Fig. 3.25 Lens forms. (A) Biconvex; (B) planoconvex; (C) convex meniscus; (D) biconcave; (E) planoconcave; (F) concave meniscus.

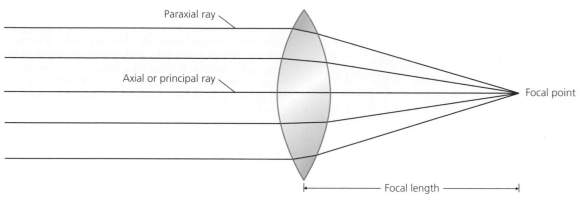

Fig. 3.26 Convergence of rays by a convex lens to a focal point.

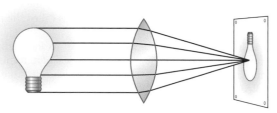

Fig. 3.27 A real inverted image of the light bulb is seen when the screen is placed at the focal point of the convex lens.

To clearly capture the image from a convex lens, a screen must be placed at its exact focal point. An example of this is shown in Fig. 3.27.

In a convex lens, the focal point always is behind the lens and therefore convex lenses are considered positive (Fig. 3.28). With concave lenses, however, the focal point always is in front of the lens, erect and virtual. Concave lenses are designated as minus lenses.

Until now we have considered point sources and point focal points. With regard to an object such as a tree, each point on the tree will have its own focal point in terms of a plus lens system (Fig. 3.29). The image behind a convex lens is always real, behind the lens, and inverted. (A real image is one that can be captured by a screen or photographic film.)

When an object is placed before a positive lens, a sharp image is formed at its focal point.

To determine the focal length and the power of the lens, one must know the distance of the object from the lens and the distance of the image from the lens. The following formula is used:

$$1/u = 1/f = 1/v$$

where:
u = Distance of object from lens
f = Focal length of lens
v = Distance of image from lens

If any two of these factors are known, then the third can easily be derived. A simpler method to determine the focal length of a lens is to use the formula:

$$U + D = V$$

where:
U = Distance in centimeters that object is in front of lens
D = Dioptric power of the lens
V = Distance in centimeters that object is behind the lens
Once one determines the D, or dioptric value of the lens, one can use the formula $D = 1/f$ and if one uses "cm," one can divide the formula $D = 100/f(\text{cm})$ to determine the focal distance in centimeters.

Spherical aberration

Because the periphery of a lens has a different curvature from its center, rays of light striking the lens at its edge do not come to the same focal point as when they strike the lens at its center (Fig. 3.30). To eliminate problems caused by this aberration, grinding techniques have been developed. Spherical aberration becomes a problem only with lenses of high power.

Chromatic aberration

The edges of spherical lenses act as a prism. However, on passing through a prism, light is broken down into its spectral components. Therefore color fringes can appear when light passes through a lens. This is particularly noticeable when dealing with lenses of high power. Chromatic aberration can be largely corrected by changes in the shape and index of refraction of the lens. Flint glass has a greater

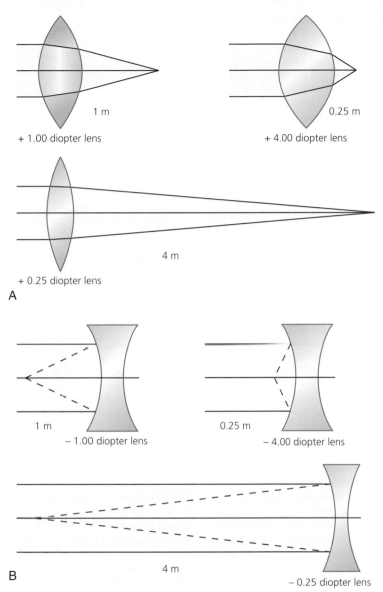

Fig. 3.28 Focal distance varies with the power of the lens. (A) Plus or convex lens: the point focus is behind the lens. (B) Minus or concave lens: the point focus is in front of the lens.

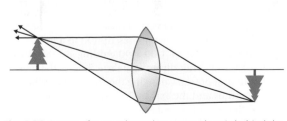

Fig. 3.29 Image of a tree through a convex lens is behind the lens, real and inverted.

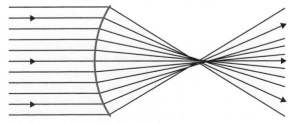

Fig. 3.30 Spherical aberration. The rays of light on refraction by the lens converge to a meeting area rather than a single focal point.

tendency to produce chromatic aberration than does crown glass. This aberration can be corrected by combining two lenses having different indexes of refraction.

1. If chromatic aberration is excessive, the image formed by the optical system will be fuzzy with colored fringes. There are ways to reduce this color distortion. A light source that has light of only one wavelength (lasers) or a narrow band of wavelengths (sodium vapor lamps) may be used.
2. A filter may be used to take out all but a few wavelengths. Good camera lenses reduce chromatic aberration with appropriate filters.
3. A doublet lens works if one lens has a low index of refraction (crown glass) and the other a high index of refraction (flint glass). This combination is called an *anachromatic lens*. The two lenses of equal dispersion value nullify each other, and the chromatic aberration that results is below that of a single lens.

Cylinders

A sphere has the same power in all meridians, whereas the cylinder has two principal meridians; one is called the *power* meridian (which has the power of the lens) and the other is called the *axis* (which is only a reference of the cylinder; it has no power).

Cylinders have the shape of a slice of a pipe or bicycle tire in that they are curved sharply in one direction but not at all in the other direction.

The curvature of a lens in one direction conveys the power of that lens and is called the *meridian* of the lens. The image of a cylinder, however, lies 90 degrees away from the meridian of power. This position is the plane of the *axis* of the lens. Therefore we have two terms: a meridian, which denotes the power of a cylindric lens; and the axis, which denotes the image of the lens, this image being always 90 degrees away from the meridian. Cylindric lenses, as in the trial case, always are denoted by the axis; for example, +1.00 axis 90 has 1.00 diopter of power at 180 degrees but it will form an image at 90 degrees.

Spherocylinders are a combination of a sphere and a cylinder. Such a lens system has two radii of curvature, each with its own focal point and image. For example, in Fig. 3.31 the rays of light from meridian x–x focus at X, whereas the rays from y–y focus at Y.

The area between the two focal points of a spherocylindric combination assumes a conoid shape, which is called *Sturm's conoid*. This optical effect is illustrated in Fig. 3.31. At A, a section of the bundle of converging rays will be in the form of a horizontal ellipse but at C, it will be in the form of a vertical ellipse. At B, the bundle forms a circle called the *circle of least confusion*. The circle of least confusion represents the dioptric average of the spherocylinder. In refraction, the

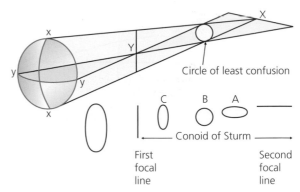

Fig. 3.31 Sturm's conoid. This represents the astigmatic interval between the two focal points of a spherocylindric lens.

conoid of Sturm is "collapsed" so that both the vertical and horizontal foci are placed on the retina. In a situation in which one focus is already on the retina, a simple cylinder will move the other focus back or forward to the retina.

A spherocylindric lens really comprises two lenses, each of different power in the two principal meridians, which are 90 degrees apart. The dioptric powers of these two components should be considered separately. For example, + 7.00 D sph − 1.50 cyl × 90 means that the spherical power is + 7.00, the cylinder is − 1.50 diopters and its axis is 90 degrees. The power of that cylinder is at a right axis to the cylinder. Thus the power in the horizontal meridian is + 5.50 D.

Transposition

Transposition is the process of changing the prescription from a plus cylinder to a minus cylinder, or from a minus cylinder to a plus cylinder, without changing its refractive value. The rules of transposition are based on the principle that when two cylinders of equal power and like sign are crossed at right angles, they produce the effect of a spherical lens of the same power as one of the cylinders.

- The rule for transposition of all compound lenses is as follows: *add the cylinder power to the sphere power algebraically, change the sign of the cylinder, and change the axis of the cylinder by 90 degrees.* The following are examples of typical transpositions:
  - transpose the following prescription to a minus cylinder: + 2.00 + 1.00 × 90. Adding + 2.00 and + 1.00 algebraically, we obtain + 3.00 as the new spherical power. Changing the sign of the cylinder to minus and the axis by 90 degrees, we find + 3.00 − 1.00 × 180.
  - Transpose the following prescription to a plus cylinder: + 1.00 − 3.00 × 70. Adding + 1.00 and

– 3.00 algebraically, we obtain – 2.00 as the spherical power. Changing the sign of the cylinder to plus and the axis by 90 degrees, we find – 2.00 + 3.00 × 160.

Practical aspects of optics

Fiberoptics

A *fiberoptic bundle* has a transparent core of material with a high refractive index surrounded by a material of lower refractive index. The core usually is plastic or glass. The rim can be glass or even air. Most fibers are tiny, being only 0.003 to 0.005 inch (0.008–0.013 cm) in diameter.

Light moves along these plastic cores because of total internal reflection. The optical effect is created by the differences in indexes of refraction. Total internal reflection occurs when light moves from a material with a higher index to one with a lower index. Light leaves the pipes at the end of tubing, where it is intense and concentrated. Most of the bundles are parallel to one another, the result being a coherent fiberoptic bundle or image conduit. Coherent fibers are used in computer output terminals as well as in many electrooptical devices.

Gonioscopy

The principle of internal reflection is a problem to an observer who has to examine the eye. Parts of the eye are not visible because light cannot get out of the eye. For instance, the angle structures of the anterior chamber are not visible because of total internal reflection.

Light has to get through the cornea for the examiner to see the angle structures. At the cornea–air interface, however, an abrupt change from a high to a low index of refraction occurs, which causes total internal reflection exactly like that of the fiberoptic tube.

If a contact lens is applied to the cornea, then light can pass through the cornea into the contact lens, which has a refractive index higher than the refractive index of corneal tissue. Once the light is past the cornea, it can travel to the eyepiece and be seen either through a mirror, as noted in the Goldmann lens (Fig. 3.32), or through simple refraction, as noted in the discussion of the Koeppe lens (Fig. 3.33).

Telescopes

There are two types of telescopes: the astronomical or inverting and the Galilean or noninverting.

Astronomical telescope

Both the objective and the eyepiece are of positive power. The primary focus of the eye lens coincides with the

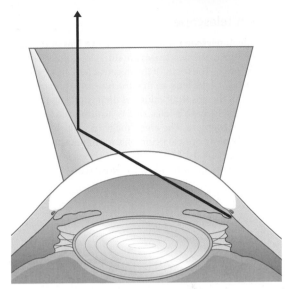

Fig. 3.32 The Goldmann lens, which gives an indirect view of the angle of the anterior chamber.

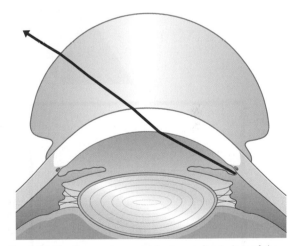

Fig. 3.33 The Koeppe lens, which gives a direct view of the angle of the anterior chamber.

secondary focus of the objective lens. They are separated by the distance equal to the sum of their focal lengths. A real image is formed in the focal plane of the objective. The image is inverted and its size is determined by the power of these lenses. The eye lens acts as a simple magnifier and forms a vertical image at infinity.

This telescope, as the name implies, is used in astronomy. Because the stars are so far away, the fact that the image is inverted is not of practical concern.

Galilean telescope

The Galilean telescope uses a negative eye lens and positive objective. Again, the two lenses are situated so that their focal points coincide. The focus of the negative lens, however, is on the other side of the lens, so that the two are separated by the difference of the absolute values of their focal length.

The image from this telescope is not inverted because of the negative eyepiece. The erect image has allowed industry to use these basic optical principles to manufacture surgical loupes. These consist of *a Galilean telescope* combined with an "add" on the front to allow for close work.

Optical illusions

Optics takes us into the fascinating field of optical illusion. In this area, geometric optics is affected by our perceptual senses and our interpretation of what we see. The saying "seeing is believing" is not always true because we are influenced greatly by background effect, as well as the effect of certain lines on each other and their interpretation by the brain. Fig. 3.34 shows examples of some of the illusions that can be created.

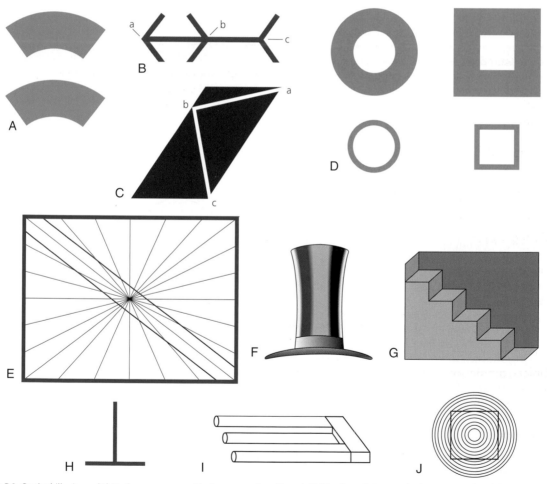

Fig. 3.34 Optical illusions. (A) Both arcs are exactly the same size. (B and C) The line ab is exactly the same as bc. (D) Upper circle and square are crowded by the large black borders and appear smaller. Both upper and lower inner circles and squares are the same size. (E) The red oblique lines are straight but they appear curved. (F) The height of the crown appears greater than the width of the brim; however, both are of the same size. (G) This may appear as a staircase or as overhanging masonry. (H) The height appears greater than the base. (I) Are there three prongs? (J) The red square is a true square and not distorted in any way.

Questions for review and thought

1. How does light travel?
2. What is the cause of the dispersion of white light produced by a prism?
3. Draw a diagram of the electromagnetic spectrum.
4. List the sequence of color hues in the spectrum.
5. What is the law of mirrors?
6. Which type of mirror magnifies: concave or convex?
7. What is a prism?
8. Draw the focal points of a concave lens and of a convex lens, respectively.
9. What is a cylinder?
10. What is Sturm's conoid?
11. What aberrations are there with high minus spectacles (greater than 5.00 diopters)?
12. What are aspheric lenses?
13. How do you find the optical center of a lens?
14. Name some common defects found in glass.
15. What is a Galilean telescope?
16. When you are looking through a prism, does the image jump to the apex or the base?

Self-evaluation questions   Q

True–false statements

Directions: Indicate whether the statement is true (T) or false (F).

1. A light entering a prism is deflected toward the apex of the prism. **T** or **F**
2. Chromatic aberration occurs when white light enters a new index of refraction and emerges broken into its spectral components. **T** or **F**
3. The speed of red light is considerably slower than the speed of white light. **T** or **F**

Missing words

Directions: Write in the missing word in the following sentences.

4. Placido's disc uses the front surface of the cornea as a _____.
5. A fiberoptic bundle works by _____ reflection, in which the light strikes the wall of the bundle at an angle greater than the critical angle.
6. Yellow lenses act as _____ filters.

Choice-completion questions

Directions: Select the one best answer in each case.

7. If the mechanical center of a lens is changed by edging, what happens to the optical center?
   a. It remains where it was on the lens.
   b. It is displaced toward the edge most shortened.
   c. It is displaced according to Prentice's rule.
   d. It shifts laterally but never vertically.
   e. None of the above.
8. Aberrations of a lens include:
   a. spherical aberration.
   b. astigmatism of oblique pencils.
   c. chromatic aberration.
   d. pincushion and barrel distortion.
   e. all of the above.
9. Convex mirrors make the size of the image:
   a. smaller.
   b. larger.
   c. larger if the object is placed within the focal point of the lens.
   d. smaller if the object is placed within the focal point of the lens.
   e. none of the above.

Answers, notes, and explanations

1. **False.** A prism is a wedge-shaped piece of glass that bends light toward its base because of a change in the direction of light waves. It creates this alteration of direction because of the change in the index of refraction between light traveling in air and light traveling in glass. When light emerges from the prism, it undergoes another change in direction toward the base.

   Although the light is deflected toward the base of the prism, the observer sees it toward the apex. By bringing together images separated in space by a heterotropia of the eyes, prisms are used diagnostically to assess the type and magnitude of a strabismus and to treat diplopia.

2. **True.** Chromatic aberration is seen naturally in rainbows. White light penetrates a suspended droplet of water and is broken up into its spectral components. Clinically, chromatic aberration is seen in patients who have corneal edema. The most common occurrences are in persons with severe or acute glaucoma or those wearing ill-fitting contact lenses. The liberated edema fluid breaks up the intact bundle of white light, and patients complain of seeing halos around lights. Frequently, a mucous blob on the cornea will do the same thing, so that not all chromatic aberration occurrences indicate pathologic conditions. Some lenses have a higher chromatic aberration than others. For instance, lenses of flint optical glass have a greater tendency to chromic aberration than lenses of barium optical glass. Flint glass has a greater tendency to chromatic aberration than does barium.

3. **False.** All the colors, whether they are reds, blues, greens, or oranges, have exactly the same speed of light, which is 186,000 miles per second. A wavelength is the distance from the top of one wave to the top of the next, whereas the frequency is the number of waves passing in 1 second. Red light may have a longer wavelength than blue but this indicates only its vertical vibration. All colors, white included, travel at the same speed.

   The speed of light depends on frequency × wavelength. When the wavelength is shorter, its frequency is increased so that the speed of white versus colored light remains the same.

4. **Mirror.** Placido's disc uses the cornea as a mirror. The disc is used to detect keratoconus. The cone-shaped deformity of the cornea is reflected in the distortion of the annular rings, which appear irregular and oblong on the cornea. Placido's disc is used in a clinical photographic system to give accurate topographic analysis of the central and peripheral sections of the cornea for contact lens fitting. The distance between the rings can be translated into radii of corneal curvature. Reflection from the cornea as a mirror is the basic principle of all keratometers. The image from the keratometer is reflected and brought into focus. A doubling device is used to keep the images aligned.

The amount of focusing required to yield sharp corneal images gives the K readings.

5. **Internal.** If light strikes any optical surface at an angle greater than the critical angle, the light, instead of passing through that surface, will be totally reflected.

   This principle is well established. Some ophthalmoscopes are based on total reflection by virtue of light striking a prism. In fiberoptic bundles the light is inside the bundle and cannot escape because the angle of incident light exceeds the critical angle and the outer coat of the light has a low refractive index. The light emerging from this fiberoptic bundle is compressed, intense, and very high in illumination. It is a pure light because none of it escapes or is broken down to its spectral components.

   Fiberoptic illumination has become an integral part of the illuminating systems used in ophthalmic microsurgery. The commercial uses of the fiberoptic system are numerous and include everything from Christmas tree decorations to illuminating systems for space travel.

6. **Haze.** Yellow lenses are basically haze filters. Skiers and hunters use yellow lenses to reduce haze and improve definition. They are not useful in night driving because they reduce the light entering the retina when lack of contrast is already a problem.

7. **a. It remains where it was on the lens.** Obviously, the center of the lens remains where it is, regardless of how the lens is edged. However, high fashion dictates the shape of the frame and with radical lens designs the optical centers can be shifted in the frame itself and in relation to the eye.

   Large frames that contain strong prescriptions, that is, − 5.00 diopters or more, frequently slide down the nose with reading. The effect of gravity drops the lens, and the vertex distance of the lens to the eye is changed. With plus lenses it increases the prescription; with minus lenses it does the reverse. Also unwanted base-up prism is added with plus lenses, with the opposite, or base-down, occurring with minus lenses.

   The optical center and the mechanical center do not coincide. The optical center of a lens is that place of the lens that does not contain unwanted prism. It is the point detected on the lens meter where the rays of light come into focus. The optical center should be in line with the eye. The mechanical center is the geographic center and in a perfectly round lens it coincides with the optical center. The optical center, not the mechanical center, concerns us.

   If the optical center is shifted in the frame, then unwanted prism will occur. If the optical center is shifted outward and the lens is a plus lens, then base-out prism will be added.

The optical centers of the lenses always should be marked and compared with the interpupillary measurements—the distance from the center of one pupil to the other.

8. **e. All of the above**.

Spherical aberration: the image from a spherical lens is never a single point because the central and paraxial rays form more concentrated images than those rays that pass through the periphery of the lens.

The degree of spherical aberration depends on:

i.   the aperture of the system; it is reduced by closing down the size of the aperture.

ii. the precise form of the lenses used; the error can be reduced, making the curvature of the anterior surface greater than the curvature of the posterior surface.

iii. the curvature of the lens; the fault can be diminished by making the peripheral curves less sloped; these are called aplanatic surfaces.

Astigmatism of oblique pencils: if light rays strike a lens at an angle instead of perpendicular to it, the image will be distorted in a form similar to that produced by a cylindric lens. Some light rays will strike the lens early and some later. The extra distance has to be traveled by the later rays to strike the lens. Moreover, a flatter section of the lens will be encountered by these rays. The resultant image will be astigmatic, sharp in one direction and fuzzy in the other. If the light rays strike a lens perpendicularly, this type of lens distortion does not occur.

Chromatic aberration: this is discussed in answer 2.

Pincushion and barrel distortion: distortion occurs when the magnification of the peripheral parts of the lens is different from that of the central area. Pincushion distortion occurs when the peripheral magnification is greater than that of the central magnification. Barrel distortion occurs when the peripheral magnification is less than that of the central magnification.

9. **a. Smaller**. Concave mirrors magnify the image of the object only if it is placed *within* the focal point of the mirror. Cosmetic mirrors always are concave, and the face has to be placed close to the mirror to have its image enlarged and in focus.

Convex mirrors reduce image size. They are commonly used as survey mirrors in retail stores where large areas of the store can be seen with the aid of a convex mirror.

Chapter | 4 |

Pharmacology

Pharmacology deals with the basic properties of drugs, their actions, their fate in the human body, and their known side effects. This chapter deals primarily with some of the drugs that act on the eye, either directly by local application or indirectly by systemic absorption.

General principles

Locally applied medication

Ophthalmic preparations placed directly in the eye are available in solution, suspension, or ointment forms. Solutions usually are instilled in the conjunctival sac and do not interfere with vision. There is very little amount of the administered drop that is retained by the eye. When a 50-μL drop is delivered, only 20% is retained (10 μL/50 L). The main disadvantage is that their duration of contact with the eye is short and therefore they require frequent instillation. Polymers often are added to solutions to enhance contact time. Although ointments remain in contact with the eye for prolonged periods, their tendency to reduce vision by creating a greasy film over the surface of the cornea limits their daily usefulness. Ointments frequently are used for bedtime therapy because of their prolonged contact time; in addition, they are less readily washed out with tears. They also are valuable for use in children who are crying (Table 4.1).

Preparations used in the eye have certain basic requirements regarding tolerance, tonicity, sterility, stability, and penetration.

Tolerance

Eye medications should cause minimal irritation or stinging of the eye. Tolerance of the medication by the eye depends on the solution's having an ideal acid–base balance. The acid–base balance is denoted in terms of its pH.

Solutions that have a pH greater than 7 are *alkaline*, whereas agents with a pH less than 7 are *acid*. The pH of tears is slightly alkaline at 7.4. A large difference between the pH of topical solution and the pH of tears may result in ocular irritation and reflex tearing. Most ophthalmic solutions have a pH that varies from 3.5 to 10.5 (Fig. 4.1).

Tonicity

The *tonicity* of a solution refers to the concentration of the chemical in that solution. Normal saline solution, or a 0.9% sodium chloride equivalent, has a tonicity approximately that of tears and is therefore well tolerated by the eye. Solutions with a high concentration of a chemical, however, are hypertonic and thus can be quite irritating. However, solutions low in concentration of a chemical (hypotonic solutions), such as water, are equally objectionable in producing irritation of the eye. Ideally, the closer the concentration of the drug to normal tears (0.9% sodium chloride equivalent), the less irritating the drug will be.

Table 4.1 Comparison of characteristics of ophthalmic solutions and ophthalmic ointments

Characteristics	Solutions	Ointments
Instillation	Easier	More difficult
Contact time	Shorter	Longer (slower movement through nasolacrimal drainage)
Irritation on instillation	Frequent	Rare
Discharge retention	No	Yes
Skin allergic reactions	Few	More frequent
Blurred vision	No	Yes (film spreads over eye)
Local symptoms (burning, stinging)	More frequent	Less frequent
Readily contaminated (requires preservatives)	Yes	No
Stability a problem with storage	Yes	Less likely

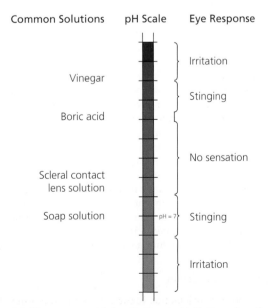

Fig. 4.1 The eye responds by stinging and irritation when the pH varies from 7. (Illustration courtesy of J. Krezanowski.)

In some cases in which a high concentration of a locally applied drug is required, this ideal may not be achievable.

Sterility

Solutions must be free from bacterial contamination. This can be achieved either by autoclaving or by passing the solution through bacterial filters. Today most solutions are manufactured in a sterile manner by drug companies. To ensure sterility for long periods, preservatives are usually added. A good preservative should be well tolerated by the eye, nonallergenic, and inhibit the growth of bacteria and fungi. About 95% of all commercially available ophthalmic products are preserved with: (1) benzalkonium chloride, (2) chlorobutanol, or (3) organic mercurials, chiefly thimerosal and phenylmercuric acetate. For eye surgery, however, the preservative drugs are usually eliminated to make the product less irritating to the open tissues. The solutions for eye surgery are available in sterile individual-dose units. For contact lens solutions, these preservatives often are too toxic to the cornea, and less irritating preservatives are incorporated.

Once a sealed bottle is opened, it is no longer considered sterile. Organisms may enter an open bottle with ease. The most notorious organism found in ophthalmic solutions, including antibiotic drops, is *Pseudomonas aeruginosa*, which can destroy an eye in 48 hours. This organism's predilection for fluorescein solution has led to the development of dry fluorescein-impregnated paper, because this organism cannot survive in a dry environment.

Stability

Solutions must be reasonably stable and not deteriorate or lose their effectiveness. Drugs such as phenylephrine hydrochloride (Neo-Synephrine) and epinephrine oxidize in the presence of air and bright light and consequently are often packaged in dark or opaque bottles. Some drugs require a special base to provide stability. Eye ointments are prepared in either a petrolatum base or a water-soluble base because these bases have proved to be stable. Drugs such as oxytetracycline (Terramycin), which are relatively unstable for any length of time in solution form, have a long shelf life in ointment form and are generally prepared this way.

Penetration

Eyedrops penetrate the eye directly through the cornea and into the anterior chamber of the eye. They do not, however, penetrate far behind the crystalline lens and therefore cannot reach the back, or posterior portion, of the eye. The cornea acts as a barrier to many drops by virtue of the lipid content of its epithelium, which functions as a barrier to all medications not soluble in fat. Eyedrops also must have water-soluble properties to penetrate the remaining portion of the cornea. Thus agents that penetrate the eye well are those that have both fat- and water-soluble properties. However, when there is mechanical disruption of the epithelial barrier in corneal abrasion or infection, there is an increase in the rate of intraocular drug penetration.

Drugs penetrate the cornea better if they are instilled directly over its surface. When corneal penetration is of utmost importance, the patient should be asked to look down and the drop should be placed above so that it will flow over the cornea.

Alternative routes of medication

Subconjunctival injections

Injections may be administered under the conjunctiva. The subconjunctival medication gains access to the eye by absorption into the bloodstream by the episcleral and conjunctival vessels. *Subconjunctival injections* are used primarily in the treatment of intraocular infection.

Continuous-release delivery

Discs impregnated with drugs permit continuous delivery of medication 24 hours a day for a full 7 days. A small membrane, sandwiching medication, is inserted into the lower conjunctiva by the patient and it gradually releases its medication. Pilocarpine can be incorporated in the Ocusert and over a period of 7 to 8 days, it is steadily released at a rate of 40 mcg/h. Lacrisert provides a continuous release of hydroxypropyl cellulose for lubrication in patients with dry eyes.

Retrobulbar injections

Drugs may be administered by injecting medication through the skin of the lower lid, the point of the needle emerging behind the eyeball. *Retrobulbar injections* of a local anesthetic are often used to paralyze the extraocular and eyelid muscles and anesthetize the eye before commencement of intraocular surgery. *Retrobulbar injections* are less commonly used for cataract surgery but are used before vitreoretinal surgeries.

Intracameral injection

An injection may be given into the anterior chamber at the start of cataract surgery to enhance patient comfort under topical anesthesia. The injection of 0.5 mL of preservative-free 1% lidocaine (Xylocaine) has resulted in a dramatic improvement in patient comfort, with a decrease in light sensitivity. This advance has led to essentially painless

cataract surgery without the use of retrobulbar or peribulbar injections. Vancomycin and other antibiotics may be used.

Systemic medication

The term systemic drugs refers to those drugs that are taken orally or by injection subcutaneously (under the skin), intramuscularly (in the muscle), or intravenously (into the vein). These routes of administration are usually chosen because of some disease in the posterior part of the eye or orbit that cannot be reached by locally applied medication. In particular, conditions such as cellulitis, uveitis, and acute allergic reactions often require systemic medication.

Complications of locally administered drugs

Allergic reactions

Many ophthalmic preparations can cause contact allergic reactions involving primarily the skin of the lids and the conjunctiva. Because hypersensitivity develops as a result of the patient's exposure to the agent, allergic reactions usually follow repeated application of the medication. Thus a delay in time occurs between the reaction to the use of a particular drug and the development of a state of hypersensitivity. This delay in time can be weeks, months, or years and is referred to as the *induction period*.

Once the hypersensitivity state is established, further instillation of the agent serves only to aggravate the allergic response. In the skin, allergic reactions may consist of edema, redness, vesiculation, scaling, and oozing, depending on the patient's sensitivity. In the conjunctiva, the most common reaction is either marked chemosis or swelling or low-grade congestion and redness of the conjunctival tissues. Differentiation should be made between an allergic response and an ocular irritation caused by the drug. Some patients with allergies complain of itchiness. In many cases, however, differentiation between the two can be made only by a smear of the discharge of the conjunctiva that reveals the typical cell of an allergic response: the eosinophil.

One of the most common ophthalmic preparations to cause allergic reactions of the skin of the eyelid is atropine. Of the antibiotics, neomycin is most likely to create a hypersensitivity state and induce an allergic response (Fig. 4.2).

Toxic reactions

Some drugs can produce irreversible damage within the eye or cause systemic disturbances within the human body. Echothiophate iodide (Phospholine Iodide), used

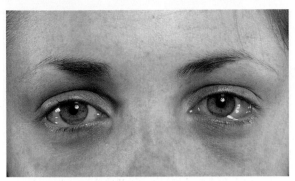

Fig. 4.2 Allergic conjunctivitis with swelling of the bulbar conjunctiva. (Reproduced from Spalton D, Hitchings R, Hunter P. *Atlas of Clinical Ophthalmology*. 3rd ed. St Louis: Mosby; 2004, with permission.)

in glaucoma, can cause cataracts, iris cysts, and retinal detachments. If this drug is absorbed systemically in sufficient quantities, it may cause nausea, vomiting, diarrhea, bladder cramps, and cardiac irregularities. One can reduce systemic absorption of eye medication by applying gentle finger pressure to the inner corner of the eyelids, over the lacrimal sac, for 1 minute when instilling drops. This will prevent drops from passing through the nasolacrimal duct to the back of the throat, where they are absorbed.

Discoloration of the eye

Pigmentation of the conjunctiva may occur after the prolonged use of epinephrine, silver nitrate, or silver–protein compound (Argyrol). Epinephrine (Adrenalin) causes black spots in the lower conjunctival sac. Silver–protein produces a slate-silver discoloration of the conjunctiva.

Undesirable side effects

Some undesirable side effects may occur. For example, topically applied steroids can:
- Raise the intraocular pressure and cause glaucoma
- Potentiate the growth of viruses, which in herpes simplex infection can cause widespread corneal damage
- Potentiate the growth of bacteria
- Cause delay in wound healing

Pigmentary changes in the macula with loss of vision may occur in patients using chloroquine (antimalarial also used in treating rheumatoid arthritis and systemic lupus erythematosus), phenothiazines (antipsychotic) or indometacin (a nonsteroidal antiinflammatory drug [NSAID]). Oral contraceptive agents may cause migraine-like syndromes, as well as retinal vascular occlusions. Cataracts can occur after the use of antiglaucoma medication such as echothiophate iodide.

Idiosyncrasy

An idiosyncrasy is a constitutional peculiarity in which an individual reacts in a bizarre fashion to a drug. For example, an unexpected reaction to cocaine may occur and the person may develop tremors, motor excitability, or convulsions and may even collapse.

Loss of effect by inactivation

Some ophthalmic solutions may lose their potency if not stored properly. For example, if exposed to light and heat, epinephrine turns brown and loses its effect. Patients receiving epinephrine derivatives should be warned of this contingency and told to keep their eyedrops in a cool, dark place, such as the refrigerator. Prostaglandins are heat sanative.

Spread of infection

In some offices, hospitals, or clinics, where a single bottle is used for a group of patients, the dropper easily can become contaminated. Consequently, infection may spread from patient to patient. This hazard can be eliminated by using small sterile disposable bottles of medication or by limiting the use of the eyedrops or ointment to one individual. When eyedrops are used, care must be exercised that the tip of the eyedropper does not touch the lashes or the eye, so that contamination of the dropper and the eye solution is avoided (Fig. 4.3). Some regulatory commissions recommend that bottles of ocular medications be discarded after being opened for 28 days.

Prescription writing

In some U.S. states, the pharmacy boards require that all prescriptions be written as printed or typed (but not as cursive) on special approved prescription paper that protects against altering. Other regulatory regulations may require that prescriptions be electronically written/transmitted. Ophthalmic assistants should be knowledgeable on their state's requirements.

Physicians use many symbols for writing prescriptions. These symbols provide a direct communication from the physician to the pharmacist. The use of Latin symbols today is an anachronism, yet several Latin symbols are retained because of tradition and for brevity (Table 4.2). The following is the format for prescription writing; the setup is shown in Fig. 4.4.
1. The patient's name, address, and date of prescription
2. The name of the drug and the percentage of concentration or the dosage of each unit (the drug usually is written out in full to avoid any confusion)

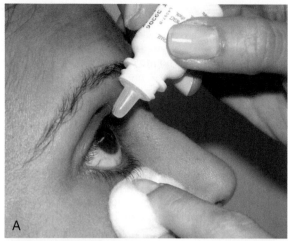

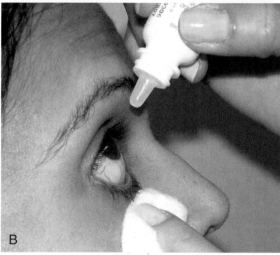

Fig. 4.3 Instillation of eyedrops. (A) Incorrect method. Note contamination of tip of bottle by lashes. (B) Correct method. Note tip of bottle is held free of globe and lashes.

3. The amount of the drug to be supplied, headed by the symbol M or Mitte, which signifies the quantity
4. Sig or S, from the Latin *signa*, "to mark," or in English, "label," which indicates to the pharmacist what directions to label on the medicine
5. The signature of the physician with notation "substitution permitted" or "dispense as written"
6. Possibly some notation at the bottom of the prescription, for example, "may be repeated 2 times," "refill prn for 1 year," or "no refill."

Table 4.2 Abbreviations and symbols used in prescription writing

Abbreviation or symbol	Meaning
RX	take thou
g	gram
h	hour *(hora)*
q	every
hs	bedtime *(hora somni)*
qs	quantity sufficient
od	right eye *(oculus dexter)*
os	left eye *(oculus sinister)*
ou	both eyes *(oculi uterque)*
mg	milligram
<	less than
>	more than
aa	equal parts *(ana)*
Sol	solution
Ung	ointment
ʒ	dram
oz	ounce
tsp	teaspoon
gt, gtt	drop, drops *(gutta, guttae)*
M	mix *(misce)*
bid	twice a day *(bis in die)*
tid	three times a day *(ter in die)*
qid	four times a day *(quater in die)*
q4h	every 4 hours
ac	before meals *(ante cibum)*
pc	after meals *(post cibum)*
non rep	do not repeat *(non repetatur)*
ad lib	as much as wanted *(ad libitum)*
ss	half *(semis)*
aq	water
prn	as the situation demands *(pro re nata)*

Dr John Doe

170 Bloor Street West
Cleveland, Ohio

Name: Miss J. White
Address: 227 Sankta Ave.

℞   Date: Jan. 4 Year

Inscription: Diamox tab. 250 mg

Subscription: M: 100

Signa: Sig.: Tab. t.i.d.

Signature: John Doe, M.D.

Substitution Permitted/Dispense as written

Repeat x2

Fig. 4.4 Example of a prescription form.

Autonomic drugs

The body contains an involuntary nervous system, which is not under our direct control. This system acts to protect the body, provide nutrition and elimination, and carry on daily regulatory activity. The autonomic nervous system is affected by our emotional behavior. The typical "fear" reaction causes our pupils to dilate, our skin to sweat, and even our hair to stand on end.

The *autonomic nervous system* is subdivided into the *sympathetic* and *parasympathetic* nervous systems. Drugs that mimic the action of these two opposing types of involuntary nervous systems are said to be *sympathomimetic* and *parasympathomimetic*, respectively. Sympathomimetic drugs such as epinephrine and phenylephrine act directly on the end organ; they are sometimes called *adrenergic agents*. Parasympathomimetic drugs either act on the end organ in a manner similar to that of acetylcholine or interfere with the action of the enzyme *cholinesterase*, which destroys the acetylcholine normally produced in the tissues. Pilocarpine acts directly on the end organ, whereas eserine, dipivefrin (DP), and echothiophate iodide represent inhibitors of cholinesterase. Some drugs act on the end organ to block the action of the parasympathetic system; they are called *parasympatholytic (cholinergic blocking) agents*. Atropine, homatropine, and cyclopentolate are representative of this group.

Autonomic drugs that affect the eyes are divided into mydriatic, cycloplegic, and miotic agents, which comprise most of the commonly used eye medications.

Mydriatic and cycloplegic agents

Mydriatic drops act on the iris musculature and serve to dilate the pupils. *Cycloplegic* drops act not only on the iris by dilating the pupil but also on the ciliary body, paralyzing the fine focusing muscles so that the eye is no longer able to accommodate for near vision (Fig. 4.5). Cycloplegic drops are essential in the refraction of children's eyes and for iritis therapy. Mydriatic agents are primarily used to dilate the pupil for intraocular examinations.

Mydriatic agents

Mydriatic agents with little or no cycloplegic effect are phenylephrine, hydroxyamphetamine, eucatropine hydrochloride, epinephrine, and cocaine.

Phenylephrine hydrochloride (Neo-Synephrine) is available in strengths of 2.5% and 10%. The latter exerts a rapid dilating effect in about 15 minutes and wears off in 1 to 2 hours. Adverse responses with 10% topical phenylephrine have occurred within 20 minutes of the last application of this drug. Some of these patients were treated with application of a cotton pledget of the drug, some by subconjunctival injection, and others by irrigation of the lacrimal sac. A number of deaths have resulted from myocardial infarction and some patients have required cardiac and pulmonary resuscitation for treatment of cardiac arrest. Another group of patients had a marked rise in blood pressure, tachycardia (fast heartbeat), or reflex bradycardia (slowing of the heart). The local ocular reaction reported was massive subconjunctival hemorrhage.

This drug should be used very cautiously or not at all in patients with heart disease, hypertension, aneurysm, or advanced atherosclerosis. Only the 2.5% solution should be used in older adults and in infants. Phenylephrine hydrochloride dilating drops are not recommended for use in low-birthweight infants. The 10% solution should not be used for irrigation. When the drug is used, a cotton pledget should be held over the lacrimal sac for 1 to 2 minutes. Patients who are taking antidepressants or monoamine oxidase (MAO) inhibitors should be treated with caution. These patients may exhibit a significant increase in heart rate.

Phenylephrine is used most commonly as an adjunct to the parasympatholytic drugs (e.g., tropicamide [Mydriacyl] and cyclopentolate [Cyclogyl]) to dilate the pupil for ophthalmoscopy. Despite these serious complications with 10% phenylephrine, no serious adverse effects have been reported with the ophthalmic use of 2.5%, although dizziness, fast, irregular or pounding heartbeats, increased blood pressure, and trembling have been reported.

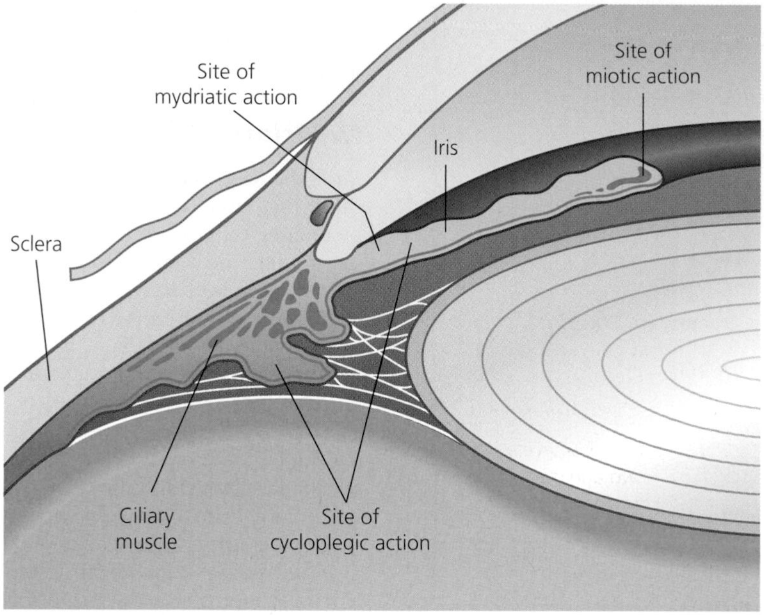

Fig. 4.5 Sites of action of mydriatic, cycloplegic, and miotic agents. Mydriatic drugs act on the dilator muscle of the iris. Cycloplegic drugs act by inhibiting the sphincter muscle of the iris and by paralyzing the ciliary muscle. Miotic drugs act by stimulating the sphincter muscle of the iris, causing the pupil to constrict.

Epinephrine (Adrenalin) exerts a mild mydriatic effect.

Cocaine is primarily a strong anesthetic agent but also exerts a mild mydriatic effect. It can be used to establish the diagnosis of Horner syndrome. It allows one to determine whether a small pupil is part of this syndrome or whether it is caused by other causes, such as a congenital asymmetry of pupil size (physiologic anisocoria).

The drugs that act as pure mydriatic agents exert their effect by stimulating the dilator muscle of the iris.

Cycloplegic agents

Cycloplegic agents act by paralyzing the sphincter muscle of the iris, and thereby producing iris dilation, and by paralyzing the ciliary muscle, which inactivates accommodation. Examples of cycloplegic agents are atropine, homatropine, scopolamine, cyclopentolate, and tropicamide.

Atropine (Isopto Atropine, Atropine-Care, generic), available as 0.5% and 1% solutions and ointment, is one of the most powerful cycloplegic and mydriatic agents. After atropine has been instilled in an adult eye, it requires 10 to 14 days for accommodation to return and the pupil to return to its normal size. With children, the local effects on the eye are similar but systemic complications are more common. The side effects of systemic absorption in children consist of rapid pulse, fever, flushing, and mouth dryness. Systemic absorption of atropine can be reduced by applying pressure over the lacrimal sac. Atropine may cause allergic manifestations in the form of an eczematoid rash around the eye and conjunctival injection. Parents should be instructed in the method of giving the drops and in observing for signs of local or systemic toxicity. Adverse reactions should be reported immediately to the ophthalmologist's office so that proper steps can be taken.

Homatropine (Isopto Homatropine, generic) is a weaker cycloplegic than atropine and is available in strengths of 2% and 5%. Its effect wears off faster than atropine and accommodation returns in 1 to 3 days.

Scopolamine (Isopto Hyoscine) is midway between atropine and homatropine in duration of action. Scopolamine produces fewer allergic responses than atropine and thus is used as a substitute for it.

Cyclopentolate (Cyclogyl, Cylate, AK-Pentolate, generic) is available in strengths of 0.5%, 1%, and 2%. It has a rapid onset of effect (30 minutes) and a duration of action of 6 to 24 hours, which makes it an ideal agent for office use. Occasionally, children can show signs of systemic toxicity not unlike that seen with atropine.

Tropicamide (Mydriacyl, Tropicacyl, generic), 0.5% and 1%, exerts its effects in 20 to 40 minutes and wears off in 4 to 6 hours. It is a relatively weak agent for paralyzing accommodation and is used primarily for its dilating ability when ophthalmoscopic examination is required.

Table 4.3 Routines for common cycloplegic agents

Drug	Strength	Frequency
Atropine	Younger than 2 years, 0.5% Older than 2 years, 1%	Under 5 years, 3 times daily for 3 days before examination
Homatropine	2%, 5%	One drop every 15 min for four applications 1 hour before examination
Cyclopentolate	0.5%, 1%, 2%	One drop every 5 min for two applications 30 min before examination
Tropicamide	0.5%, 1%	One drop every 5 min for two applications 20 min before examination

Cycloplegics are used in the treatment of iritis to relieve ciliary muscle spasm and produce pupillary dilation. The latter is important in preventing the iris from binding down to the lens to form posterior synechiae. These agents are commonly used to inactivate the ciliary muscle for the purpose of objective refraction (Table 4.3). The eyes of darkly pigmented persons dilate with difficulty and hence require stronger concentrations and repeated instillations to obtain an adequate effect. Drugs, such as atropine and homatropine, are not used routinely in adult eye refraction because of the prolonged delay in accommodation and pupillary function.

Miotics

Miotics act by stimulating the sphincter muscle of the iris, which in turn causes constriction of the pupil (see Fig. 4.5). These agents are used in:
- The treatment of open-angle glaucoma because they improve the outflow of aqueous humor from the anterior chamber of the eye
- Angle-closure glaucoma because they withdraw the congestion of iris tissue from the angle structures
- The management of convergent strabismus by reducing accommodative effort (used in place of glasses, especially for children younger than 2 years)
- The treatment of accommodative insufficiency, in which they may play a small role

Direct-acting miotics

Pilocarpine hydrochloride (Isopto Carpine, Pilopine-HS Gel, generic) may range in strength from 0.25% to 6% and have

a duration of action of 4 to 6 hours. Pilocarpine is a stable, inexpensive, and reliable drug. The local side effects may consist of:
- Ciliary spasm, which may produce a headache, especially in young patients
- Decreased vision in patients with cataracts inasmuch as the pupil is made smaller, which allows less light to enter the eye
- Allergic or toxic reactions that involve the lids and conjunctiva

Systemic side effects are uncommon. Pilocarpine is most commonly used in the chronic care management of open-angle glaucoma and acute care treatment of angle-closure glaucoma.

Carbachol (Isopto Carbachol) is available in strengths of 1.5% and 3% and has a slightly longer duration of action than does pilocarpine. It is absorbed poorly through the cornea and is usually prescribed for patients who are allergic to pilocarpine or for those whose condition cannot be adequately controlled by pilocarpine.

Cholinesterase inhibitors

Cholinesterase inhibitors are drugs that inactivate an enzyme in the body called *cholinesterase*. As a result, another chemical, called *acetylcholine*, which is normally inactivated by cholinesterase, is freely permitted to exert its effects. The effect of acetylcholine is similar to that of the direct-acting miotics.

Physostigmine is found in strengths from 0.25% to 0.5%. It is used more frequently in the ointment form because drops are unstable and irritating to the eye. It is a fairly powerful miotic and is frequently combined with pilocarpine in resistant cases of glaucoma. There is a high incidence of allergy to physostigmine. Combinations of miotics are generally not recommended. However, the combination of pilocarpine and physostigmine medication is sometimes advocated because these two drugs are able to reinforce each other. Physostigmine is not commercially available in the United States.

Echothiophate iodide (Phospholine Iodide), 0.03% to 0.25%, is a powerful and long-acting agent. It has been shown to produce cataracts and iris cysts with prolonged usage. It should be kept refrigerated because it deteriorates at room temperature.

Side effects

The long-acting anticholinesterase agents are the most likely to produce side effects both locally (in the eye) and systemically. *Local effects* include:
- Ocular discomfort and pain resulting from ciliary body spasm (most apparent during the initial phase of treatment, usually subsiding as treatment continues)

- Induced myopia with blurred vision for distance
- Cataracts
- Retinal detachment
- Iris cysts
  Systemic effects include:
- Headaches
- Sweating and salivation
- Nausea, vomiting, and diarrhea
- Lethargy and fatigue
- Cardiac arrest and fall in blood pressure

Drugs that lower intraocular pressure

With the introduction of *timolol maleate* (Timoptic, generic) in 1978, new programs of research toward pharmaceutical agents that do not affect the pupil or accommodation began. Timolol is a nonselective beta-adrenergic receptor blocker that acts to decrease the formation of aqueous humor. The drug is available in 0.25% and 0.5% strengths, and dosage ranges from 1 drop daily to 1 drop twice daily with or without other antiglaucoma medication.

Adverse reactions are generally uncommon, but if they are present and significant they may lead one to discontinue the medication. Ocular side effects include corneal anesthesia, a punctate keratopathy, and an allergic blepharoconjunctivitis. Systemic reactions consist of bronchospasm in those with underlying pulmonary disease, bradycardia, hypotension, central nervous system disturbances (e.g., confusion and hallucinations), and gastrointestinal disturbances (e.g., nausea and diarrhea). Timolol should be used with caution in patients with known contraindications to systemic use of beta-adrenergic receptor blocking agents, such as patients with obstructive pulmonary disease (e.g., asthma and emphysema) and cardiovascular disease (e.g., congestive heart failure, bradycardia, heart block, and hypotension).

Because of its excellent therapeutic response, its low frequency of application, and its generally uncommon adverse reactions, timolol has gained widespread use in the ophthalmic community. Levobunolol (Betagan, generic) is equivalent to timolol. Carteolol (generic) is also available and has fewer adverse effects on lipids.

In an attempt to decrease the systemic side effects so that it can be used in patients with asthma and emphysema, betaxolol (Betoptic S, generic), a selective beta-blocker, was developed. Although fewer pulmonary effects are seen with this drug, they have not been totally eliminated. In addition, the fall in intraocular pressure is not as great with betaxolol as with timolol, a nonselective beta-blocker.

A sympathomimetic agent, *dipivefrin hydrochloride* (Propine, generic), is available in a 0.1% concentration for application of 1 drop twice daily. The drug has a 17 times greater penetration through the cornea than epinephrine alone; therefore the amount necessary to achieve a similar therapeutic response is significantly less. This reduces the systemic side effects, which may include an elevation in blood pressure, tachycardia, and headache. Ocular side effects may consist of an allergic blepharoconjunctivitis, a punctate keratopathy, and cystoid macular edema. The latter condition is seen in aphakic patients and has been reported to occur in up to 30%. The macular edema is reversible when the medication is discontinued.

Other drugs used to lower intraocular pressures include apraclonidine hydrochloride (Iopidine), which is available in 1% strength for postlaser intraocular pressure spikes and 0.5% for long-term use. Topical dorzolamide 2% (Trusopt) is a major advance in decreasing aqueous inflow. Its side effects are few. A newer group of prostaglandins is available and effective in one-time daily doses. Latanoprost 0.005% (Xalatan) increases uveoscleral flow, but at the risk of changing iris color. Others that have followed in this group include travoprost (Travatan, Travatan-Z) and bimatoprost (Lumigan). They are available in 2.5 mL, 5 mL, and 7.5 mL sizes. By using once daily, there is less toxicity to the cornea. Cosopt is a combination of dorzolamide hydrochloride and timolol maleate. Combination drugs that are on the market include Combigan (brimonidine tartrate 0.2% and timolol maleate) and Simbrinza (brinzolamide 1.0% and brimonidine tartrate 0.2%).

The drug armamentarium against glaucoma has been greatly aided by the use of drugs, taken orally or intravenously, that lower the intraocular pressure. Those commonly used are the carbonic anhydrase inhibitors, glycerol, urea, and mannitol.

The *carbonic anhydrase inhibitors* block the formation of aqueous humor and thereby lower the intraocular pressure. Examples include acetazolamide (Diamox, generic), 125-mg, 250-mg tablets, and 500-g timed-release capsules; dichlorphenamide (Diclofenamide Daranide), 50-mg tablets; and methazolamide (Neptazane, generic), 25- to 50-mg tablets. Side effects of these drugs are:

- Numbness and tingling of the hands, feet, and tongue
- Drowsiness and fatigue
- Kidney stones
- Gastrointestinal upsets (nausea and vomiting)
- Mild skin eruptions
- Blood disturbances

Glycerin is a thick, viscous liquid in a 50% solution given in an oral dosage of 1 to 1.5 g/kg of body weight and is used to lower the intraocular pressure in acute narrow-angle glaucoma and before intraocular surgery. Because of its overly sweet taste, it is mixed with orange juice or lemon juice to make it more palatable. It can cause nausea, vomiting, or headaches.

Mannitol (Osmitrol) is administered intravenously in 5% to 20% solution, with a total dosage of 0.5 to 2 g/kg of body weight given over a period of 30 to 45 minutes. It is used interchangeably with urea. Along with urea and glycerol, mannitol has a large molecular structure that draws fluid out of the eye and other tissues into the vascular tree of the body.

Anesthetics

Topical anesthetics

Topical anesthetics in drop or ointment form are applied directly to the eye to abolish corneal sensation. Surface anesthesia of the cornea permits the application of instruments, such as the tonometer for the measurement of intraocular pressure. Topical anesthetics are also used to perform surgery on the eye, remove foreign bodies, and facilitate examination with lenses, such as the goniolens. Cocaine, the prototype of the group, is a naturally occurring drug. The remainder of topical anesthetics are synthetic. Cocaine is rarely used as an anesthetic because it causes damage to the corneal epithelium and produces pupillary dilation. However, it is considered useful when removal of the corneal epithelium is desired, as in epithelial debridement for dendritic keratitis. Commonly used topical anesthetics are proparacaine hydrochloride (Proxymetacaine, Alcaine, Paracaine, Ophthaine, Ophthetic, generic) 0.5%; tetracaine hydrochloride (Altacaine, Pontocaine, Tetcaine, generic) 0.5%; cocaine 1% to 4%; benoxinate hydrochloride. The suffix "-caine" appended to the name of the drug usually indicates that the drug is an anesthetic.

An inflamed eye is much more difficult to anesthetize because the blood vessels carry away the anesthetic. For mild anesthesia, such as tonometry, one or two drops are sufficient, but to remove a foreign body deeply embedded in the cornea, more drops may be required at 1-minute intervals.

To avoid a self-inflicted corneal abrasion, it is important that the patient be cautioned against rubbing the eye for a short period after topical anesthesia.

Side effects

Local anesthetics are capable of producing contact allergy. Some anesthetics, such as butacaine, have fallen into disfavor because of a frequent tendency to produce allergic reactions. Side effects do occur, although they are minimal with proparacaine and tetracaine, but cocaine has significant side effects, including:
- Irregularities in the corneal epithelium
- Restlessness and delirium
- Irregular respiration, chills, and fever
- Convulsions
- Cardiovascular disorders

Toxic reactions to cocaine result from central nervous system stimulation and may require the rapid administration of a short-acting sedative to counteract them.

Injectable anesthetics

Local anesthetics by injection are used in ophthalmology to produce:
- Anesthesia of the globe
- Anesthesia of the eyelid
- Paralysis of the muscles that move the eye and the eyelid
- Paralysis of the facial muscles

Commonly used agents are procaine hydrochloride (Novocain) 1% to 4%, lidocaine hydrochloride (Xylocaine) 1% to 2%, and prilocaine hydrochloride (Citanest) 1% to 2%. These agents may be combined with epinephrine, which constricts the blood vessels. The purpose of producing vasoconstriction is to reduce the vascularity of tissues and minimize bleeding. These agents also reduce the amount of local anesthetic absorbed by the blood vessels, thereby prolonging the duration of anesthesia. In addition, local anesthetics may be combined with hyaluronidase, which spreads the anesthetic throughout the tissues, thereby producing more prompt and widespread anesthesia.

Side effects

Injectable anesthetic agents may cause:
- Depression of blood pressure
- Depression of respiration
- Stimulation of the central nervous system, leading to nervousness, dizzy spells, nausea, and convulsions
- Depression of the central nervous system, leading to respiratory or circulatory collapse

Management of toxic side effects

The ophthalmic assistant should be prepared to render assistance in the event of a reaction to a local anesthetic.

Fainting

The following action should be taken when a patient faints. Check the airway and breathing. If indicated, call 911 and begin rescue breathing and cardiopulmonary resuscitation (CPR) (see Ch. 45). Loosen tight clothing around their neck. Raise the person's feet, about 12 inches, above the level of the heart. If the person has vomited, turn the head to the side to prevent choking. Keep the person lying down for a minimum of 10 to 15 minutes in a cool and quiet area. If this is not possible, sit the person forward with the head between the knees.

Central nervous system stimulation

If tremors or convulsions occur, the ophthalmic assistant should attempt to restrain the patient to avoid self-injury. Again, encumbrances around the neck should be loosened. The ophthalmologist may wish to give the patient diazepam (Valium) to control the reaction, so this should be available and ready to use.

Respiratory emergency

A patient who has difficulty in breathing should be watched carefully. If respiration ceases, artificial resuscitation may become necessary. Today, mouth-to-mouth resuscitation is the treatment of choice. Human immunodeficiency virus (HIV) precautions should be adhered to.

Allergic reaction

Severe allergic reactions or idiosyncrasies to drugs may occur that require immediate specific therapy. This is particularly important to the ophthalmologist in view of the increasing number of surgical procedures and fluorescein angiographic examinations being performed in the physician's office. Any patient developing generalized itching, skin rash, difficulty in breathing, or a rapid and weak pulse after administration of a drug should be considered as having an allergic reaction.

Once an acute allergic reaction is suspected, the following prompt treatment is indicated:
- Epinephrine injected subcutaneously or intramuscularly
- Oxygen
- Corticosteroids injected intravenously
- Tracheostomy for laryngeal edema not responding to the aforementioned methods

The ophthalmic assistant should know where to immediately procure and have available for the ophthalmologist:
- Oxygen
- Epinephrine
- Diazepam
- Intravenous cortisone
- Spirits of ammonia or smelling salts
- Syringes with needles

Antiallergic and antiinflammatory agents

Corticosteroids

Corticosteroids are hormones that either are derived from the adrenal gland or are synthetically produced. Cortisone

Table 4.4 Topical steroid preparations

Drug	Concentration (%)
Cortisone acetate suspension	0.5
Cortisone acetate ointment	1.5
Hydrocortisone acetate suspension	0.5, 2.5
Hydrocortisone acetate ointment	1.5
Prednisolone acetate	0.12, 1
Prednisolone phosphate	0.125, 1
Dexamethasone phosphate	0.1
Dexamethasone ointment	0.5
Betamethasone solution	0.5

Table 4.5 Systemic steroids commonly used and their equivalent dose

Drug	Dose (mg)
Cortisone acetate	25
Hydrocortisone	20
Prednisone	5
Prednisolone	5
Triamcinolone	4
Methylprednisolone	4
Paramethasone	2
Dexamethasone	0.75
Betamethasone	0.5

was the first hormone to be isolated. Other steroid preparations are modifications of cortisone, developed to improve and minimize the side effects. For diseases of the eye, steroids are used primarily because they reduce the inflammatory and exudative reaction of diseased tissues. In this regard, they are invaluable because they reduce swelling, redness, cellular reaction, and the final stage of tissue repair, scarring.

Steroids may be given topically or systemically (Table 4.4). Topical steroids are generally used for disorders involving the anterior segment of the eye. Systemic steroids are used for diseases of the posterior segment of the eye and for acute allergic reactions of the eyelids (Table 4.5).

Temporal arteritis

Although steroids are useful in a large variety of ocular conditions, they must be administered with good indication, by the proper route (Table 4.6) and under the supervision of a physician. These precautions are necessary because of the sinister complications of these agents both in the eye and in the body (Table 4.7).

If a patient is receiving steroids, the ophthalmic assistant should inquire into his or her medical background. Patients with conditions of diabetes, hypertension, tuberculosis, and peptic ulcers, if given steroids systemically, often will have an exacerbation of their disease.

Steroid therapy is used in the following eye diseases:
- Contact dermatitis of the eyelids and conjunctiva
- Blepharitis
- Phlyctenular conjunctivitis and keratitis
- Ocular pemphigus
- Vernal conjunctivitis
- Acne rosacea keratitis
- Interstitial keratitis
- Sclerosing keratitis
- Chemical burns of the cornea and conjunctiva
- Marginal corneal ulcers
- Iritis
- Iridocyclitis
- Most forms of posterior uveitis
- Sympathetic ophthalmia
- Herpes zoster ophthalmicus
- Scleritis and episcleritis
- Pseudotumor of the orbit
- Temporal arteritis
- Optic neuritis

Table 4.6 Common routes of steroid administration for ocular inflammation

Condition	Route
Conjunctivitis	Topical
Blepharitis	Topical
Episcleritis	Topical
Keratitis	Topical
Scleritis	Topical and systemic
Anterior uveitis	Topical and subconjunctival
Posterior uveitis	Systemic and subconjunctival
Endophthalmitis	Systemic and subconjunctival
Optic neuritis	Systemic
Temporal arteritis	Systemic
Sympathetic ophthalmia	Systemic and topical

Table 4.7 Side effects of steroids

Ocular effects		Systemic effects
From local application	From prolonged systemic use	
Glaucoma	Decreased resistance to infection	Water and salt retention
Proliferation of bacteria	Delayed wound healing	Mental disturbance
Overgrowth of fungi	Papilledema	Hypertension
Proliferation of viruses, especially herpes simplex	Edema of face and eyelids	Sweating
Decreased wound healing	Cataracts	Generalized weakness
Cataracts	Glaucoma	Wasting of skeletal muscles Demineralization of bones Thrombophlebitis Delayed wound healing Bleeding problems Menstrual irregularities Acne Decreased resistance to infection Growth retardation in children

Table 4.9 Some adverse effects of systemically administered antimicrobial drugs

Drug	Possible toxic effect
Ampicillin	Anaphylactic reactions
Clindamycin	Pseudomembranous colitis
Erythromycin	Stomatitis; gastrointestinal disturbance
Gentamicin	Hearing defect; kidney damage
Meticillin	Allergic reactions; rarely bone marrow depression and renal damage
Nafcillin	Similar to those of meticillin
Oxacillin	Similar to those of meticillin
Sulfisoxazole	Allergic reactions; bone marrow depression
Sulfacetamide	Similar to those of sulfisoxazole

Ideally, an antiviral should have properties that can work on viruses without causing damage to human cells, is cost effective, and is readily available. As we learn more about virus behavior this may come about.

The first antiviral agent, 5-iodo-2-deoxyuridine, although no longer available in the United States, had been invaluable in the treatment of herpes simplex infections of the cornea. This drug, like the other antivirals, interferes with deoxyribonucleic acid (DNA) synthesis of the virus to produce a virus that cannot function as an infective agent. This drug frequently is referred to as idoxuridine (IDU), or its manufacturing trade names of Herplex or Stoxil may be used.

IDU is used topically for the treatment of herpes simplex and vaccinia keratitis. It is of greatest benefit against the epithelial forms of herpes simplex infections. No serious side effects or contraindications are known in the use of IDU as an ophthalmic solution. This drug is given by instilling one drop in the affected eye every hour during the day and every 2 hours during the night until the lesion has cleared. It should be stored in a cool place.

Vidarabine (Vira-A) 3% is an antiviral ophthalmic ointment, specifically for herpes simplex. It is useful for early cases of herpes simplex of the cornea and can be used in cases of herpes resistant to IDU. It does not appear to have any effect on other viruses.

Trifluorothymidine (TFT) or trifluridine (Viroptic), is an antiviral agent used in the treatment of herpes simplex keratitis. It is available as a 1% solution, and the usual dosing schedule is a frequency of every 2 hours when the patient is awake. TFT has been shown to effectively heal 97% of ulcers and to be highly effective in treating diseases resistant to IDU and adenosine arabinoside (Ara-A) or vidarabine. The drug's penetration of the cornea and anterior chamber has been shown to be superior to that of other antivirals.

Acyclovir (Zovirax) is a newer antiviral agent that is administered in oral form. The drug can be metabolized only in cells that have been infected by the herpes virus, and therefore uninfected human cells will not be affected by the drug. Acyclovir has been shown to be effective in shortening the course of disease in herpes zoster (shingles) and in severe cases of herpes simplex.

Other current antiviral agents for systemic or intravitreal administration include cidofovir—intravenous, foscarnet—intravenous, valacyclovir—oral, and valganciclovir—oral.

Antifungal agents

Fungal infections of the eye are uncommon, but when they do occur they can be devastating, especially when treatment is delayed. Antifungal agents generally act by binding to the fungal cell wall. This leads to changes in permeability that result in death of the organism. The most commonly used antifungal agents include the following three:

- Natamycin (Natacyn), or pimaricin, is available in a 5% suspension. Because this drug penetrates tissues very poorly, it is useful only when applied topically
- Amphotericin B (Fungizone) also can be administered topically, subconjunctivally, intravitreally, or intravenously. The drug is highly irritating when used topically and may be toxic to the kidneys when administered intravenously. Use of this drug should be reserved for severe infections or resistant organisms
- Ketoconazole (Nizoral) is available for oral administration. Unlike amphotericin, however, it is generally well tolerated. Significant adverse reactions include liver toxicity.

Antiparasitic agents

Acanthamoeba, a ubiquitous parasite found in soil and water, is capable of causing severe keratitis. The infection is most common as a complication of contact lens wear. Agents that have provided some success in the treatment of this parasite include dibrompropamidine 0.15%, polyhexamethylene biguanide (PHMB) 0.02%, chlorhexidine, and neomycin. Corticosteroids are contraindicated.

Decongestants

Decongestants are solutions that shrink the size of the conjunctival blood vessels and in doing so eliminate excess eye redness. These solutions are used to provide symptomatic relief of eye irritation and watering caused by hay fever,

Table 4.10 Pharmaceuticals used in the treatment of seasonal allergic conjunctivitis

Drug category	Trade name	Generic name
Antihistamine	Optivar	Azelastine
Mast cell stabilizer	Crolom	Cromolyn
Antihistamine	Emadine	Emedastine
Antihistamine/ mast cell stabilizer	Elestat	Epinastine
NSAID	Acular	Ketorolac
Antihistamine/ mast cell stabilizer	Zaditor	Ketotifen
Antihistamine	Livostin	Levocabastine
Mast cell stabilizer	Alomide	Lodoxamide
Antihistamine/ decongestant	Vasocon-A	Naphazoline/ antazoline
Antihistamine/ decongestant	Naphcon-A, Visine-A	Naphazoline/ pheniramine
Antihistamine/ mast cell stabilizer	Alocril	Nedocromil
Antihistamine/ mast cell stabilizer	Patanol	Olopatadine
Mast cell stabilizer	Alamast	Pemirolast

NSAID, Nonsteroidal antiinflammatory drug.

smog, and smoke and to relieve eye fatigue resulting from driving, excessive reading, and close work.

Some common decongestants are phenylephrine (Zincfrin solution, Prefrin, Neo-Synephrine), tetrahydrozoline (Visine), and naphazoline (Vasocon, Privine). A common result of use of these drugs is rebound hypersensitivity with recurring redness.

Decongestants are often called vasoconstrictors (such as phenylephrine) and may be contraindicated in infants and adults with narrow angles. They may bring on an attack of narrow-angle glaucoma. Also, a 10% dose may cause an increase in blood pressure or ventricular arrhythmia and even death.

Antiallergic agents

A number of pharmaceutical agents are specifically used during the allergy season (Table 4.10). Some are combinations of the previously mentioned decongestants and histamine blockers.

Contact lens solutions

With the proliferation of contact lens solutions, three important factors should be considered in choosing a system: safety, efficacy, and cost. Most contact lens solutions contain more than 95% water. The solution formation depends on the addition of preservatives, wetting agents, buffers, surfactants, cleaners, and disinfectants.

Contact lens requirements call for disinfection but not sterilization; although the incidence of eye infection from contact lenses is low relative to millions of wearers, the hazard is always present. Sterilization is the complete destruction of all forms of microbial activity. Disinfection is the destruction of all vegetative bacterial cells, but does not include spores. Common contact lens solution preservatives include organomercurials (e.g., thimerosal, chlorhexidine, and ethylenediaminetetraacetic acid [EDTA]).

Contact lens solutions can cause toxicity or hypersensitivity reactions manifested as conjunctival redness, punctate keratopathy, or corneal infiltrates. Therapy consists of recognizing the potential cause of these symptoms and switching contact lens solutions.

Stains

Fluorescein is an ocular stain used to show defects or abrasions in the corneal epithelium. The pooling of fluorescein on small corneal defects is best seen by means of ultraviolet or cobalt blue light for illumination. The danger with this agent in solution form is contamination with *P. aeruginosa (Bacillus pyocyaneus)*, which appears to flourish in fluorescein. Sterile dry fluorostrips are available commercially to prevent this complication. High-molecule fluorescein has been used with soft contact lenses. The high molecule of fluorescein does not penetrate the pore structure of the soft lens and consequently does not ruin the contact lens during examination.

Rose bengal is a red dye that has an affinity for degenerating epithelium. Similar to fluorescein, it will stain areas in which the epithelium has been sloughed off. The dye also stains cells that are damaged or unprotected by native mucoproteins. Unlike fluorescein, however, intact nonviable epithelial cells of the conjunctiva or cornea will stain brightly with rose bengal. The stain is helpful in making the diagnosis *of keratoconjunctivitis sicca* or other conditions associated with dryness of the conjunctiva and cornea.

Answers, notes, and explanations—Continued

drops that are low in salt concentration or "hypotonic," such as water, also will produce irritation of the eye.

8. **a. Blepharitis**. Systemic administration of steroids is not without hazard and its use is confined to those conditions in which the benefits of steroid therapy cannot be achieved by a local topical route. By systemic administration, the adverse effects may result in water and salt retention, swelling in and about the face and eyelids, mental derangements, hypertension, gastric disturbances, accentuation of diabetes, increased blood glucose level, delayed wound healing, and a number of other medical problems.

9. **c. Valcyclovir** (Valtrex). Valcyclovir has been effective in inhibiting the herpes simplex virus by interfering with the early steps of DNA synthesis. It can be used in cases resistant to IDU or vidarabine.

Chapter | 5 |

Microbiology

*Michael A. Ward**

Microbiology is the branch of science that deals with microscopic, unicellular, and cell-cluster organisms. The major microbial categories that may be associated with eye infections are *bacteria, viruses, fungi,* and *parasites*. A basic understanding of microbiology is helpful for the ophthalmic assistant, who may be required to take smears, stain the appropriate slide, and assist in taking a culture.

In everyday life, we are constantly in touch with microbes. We wash our hands to lower the number of microbes on our outer skin. We disinfect wounds for the same reason. We cover our sneezes and wash our fruit to prevent getting or spreading infectious diseases. We add chlorine to our water supply to inhibit the growth of *pathogenic* (disease-causing) bacteria. We do many things to control the growth of bacteria, but most bacteria are helpful in our daily lives. In fact, we could not live without the help of certain bacteria that exist in and on our bodies. For example, bacteria in our gut are necessary for absorption of certain vitamins.

Some bacteria actually educate our immune system and help to protect us against pathogenic microbial invaders. Certain species of bacteria are normal inhabitants of specific geographic areas of the body and their numbers are controlled by the local environment's moisture, temperature, and available nutrients. However, when such bacteria (say from the gut) get into the wrong place (like the eye) they have the potential to cause disease.

The eye is subject to the same types of infections that may occur in other parts of the body. Microorganisms are everywhere in our environment, and fortunately the eye is very resistant to infection. Our intact epithelial skin surface resists most microbial invaders. Any break in the skin of the outer eye can act as a portal of entry for microbes, at which point if a significant concentration of microbes, an *inoculum*, is present it may overcome our ocular defenses and cause an infection. Ocular trauma, surgery, radiation, severe surface dryness from exposure or inadequate blinking, lid abnormalities, and corneal degenerative changes may create surface disruptions that leave the eye more susceptible to infection. Persons with normal ocular surface structures may still be susceptible to diseases if their ability to defend against infectious agents is compromised. A compromised immune system can be present in patients with diabetes, acquired immunodeficiency syndrome (AIDS), and those taking immunosuppressive agents, such as oral steroids.

A variety of organisms can cause ocular disease of the eye (Box 5.1). These infectious agents have a predilection for certain sites of the eye and usually vary in their severity in causing ocular disease. By far the most common infections result from bacterial and viral organisms. Bacteria are larger than viruses and may easily be seen under magnification by a light microscope. Bacteria range in size from 0.2 to 5 μm and viruses from 0.005 to 0.1 μm. Viruses cannot be seen with a light microscope but can be indirectly viewed with electron microscopes.

*Images in this chapter are courtesy of Michael A. Ward, unless otherwise stated.

Answers, notes, and explanations

A

1. **True**. The herpes simplex virus is one of the most common viruses affecting the eye. The virus invades the corneal epithelium and gives rise to a dendritic ulcer, which usually affects the central portion of the cornea. The ulcer is almost always unilateral and may affect any age group. A history of cold sores on the face can be elicited in approximately 55% of cases. The infection often recurs in the same eye, and the lesion may be precipitated by the following triggering factors: fever, menstruation, cold, emotion, and overexposure to sunlight. Herpesvirus can be cultivated on the chorioallantoic membrane of a developing chick embryo. The virus also has a typical cytopathic effect on HeLa cell cultures.

2. **False**. It is not usually possible to positively identify an organism by means of microscopic shape and staining characteristics, and often it is necessary to obtain a smear and culture the bacteria. A presumptive diagnosis, however, may be made by considering the clinical picture along with the microscopic shape and staining reaction.

3. **False**. Viruses are the smallest organisms that invade the body. Most cannot be seen by present-day forms of light microscopy, and special techniques, such as electron microscopy are necessary for diagnosis.

4. **Wright and Giemsa**. The routine stains used to determine cell structure and the presence of inclusion bodies are Wright and Giemsa stains. These allow the cellular response to a particular agent to be determined. Classically, in acute bacterial conjunctivitis the predominant cells would be polymorphs; in viral conjunctivitis, lymphocytes; and in allergic conjunctivitis, eosinophils. The detection of inclusion bodies is of importance in the diagnosis of inclusion conjunctivitis. Gram stain is used mainly for the detection of bacteria.

5. **Endophthalmitis**. Endophthalmitis is a rare condition that usually manifests as a decrease in vision, pain, conjunctival redness, and vitreous haze. In most cases, the infection follows a penetrating eye injury or surgery for glaucoma or cataract. In rare instances, it is the result of a blood-borne infection. If all three coats of the eye, as well as the vitreous, are involved by the inflammatory process, the condition is called a *panophthalmitis*. It is very difficult to determine clinically whether the patient has an endophthalmitis or a panophthalmitis.

6. **Blood agar**. Cultures are used to determine which infective agent is responsible for a lesion and the sensitivity of the organisms to various drugs. Blood agar is the basic medium used in ophthalmology. Other media used are as follows:
   a. Chocolate agar: gonococci, *Haemophilus influenzae*
   b. Blood agar enriched with vitamin K: *Actinomyces israelii*
   c. Löwenstein-Jensen: *Mycobacterium tuberculosis*
   d. Sabouraud-dextrose agar: fungi
   e. Culture specimens from both eyes should be obtained, even though only one eye is involved. When the specimen is obtained, contamination of the applicator by the lashes and lid margins should be avoided.

7. **d. Adenovirus**. Viral conjunctivitis is characterized by generalized injection of the conjunctiva, minimal discharge, and profuse tearing. The preauricular lymph node is commonly enlarged in adenovirus infections, and occasionally, the patient may have an associated sore throat and fever. Bacterial conjunctivitis is associated with a profuse discharge, which may cause the lids to adhere, and the patient may have difficulty in opening the eyes on awakening. In addition, a history of a sandy, scraping feeling often is obtained. The conjunctiva is diffusely injected and it is rare for the preauricular lymph node to be enlarged. Answers *a, b, c,* and *e* are all common bacterial causes of conjunctivitis.

   In summary, the following table aids in differentiating viruses from bacteria.

	Viral	Bacterial
Tearing	++	–
Discharge	–	++++
Injection	++	+++
Preauricular node	+++	–
Sore throat and fever	+++	+

8. **a. Finger-to-eye transmission**. This question emphasizes the fact that medical personnel who touch lids, conjunctiva, and other ocular tissues must wash their hands between patients when patients with ocular infections are examined. The physician's office is the source of many epidemics of adenovirus infection. In many epidemics, the spread has been traced to finger-to-eye transmissions; many patients with the infection have not had applanation tonometry.

9. **d. Make a smear and take specimens for culture, start antibiotics appropriate for gram-negative and gram-positive organisms, and reevaluate patient in 24 hours**. This patient in all probability has a bacterial corneal ulcer and requires urgent treatment with antibiotics that will be effective against both gram-positive and gram-negative bacteria. Once the organism has been cultured, the antibiotic can be modified appropriately. The presence of the hypopyon does not necessarily imply an endophthalmitis. In all probability, it is a "sterile" reaction to the infected corneal ulcer.

Chapter | 6 |

Office efficiency and public relations

Harold A. Stein, Melvin I. Freeman, and Melissa A. Jones

A well-run office is important not only for the efficiency of the staff but also because it keeps patients essentially happy. The roles of the secretary, bookkeeper, receptionist, and all other staff in a busy office are important. Familiarity with the overall practice is necessary: not only the handling of patients but also the backup services required, such as completing insurance forms, reports, collecting, billing, and accounting.

How to make patients happy

Making patients happy is not just good practice; it may even prevent lawsuits. Patients are ambassadors of goodwill for the practice. The secret to making patients happy lies in developing good communication skills. These communication skills start with an attitude of empathy and caring and letting patients know directly and indirectly that they are important. This attitude is reflected not only by what the physician says and does but also by what the office staff say and do and how psychologically comfortable the patient is made to feel in the office environment. There are a number of ways in which the office staff can show their caring.

1. Do not keep patients waiting for long periods. One of the key factors affecting patients' overall rating of a practitioner is the time spent waiting in the reception area. Waiting time is a major cause of patient dissatisfaction, which increases dramatically when waiting time exceeds 30 minutes. Office schedules cannot always be controlled, especially if emergencies occur. For those physicians who are chronically behind schedule, the staff should take a close look at how appointments are made

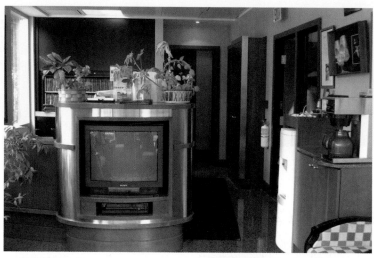

Fig. 6.1 The waiting room should be pleasant and well decorated to make the patient comfortable.

and try to prevent snarl-ups in the schedule. If delays are unavoidable, patients should be told why they are waiting and how long the wait may be; this helps minimize the aggravation. Also, give them options. They may wish to reschedule if an emergency has made the physician significantly late. A Service Recovery Toolkit can also be valuable. It may contain things, such as coloring books with crayons for children or a small gift certificate for a cup of coffee and dessert at a local restaurant. In addition, interesting materials should be available to help patients pass the time. These include topical and current magazines or video educational material with television sets in the waiting room (Fig. 6.1). While waiting, free wi-fi access is an expected service.

2. Make patients feel important. The first contact the patient has with a physician's office should be courteous, respectful, and personalized (Fig. 6.2). This can include little gestures of kindness, such as the nurse asking after a recent baby, the receptionist asking for a preferred appointment time, or the physician inquiring after an ailing family member or recalling some details of an earlier conversation. In the past, it was appropriate for physicians to stand up and shake a patient's hand when first greeting a patient and to touch patients in a neutral manner (on the arm, shoulder, or hand) during the course of a consultation. These gestures convey empathy, friendliness, and concern. Unfortunately, with the recent worldwide pandemic, these gestures are no longer a safe practice. Nevertheless, it is critical to convey information in a tone that is neither patronizing nor too technical so that the patient understands the basic problem and what is going to be done to help correct it. The physician should make eye contact with the patient being examined. Older adults often find it offensive if

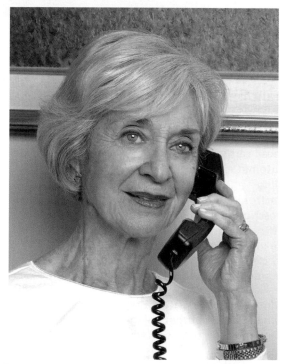

Fig. 6.2 An ophthalmic assistant should be warm and courteous and make the patient feel at ease.

the physician directs advice to the younger person who may be accompanying them. Patients are often reluctant to ask questions, and it is better to err on the side of too much information rather than give insufficient information. Finally, physicians should not make patients feel they are too busy to listen to their problems, because patients may not only go elsewhere but also be thoroughly dissatisfied and litigious.

3. Create space for comfort. Surprisingly small details, such as how the furniture is arranged, can make a difference in overall patient response. In an eye practice, a desk intervening between a patient and the ophthalmologist often serves as a barrier to communication. It is much better to have a direct, closer interaction with the patient. Both intimacy and empathy are given a head start by placing the chairs near each other to eliminate any broad expanse of space between physician and patient.

4. Respect a patient's right to privacy. Any discussions of fees with the physician or receptionist should be conducted privately so that details of these conversations are not overheard by a room full of strangers. Confidentiality is important.

5. Look the part. Some patients do not respond well to individuals with long hair or those dressed in blue jeans, sports shirts, athletic shoes, and sports socks. To earn patient respect, the physician and staff members should wear conservative business attire or the practice uniform. A consistency in color among the staff or laboratory coats may serve the purpose of professionalism. Nametags of the staff are a friendly gesture.

6. In the examining room, pay attention to detail. Unclean examining rooms make patients uneasy, especially when evidence from previous examinations is clearly visible. Cleanliness is an important image for patients, so provide hand sterilizers, for example, Fig. 6.3. Interruptions during an examination can be particularly annoying.

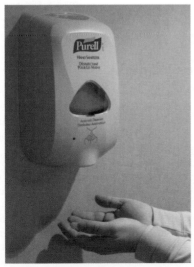

Fig. 6.3 A hand sanitizer for staff and patients is useful to show that the office cares.

A loud intercom system undermines privacy and is unprofessional except for emergencies. Small conveniences, such as a coat rack in the waiting room, along with soothing decor, plants, and art prints, all help to create the impression of a pleasant, welcoming environment and a caring physician. Redecorating every so often may be a good plan. Old or worn-looking magazines is a definite no. Putting magazines into clear plastic holders will keep them looking fresh.

7. Master communication skills. Conversation is an important factor in making or breaking the physician–patient relationship. Here are a few tips:

   • Be upfront. Give information right at the beginning of the visit and not at the end. One can talk while examining with a slit lamp, retinoscope, and so on. Friendly conversation is appreciated

   • Be creative. Use everyday language to explain what is wrong and how you are planning to correct it

   • Be personal. Ask questions about patients' families, social life, and work situations so that they feel they have not been forgotten from one visit to the next. Make notes on charts about patients' interests and concerns for recall at future visits

   • Be prepared. If you have something that needs to be shared with a patient's family, ask them to come in from the waiting room and share the information with them

   • Solicit patient feedback. Confirm that what you have told the patient has been understood by asking the patient to relay the information back to you. This is particularly important for educating patients about care systems for contact lenses. Too often patients leave the office unable to manage their contact lens care systems. Written information will ensure that the message gets across. Handouts are very important and are even more effective if they are personalized. Keep the materials fresh. Update often and do not make copies of copies that end up looking unprofessional and show a lack of attention to detail.

   • Be human. Patients want human beings looking after them. It is perfectly acceptable to tell patients that you also feel bad when the news you have for them is bad.

8. Be fair in all matters of finance. Charge fairly for your professional services but do not overcharge. Be fair in providing refunds to patients who prove to be unsuited for contact lens wear. Always look at the situation from the standpoint of the patient. Maintain goodwill at all costs. It is a truism that one happy patient will let one other person know of your great service but one unhappy patient will tell ten about their bad experience.

9. Never ever put anything on the records that would be damaging if the records appeared in a court room, for example, the patient is crazy.

New patients and returning patients

Normally in an eye practice, there is a 10% to 20% annual increase in new patients. This is important for growth of a practice and for interest. One should record on a month-to-month basis this ratio compared with old patients returning. If the trend of new patients is downward, one has to look at internal marketing. Is everyone being asked for a referral? Is the telephone answered by a recording? Is the call abandonment rate high? Is the telephone voice bright, cheerful, and welcoming? The best marketing is providing the patient with an exemplary experience. One may even consider more external marketing and promotional items. Is a definite percentage of revenues allocated to this?

The telephone

The telephone is usually the first contact the patient makes with the office. These calls must be handled in a manner that will reassure the caller, provide confidence in the office, and at the same time protect the doctor from unnecessary interruptions. The receptionist who answers the phone must have the wisdom of Solomon to permit access to the services on the basis of priority. The staff should answer the phone personally most of the day.

Use of answering machines should be kept to a minimum. Having to respond to a "Press 1, Press 2" command is a turn-off to many.

Basically, two symptoms require immediate attention: pain and loss of vision. Pain can mean anything from acute glaucoma to a corneal abrasion. Whatever the cause, it requires attention. Loss of vision is more difficult to assess. Sudden loss of vision can be a result of a central retinal artery occlusion and should be seen immediately. Other symptoms to be given top priority include transient loss of vision in one eye (carotid artery disease) or flashes of light (retinal detachment).

The telephone should be operated efficiently. Current systems include call forwarding, digital punch systems, conference call systems, and music or information that comes on when the patient is placed on hold. Telephone equipment provides for on-hold messages. This is an ideal opportunity to improve public relations and add some form of promotion for your practice, for example, an on-hold message such as, "We appreciate that your time is valuable. We will be with you as soon as possible. Thank you for holding." This is an important service for busy lines. An adequate number of telephone lines is needed so that the patient does not spend an excessive amount of time listening to busy signals. The use of physician lines, "hotlines," and outgoing unlisted lines is valuable for a busy office.

Frequently called numbers need not be dialed if memory call-through systems are used. Video display units make dealing with a caller easier. For example, if the caller has a swollen red eye, that patient will be seen immediately even if there is a language or articulation problem that prevents understanding the patient's complaints. Services such as Skype and ZOOM allow telehealth visits which is now an expectation.

When the telephone rings, it should be answered at once. The receptionist should not permit the line to ring and ring while completing bookkeeping or other duties. The patient becomes more impatient and difficult to handle with each ring. It is an act of courtesy to permit the caller to hang up the phone first when the conversation is finished. Otherwise, it might seem as if the receptionist is trying to get rid of the patient.

Patience, finesse, and tact are needed to handle many patients on the telephone. The ophthalmic assistant should try to wear a smile at all times. Although callers cannot see the person to whom they are speaking, they can readily sense an attitude over the telephone. The ophthalmic assistant will be called on to help, advise, and sympathize with many patients. Calls should be screened carefully so that the ophthalmologist may answer non-urgent calls at a convenient hour. Sometimes the physician will want the ophthalmic assistant to take calls from patients reporting on their condition or requiring information, or the physician may want to receive all calls from patients personally. Tasking the physicians and nurses through the electronic medical record (EMR) application ensures that patient requests are not lost or misplaced. If this is not part of your EMR, it is important that all telephone messages be recorded on a pad. Memory should never be trusted; a busy schedule often makes memory very short. It is a good idea to use a telephone message pad with a duplicate or carbon copy. If the physician wishes a call returned, the assistant has a copy of the name and number. It also is a handy record of incoming messages and telephone numbers.

Memory joggers

Some individuals remember names well; others remember numbers. Some forget appointments and social dates quickly. There are activities that minimize forgetfulness and can make one more efficient. The old concept of "write it down" applies to all of us.

1. Make notes of everything that you think you may forget. These can be made on a notepad, an Android, or iPhone but should be transcribed into an active memory list sometime later.
2. Keep a daily calendar that is all in one place for writing down appointments, entertainment events, and other personal events. Begin early not to trust to memory.
3. Try to learn at least one new thing daily. If it is an eye disorder or new disease, then write it down and look it up later when time permits.

4. Repeat information to yourself a couple of times. As the day progresses, repeat the information once again.
5. Attend local seminars and record vocabulary you find unfamiliar to look it up later. Online classes or learning modules are a great way to stay current with advances in ophthalmology.

Risk management

The telephone is an important vehicle for interviews and assessment of the patient's problems. Many patients will telephone with emergency problems. Remember that the caller may be confused, distraught, rude, or even unable to give a clear account of what is occurring. Skillful management by the telephone receptionist may be sight saving and perhaps even lifesaving. Therefore the staff member should be courteous, compassionate, efficient, and informative in telephone conversations.

The Board of Directors of the American Academy of Ophthalmology has offered the following guidelines to reduce litigation risks:

* Always confer with the doctor if you have questions relating to the call.
* Take down the caller's number and promise to call back if in doubt about the correct answer to a question.
* Avoid giving general medical advice or discussing diagnoses.
* Answer questions in a friendly but noncommittal manner and refer to the ophthalmologist for definitive answers.
* Do not forget to return the call as soon as possible because often the patient is extremely anxious.
* Try to determine the following:
  * The caller's name, address, and telephone number
  * The essence of the problem
  * When the symptoms first occurred and their duration.

The following list includes typical emergencies that require immediate attention:

1. Chemical contact with the eyes and face. Alkali burns are extremely urgent matters. Patients should have emergency care at the scene of the accident by copious washing before they are brought to the ophthalmologist's office. An acceptable measure would be to fill a basin or bucket with tap water and immerse the patient's head into the water with the eyelids open under water
2. Severe eye, head or face injury, particularly a perforating eye injury
3. Acute or partial loss of vision
4. Recent onset of pain in or around the eye
5. Postoperative pain, infection, or increased redness or decreased vision
6. Recent bulging of an eye
7. Recent onset of flashing lights, floaters, curtains, or veils across the vision
8. Recent onset of double vision
9. Recent change of pupillary size
10. Recent onset of droopy eyelid
11. Foreign bodies in the eye
12. Urgent consultations requested by other physicians.

If the patient has an emergency problem and the physician is unavailable, it is best to advise the patient to see another physician or obtain emergency room care immediately. One outstanding admonition that hangs over the head of every physician is that of "abandonment." One cannot abandon patients, particularly those in the immediate postoperative period. This carries sensitive legal implications.

It is important not to release any information regarding a patient without a legally valid written authorization. A caller who identifies him- or herself as a close relative desiring information should be asked to speak to the physician in the patient's presence.

Remember that all recommendations by the American Academy of Ophthalmology are only examples of important considerations. They should be supplemented by instructions from the ophthalmologist and experienced staff members.

Returning telephone calls

Patients' telephone messages should be responded to on the same day and within a reasonable period of time if possible; otherwise the office staff may have to deal with aggravated patients. Waiting until the end of the day to return patients' telephone calls can be a burdensome task; staff members are fatigued and it may be difficult to reach the patients. In addition, while waiting for their call to be returned, patients have had an opportunity to think about their problems more and become anxious.

Patients appreciate a quick response. Further, the patient who knows that the call is being made between patient appointments may be less likely to waste time with casual questions. If it appears that the call will take a long time, the staff member can arrange to call the patient back at a later time or encourage the patient to make an appointment to come into the office.

Telephone manners

A telephone call is usually the first contact a patient has with the ophthalmologist's office. The following rules ensure a good impression:

1. Personality is revealed by voice and language. How you speak and what you say are the two most important factors in handling telephone calls. The voice should be clear, courteous, friendly, alive, and precise.

Pronunciation should be clear, with lips placed about half an inch from the mouthpiece. Cultivate an attractive, well-modulated voice with pleasing inflections. You should try to make your voice attractive, just as you would try to make your appearance attractive. The impression that is created for the person calling depends on the inflection and tone of your voice. The impression you make—good, poor, or indifferent—reflects on the ophthalmologist and the office. You are the ophthalmologist's representative.

2. Use well-selected, appropriate words and phrases (Box 6.1). Express yourself with a business-like conciseness in a courteous manner. Use the terms "please," "thank you," "I am sorry," and other expressions of appreciation and regret with a tone of sincerity, which will be quite obvious to the listener. Do not try to cut the person off with constant interjections. Above all, be understanding.

3. Ask who wishes to speak to the doctor. The doctor may not wish to speak to a brother-in-law or a stockbroker but may be receptive to calls from an industrial nurse.

4. Tell patients that the doctor can best answer a call after hours. There is more time and less disruption of normal service. Make sure the doctor receives all patient calls. It is good public relations to ensure that those calls are returned by the doctor on the same day.

5. The office should have enough lines so that busy signals are kept to a minimum. Use a *private line* for any outgoing calls and keep these to an absolute minimum. Avoid personal calls. Cell phones should be put away and only used during breaks and emergencies.

6. Avoid putting people on hold unless absolutely necessary. If you must put someone on hold, explain the situation and ask if the person would like to hold or would prefer that you return the call in a few minutes. If the choice is to hold, *thank the person for being patient* as soon as you return to the line. Remember, courtesy is very important.

7. Be calm and steady and avoid excitement or abruptness even when the lines become busy. Keep your remarks short. The longer you talk, the more irritable the person on the line or on hold becomes.

8. It has been said that people prefer to talk to those who speak at roughly the same speed as they do, that is, a fast-speaking caller is happier being dealt with by a fast-speaking person. They seem to bond. Therefore match the speed of your voice as well as the tone to the caller.

9. Try not to abandon the telephone at lunch to an answering service. Rotate the incoming calls among staff members. An answering service should be used sparingly because personnel are not skilled in handling patient questions nor do they have access to the appointment book for schedules.

10. Never repeat personal information you may hear, no matter how unimportant it may seem to you.

11. If answering services are used after hours, train them well in what to say in response to a few basic questions that might be asked. Typed script responses can be helpful.

12. Do not hesitate to ask for the repetition of words or names if you are in doubt. Many names sound very much alike but are quite different. Foreign names given by persons with an accent should be repeated or spelled slowly until they are understood. To ensure accuracy, repeat numbers, amounts, addresses, and other important items. Always remember to get two identifiers when speaking with a patient.

13. Have paper and pencil ready for messages and obtain accurate and complete information, including correct name, address, and telephone number in duplicate.

14. Keep a list of frequently called telephone numbers. Those used regularly can be programmed into your phone system.

15. Sit properly. Poor posture produces fatigue early in the day, and fatigue becomes reflected in your voice.

16. Do not photocopy a medical chart and give it to a patient unless authorized by the ophthalmologist. There may be a lawsuit pending.

17. Avoid discussion of fees unless so instructed.

Box 6.1 Telephone techniques

Do not say	Say
When do you want to come in?	Would you prefer a morning or afternoon appointment?
The doctor is booked up until____.	The doctor is scheduled at that time. He can see you at_____.
The doctor is running late.	The doctor was interrupted in his schedule today.
I called to remind you that_____.	I called to confirm or verify_____.
Cancellation.	Change in schedule.
Checkup.	Examination.
Are you an old patient of Doctor__?	Are you a former or established patient of Doctor_____?
You misunderstood.	There was a misunderstanding.
Are you a patient here?	When did we see you last?
Are you on welfare or Medicare?	What type of health insurance coverage do you have?
What is your problem?	Can you tell me what your problem is so we can schedule you properly?

<table>
<tr><td>

Box 6.2 **Pet peeves of callers**

1. Receive a recording too many times
2. Doesn't introduce oneself. Doesn't use their name. Treats them like a number
3. Put them on hold before they have had a chance to speak
4. Keep them on hold too long without returning to the telephone
5. Transfer them to people who can't help them: "the runaround"
6. Promise to call them back and never do
7. Accidentally disconnect them, particularly a long-distance call, without getting their name or telephone number

</td><td>

Box 6.3 **Establishing rapport with patients**

Sentences of goodwill

"Thank you for holding, Mrs. Brown."
"How may I help you?"
"It's very important that you come in right away."
"I'd like to verify some information to ensure that your medical record is current."
"Could you please repeat the appointment information to me, Mrs. Jones, so I can make sure I communicated clearly?"

Responding to angry patients

"I understand how you feel.'
"Hello, Mrs. Jones. This is Tammy Smith, Dr. Brown's assistant."
"That's understandable, Mrs. Jones."
"I'll be happy to see that the doctor calls you by 5:00 PM. How can we reach you?"

</td></tr>
</table>

18. Avoid any discrimination. Everyone has the right to receive equal treatment to services regardless of race, ancestry, color, place of origin, citizenship, creed, sex, sexual orientation, age, marital status, or disability. This discrimination may be an act, decision, or communication that imposes a burden on them or denies them a right or benefit that others may enjoy.

19. Ophthalmologists may restrict their practice to a subspecialty but should make recommendations or suggestions for ongoing care to a colleague. The referral should be made in a timely manner. The ophthalmic assistant may aid in this referral.

Office personnel should always remember when answering the telephone that they are important representatives of the doctor and can assist immensely in the building of a reputation. They must be master psychologists tuned in to the emotional ills and pressures of the public. In many cases, a voice is the only contact that the telephone patient has with the office. Therefore the office must be represented with courtesy, dignity, and a spirit of service, with personnel giving clear and complete answers promptly.

Kim Fox, in her book *Telephone Power*, suggests the seven pet peeves of callers. She also outlines ways of establishing rapport with patients (Boxes 6.2 and 6.3).

Scheduling appointments

It is difficult in an ophthalmology office to be on time. Because many patients require dilating eyedrops, it means everyone must wait at least 30 minutes. Therefore waiting patients are always present. If emergencies or difficult cases are added, then the normal waiting time can be extended to 1 hour. Waiting is tedious. No one likes to sit beside a total stranger for prolonged periods. Patients become irritated and their tempers grow short. The irritability spreads and affects the entire staff. A hostile patient does not foster good doctor–patient relations.

If waiting is a fact of the office environment, the best way to prevent a potentially disruptive situation is to explain on the patient's arrival that a wait of 30 to 45 minutes may be required to allow for eyedrops and a preliminary examination before the patient sees the ophthalmologist. It does not change the reality of waiting but at least the person knows what to expect and, more important, the reason for the delay. If it is a reasonable explanation, most patients will understand and accept the distress of sitting around. Occasionally, a patient will be unreasonable and short-tempered but one cannot satisfy everybody. The assistant should always forewarn patients about the necessity of waiting for the doctor and explain why. Available coffee, tea, or soft drinks along with a TV monitor help goodwill. For those waiting, free wi-fi access is a must.

The waiting game can produce bitterness on both sides. For the physician, the patient who does not show up for an appointment, or shows up late, has kept the clinician waiting. Some physicians charge for missed appointments. A valid case can be made for doing so, because time is the major commodity for the professional. Many patients feel the same way. Who is to say that a physician's time is more important than anyone else's? Some patients have billed their physicians for lost time spent uselessly in a waiting room. Of course, these views represent the extremes of the doctor–patient dispute.

It is difficult to control the size of an eye practice and simultaneously retain patient goodwill. A well-trained ophthalmic assistant can be the solution, in whole or in part, to the doctor's dilemma. The ophthalmic assistant responsible for telephone appointments acts in the role of doorman to the practice. The assistant is, after all, the first contact the patient has with the office. He or she can attract or discourage new patients or drive away old ones.

The ophthalmic assistant may not be primarily responsible for the scheduling of appointments but should act in a supervisory capacity to see that the physician's appointment schedule is not overcrowded. Any appointment system must be formulated to suit the particular working habits and peculiarities of the physician involved. Appointments must be generously spaced and an adequate amount of time allocated for any special procedures that are to be performed. An efficient appointment system makes allowance for the fact that many patients will require eyedrops. Special consultations for problem cases will require additional time apportioned to the patient's visit. Emergencies often arise during the course of the day and blocks of time may be set aside to permit the efficient, smooth handling of these emergencies with minimal disruption of the existing schedule. A routine daily huddle with the physician and assistants allows schedules to be refined. Knowing what worked, or did not work, yesterday allows scheduling mistakes to be minimized and leads to a continual improvement of the schedule. We can learn from our mistakes and successes.

No one should rely on memory in recording an appointment. All appointments must be marked in the appointment book, preferably in pencil so that they can be erased in case of cancellation. A more efficient way to handle appointments is a computerized scheduling system. This allows instant recall if someone calls in about a future appointment. This is now the most common way, but it depends on a staff person who is computer literate.

In making an appointment, it is important to spell the name of the patient correctly. The telephone numbers, both home and business, should be obtained in case it is necessary to contact the patient to alter the time of the appointment. The appointment time should be repeated to the patient at least once, so that there is no misunderstanding about the date and time. Whenever possible, patients should be given the first available appointment time suitable for their needs. Tactful questioning of the patient should reveal who referred the patient, whether it was a physician, an optical house, an optometrist, or another patient. It is a matter of good public relations to note this person in the appointment book, as a reminder when the patient arrives.

More time should be allowed for first visits because the doctor will require and usually will wish to spend more time examining new patients. When special tests or procedures are anticipated, such as visual fields or minor surgery, they should be noted and suitable time permitted. The appointment schedule should be marked in advance whenever the physician is attending meetings or conferences so that double bookings do not occur, to avoid cancellations and rescheduling.

It is false economy to book patient appointments too close together and not leave adequate time for individual staff, department, and all-staff meetings, or to fail to put major policies and group decisions in writing. Hallmarks of the most successful practices include:
- Doctor breakfast or lunch meetings to communicate as colleagues
- Roundtable sessions to solve specific problems at a set time
- General staff meetings
- Suggestion boxes strategically placed
- An annual retreat
- A written procedure and policy manual
- Weekly staff bulletins
- Email communication to staff
- Routine physician/staff huddles

Booking the arriving patient

When a patient arrives at the office, certain documentation procedures must be performed to obtain the vital information necessary for the complete charting of the patient. The area of introduction of the patient to the staff should be pleasant. Records should be readily available.

If the receptionist has a good memory, greeting the patient by name on arrival is good public relations. If not, tact in obtaining vital information is important. Many patients will be reticent about giving their age, particularly in front of other patients. Insurance numbers and statistics on financial affairs must be tactfully handled. If a verbal request for information does not provide sufficient confidentiality, a blank information card on a clipboard can be given to patients to complete while they are seated and then returned to the receptionist. This is preferable to asking for confidential information in front of others. Ensure Health Insurance Portability and Accountability Act (HIPAA) confidentiality requirements are maintained. Always use two identifiers to ensure that you are speaking with the patient whose chart you are reviewing.

All patients should be given a warm welcome, just as if they were being received into a home. They should feel wanted and comfortable no matter how busy the office situation at the time. Each person should be treated as an individual. Some personal detail that may have been noted previously should be inquired after if the receptionist knows the patient.

Records of patients seen previously will be obtained from the files. If the patient has never been seen before, a new record is opened and all the vital information recorded. This process should be part of a written policies and procedures manual.

Once the day begins with the scheduled appointments, it is important that there be minimal delay in the processing of each patient. Before the patient is seen by the ophthalmologist, politeness, kind words, and a cheerful "hello" will go a long way in promoting goodwill for the ophthalmologist and the office. The office assistant should always speak to the patients and assure them that they will be seen shortly by the doctor.

In ophthalmology, because eyedrops are usually instilled and the patient must wait a given length of time, a proper flow of patients into different rooms should be planned. The placing of patients into designated rooms by the ophthalmic assistant will ensure proper attention by the ophthalmologist with minimal delay. Patients with sore or painful eyes should be seated in the waiting room in such a position as to avoid facing glaring lights.

The reception room

Once in the office, the patient should not have to wait more than 15 minutes before being shown into an examination room. Those 15 minutes in the reception room should be comfortable and pleasant.

A wide variety of current reading material will occupy patients as they wait. Chairs should be spaced so that each patient has elbow room and does not feel cramped up to another person. As a courtesy to patients who find cigarette smoke irritating, you might post a sign that reads "Smoking not permitted in this healthcare facility."

Many offices have educational brochures available that explain common eye ailments. The reception room is a perfect place to circulate patient information brochures or past newsletters and to dispense information about the practice. Brochures might contain information on office hours, insurance, emergencies, and new medical developments for eye conditions. Ensure these are updated regularly.

The decor of the reception room should create a bright, cheerful atmosphere. Artwork, photographs, plants, and fresh-cut flowers will assist. Depending on the doctor's wishes, the assistant may choose to have coffee, juice, or water available to patients on request. A TV monitor with low or no sound may be of help.

Avoid personal conversations with other staff members or on the phone with friends because these often can be overheard by patients. It is not always apparent when a patient is just around the corner. Staff must be professional at all times.

Running late

No matter how carefully an appointment system is planned, delays and waiting periods will occur in a busy ophthalmic practice. Unlike other specialists, who can control to a certain extent the number of return visits, ophthalmologists,

because of the number of emergencies encountered coupled with demands from referring physicians, have difficulty in adhering to a fixed schedule. Ironically, the qualities that make them run late are the qualities that make them available to patients. When an emergency patient calls, an ophthalmologist says, "Yes, come in and I will take care of you." When a patient talks about ailments (or problems that may be causing the illness), a good doctor will not shove the patient out the door just to stick to a schedule. When confronted with a complicated eye problem requiring extensive testing, a competent ophthalmologist, no matter how busy, will take the time to arrive at the diagnosis that sometimes may be not only sight saving but also lifesaving.

When the doctor is running late, if the waiting patients begin complaining, the ophthalmic assistant should give them a little insight into these facts.

Scribes

Scribes are a major time saver for an ophthalmologist in the recording of information. They can increase the productivity of the office and reduce patient waiting time.

Some ophthalmic assistants train to be a scribe for the examining ophthalmologist. They must be familiar with ophthalmic vocabulary, as well as vocabulary shortcuts, symbols, and testing equipment. They should have legible handwriting or excellent typing skills. Ophthalmic scribes can save time in an office not only by recording the examination details but also by prewriting prescriptions for drugs and spectacles for the licensed doctor's signature. They also assist when reemphasizing instructions while the doctor sees the next patient. Ophthalmic assistants' knowledge will increase by virtue of the fact they will eventually see and hear about every ophthalmic disease, disorder, and treatment.

Another advantage of a scribe to an eye practice is that it allows the physician more face-to-face time with the patient. Forms are often delegated to the scribe to fill in then return to patients immediately, rather than by mail.

The ophthalmologist should verify that clinical notes and forms are completed accurately.

Scribes' signatures should be placed for medical-legal purposes, and on electronic records, scribes should have their own password.

Making future appointments

If a repeat appointment is required within the next 2 to 3 weeks because of iritis, conjunctivitis, glaucoma, or postoperative care, this appointment should be made at a designated time that does not overcrowd an already crowded appointment schedule. Usually these repeat visits are short so they can be scheduled before other regular appointments or integrated into the appointment system by a reserved block of time at the end of the appointment system.

It is also important for working patients that repeat appointment times be given early in the day. A minimal amount of delay is expected in the appointment system at that time because unexpected emergencies tend to occur as the day progresses.

Financing

There are a number of financing companies that provide excellent resources to finance expensive procedures for the uninsured or underinsured surgical patient. These companies also provide handouts, newsletters, emails, and support staff to inform patients of the availability of financing for surgery.

Recall cards

Recall cards probably are the single most important vehicle an office has to maintain a regular, steady flow of patients. Many patients need to see an ophthalmologist only every 3, 6, or 12 months. Keeping a record of when they are due for their next examination is a method of ensuring that they receive continuing eye care, particularly for glaucoma or postoperative patients. It is difficult to provide the quality of eye care necessary if people forget or neglect to check their eyes. A recall card is a friendly reminder inviting them to call the office to schedule an appointment at their earliest convenience.

If your EMR does not provide for an automated recall system, the best way to establish a recall card system is to set up a tickler file and keep it near the last person to speak with the patients before they depart from the office. At that time, the physician's notes can be read and a recall postcard addressed with the month of suggested return on it. It is then filed in the tickler file according to month. At the beginning of each month, the recall cards that are in the file for the following month should be sent out. Some offices like to follow up the recall card with a personal telephone call. Future appointments may be made as far ahead as 1 to 2 years in an appointment book or computer. It is important to remind these patients by SMS (text), email, postal card or by telephone at least 1 to 2 weeks and also 1 to 2 days before the appointment. Rescheduling may be required if the date selected is no longer convenient for the patient.

Automated voice machines

There are several companies offering telephone assistance for offices to optimize patient communication. We are familiar with the TeleVox system, which provides caller ID on all incoming calls, prompts the caller to transfer to specific departments—such as to schedule appointments—and provides extensions to speak to live personnel. The system messages can be customized and changed to suit the priorities of the office.

The system can also be used for appointment reminders for scheduled patients, at an appropriate time 2 to 3 days ahead of their appointment. This can be achieved by simply entering the database of upcoming patients and can essentially reduce the "no show" rate by 35%. This also provides an opportunity to fill the appointment holes with transfers, emergencies, referrals, and so on, and helps raise the overall efficiency of the office.

The recall message can be produced in several languages, a nice touch for some, which may help to reach out to patients who have never returned.

Filing

Filing is an important aspect of everyone's everyday practice. If a file is lost or misfiled, a great deal of valuable information may be lost, including measurements that may be impossible to obtain again. The doctor may have to spend considerable time trying to recover information. Anyone may remove files from the filing system, but only one person should be delegated the responsibility of refiling. When a file is misplaced, everyone may be called on to aid in the search for the file. Often the file may have been removed for reports, letters, surgery, and so on.

Most ophthalmic offices have a central filing system, with files placed in alphabetic order. These systems may be further subdivided by an active drawer, which includes files of patients who are under active treatment and who will be returning within the next 4 weeks. Some hospitals and offices file their charts under a numeric system. This is more efficient and minimizes lost files, but it requires additional work. Each chart is numbered in order of being opened and it is filed accordingly. Cross-references are made of all names, in alphabetic order, and even double cross-referenced so that any special foster names or married names are indexed. In an alphabetic system of filing, the controversial order of names, such as those beginning with Mac and Mc and names such as DeForest are filed according to an agreed-on procedure, which must be known to all. In addition, common names, such as Brown, Smith, and Lee should be arranged in the order of the initial of the patient's first name. The numeric filing system eliminates these challenges and minimizes the number of misfiled records.

It has been our practice to separate the financial from the clinical records for each patient seen. With the advent of Medicare, we have found it expedient to change our patient processing routine so that the financial records, including billing and posting, are prepared at the time of the patient's office visit. The first statement and an account for submission to the insurance company can be given to the patient at this time.

Laboratory and x-ray reports, along with letters from other physicians, must be appended to the patient's chart and brought to the attention of the eye doctor. It is unacceptable to simply file such letters with the chart until the next patient visit without them being seen by the eye doctor.

Missed appointments and cancellations should be noted on the patient's chart and brought to the doctor's attention. Sometimes important litigation hinges on this type of information.

Files should be purged at least annually to allow more space. Outside storage is an option if space is limited. Files of known deceased patients and very old files should be purged regularly and sent to a shredding service or shredded onsite if available. One should establish a year date for the last visit (e.g., 7 years, 10 years) before deleting a file. The practitioner's office should have a policy for length of retention of medical records that follows state or provincial laws and advice of the practice's malpractice insurance company.

Electronic medical and health records

EMRs and electronic health records (EHRs) are a computerized medical records system created in organizations that deliver health care, such as hospitals, integrated delivery networks, clinics, ambulatory surgical centers, and healthcare provider offices. These records make up a healthcare information system that allows for storage, retrieval, and modification of the healthcare record.

The terms EMRs and EHRs are often used interchangeably, although technically EMRs represent a duplicate of a paper-based charting, whereas EHRs are electronic records with the ability for electronic exchange of patient data from practice setting to practice setting. These electronic records can contain a wide range of patient data including patient demographics, medical history, medications, allergies, immunizations, vital signs, physical examination findings, laboratory tests, radiologic images, photos, prescriptions, and billing and insurance information.

EHRs are being heavily promoted by federal and state governments, insurance companies, and large medical institutions as a system to help physicians and office staff better care for patients before, during, and after healthcare encounters. Because of these promotions, EHRs are being incorporated into the vast majority of healthcare provider offices. They are ways to improve efficiency, promote quality improvement, overcome poor penmanship that contributes to medical errors, and offer standardization of forms, terminology, and abbreviations. They allow for data input for collection of epidemiology and clinical data. Barriers to adoption of electronic records include start-up costs, system maintenance costs, and training costs. Patient privacy issues are of concern with electronic records because of their portability and potential access by unscrupulous users and unauthorized individuals. It is necessary that all HIPAA requirements be met.

Prescription pads

Each prescription for a medication should be signed by the prescribing doctor. For most of those with EMRs, the prescriptions should be created in the application and sent electronically to the patient's pharmacy of choice. Blank prescription pads should be kept in a drawer so a patient (or staff member) is not tempted to steal a pad and self-prescribe a narcotic or other medication.

Office equipment

Equipment is an important factor in office efficiency. The ophthalmologist or office manager must constantly be on the watch for new business machines that may improve office efficiency. These include calculators, postage meters, and multifunctional devices, which normally include the copier, scanner, e-mail, and fax functions. One also must watch for new ideas in billing procedures and form procedures that will be helpful. Floor and wall coverings that reduce noise should be used. Seats should be arranged to relieve back strain. Stamping and sealing envelopes by machine greatly facilitate the speed of these procedures. The telephone system should be regularly reviewed to ensure that one has the most efficient system available and that proper lines of communication are established between rooms, through either the telephone or an intercom system.

The personal computer, which is now standard in the ophthalmic office, is discussed in detail in Chapter 20.

Ophthalmic equipment is very precise and must be kept in perfect working order. Basic principles to consider include the following:

1. Keep the machines (slit lamp, keratometer) covered when not in use.
2. Regularly check the accuracy of such devices as the radioscope, keratometer, and lensometer.
3. Learn to maintain the instruments, from changing a bulb in the projector to attaching a topogometer.
4. Make sure regular maintenance is performed for such instruments as the automatic refractor, keratometer, pneumotonometer, visual field, and corneal topography machines.

apply oneself. The ophthalmic assistant must be orderly, accurate, and careful in conduct, show an ability to intelligently and quickly answer the many questions that patients ask, and above all show a good sense of humor.

Moral qualities, the foundations of character underlying everything else, include honesty, sincerity, loyalty, and trustworthiness. The ophthalmic assistant should have the courage and determination to do the right thing, regardless of the consequences. Considering the welfare of the patient is always the best starting point. These qualities provide an important guideline to the daily behavior of the ophthalmic assistant who works with the public. An assistant can review the effectiveness evaluation to see how he or she rates (Box 6.4). Self-evaluation can be important.

Personal qualities for improved office efficiency

Avoiding interruptions

Before leaving the office at night, create a to-do list for the next day and prioritize the order. Organize a special me or personal hour (preferably early in the morning) and turn all phones and distractions off. Tell your coworkers you want "peace and quiet" to do a special project. You will probably complete this in half the time! Do not become distracted by other tasks or emails on your computer; if you have a door, close it. If you work in a cubicle, put up a "do not disturb" sign, and if appropriate devote at least 1 to 2 hours a day to uninterrupted work. Tell other assistants what you are doing and they will probably do the same.

The attitudes of each of us are based on our likes and dislikes and are expressed in our words, our actions, and our behavior. Some of these attitudes become habits, some of which are helpful and some harmful to ourselves, the people we work with, and the patients we greet. The ophthalmic assistant should analyze these attitudes and try to eliminate those that are inappropriate.

An attractive personality depends on an expression of physical, mental, social, and moral qualities. Physical qualities give first impressions to people we meet. Our appearance, voice, manner, energy, and bearing portray a first impression to the patient. Social qualities are developed through our everyday contacts with people. To make a favorable impression one must be considerate of others, cooperative, and courteous and show tact, cheerfulness, and kindness. In addition, patience and sympathy must be part of one's personality. These attributes create a pleasant and stimulating atmosphere in the office.

Mental qualities include intelligence, a keen observation, a retentive memory, and an ability to concentrate and

Improving the patient experience through service recovery

It has been said that "a happy patient will tell one other person of their great experience. An unhappy patient will tell five." This adage is no longer accurate. With the widespread use of Twitter, Facebook, Instagram, and sites such as YouTube, an unhappy person can now connect with literally millions of others with very little effort and in a very short time. This highlights the need to ensure the best possible patient experience, especially if some type of service issue occurs.

There are two types of service issues: expected and unexpected. The expected is handled by proactive methods and established triggers that start the service recovery process. These mishaps include the usual examples of the doctor being late and emergencies arising in the clinic. Communicate early with patients about problems or delays, and offer sincere apologies. A tool kit with gift cards for coffee or a nearby restaurant, taxi vouchers, and other goodies also can be useful.

The unexpected mishaps are a bit more complicated, such as patients arriving on the wrong day or making unreasonable requests. First, one needs to know how to recognize these situations through tell-tale signs; patient body language, tone of voice, anger, or silence. Then one must be prepared to listen, ask questions, and listen again.

Respond with HEART, which stands for:

Hear. "Please tell me what has happened. I'd like to know how I might help you today." Hear what the patient has to say by truly listening. The biggest gift you can give another is your full attention. Try not to formulate a response while the patient is speaking; just work to understand his or her point of view.

Box 6.4 Rating effectiveness as an ophthalmic assistant

Dependability

Trustworthiness in carrying out instructions and assignments
Excellent
Above average
Average
Below average
Unsatisfactory

Productivity

Achievement of satisfactory quantity of work
Excellent
Above average
Average
Below average
Unsatisfactory

Adaptability

Reception of new ideas and methods; adjustments to
    changes in work
Excellent
Above average
Average
Below average
Unsatisfactory

Cooperation

Tact: willingness to assist; agreeable compliance
Excellent
Above average

Average
Below average
Unsatisfactory

Accuracy

Exactness, professional skill
Excellent
Above average
Average
Below average
Unsatisfactory

Initiative

Performance in analyzing problems, accepting responsibilities,
    planning necessary action, and following through
Excellent
Above average
Average
Below average
Unsatisfactory

Individuality

Personal appearance, neatness, behavior on job
Excellent
Above average
Average
Below average
Unsatisfactory

Empathize. "I know what you mean. It can be difficult. I understand what you might be feeling." People want to have their feelings validated. Expressing understanding goes a long way toward helping defuse a tense situation.

Apologize. "I'm sorry that this happened. Please accept our apologies for this delay. I know that your time is valuable." Give a simple apology without blame. Be sincere.

Respond. "How would you like it resolved? We'll be addressing this by…" Make sure to follow up with the patient. Set a timeline for any responses or additional actions, and be sure to stick to it. Give the patient your contact information so that you can be contacted if further questions arise.

Thank. "Thank you for bringing this to my attention. I appreciate you letting me know about this." No one wants to be considered a problem, and these occasions should be looked at as opportunities for improvements. Without someone pointing out issues, larger problems can occur in the future.

What can be expected from patients? Three possibilities are:

Those who have had a great experience: no problem, they are happy

Those who have had a bad experience and no one responds to it: they are unhappy

Those who have had a bad experience that is resolved: these patients are the happiest of all

This is not meant to be a case for making patients unhappy, but a case for the power of service recovery. Complaints are a gift and the schoolbook from which we can learn. Handling complaints skillfully can actually lead to staff satisfaction. It feels good to resolve a conflict, and the payoff of a happy patient is priceless. Responding with HEART will pay great dividends to patients, staff, and the practice.

Administrative assistant duties

The ophthalmic assistant may be required to compose or type letters to insurance companies, physicians, or suppliers. Although the dictator of the letters is responsible for clarity, thought, and completeness, the typist must be given credit for proper setup and form of the letter. Margins must be clearly laid out, paragraphs introduced properly, and punctuation correctly placed. The visual setup of the letter is as important as the wording: both contribute to the impression the receiver will form about the office. Programs, such as Microsoft Word, help ensure that correspondence looks professional.

As time goes on, many types of forms will become routine and standardized. Even letters will have a standard form of setting up introductory paragraphs and conclusions. The best way of doing things becomes standard. No matter what it may be, there is a best way of doing it, whether it is folding and sealing a letter, putting on a stamp, setting up a letter, or saving a copy. Once these standards are discovered and established, the wasteful and useless movements are eliminated.

Handling the ophthalmologist's schedule

Eye doctors are usually busy people; consequently considerable demands are made on their time in the office, in the hospital, and in extra activities. They may be required to fulfill teaching roles and speaking engagements and become involved in community work. From time to time these additional involvements will be made known to the ophthalmic assistant. When they interfere with existing schedules, the assistant should try to ensure that the office and the hospital are organized to accommodate these changes.

The assistant must ensure the appointment book is not overcrowded so that the physician is not constantly delayed in attending meetings or giving lectures. There are times when the ophthalmologist will have to cancel appointments for an emergency, a court case, or an illness. If the physician will be unable to be at the office for an appointment and knows beforehand, the patient should be notified by telephone or text. Texting information, such as reminders or cancellation of appointments, has become the preferred mode of communication for many. This requires that all phone and email information be collected as part of the new patient intake form or general update of patient demographics. It is good practice to always ask the patient if any of their personal information needs to be updated.

Canceling a patient appointment will be costly but it is necessary to prevent putting the patient to the inconvenience of coming to the office. The catch word is "rescheduling" and not canceling.

Handling sales representatives

Sales representatives from the various drug and optical firms attempt to bring the latest information on new products and changes in products to the physician. Some come only occasionally to the ophthalmologist and some come frequently. No matter how busy, the doctor usually prefers to see these salespeople. A few minutes spent with a sales representative may make the ophthalmologist knowledgeable on a valuable new therapeutic tool. Sometimes, however, the physician may be too busy to see a salesperson and may wish the ophthalmic assistant to obtain all the pertinent information and to summarize the contents of the individual reports or to obtain summaries and abstracts of these. Practical experience can teach the assistant how to make a good abstract and then present it to the ophthalmologist at a more leisurely moment or at the end of the day.

The ophthalmic assistant will soon become familiar with the various representatives from the pharmaceutical and optical firms who visit the ophthalmologist. All physicians are interested in receiving firsthand information about their products. One must, however, discriminate between these sales representatives and magazine salespeople, peddlers, and the like. Sales representatives always present cards, are never abusive, and never attempt to get into the doctor's office under false pretenses. Accordingly, they should be greeted graciously. When seeing the representatives, the assistant should explain how busy the doctor is at the given time and how much of the practitioner's time they may have. The doctor is then in a position to close the interview when he or she chooses. If it is inconvenient for the clinician to see a sales representative at the time of his or her call, the caller is entitled to an explanation and should be asked to return at a more convenient time when the physician will be able to see him or her.

In addition to these individuals, there may be many callers who take up the doctor's time unnecessarily. The ophthalmic assistant may be very useful in graciously handling these callers, talking to them, and diverting them. For example, insurance salespeople and those who sell stocks and bonds can be diverted from office hours to a more convenient time, if the doctor wishes to see them. If the caller does not wish to state the nature of business and the ophthalmic assistant knows that the doctor does not wish to be disturbed by such visitors, the caller should be asked to write a letter to the clinician about the matter.

Handling mail

The doctor should receive mail in an orderly fashion. Personal correspondence is kept together, as is correspondence relating to patients, such as x-ray and laboratory reports and consultation letters. Drug company correspondence is compiled and kept separate from advertisements and medical journals. Such organization expedites the doctor's review of the mail. The accounts should be given to the personnel primarily responsible for them. Before the doctor is presented with an insurance form to complete, the patient's record should be obtained and a certain amount of the form completed by the administrative or ophthalmic assistant.

Medical ethics

Physicians are bound by a code of rules and customs to which they are expected to adhere. The background for this code is the Hippocratic Oath, named after Hippocrates, a Greek physician of the fifth century BC who is called "The Father of Medicine." Hippocrates gave sound and shrewd descriptions of many diseases and thus raised the ethical standards of medical practice. The classic version of the Hippocratic Oath is a beautiful and inspiring statement that was demanded of the young physician about to enter the practice of medicine (Box 6.5). It placed medicine on a scientific foundation, freeing it from superstition, philosophy, and religious rites. Today, the Hippocratic Oath and its modern versions serves as a foundation on which the highest standards of medicine are practiced.

The principles of medical ethics have been developed over the course of centuries as medicine has evolved. Many of these writings may seem old-fashioned now because they are no longer needed, but others have never varied. Although the Hippocratic Oath concerns itself only with the relationship between the physician and the patient, modern medical ethics also govern the relationship of the physician to the community and to fellow physicians. Even though the overall knowledge and technology of modern medical science are vastly superior to those of ancient times, the universal theme of "self-discovery"' has not changed since the days of Hippocrates. The ophthalmic assistant should be acquainted with the fundamental rules of medical ethics, because his or her actions will reflect on the ophthalmologist.

One of the principles of medical ethics is strict secrecy, which must be observed regarding all matters pertaining to the patient. It is not ethical to criticize the work of another physician to a patient. If a physician has inadvertently

---

Box 6.5 Oath of Hippocrates (Classic Version)

I swear by Apollo the Physician, by Aesculapius, by Hygeia, by Panacea, and by all the gods and goddesses, calling them to witness that according to my ability and judgment I will in every particular keep this, my Oath and Covenant: to regard him who teaches this art equally with my parents, to share my substance with him and, if he be in need, to relieve his necessities; to regard his offspring equally with my brethren; and to teach them this art if they shall wish to learn it, without fee or stipulation; to impart a knowledge of the art by precept, by lecture, and by every other mode of instruction to my sons, to the sons of my teacher, and to pupils who are bound by stipulation and oath, according to the Law of Medicine, but to no other.

I will follow that regimen which, according to my ability and judgment, shall be for the welfare of the sick, and I will refrain from that which shall be baneful and injurious. If any shall ask of me a drug to produce death, I will not give it, nor will I suggest such counsel. In like manner I will not give a woman a destructive pessary.

With Purity and Holiness will I watch closely my life and my art. I will not cut a person who is suffering from a stone, but will give way to those who are practitioners in this work. Into whatever houses I shall enter, I will go to aid the sick, abstaining from every voluntary act of injustice and corruption, and from lasciviousness with women or men, with freemen and slaves.

Whatever in the life of men I shall see or hear, in my practice or without my practice, which should not be made public, this will I hold in silence, believing that such things should not be spoken.

While I keep this, my Oath, inviolate and unbroken, may it be granted to me to enjoy life and my art, forever honored by all men; but should I by transgression violate it, be mine the reverse.

---

expressed some opinion to the ophthalmic assistant in private, the assistant may, out of loyalty to the ophthalmologist, wish to show superiority to the patient by voicing criticism of the other physician's treatment. This is strictly against medical ethics.

A physician must be careful to avoid exaggerated publicity or connection with any incident that has news value, especially of a sensational kind. When newspaper reporters call at the office for information or a statement by the physician, they should be transferred directly to the ophthalmologist, who is fully cognizant of responsibilities both to the public and to fellow medical colleagues. Discretion in this area belongs solely to the doctor.

Each physician has occasion to refer patients to outside agencies for some form of service or for the purchase of optical or medical supplies. Patients often ask for the name of an individual or organization from whom they may obtain these services. Their confidence in the opinion of their ophthalmologist is an important consideration in deciding whom to consult and where to go. The names, addresses, and telephone numbers of those physicians or optical firms in whom the ophthalmologist has a measure of confidence and to whom he or she might refer patients must therefore be known to the ophthalmic assistant and must be kept in such a way that the list can be consulted readily. A list should be kept available of agencies, such as the local institute for the blind, diagnostic laboratories, and organizations that deal with the perceptually handicapped child.

In the physician's absence

The ophthalmic assistant can be of immense help to a physician who presents papers at meetings of medical societies, writes articles or books, or undertakes research work. Physicians who communicate findings to the scientific world usually do extensive writing. The assistant can be of invaluable aid in assembling research or reference material and in editing manuscripts. The time when the physician is away from the office for meetings or holidays can be put to good use in this area. The ophthalmic assistant with a leaning toward writing may prefer this phase of work to all others and be instrumental in obtaining reference materials, in searching the Internet, cumulative indexes and libraries for material on the pertinent subject, and in assembling these for the attention of the ophthalmologist. This work, whether it is for a lecture, article, or book, will provide insight into many new facets of ophthalmology.

Aids in public relations

1. At one time or another, every ophthalmic assistant will be confronted with an office full of patients waiting at their appointed times while the ophthalmologist has been delayed. The assistant should attempt to reappoint patients who do not have an urgent problem and those who cannot afford to wait. If reappointments or delays are required, the patient is entitled to an explanation of this inconvenience. Because the physician's day is usually devoted to providing service to others, such explanations can be freely candid if they do not violate HIPAA regulations. Most patients appreciate the demands constantly made on the physician's time and are usually quite fair in thoughtfully considering these delays. For those patients who prefer to wait in the office, refreshments should be offered if the facilities are available.

2. The waiting room should be kept clean and neat at all times. Magazines without covers should be removed and broken toys removed or repaired. Ensure that all toys are of the type that can be sanitized between use.

3. The ophthalmic assistant should always be neat, fresh, and well groomed. Extreme styles of clothing should be avoided; make-up should never be excessive. Colognes/perfumes and scented lotions should be avoided as some patients may be sensitive/allergic. Uniforms may be worn. Nametags are desirable.

4. As much as possible, have the same member of staff deal with the same patient. Maintain eye contact and a pleasant expression. Smile! Separate work duties from home and personal duties.

5. Patients should be called from the waiting room with a soft and friendly voice that rings with hospitality. If a patient has poor vision, the tone of voice should remain unchanged. Many people approach the partially sighted as though they had lost their other sensory functions and tend to speak in a loud voice or even shout.

6. However, not all patients are blessed with good hearing. The ophthalmic assistant may be required to speak in louder tones in communicating with the hard-of-hearing patient.

7. The ophthalmic assistant should attempt to have patients remove overshoes, overcoats, and scarves before entering the ophthalmologist's inner office. Coat racks should be available. This invariably saves time and allows patients to be more comfortable for the examination.

8. Children may be led by the hand to the examining room (Fig. 6.4). A small toy or gift may establish better rapport with the child.

9. Personalizing a practice can be done in many ways. Look around the office. Is everyone wearing a name badge? Do the nurses, assistants, and technicians have cards with their name and title on them so patients can call directly and ask them questions? When the physician enters the examining room, does the technician introduce the patient to the ophthalmologist? Are visual aids available (Fig. 6.5)? Hearing aids can be helpful for the hard of hearing (Fig. 6.6).

10. Because of the increasing number of senior citizens who come to ophthalmology offices, some doctors are beginning to offer some form of transportation within a certain radius. This is a great service to seniors who might not drive or surgery patients who are temporarily unable to drive. A limousine or van that seats six to eight people can be used to pick patients up and return them to their homes. When patients call to make an appointment, the assistant can tell them that on Tuesday and Thursday mornings, for example, a transportation service is available to those living within

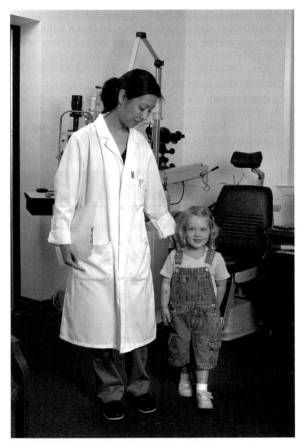

Fig. 6.4 Handling the young child.

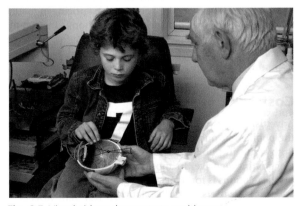

Fig. 6.5 Visual aids to demonstrate problems.

a 5-mile radius of the physician's office and are having surgery. Would they like to take advantage of such a service? Scheduling transportation requests ahead of time will allow the driver to plan an effective route for picking up patients. The driver should be a patient,

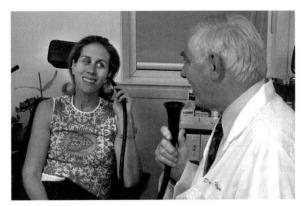

Fig. 6.6 A hearing ear trumpet can be used for the hard of hearing.

courteous person with an excellent driving record and a personality that will make the passengers feel comfortable and safe. Advertising a service, such as free transportation is bound to increase telephone requests by new patients for further information about your office and its services. At a time when more and more new patients are "shopping" for physicians, a service, such as free transportation will draw attention.

11. No matter how minor or short a surgical procedure or hospitalization is according to medical standards, it is of major importance to the patient and should be acknowledged as such by the office personnel. Following up surgical procedures with a call from someone in the office or sending a gift, such as a plant to a recuperating patient is an extremely courteous and personal gesture. Often a personal note from the physician will boost the patient's morale beyond anyone's expectations. Surgical patients always should be given priority scheduling for follow-up appointments, and any questions they may call in with should be answered quickly. Patients should never feel that the physician or office personnel are ignoring them now that the surgery is over! Developing a special protocol for handling surgery patients will, in the long run, boost the physician's practice. Patients love to talk about their surgeries; let what they say about your office be positive and flattering.

12. Keep records of where new patients are coming from. Have a tracking form that you keep next to the appointment book. With EMRs, it may be possible to do a regular report showing the new patient zip codes. This can be very helpful if a newsletter or marketing piece of any type is desired. When new patients call for an appointment, ask them who referred them to the office. If they are responding to an advertisement and your office runs more than one advertisement, ask them *specifically*

Self-evaluation questions

Q

Office problems to solve

Office efficiency is promoted through the work of intelligent, responsible people using the faculties of cooperation, creativity, industry, interest, and sensitivity. Problems that may arise in the office often do not have a cut-and-dried solution. Each situation is unique and requires individual attention. The following problems and brief discussions on how to handle them touch on some areas of difficulty that might be encountered. We have included some of our ideas, but there are a multitude of others that we encourage you to explore.

Problem 1. A patient calls and demands an immediate appointment because he is having a problem with his eyes. He sounds quite hysterical to you and the symptoms do not seem to indicate an emergency. What do you do?

Problem 2. The doctor is away for 2 weeks. Shortly after his or her departure, an important letter arrives in the mail and requests a speedy acknowledgment or reply. What should you do?

Problem 3. The doctor has asked you to reschedule some appointments because of a change in his or her surgical schedule. You have been unable to reach a patient by phone and the appointment is a week away. How should this be handled?

Problem 4. A patient arrives for an appointment and you are unable to locate her chart. How do you handle this situation?

Problem 5. The doctor is running late in his or her appointments. How would you handle the delay with newly arriving patients?

Problem 6. A sales representative arrives and insists on seeing the doctor even though the waiting room is crowded. How do you handle this situation?

Problem 7. What information should you obtain from patients or referring physicians' offices when they call to make an appointment?

Problem 8. It is sometimes difficult to see our own surroundings objectively. It is an interesting and informative exercise to imagine that you are a patient coming into the ophthalmologist's office for the first time. What is your initial reaction to this office? Is it clean, bright, and pleasant or stuffy and forbidding? Was your initial contact with the receptionist pleasant? Did you feel relaxed and comfortable with his or her manner, or did he or she seem harassed, overworked, or hostile? Did you find the waiting room to be well lit, with an interesting assortment of neatly displayed magazines, inviting you to enjoy your wait? Or did you find yourself peering at a tattered 3-month-old periodical in an overheated, overcrowded waiting room?

Problem 9. It has been the assumption throughout these questions that you are an employed ophthalmic assistant. Perhaps you are not. Perhaps you are embarking on a search for employment in this field. You will, then, have to prepare a résumé of your skills, experience, and training. You also will have to be prepared for an interview (or several interviews) with ophthalmologists. Consider the initial impression you want to make on them and the qualities and abilities you want to convey. Do you present yourself as a dependable, cooperative person who can meet challenges and accept responsibilities? Is your appearance neat and professional? You want to go into an interview feeling good, looking good, and emanating confidence in your ability to do the job and your eagerness for the opportunity to do so. How do you plan on doing this?

Answers, notes, and explanations

Answer 1. There are a few ways to handle this situation. You could tell the patient that you are fully booked and that he can try to reach another physician who might be able to see him on a more immediate basis. You are, however, risking feelings of ill will by turning away this patient. You could inform the patient that he can be placed on a cancellation list and will be notified when an opening becomes available. This means you have taken the responsibility of diagnosing this problem as not urgent. Can a telephone conversation with an upset and frightened patient tell you this?

A third alternative is not to take it upon yourself to diagnose the patient's condition. Take down all the symptoms he is experiencing, get his phone number, pull his chart, and give the message to the doctor. The physician knows his or her patients, as well as possible serious potential problems, and should make the final decision as to what should be done.

Answer 2. The letter should not be left to vegetate for 2 weeks. If the matter is very pressing, contact the doctor. However, even important correspondence may not be extremely urgent. A courteous and considerate way to

Answers, notes, and explanations—Continued

A

handle this would be to send the correspondent a brief note explaining that the doctor is away until a certain date and the letter will be answered promptly on his or her return.

Answer 3. You can make a note to call the patient the following day; the person may be out just for the day. This means that you must not forget to place this call on the next day. However, chances are that the patient has given you only a home number and cannot be reached there during the day. Therefore if you are relying on this single mode of communication, you will have an irate patient to handle 1 week, hence if the person arrives for the appointment. Also remember that text messaging is now a preferred method of contact by many patients. To prepare for this, ask your patients when they check in, how they wish to be contacted in the future. Many office systems will allow the patient to respond with a Y if they have received the text.

It is probably best to send a note as soon as you find it difficult to reach the patient by phone or text. Rather than leave it another day and waste precious time, post a note advising of the canceled appointment and provide an alternative date. This is easy and convenient and saves patient anxiety and the feeling of having been overlooked.

Answer 4. You could ask her to sit in the waiting room while you look for the chart. However, if you cannot find it within a reasonable time, you are delaying the patient. If you put her name on a blank chart, you would leave the doctor with an embarrassing problem.

It is best to explain to the patient that you are unable to locate her chart at the moment (this should be said after you have thoroughly searched the various areas where it might be). You should tell her that it will take a bit of time to check the files and make up a duplicate chart for today to keep her from waiting. Reassure her that her chart will be located. Not having to locate physical charts is an advantage of the electronic medical record. Of course, in the event that your computer system is down, you will need to ensure that your office has a standard policy and process for downtime procedures.

Answer 5. It is easiest, but most unwise, to avoid the situation and hope that no one will complain about the delay. This is inconsiderate to the patient who may have another appointment to keep, who must get back to work, or who simply does not appreciate being kept waiting a disproportionate length of time.

One can directly inform an incoming patient that the doctor is running late (because of emergencies, a delay at the hospital, or whatever the case may be) and, unfortunately, there will be a longer than usual wait. Because the patient is being inconvenienced, offer a choice of waiting or rescheduling the appointment. A Service Recovery Toolkit can come in handy when this situation presents.

Answer 6. Some doctors will see sales representatives when they drop by; others prefer to have the ophthalmic assistant make an appointment for these brief visits or have the representative come at the end of the day.

If the practice is busy, as the crowded waiting room would indicate, it is best to form a consistent policy with sales representatives. The pharmaceutical representative will quickly learn when and how the ophthalmologist is available.

If a representative insists on seeing the doctor, present the doctor with his or her card and let the doctor decide what to do. You will find, however, that most sales representatives who come to your office will be courteous and cooperative. It is up to the ophthalmic assistant to set a mutually accommodating manner for visits to be made with maximum efficiency and minimal time lost.

Answer 7. You will need the patient's full name and phone numbers, home and business. Ask if the patient has been to the office previously; if not, you should record the person's mailing address. This is needed if you have to change the appointment and the patient cannot be reached by phone.

It is also helpful to know the basic nature of the problem or the reason for the appointment; that is, a postoperative check, a complete eye examination for a driver's license, a minor surgical procedure, an ocular injury, a contact lens problem, and so on. This information will help you in the scheduling of time for the appointment and in your preparedness for the patient.

When scheduling a consultation appointment, you will need the referring physician's name and, preferably, the nature of the patient's problem. If the patient has undergone any tests related to this particular problem, request that copies be forwarded to you before the appointment date.

Answer 8. Try to go through this mental experiment. Chances are you might see some things you had never before realized existed and that are in need of change or improvement.

Answer 9. This is a personal evaluation and an exercise well worth doing as a method of providing yourself with a self-assessment, as well as learning to put your best foot forward.

Name:	Norman Deer
Address:	39 Roxborough Road
Telephone:	923-4117
Referred by:	Dr Peters
Family doctor:	Dr Peters
Employed by:	Westinghouse
Occupation:	Clerk
Type of insurance:	Blue Cross
Insurance No.	464-347-213
Age:	50 – Birth date 4/6/1972
Chief complaint:	Difficulty with fine print
History of present illness:	Past 6 months difficulty in reading stock reports. Distance vision fine. No other eye complaints.
Past health:	Diabetes 12-year duration
Medications:	Metformin 500 mg BID
Allergies:	Penicillin, sulfa
Family history:	Glaucoma in mother

Fig. 7.1 Typical history.

Chief complaint

The chief complaint constitutes the reason for the visit. In a sentence or two, the ophthalmic assistant should write down the main reason for which the patient has come to the ophthalmologist for advice and help. In this context, the prime question should be direct, simple, and forthright: "What brings you here today?" Many times the patient responds, "That's what I'm here to find out!" The patient may reply concisely or give a long, rambling account of various symptoms. If the patient cannot provide focused answers on the main issue after repeated questioning, the ophthalmic assistant should record what he or she regards as the most serious problem among the patient's symptoms. Commonly described chief complaints are *pain, loss of vision, eye fatigue,* and *blurred vision for near.* One must

then proceed to pin down the specifics of the complaint, such as date of onset, cause, severity, and duration.

History of present illness

After the chief complaint is recorded, the patient should be questioned in greater detail about the main symptoms. These descriptive terms can be summarized using the mnemonic "FOLDARS" which stands for frequency of symptoms, onset, location, duration, associated signs and symptoms, relief, and severity. For example, asking the patient when the symptoms began and how often they noticed them, as well as if the symptoms come and go or are continuous. Was the patient doing anything that seemed to bring on the symptoms and have they taken any medications or used any items to relieve the symptoms. If the patient is describing pain, use the pain scale of 1 to 10, with 10 being the most severe, and if the pain is interfering with their activities of daily living.

The pertinent points regarding the most common ophthalmic complaints are reviewed in Table 7.1 to aid the ophthalmic assistant in evaluating symptoms and possible causes.

Loss of vision

Very few patients will state that they have lost vision, unless, of course, they have become blind because of a serious ocular disease or accident. Most patients complain of blurred vision and state this problem in terms of a limitation of function, such as, a decrease in ability to read at near. Blurred vision may have many causes and assume different forms.

Blurred vision secondary to an error of refraction

Hazy, foggy, or blurred vision, if it occurs at a particular distance, usually indicates a refraction error. The myope cannot see in the distance and the hyperope may have difficulty at near. It is the patient with astigmatism who has difficulty seeing both in the distance and at close range. Even with astigmatism, however, poor visual acuity is not evenly distributed, inasmuch as this type of patient will generally see better at close range because of the magnification afforded by proximity. Most patients with refractive errors have a specific visual disability limited to specific activities.

Blurred vision for close work

A patient whose vision is blurred for close work is usually a presbyope and may complain of an inability to read a menu, see their cell phone screen, work on their computer, or read the stock market report.

t0010

Table 7.1 Ocular symptoms and their possible causes

Symptom	Possible causes	Symptom	Possible causes
Symptoms indicating urgency		Blurred vision in the elderly	Macular degeneration Cataracts Ischemic optic neuropathy
Pain in the eye	Chemical burn Flash burn to cornea Keratitis Glaucoma Iritis Temporal arteritis Retrobulbar neuritis	Persistent tearing in one eye	Dacryocystitis Blocked tear duct Entropion, ectropion Trichiasis Chalazion Bell's palsy
Sudden loss of vision	Macular degeneration Retinal artery occlusion Retinal detachment Retinal vein occlusion Retrobulbar neuritis	Enlarging nodule on lid	Basal cell carcinoma
		Foreign body sensation	Corneal foreign body Corneal abrasion Herpes simplex keratitis
Transient loss of vision	Carotid artery disease Migraine Papilledema Severe hypertension	**Significant symptoms that should be seen as soon as possible**	
		Gritty feeling	Dry eye syndrome from any cause Conjunctivitis Ocular irritation: dust, wind, ultraviolet lights
Diplopia	Myasthenia gravis Thyroid disorders Diabetes Third nerve palsy from any cause	Headaches	Often tension Hypertension Brain tumor Migraine, cluster headaches, etc.
Ptosis	Third nerve palsy Diabetes Myasthenia gravis	Blurred distance vision in adult	Diabetes Cataract Macular edema
Flashes of light	Retinal detachment	Spots before eye	Retinal tear Vitreous detachment
Trauma	Blow-out fracture of orbit Hyphema	Pain behind eye	Sinus disease Thyroid disorders Orbital tumor (rare) Aneurysm of the carotid artery (rare)
Symptoms requiring prompt attention			
Discharge and matting of lids in morning	Conjunctivitis		
Red eye	Any external disease of eye	Eruption on skin	Atopic allergy Seborrhea Herpes zoster Drug reaction
Swelling of lids	Bilateral blepharoconjunctivitis Acute allergies Thyroid disease		
Halos around lights	Angle-closure glaucoma Cataracts		

Blurred vision for distance work

In this instance, the patient is not apt to be a young adult for whom a fresh diagnosis of myopia is about to be made. The patient who is in school most often will complain of inability to see the PowerPoint screen, whiteboard, or blackboard. The patient who drives an automobile will state that road signs appear to be fuzzy, especially at dusk. Occasionally, a patient will recognize this problem by noting that the television set appears fuzzy only to him or her. With regard to television, mothers often become very alarmed when their children sit close to the television screen. This is not usually a symptom of myopia because children like sitting close to the screen for two reasons. First, they enjoy the magnification because big things are easier to view and second, the closer they are to the screen, the greater is their sense of involvement with the story being told.

Blurred vision secondary to organic disease

The patient with organic disease has difficulty seeing things at all times regardless of the activity. The patient who has a cataract or macular degeneration will be limited in both distance (driving) and at near (reading). The patient with a cataract sees as though looking through a frosted glass window and the patient with macular disease finds things missing when looking straight ahead and so must look at them askew.

Loss of central vision. With loss of central vision patients discover that they are unable to see clearly straight ahead but that they have retained peripheral vision (Fig. 7.2). When looking at a face, they may state that the face appears gray or indistinct, whereas the background around the face appears to be clearer. Such a patient commonly sees better in dim illumination. The visual acuity in the affected eye is usually poor. This symptom, if sudden in onset, usually means a disorder of the macula or the optic nerve. If a patient describes a new loss or change in central visual acuity, most physicians will want the assistant to performing an Amsler Grid test (see Ch. 18) and color vision testing (see Ch. 8).

Distorted vision. Distortion of vision is most commonly a sign of macular edema. The patient with this symptom usually complains that objects appear minified and slightly fuzzy and that lines appear wavy rather than straight. Visual distortions are also common in patients, such as high refractive errors, whose glasses lenses are very thick lenses. A new onset of distorted vision should prompt the ophthalmic assistant to perform the Amsler Grid Test (see Ch. 18).

Night blindness. The patient with night blindness finds difficulty in seeing things in the early evening, and this difficulty becomes worse as night falls. Such a patient has difficulty in movie theaters, dark rooms, and so forth, yet can see clearly straight ahead in daylight. Some patients may eventually suffer visual field restrictions, which make driving and, later, normal ambulation difficult even during the day (Fig. 7.3). This symptom may be a manifestation of retinitis pigmentosa or vitamin A deficiency.

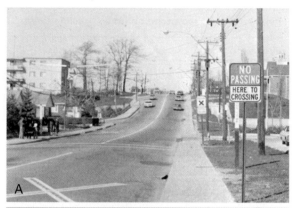
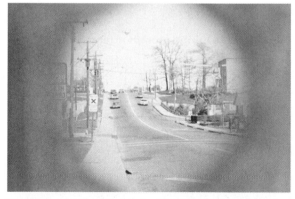

Fig. 7.2 (A) The road as it appears to a person with normal central and peripheral fields of vision. (B) Loss of central field. The central field of vision is indistinct, whereas the peripheral field of vision remains clear.

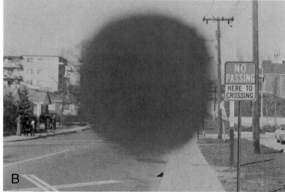

Fig. 7.3 Restricted peripheral visual field. The central field is clear.

Transient gray-outs or blur-outs of vision lasting several seconds in one or both eyes. Although this symptom appears to be inconsequential, it often is of great importance. This obscureness of vision may be a symptom of papilledema (swelling of the disc as a result of increased intracranial pressure), carotid insufficiency, or arteriosclerosis.

Inability to see to the right or to the left. This symptom follows a profound field loss in which the patient loses half the field of vision. Such a patient, when reading the visual acuity chart, sees letters on half the chart only and sees them clearly to the 20/20 line of the unaffected side. Usually, the patient has difficulty in any visual tasks, such as driving, reading, or even ordinary ambulation (Fig. 7.4). When this occurs on the same side in both eyes, one has to be suspicious of brain involvement of the opposite side.

Ascending veil. The patient may see a dark shadow ascending like a fog arising in the lower field of vision. This symptom is frequently an ominous indicator of a retinal detachment occurring in the superior retina (Fig. 7.5).

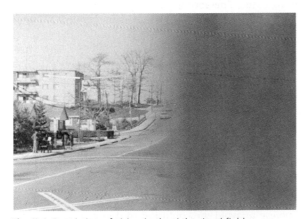

Fig. 7.4 Restriction of vision in the right visual field.

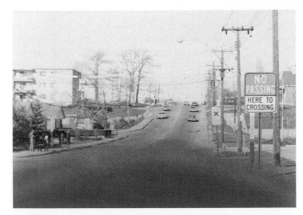

Fig. 7.5 Ascending dark veil from below, which may indicate a retinal detachment from above.

Headaches

Headaches are a challenge for all medical personnel. Commonly, the patient with a headache has been referred by the family physician, who, unable to find an organic cause for the complaint, to an ophthalmologist for further assessment. Unfortunately, most headaches are not caused by a refractive error or a correctable disorder within the eye, and the ophthalmologist must often report to the family physician that there appears to be no ocular cause for the patient's headaches. Although the symptom of headache is difficult to evaluate, it must be treated with respect because this complaint may indicate many sinister conditions, such as severe hypertension or brain tumor. Of importance in the assessment of any headaches are the following:

1. *Family history of headaches*. In many of the vascular headaches, such as migraine, a positive family history is frequently obtained.
2. *Onset and duration*.
3. *Severity* (using the pain scale).
4. *Associated symptoms*. In this regard the ophthalmic assistant is really searching for other findings associated with the headache. For example, the patient with a migraine headache sometimes sees an aura before the onset of the headache. This aura usually consists of flashing lines in zigzag formation, extending from the central area to the periphery and lasting approximately 20 minutes. Other important associated symptoms that should be noted are nausea, vomiting, blackouts of vision, fainting spells, weakness of an arm or leg, numbness of the fingertips, and difficulties with coordination.
5. *Relationship of the headache to visual activity*. Do the headaches follow prolonged periods of close work or do they appear when the patient rises in the morning? Obviously, headaches caused by errors of refraction will not appear at night, during sleep, or on awaking.
6. *Character of the headache and its location*. A notation should be made of the nature of the patient's headache, whether it is vice-like, throbbing, or dull, as well as its location, that is, in or above the eyes or in the temple regions.

Asthenopia

Asthenopia is a wastebasket term denoting a number of sensations that accompany uncorrected refractive error and problems in ocular motility. Included in this ocular wastebasket of symptoms are the complaints of:

- General eyestrain
- Eye fatigue after reading
- Pulling sensations
- Inability to focus
- Heaviness of the lids after reading

- Sensitivity to sunlight or fluorescent light
- Tendency to fall asleep after reading one or two pages
- Burning, itching, and watering of the eyes with reading

In addition to refractive errors, these symptoms may be a result of chronic conjunctivitis, allergy, lack of tears, an emotional disorder, or fatigue. The patient with asthenopic complaints is apt to be vague and elusive in describing symptoms. Because the disability tends to be minor, the patient is often reduced to repeating that "the eyes just don't feel right."

Red eye

The most common cause of a red eye is acute conjunctivitis. The salient features of conjunctivitis are discharge, pain, and blurred vision.

Discharge

The discharge of conjunctivitis can vary from being profuse and watery to being rather scant or purulent. During the day, of course, the discharge tends to drain and is wiped away with tissues, but during the night it tends to accumulate and dry. Thus the patient with conjunctivitis complains that the lids are stuck together in the morning, the lashes being matted together in the dry discharge.

Pain

Normally there is no pain with simple conjunctivitis unless the cornea is involved. A secondary keratitis is a common accompaniment of conjunctivitis, especially if the offending organism is *Staphylococcus aureus*. The patient usually complains of a sandy or scratchy feeling or of the sensation of a foreign body in the eyes.

Blurred vision

Because the clarity of the optical media is not affected by conjunctivitis, visual loss is not a prominent complaint in this condition. Because of the discharge over the surface of the cornea, however, the vision in the affected eye may be hazy. Occasionally, such a patient even complains of seeing halos around lights.

In cases of conjunctivitis, it is helpful to gain information regarding the source of the infection. Inquiry should be made into the presence of a similar disorder appearing in relatives or friends. Detection of the source of the infection may be very important, especially in crowded institutions, such as childcare facilities, schools, camps, dorms, or military barracks, where infection can travel through an entire group. It is also important to ask the patient if treatment has been started either by the family or primary care physician or by the patient.

Other causes

The red eye is also a manifestation of *acute iritis* and *acute narrow-angle glaucoma*, although the incidence of these two conditions is far less than that of *acute conjunctivitis*. The diagnosis of *acute glaucoma* can virtually be made over the telephone. The onset of this condition is sudden and dramatic, with the entire triad of pain, loss of vision, and congestion of the globe occurring within a matter of 30 minutes. The pain of acute glaucoma, unlike that of conjunctivitis, is intense, and the patient may have associated nausea and vomiting. Also the visual loss is profound and frequently the vision is reduced to hand movements or counting fingers. The only real distinguishing feature between acute glaucoma and acute iritis, in terms of symptoms, is the difference in the onset of the two conditions. Iritis takes hours or days rather than minutes before it becomes fully developed.

The differential diagnosis of the common causes of an inflamed eye is outlined in Table 7.2.

Double vision or diplopia

The patient with true diplopia reports seeing two objects instead of one. This symptom occurs when there is an acquired loss of alignment of the eyes, so that each eye does not project to the same place in space. Loss of ocular alignment is a common finding in children with strabismus. Children with strabismus, however, do not see double because they are capable of suppressing the vision in one eye to avoid the confusion of double images. Adults are not as adaptable as children and are disabled by double vision (Fig. 7.6). They have faulty spatial orientation and projection and complain of dizziness, inability to walk straight, and inability to reach accurately toward an object in space. If the diplopia results from the loss of alignment of the eyes, then covering one eye will always eliminate the second image.

Occasionally, the patient may have monocular diplopia. With monocular diplopia, the double vision persists when one eye is closed. It is important to make this distinction in the history. Binocular double vision is always caused by the development of a weak or paralyzed extraocular muscle. The loss of alignment results from the fact that an opponent muscle carries the eye over to one side, being unopposed by the palsied muscle. For example, if the right lateral rectus muscle (6th cranial nerve) becomes paralyzed, the left medial rectus muscle would carry the eye inward toward the nose (esotropia; Fig. 7.7).

Table 7.2 Common causes of the red eye

	Acute conjunctivitis	Acute iritis	Acute glaucoma	Corneal injury
Symptoms	Redness, tearing, possible discharge	Redness, pain, photophobia	Redness, severe pain nausea, vomiting	Redness, pain
Appearance of conjunctiva	Injection	Ciliary injection	Defuse injection	Defuse injection
Vision	Unaffected—can be blurred by discharge	Moderately reduced—blurred	Markedly reduced—haloes	Blurred
Cornea	Clear	May observe precipitates	Edema—hazy	Defect seen with or without stain
Pupil	Normal size	Constricted	Semi dilated/fixed	Normal or constricted
Pupil light response	Normal	Sluggish	Fixed unresponsive	Normal
Secretions	Clear to purulent	Tearing	Tearing	Tearing
Intraocular pressure	Normal	Reduced to elevated	Very high	Normal
Laboratory tests	Smear for organisms	No organisms	No organisms	No organisms

Note: Other causes of a red eye are detailed in the text.

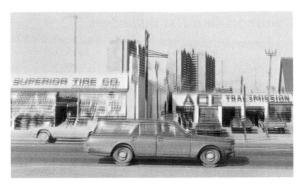

Fig. 7.6 Double vision. The images are just slightly displaced vertically.

Monocular diplopia is quite uncommon and may be caused by an extra pupil or cataracts, or it may appear in the recovery phase after strabismus repair.

Floating spots and light flashes

Virtually everyone has seen, at some time or another, small spots before the eyes. They may appear singly or in clusters; they may be punctate or linear; they may travel with the movements of the eye or against them. These floaters are most apparent when the illumination is high and when one is gazing at a clear surface. The most common situations in which they are seen include looking up at a clear summer sky, gazing against a blank white wall, and reading.

These floaters usually are caused by the formation of small particles in the vitreous body and are generally innocuous. However, floaters may, on occasion, be indicative of a more serious derangement within the eye. They may be caused by cells in the vitreous from an active iridocyclitis or they may be secondary to a retinal tear, hemorrhage, or a detachment.

Tearing

Tearing as an isolated event occurs most commonly as a result of a blockage of the nasolacrimal duct. In infants, it results from failure of the duct to become completely canalized. Although tearing is most often a sign of a blocked nasolacrimal duct, it can also be caused by congenital glaucoma, foreign bodies on the cornea, or in turned lashes. Every child with tearing should be assessed carefully.

In adults, tearing is a less specific symptom. It may occur as a result of entropion, chronic conjunctivitis, allergy, dry eyes, or obstruction of the nasolacrimal duct. In taking the history of a patient whose primary complaint is tearing, one must note the duration of tearing, whether it appears to come from one eye or both, and associated findings, such as redness of the eye or discharge.

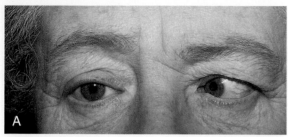

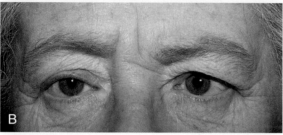

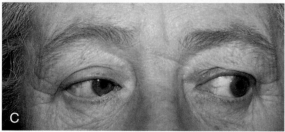

Fig. 7.7 Right esotropia. (A) Right eye does not move to left; (B) right eye moves only partially out to left; (C) right eye turns left normally. (Reproduced from Spalton D, Hitchings R, Hunter P. *Atlas of clinical ophthalmology*, 3rd ed. St Louis: Mosby; 2004, with permission.)

Past health, medications, and allergies

Patients should be asked about their general health at present, usually using a "Review of Systems" form filled out by the patient before the exam, as well as their past health status. In particular, diabetes, hypertension, cardiac disorders, autoimmune disorders, and arthritis should be mentioned. Many systemic disorders have ocular manifestations. If a positive history is obtained, the ophthalmologist can direct the examination with greater purpose.

Equally important is obtaining a history of any medications the patient may be taking. Often the patient will not know the name of the medication but will refer to the reason for taking the medication. With many electronic medical record systems, the names of medications prescribed by other physicians are readily available. One should confirm with the patient that they are still taking the medications on the list. One may also ask the patient to call their pharmacy to get this information.

Inquiry should also be made into the presence or absence of allergies. In general, five types of allergic responses should be inquired about:

1. Allergy to drugs (taken internally or applied topically)
2. Allergy to inhalants (dust, pollens, molds, etc.)
3. Allergy to contactants (cosmetics, woolens, soap, etc.)
4. Allergy to ingestants (food allergies, including lactose intolerance)
5. Allergy to injectants (tetanus antiserum, etc.)

Family history

It is helpful if inquiry is made into the familial history of the more common ocular disorders. In particular, the presence or absence of such familial diseases as myopia, strabismus, and glaucoma should be asked about. A negative family history does not rule out a genetic familial propensity. Many patients really do not know the ocular status of their relatives, and others may be reluctant to share such information.

Common familial disorders

- Migraine
- Retinitis pigmentosa
- Retinoblastoma
- Color blindness
- Nystagmus
- Albinism
- Sickle cell anemia
- Choroideremia
- Keratoconus
- von Recklinghausen disease (elephant man disease; neurofibromatosis)
- Marfan syndrome
- Diabetes
- Hereditary macular degeneration (Stargardt disease)

Tips in history taking

The ophthalmic assistant should follow a systematic order in taking an adequate history:

1. Identify the chief reason why the patient has sought an eye examination.
2. Identify any secondary problems the patient has that are referable to the eye.

3. Identify any systemic or general illness the patient presently has, and any medication being taken.
4. List past ocular disorders or operations including lasers and refractive surgeries.
5. Determine whether the patient is wearing contacts or spectacles and, if so, how old they are and when the last eye examination occurred.
6. Be concise but also go into detail about any specific ocular problem that arises. General questions regarding any abnormality may be important, such as time and duration, family involvement, etc.
7. Record any previous therapy and the response.
8. Find out what your physician wants and expects from your history. Some physicians want very brief histories and others want all the details. Some are sticklers about spelling, complete sentences, and grammar and others are less particular on these details.

Scribes

Scribes are a fairly new subspecialty interest among ophthalmic assistants. They work closely with their employing ophthalmologist and are in the room with the patient and doctor while the patient history and examination are being performed. They are the official recorder of what transpires. He or she should sign the records as noted at the end of this section. Sometimes records end up in the hands of lawyers, and legible writing or typing and correct information are a must.

Scribes are a valuable asset because the specific details in recording are often overlooked by the doctor, who is busy responding to the patient's questions or giving specific instructions. Scribes can record details on the go. In addition, the patient may forget some aspect of the instructions, and the ophthalmic assistant can explain or repeat them. The scribe may become the best known contact for the patient to call back a few days later.

Scribes have become vital to many ophthalmologists. Although scribes were often used before the implementation of EHRs, the use of scribes in ophthalmology in recent years has exploded. Trained scribes, or medical assistants or technicians acting as scribes, allow the physician to see patients more efficiently, with the added bonus that paper charts are often more legible!

"Let me introduce my scribe _____, who will type or write while I review your chart and complete your examination. Then we will discuss our plan." This sentence is a quick and elegant way for the physician to convey to the patient who the "extra" person in the examination room is and that person's role in the patient's care. A scribe allows face-to-face interaction between the provider and the patient that is lacking when the physician must turn his or her back on the patient to write or type.

It is crucial for scribes entering data in the EHR to be computer savvy—the best scribes type more than 70 words per minute—and familiar with medical and ophthalmic terminology and abbreviations. Like all medical personnel, scribes must abide by HIPAA privacy rules, and as an unlicensed individual, cannot practice independently. The scribe is present during the patient encounter and records the actions and words of the physician as they occur. Scribes may not interject their own observations or impressions into the medical record, but with time and training, often anticipate and respond to the physician's needs in the clinic.

Physicians and other licensed providers may rely on the review of systems (ROS) and past, family, and social history (PFSH) obtained and recorded by the scribe; however, this task is often assigned to the certified ophthalmic medical technician. The technician who does the workup for a patient should not also be the scribe for that patient, because it is not clear in the electronic audit trail when that person was functioning as a technician or as a scribe. Technicians, scribes, and physicians must use their own logins in EHRs, which can sometimes slow down the examination; however, there are electronic swiping devices that may be used to quickly change personnel logins. It is crucial that scribes do not document findings under the provider's login.

Scribes serve as a physician extender in EHRs or on paper. Some examples of other duties commonly performed by a scribe include:
- Input of examination into EHR while the physician dictates
- Edit note per physician request
- Pend medications, tests, orders (for provider to sign)
- Retrieve printouts of refractions, medications, and orders
- Input return visits or follow-up appointments as needed
- Instill eyedrops under the physician's or other licensed provider's order
- Upload test and imaging results
- Fill out surgical consent forms and witness consent signature
- Hold eyelids and retrieve instruments and drops for physician
- Direct patients to "in-process" waiting, photography, laboratory results, or check-out areas

Scribes typically do not:
- Assist with procedures
- Triage
- Draw up medications
- Schedule patients

When a scribe enters information on a paper medical record and correction is needed, the provider must add and sign an addendum to the scribe's note, rather than cross out or alter what the scribe has written or typed. On electronic records, the physician may override the scribe's documentation. The provider must sign an attestation that he or she has reviewed and supervised the scribed chart, whether paper or EHR, and attest to its accuracy and completion. The scribe's attestation may be as simple as "Scribed for Dr. _____ by _____ date/time," and must be legible!

In March 2015 the International Joint Commission on Allied Health Personnel in Ophthalmology (IJCAHPO) announced the release of a new Ophthalmic Scribe Certification (OSC). The certification examination is designed to test the knowledge of ophthalmic scribes and ophthalmic medical personnel who create and maintain patient medical records under the supervision of an ophthalmologist. These records include the documentation of a comprehensive patient history, physical examination, medications, laboratory results, and other pertinent patient information.

In addition to recognizing IJCAHPO's certification of ophthalmic assistants, technicians, and medical technologists, the Centers for Medicare & Medicaid Services (CMS) includes certified ophthalmic scribes to enter electronic medication, laboratory, or radiology orders into EHR systems. The examination content covers history taking, ophthalmic patient services and education, ophthalmic terminology, medical ethics and legal issues, and medical notes/records.

A scribe's responsibilities are ultimately controlled by the regulatory requirements and policies established by their healthcare setting, and the level of risk an employer is willing to accept. As the use of scribes becomes even more prevalent, the potential for expanded legal guidance and direction grows. Practices should monitor federal, state, and regulatory changes to ensure their practices consistently meet compliance with standards.

Acknowledgment

Contributed by Carol J. Pollack-Rundle, BS, COMT.

Summary

The role of the ophthalmic assistant in obtaining a history will, of course, vary with the policies of the supervising ophthalmologist or institution. Some ophthalmologists prefer to expand on a skeleton history, whereas others prefer to do the entire questioning themselves. Whatever duties are assigned to the ophthalmic assistant should be performed as efficiently and expeditiously as possible. A few short sentences under each heading usually are sufficient to cover an office history. It is neither appropriate nor efficient for the ophthalmic assistant to spend an hour documenting the patient's complaints.

The analysis of the importance of symptoms is a difficult task because a symptom is merely an expression of disordered function. It depends not only on the patient's condition but also the person's ability to define the trouble with clarity. Exaggerations, distortions of complaints, irrelevancies, vagaries, and lapses of memory tend to lead the examiner astray. A good historian should not interpret for the patient. If a given history is not precise, a statement of the patient's actual complaints should be recorded. The interpretation of the history is the domain of the physician, who will assess all the findings from the history, physical examination, and pertinent laboratory or radiologic studies to arrive at a final diagnosis.

The ophthalmic assistant, in obtaining a history, should try to combine the qualities of a good police detective and teacher. The patient's questioning should be directed toward obtaining the facts. The spirit of that questioning should be calm, sympathetic, and patient. If possible, the ophthalmic assistant should try to make some notation on the chart of a personal nature, such as the patient's interests and hobbies, occupation, recent accomplishments, or recent tragedies. Such notations are helpful to the ophthalmologist in establishing rapport with the patient and setting the mood for the examination. Of course, on revisits, it is gratifying to the patient to be recognized as a human being rather than as an eye problem. If time allows, office can ask patients about their personal interests. It is all part of a good history. A happy patient will be more cooperative and eager to share information than one who does not feel valued as a person.

Questions for review and thought

1. A patient complains of sudden loss of vision in one eye. Outline a series of questions that will bring out the essential features of the problem.
2. Double vision may indicate a paralysis of one or more muscles of the eye. What factors are important in identifying the seriousness of the condition? What muscles might be affected?
3. List the factors that will strengthen the professional components of the ophthalmic assistant's behavior.
4. List the various factors necessary to complete a proper insurance claim in your area.
5. A patient complains of seeing small floating objects in his vision. Outline a series of questions that will bring out the highlights of the history.

6. What is eyestrain?
7. For what conditions is the family history important?
8. Outline a useful sequence to follow in obtaining a good history.
9. What common systemic illnesses have an effect on the eye?
10. What medications should be recorded that affect the eye?
11. What cap color coding is used on miotics and mydriatic eye medications?
12. List and describe the essential elements of a complete problem-oriented medical case history.

Self-evaluation questions   Q

True–false statements

Directions: Indicate whether the statement is true **(T)** or false **(F)**.

1. History taking is a confidential experience between the patient and the technician who is involved in the questioning. **T** or **F**
2. The most significant question to be asked is, "What medications are you taking?" **T** or **F**
3. The patient should be allowed to speak freely of all his or her problems while the technician is taking a history. **T** or **F**

Missing words

Directions: Write in the missing word(s) in the following sentences.

4. The most common cause of blurred vision is a
   _____.
5. Patients who are unable to see in movie theaters or in the evening are said to have _____.
6. An ascending veil in the lower portion of one's vision is an indicator of a possible _____.

Choice-completion questions

Directions: Select the one best answer in each case.

7. Which of the following is not normally considered in the differential diagnosis of an inflamed, red eye?
   a. Acute conjunctivitis
   b. Acute iritis
   c. Acute glaucoma
   d. Keratitis
   e. Dacryocystitis
8. Which of the following is not part of a history?
   a. Chief complaint
   b. History of past health
   c. Family history of eye disease
   d. Visual assessment
   e. Medication currently used

Answers, notes, and explanations   A

1. **True**. The confidentiality of the patient's identity, history and symptoms is paramount (see Ch. 20; HIPAA and patient privacy).
2. **False**. The most significant question is, "What is your chief complaint?" It is essential to select efficiently the key problem for which the patient has sought help from an ophthalmologist. Once the essential problem or problems have been identified, then the nature of surrounding involvements can be more effectively detailed. The recording of the history becomes important because if it is clearly itemized, the ophthalmologist can minimize time spent in finding the essential facts and avoid the confusion of a mass of disorganized information. Complaints should be reduced to concise and compressed expressions related to the character and date of onset.
3. **False**. Allowing patients to ramble in a disconnected way serves no purpose except to allow them to get things "off their chest." The most effective way to take a history is for the examiner to guide the direction of the interview so as to bring out the salient features and to jog the memory of the patient for details pertaining to the relevant complaint. In addition, the interviewer must detail other areas in the interview that the patient normally would not have considered. In this way, one can arrive at an accurate and significant history that will have a meaningful and reliable effect in determining the diagnosis.
4. **Refractive error**. In an ophthalmologist's office, the most common thing people complain about is some blurring of vision for either distance or near. For most people who seek eye attention, it usually is the myopia that leads to the visit, whether the person has been referred by school or the department of motor vehicles or has just noticed a tendency to squint. In older adults, it is the presbyope who requires glasses for reading and seeks attention for blurred vision at near. Although numerous organic diseases affect loss of vision, these are in the

Answers, notes, and explanations—Continued

minority in an ophthalmologist's practice; however, they always have to be considered when the eye cannot be refracted to a normal visual acuity or when the history suggests more detailed organic loss.

5. **Night blindness**. A number of tests have been developed to determine the levels of light sensitivity and dark adaptation. The term *mesopic acuity* refers to vision under reduced illumination. A number of disease processes affect dark adaptation and produce night blindness. Such conditions as retinitis pigmentosa initially affect the rods that are abundant in the periphery of the eye and are responsible for mesopic vision by gradually obliterating them so that the patient is unable to navigate in the evening, in movie theaters, and in dimly lit rooms. Other diseases affecting vision under reduced illumination include retinal and choroidal arteriosclerosis, retinal abiotrophies, choroideremia, Oguchi disease, and hypovitaminosis. The test equipment for dark adaptation and mesopic vision is usually complex and expensive compared with equipment for visual field studies or color discrimination, and consequently it is often unavailable in most practitioners' offices.

6. **Retinal detachment**. When the retina separates from its underlying base, the sensory component is lost and a field of vision that is proportionate to the detached retina becomes diminished. To the patient this manifests as a loss in one or another portion in his or her field of gaze. It may go unnoticed until it begins to affect the macular area of the eye. The patient then responds by complaining of an ascending veil.

7. **e. Dacryocystitis**. This is an inflammation of the lacrimal sac or tear sac that results in a swelling over the tear sac portion. It occasionally spills bacteria into the conjunctival sac, resulting in a secondary conjunctivitis. It is frequently a painful condition that requires antibiotics, hot compresses, and occasionally, surgical intervention for resolution to occur.

8. **d. Visual assessment**. Visual assessment is part of the patient's physical examination and is part of the objective measurements. The history is related to the person's complaints and past and present health, along with medications and family history. Any objective measurements are part of the physical examination. The diagnosis of any condition depends on both the history and the physical examination.

Chapter | 8 |

Preliminary examination

Harold A. Stein, Raymond Stein, and Sara M. AlShaker

Preliminary examination saves the doctor time in assessment of the patient. A preliminary examination of the eyes trains and alerts the ophthalmic assistant to the numerous variations and abnormalities that occur around the eye and the eyelid. It provides a fascinating change from routine duties and challenges the assistant to sharpen diagnostic acumen and develop an interest in the many major and minor diseases and disorders of the eye.

Vision assessment

Vision should be assessed both with and without glasses on a standardized chart, and each eye should be tested independently. It has been found that the normal eye can easily distinguish two points separated by an angle of 1 minute to the eye. By convention, most visual acuity charts are constructed so that the sections of a letter subtend 1 minute of arc. Each letter is printed on squares made up of five parts in each direction so that the whole letter to be identified subtends a 5-minute angle to the eye (Fig. 8.1).

Visual acuity (VA) is determined by the smallest object that can be clearly seen and distinguished at a distance. The commonly used Snellen charts consist of letters carefully designed to subtend a 5-minute angle to the eye at certain specified distances (Fig. 8.2). Generally speaking, 20 feet (6 m) has been considered a practical distance for assessing vision for distance, and the charts have been calibrated with this in mind (Fig. 8.3). At 20 feet, the distant rays of light from an object are practically parallel and very little effort of accommodation is required. In rooms that are shorter than 20 feet, mirrors may be used to achieve the required distance. Also charts may be proportionally reduced in size to compensate for a room with a shorter working distance.

The results of vision testing are expressed as a fraction. The numerator denotes the distance the patient is from the chart letters and the denominator denotes the distance from the chart at which a normal person can see the chart letters. For example, if a person reads the 20/20 line at 20 feet, visual acuity is 20/20 (VA = 20/20). If the person reads the 20/60 line at 20 feet, visual acuity is 20/60 (VA = 20/60). This actually means that the person can see at 20 feet a letter that a normal person can see at 60 feet (18 m).

In general, in the western hemisphere, visual acuity charts are designated in feet, whereas in Europe the metric system is used (Table 8.1).

A quiet area should be selected for testing visual acuity. The chart should be fastened at eye level on a light, uncluttered wall that has no windows nearby to avoid glare. The recommended illumination on the wall chart is 10 to

30 footcandles, but many offices use projected types of vision charts or retroilluminated charts (see Fig. 8.3). The general illumination in the room should not be less than one-fifth the amount of illumination on the chart.

In assessing vision, the examiner places an occluder over one of the patient's eyes without exerting any pressure on the eye. The patient is then asked to read the chart. The smallest line of letters identified is noted. Adjacent to the line is a notation, such as 20/20 or 20/40. The line read clearly is recorded as 20/20 or whatever the case may be. If one or two letters are missed in the line, this may be recorded. For example, if the patient sees the 20/20 line but misses one letter, visual acuity should be recorded as 20/20 − 1.

The patient who is unable to read the largest letter is asked to walk toward the chart; the distance at which he or she begins to read the large letter is recorded as the numerator. For example, 4/200 indicates that the patient was 4 feet from the 20/200 letter. If it is impossible for the patient to distinguish the large letter, the examiner holds his or her fingers before the patient's eye in good light and the vision is recorded as the farthest distance at which the fingers can be counted. For example, if the patient can accurately count the number of fingers the examiner is holding up 3 feet (1 m) away, this is recorded as counting fingers at 3 feet. If

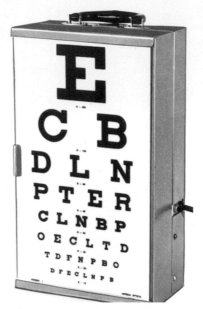

Fig. 8.3 Snellen visual acuity chart.

Table 8.1 Conversion table of visual acuity

Meters	Feet
6/6	20/20
6/7	20/25
6/9	20/30
6/12	20/40
6/18	20/60
6/24	20/80
6/30	20/100
6/60	20/200
6/90	20/300
6/120	20/400

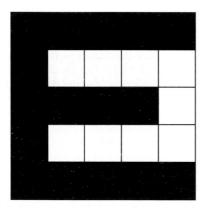

Fig. 8.1 The letter E. Each section of the letter subtends 1 minute of arc. Whole letter subtends 5 minutes of arc.

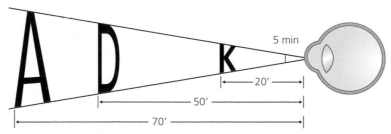

Fig. 8.2 Each letter on visual acuity chart subtends a 5-minute angle to eye independent of distance.

the patient cannot distinguish fingers, the examiner should wave a hand in front of the eye. If the patient perceives hand movements, the vision is recorded as HM, or hand movements. If the patient cannot even detect hand movements, the room is darkened, a test light is shone into the eye from the four quadrants, and the patient is asked to point in the direction of the light. If the patient can accurately point to light, vision is recorded as light projection. If the patient cannot distinguish the position but is able to just detect the light, the visual acuity is recorded as light perception. If the patient is unable to detect light at all, the vision is recorded as absent light perception.

Illiterate patients and preschool children (ages 2–5 years) may be tested by charts made up of numbers, pictures (Figs. 8.4 and 8.5), tumbling E's (Fig. 8.6), or Landolt's broken rings. HOTV (Fig. 8.7) and LEA symbols (see Fig. 8.4) are reliable tests for preschool children. The child can either match the projected optotype to a handheld chart or name the letter or shape, depending on their developmental level. In the tumbling E test, the child points in the direction of the E either with a finger (Fig. 8.8) or with a handheld cutout E. With Landolt's broken-ring test, the child merely identifies where the break in the ring occurs (Fig. 8.9). Other optotypes, such as Allen figures, do not conform to accepted parameters of optotype design and are less used nowadays.

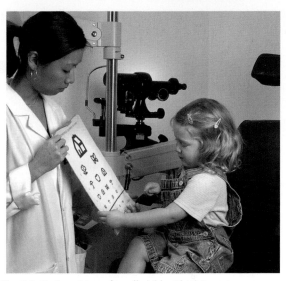

Fig. 8.5 Testing vision of small child with pictures.

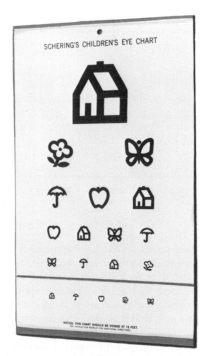

Fig. 8.4 Picture visual acuity chart.

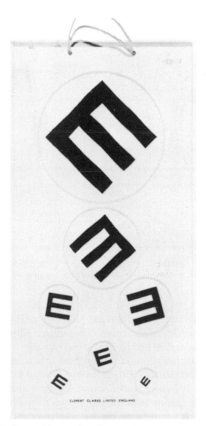

Fig. 8.6 E chart with rotating E's.

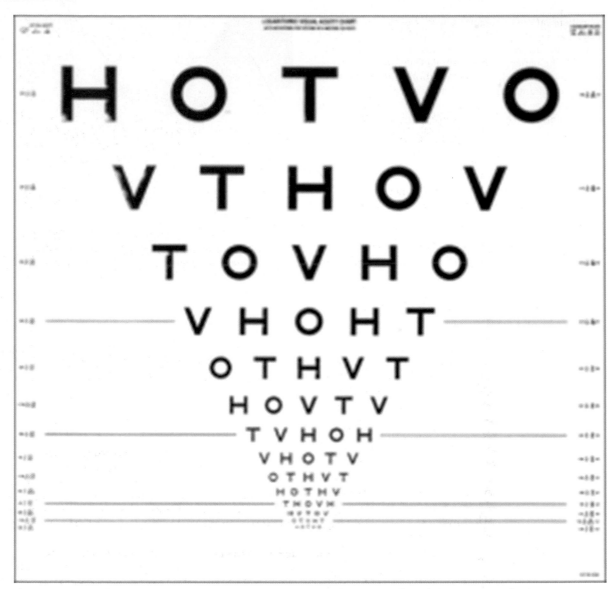

Fig. 8.7 HOTV test. (From Hartmann EE, et al. Preschool vision screening: summary of a task force report. *Pediatrics*. 2000;106(5):1105–1106.)

For near vision, the examiner holds the near vision card at normal reading distance, and the patient indicates on the key card the letters that he or she can identify.

Preverbal children are tested by preferential looking tests, such as Teller Acuity Cards II (Stereo Optical Co, Chicago, IL) (Fig. 8.10) and Cardiff Acuity Cards, if available. The basis of these tests is that a child presented with two different patterns will fixate on the pattern or picture rather than on a plain stimulus. Each eye is tested at a time and the child's preferential looking at the stimulus is observed by the experienced examiner and recorded. If these tests are not available, more crude methods of visual assessment can be used, such as monocular fixation, following of a moving object and objection to monocular occlusion. Simply flash a light into each eye consecutively. If the child is able to fixate on the light centrally and steadily, vision may be assumed to be grossly normal. If the child's fixation is eccentric but steady, the child's vision is probably below

THE 'E' GAME

1. First ask the child to point three fingers in the same direction that you point your fingers:

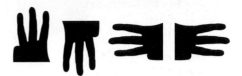

2. Then tell him to consider the E as a table with the arms of the E representing the "legs of the table".

3. Show the E in different positions and ask the child to point his three fingers in the direction of the "legs of the table".

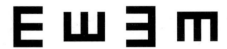

4. Vary direction in which the fingers point. Be sure the child understands the game before testing.

Fig. 8.8 Three-finger E test.

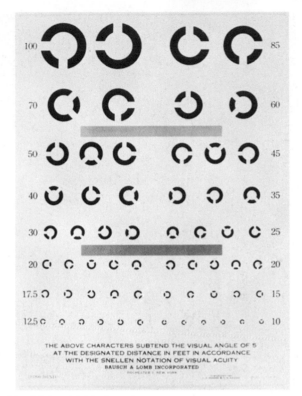

Fig. 8.9 Landolt's broken-ring test.

normal. If the fixation pattern is unsteady and eccentric, vision is probably extremely poor and the eye defective. An infant should be able to follow a light by the age of 3 months and reach for toys by the age of 4 to 6 months.

When visual acuity is tested, the following points should be noted:

1. For the preliterate child, most pediatric ophthalmologists consider Snellen or Sloan optotypes to be the most accurate, followed in decreasing order of accuracy by HOTV and LEA symbols, tumbling E, Allen figures, and fixation behavior. The examiner should use the most sophisticated test a child can perform.

2. A false idea of visual acuity will be obtained if an isolated letter is presented to the patient rather than a line of letters. This is particularly true in persons with amblyopia, who may have 20/40 or 20/50 vision when tested with isolated letters and only 20/200 vision when asked to identify letters in a series. This is known as the *crowding phenomenon*. Single optotypes can be surrounded by *crowding bars* to overcome this problem.

3. There can be differences in recognition of letters in the same line. The letter L is considered the easiest letter in the alphabet to identify and B the most difficult. The letters T, C, F, and E are progressively more difficult.

4. Vision should always be tested with and without the patient's glasses so that a comparison between the two can be made.

5. In children, visual acuity testing should not be prolonged and fatiguing. Children are easily distracted and may fail to respond to conventional visual acuity tests because of loss of interest or short attention span.

6. In all visual acuity measurements, the assistant should note any consistent pattern in the letters missed by the patient. For example, failure to see the nasal or temporal half of the chart may indicate a serious field defect, with loss of vision of half the visual field of each eye.

7. If both eyes are tested together, it is usually found that each eye reinforces the other, so that binocular vision tends to be slightly better than the vision of each eye tested separately.

8. A false visual acuity will be obtained if the patient partially closes an eye or squints. This causes a decreased pupillary aperture and thus allows only central rays to

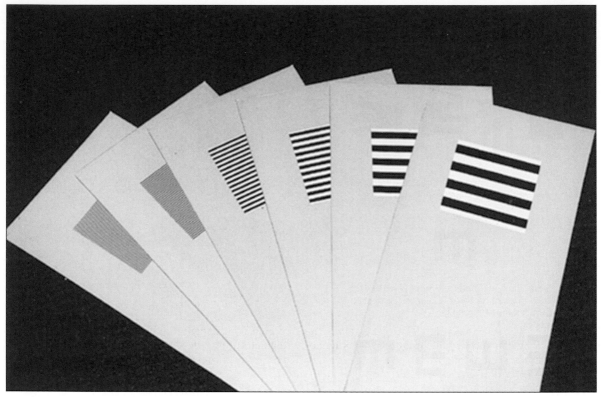

Fig. 8.10 Teller acuity cards. (From Yanoff M, Duker JS. *Ophthalmology*. 5th ed. Elsevier; 2019:1196, Fig. 11.2.5.)

enter the eye, giving much better vision than the patient would normally have. It is important for the patient to keep the eyes wide open.

9. The patient should be observed during testing to prevent peeking around the occluder. Illiterate patients often say they cannot see rather than admit ignorance. It is important to obtain their confidence and coax them to read a number or illiterate E chart.

Early treatment diabetic retinopathy study chart

The early treatment diabetic retinopathy study (ETDRS) chart was developed in 1982 and then revised in 2000 by the National Eye Institute for use in the Early Treatment Diabetic Retinopathy Study. The chart (Fig. 8.11) comprises a set of letters originally created by Louise Sloan, using the design of the LogMAR visual acuity chart that consists of letters (optotypes) arranged in standardized typeface, spacing, and size. It differs from the Snellen chart in that there is an equal number of letters per row, the rows and letters are equally spaced on a log scale, and the individual rows

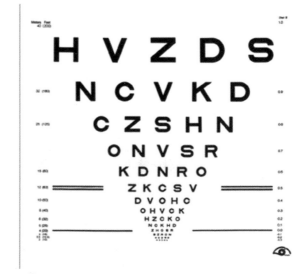

Fig. 8.11 Early treatment diabetic retinopathy study visual acuity chart. (From www.nei.nih.gov by National Eye Institute, National Institutes of Health. https://nei.nih.gov/photo/visual-acuity-testing.)

are balanced for letter recognition difficulty. Experts believe that the chart provides a more accurate and reproducible measurement of visual acuity than Snellen chart testing. The ETDRS chart has the same number of letters on each line (five), but the size of the letters on a line decreases based on a geometric progression. The ETDRS chart has become the preferred or required chart used in most clinical trials. The standard test is performed at a distance of 4 meters.

Use of pinhole

The pinhole disc, if placed before the eye, eliminates peripheral rays of light, improves contrast, and generally improves vision to almost within normal limits if the patient has a refractive error. The pinhole disc thus serves to differentiate visual loss caused by refractive errors from poor vision resulting from disease of the eye. In the latter condition, vision is not improved when a pinhole disc is placed before the eye (Fig. 8.12).

Dynamic visual acuity

Visual acuity measured in an office setting is artificial. The eyes are steady, the body is still, and the target is immobile. In real life, as we walk down a street, the eyes are in motion, the body is displaced both forward and vertically, and the object of regard is rarely still. We look at things in action. This type of acuity is sometimes called kinetic vision or dynamic visual acuity.

Kinetic vision, or moving vision, cannot be measured but it is known that acceleration reduces acuity. The faster one travels, the worse one's vision becomes. Body displacement spoils good vision. Try reading on a truck with poor shock absorbers. Fast eye movement is also a detriment to seeing clearly. It is impossible to follow a tennis serve traveling at more than 100 miles (160 km) per hour.

Contrast sensitivity

Another aspect of vision that has proven of interest is contrast gradient visual acuity. This is a measure of the acuity when hampered by poor contrast. A person can have 20/20 Snellen acuity and complain of poor vision. Snellen acuity measures only an individual's ability to see small, high-contrast images. The visual contrast test can assess the entire spectrum of images and contrast. An individual with cataracts or night blindness may see well in daytime but see poorly at night or on cloudy days when there is little contrast. Vision in the real world can be evaluated more realistically.

Contrast sensitivity testing measures vision that resembles real-life situations more closely than the Snellen chart. Contrast sensitivity could probably be detected with photographs of real-life situations with different variations in their contrast; however, this is not practical and reproducible. Consequently, contrast sensitivity charts or machines are used. The contrast sensitivity chart presents a pattern of stripes of varying contrast, size, and orientation. The patient is asked to describe the orientation of the stripes.

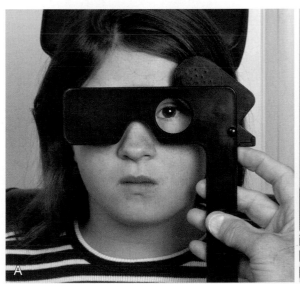 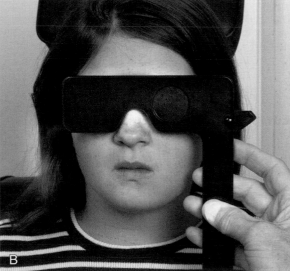

Fig. 8.12 Assessment of pinhole vision. (A) Left eye open. (B) Pinhole inserted.

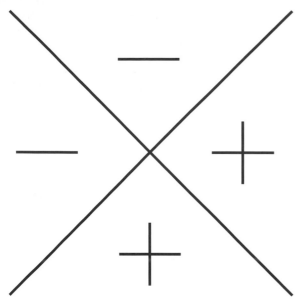

Fig. 8.13 Pelli-Robson contrast sensitivity chart. (From Bowling B. *Kanski's Clinical Ophthalmology*. 8th ed. Philadelphia: Elsevier; 2016.)

If the patient answers correctly several times, it is assumed that he or she is able to see these objects at that particular size and contrast. Many sizes and contrasts are presented to determine whether the patient has normal or decreased contrast sensitivity.

Contrast sensitivity tests may be presented as a wall chart with grids of varying size and contrast and a recording pad and instruction for analyzing the results. A smaller chart for near vision testing is also available. The Pelli-Robson chart (Fig. 8.13) determines the contrast required to read large letters of a fixed size. In this chart, the contrast varies but the letter size remains the same. In the Regan contrast sensitivity chart, low-contrast letters of different sizes are shown to the patient. In the Ginsburg Functional Acuity Contrast Test chart, sine-wave gratings tests special frequency (sizes), and levels of contrast are used to plot a contrast sensitivity curve.

In some practices, patients are evaluated for contrast sensitivity before and after fitting contact lenses. If the fit is incorrect or the lens is not properly designed, the contrast sensitivity may decrease. This may be even truer with bifocal contact lenses. In addition, lenses often spoil with protein accumulation. Protein deposition reduces their contrast sensitivity while providing good Snellen acuity. In addition, contrast sensitivity testing can help to determine improvement in macular degeneration after use of nutritional supplements and to evaluate treatment response in patients with glaucoma.

The use of contrast sensitivity tests has become important in refractive surgery. The use of lasers to alter the shape of a normal eye so that there is a reduction in myopia must be accompanied by an evaluation. Contrast sensitivity is an important hallmark of the final visual acuity in a person and is much more reliable than Snellen acuity.

Glare testing

Visual acuity may degrade considerably in the presence of bright light. This is particularly true if there are opacities in the media, such as a posterior polar cataract. A number of glare test devices are available on the market (true visual acuity [TVA], brightness acuity tester [BAT], Eye Con) that create a dazzle effect and identify the person whose vision is reduced by glare. The BAT (Fig. 8.14), developed by Jack Holladay, delivers three controlled degrees of light when the eye is viewing a Snellen target. Vision with opacities in the ocular media, cornea, lens, posterior capsule, and vitreous, when under the effect of bright light, degrades considerably and provides a true visual acuity in ambient lighting.

In glare testing, the patient looks into the machine or at some Snellen letters arranged on a wall chart. The examiner then turns on lights that shine directly into the patient's eyes. The lights have been calibrated to imitate the brightness of headlights coming toward the patient at night, both high and low beams. With the lights on, the patient is instructed to read the letters on the chart. The acuity is measured after glare testing is recorded. With high-beam light, this usually falls off considerably if lens opacities are present.

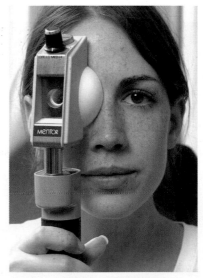

Fig. 8.14 Brightness acuity tester developed by Jack Holladay to test visual effect of bright sunshine on patient with cataracts.

The Miller-Nadler glare tester is commonly used to test for visual discrimination during bright daylight conditions. It consists of a tabletop viewing screen and a slide projector with 17 slides of varying sizes of land, dot, sea, and rings. The slides are projected onto the viewing screen. With each successive slide, the background is made progressively darker, thus decreasing contrast. The projector screen acts as a glare around the edge of the slide and shines into the patient's eyes. The ability or inability of a patient to detect breaks in rings of smaller size and lower contrast correlates with loss of functional vision outdoors in bright sunlight.

Macular photostress test

This is a sensitive test for detecting macular dysfunction, such as cystoid macular edema, central serous retinopathy, and senile macular degeneration. Under conditions of bright light, such as produced by the BAT (see Fig. 8.14), these disorders are slow to recover vision. Normal recovery to bright light is 0 to 30 seconds but it becomes prolonged to more than 1 minute in patients with maculopathies.

Potential acuity

Potential acuity meter

It is often difficult to see behind a dense cataract, or even an early cataract, to give a good estimate of the potential visual acuity of any particular eye. The cataract often partially obscures the fundus so that evidence of optic atrophy, retinal detachment, and macular disease cannot be determined. Although B-scans can sometimes determine retinal detachments, the subtle retinal defects, such as macular edema, macular degeneration, and other vitreoretinal defects are often difficult to determine.

The Guyton-Minkowski potential acuity meter (PAM) is a small apparatus that attaches to a slit lamp. The patient looks into a small aperture in the machine and sees the Snellen acuity chart. The examiner can control the position of the acuity meter, shine it through the pupil, and direct it through particular sections of the patient's crystalline lens. Even patients with mild to moderate cataracts are not totally dense to this light and there are small breaks between opacities. The examiner shines the light through one of these small breaks; the patient can see it unobstructed by the cataract and can then read down the Snellen chart. This has important prognostic significance for determining what the acuity will be following cataract surgery. It lets the physician know that the retina and media are intact and gives an estimate of potential visual acuity.

Interferometer

The interferometer is an apparatus similar to the PAM. Instead of a Snellen chart that is imaged on the retina through breaks in the cataract, the interferometer shines red laser light or white achromatic light directly through the opaque portion of the cataract. The light is not blocked by lens opacity and passes through unchanged. Laser light in a pattern of stripes, either red or white depending on the type of machine, is separated by black stripes of equal size. The width of the stripes can be changed. The patient is asked to name the orientation of each grid as the width is changed, to estimate acuity. As the stripes become smaller, it becomes more difficult to detect which way they are pointing. If the patient can name the orientation of several grids with very thin stripes, it is assumed that the retina can resolve images at that visual level and should approximate good postoperative acuity.

Retinometer

The Heine (Heine Optotechnik GmbH & Co., Germany) Lambda 100 Retinometer (interferometer) operates on the principle of the Maxwellian view: a microaperture is illuminated by a halogen bulb through a red filter and imaged by an optical system into the patient's pupil. The optical system consists of two lenses between which optical grids with variable spacing can be positioned in the parallel beam that passes through them. The resulting diffraction forms a circular test pattern with equally spaced red and black lines on the retina. The distance between the lines corresponds to that of the Snellen E (Visus 1 = 33 lines/degree of visual angle). The orientation of the lines can be selected by means of a prism in 45-degree steps. Because the beam in the pupillary plane is very narrow (a few tenths of a millimeter), a tiny "window" in the opacity of the lens is enough to allow the light to pass through for a successful examination.

The PAM, the interferometer, and the retinometer give only an estimate of the potential acuity. A patient's acuity may be much better or worse than what was expected.

Near vision testing

Near vision charts are designed to be read at 14 to 16 inches. In patients with accommodative loss, as in patients with early presbyopia, a corrective lens is required to record the near vision. The near vision is recorded as the smallest type that can be comfortably read at the distance at which the card is held. Test cards are available in a wide variety of forms, such as printed paragraphs, printed words, music, numbers, pictures, and E's (Fig. 8.15).

Near vision for normal individuals may be recorded as 14/14, J2, or N5. The term 14/14 has the same meaning as the Snellen fraction in that the patient is able to read, at 14 inches (35 cm), small print that is easily seen by a normal individual. The term J2 refers to the Jaeger system. In the latter part of the 19th century, Jaeger designed a system

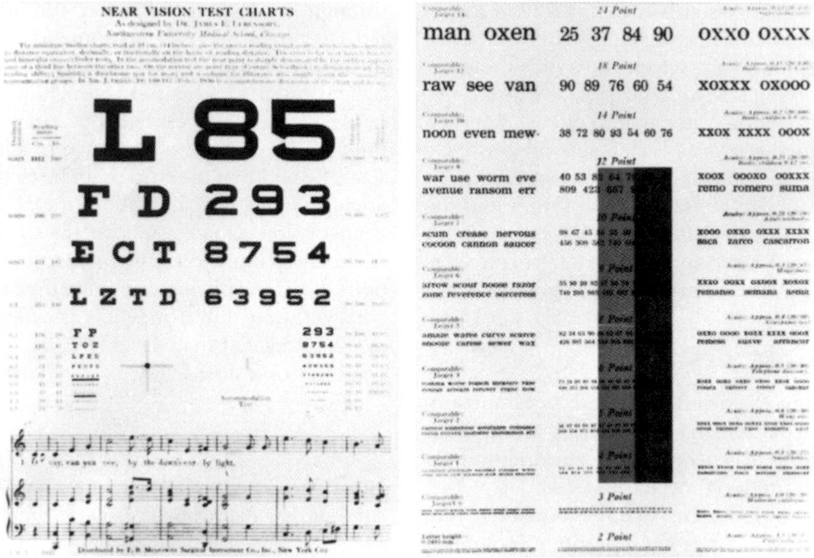

Fig. 8.15 Lebensohn reading chart.

of readable print and arbitrarily assigned numbers, beginning J1, to the various sizes. The term *N5* refers to the printers' point system; the print ranges in size from N5 to N48.

Near vision in children does not always correspond to the vision taken in the distance. Children can usually read despite significant refractive errors because they can hold reading material close to their eyes and thereby obtain magnification by the powerful range of accommodation.

Measurement of glasses

Before the refractive status of a patient is evaluated, it is important to know the previous prescription. The ophthalmic assistant should be very familiar with the technique of neutralizing lenses and arrive at the prescription of the glasses the patient is wearing.

The lensmeter is an instrument designed to measure the prescription of an optical lens (Figs. 8.16 and 8.17). (Lensometer is the trade name of the American Optical Company. All other manufacturers refer to lens-measuring equipment as lensmeter, Vertometer, Vortexometer, or Focimeter.) Lenses are made up of either spheres or cylinders or a combination of both. By using a target area on the lensmeter, one can determine the exact prescription of any lens. All targets have some means of identifying two meridians that are at right angles to each other.

Many types of lensmeters are available. Each manufacturer publishes a manual showing how their instrument

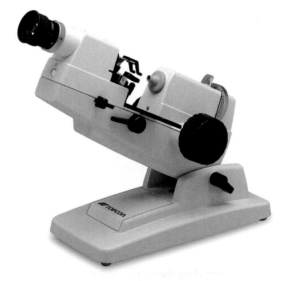

Fig. 8.16 Topcon lensmeter. (Courtesy Topcon Europe Medical BV; www.topcon-medical.eu.)

is used because the instruments vary in approach. Some work in minus cylinders with plus spheres. Some manual instructions are in plus cylinders for all readings; others are in minus. Therefore the user may be confused when confronted with an unfamiliar instrument.

Although the instruments vary, the eyepiece on all lensmeters (except the projection type) must be adjusted to compensate for the user's refractive error, if any exists, or all

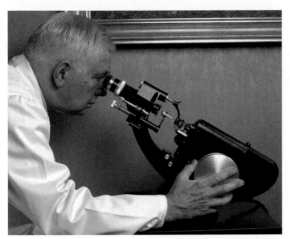

Fig. 8.17 Measurement of spectacles with a lensmeter.

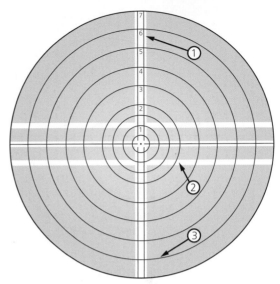

Fig. 8.18 American lensmeter target. 1, Single line; 2, triple lines; 3, rings to measure prism in lens.

readings will be inaccurate. The examiner should perform the following procedure:

1. Turn the power-focusing wheel until the target is not visible.
2. Turn the eyepiece fully counterclockwise.
3. Look through the eyepiece and turn it slowly clockwise until the grid or reticule just comes into focus. The correct position is the place where it first comes into focus. If in doubt, repeat.
4. Bring the target into sharp focus. The reading should be zero. If it is not, repeat. If zero cannot be obtained, set the power wheel to zero, turn the eyepiece counterclockwise to blur the reticule, then clockwise until the target and reticule just come into clear focus. Note the number on the scale around the eyepiece for quick, future adjustment.

If the examiner wears distance glasses while making this adjustment of the eyepiece, they should be worn every time the lensmeter is used. If the examiner prefers to use the instrument when not wearing glasses, then the eyepiece adjustment should be made without them. It is important to be consistent.

Lensmeters fall into two categories: those using the American crossed-line-type target (Fig. 8.18) and those using the European dot-type target (Fig. 8.19). Both types are accurate, providing the correct technique is used. The target type therefore is a matter of individual choice and of the operator's familiarity with a specific type.

The American crossed-line-type target consists of solid straight lines at right angles to one another. A single line runs in one direction and three parallel lines run in the opposite direction (Fig. 8.20). The whole target can be rotated 360 degrees for determining cylinder axis. At the beginning, it is easiest to measure a lens with this type of lensmeter by following five simple rules:

1. Place the spectacles on the base so that both left and right lenses are resting on the holder. This prevents rotation of the lens and inaccurate axis reading.
2. Focus the single line. Rotate the lines by using the axis wheel so that the single line gives readings closest to zero for both the plus and the minus spheres. This is then marked down as the sphere component.
3. Focus the triple line and record the difference from the single line to the triple line. This is the cylinder portion. For example, if the single line is at +1.00 and the triple line is at +3.00, the prescription will be + 1.00 + 2.00.
4. Rotate the axis wheel so the target is on axis when the triple lines are continual. Mark down this axis; this is the axis of the cylinder (e.g., +1.00 +2.00, axis 90). If the single line and the triple line are in focus at the same time, the lens is a sphere.
5. In determining the reading addition in a bifocal lens, move the lens up to the reading segment and then focus again on the triple lines. The difference from the recording of the last triple line to the new triple line in focus is the reading addition. This is always recorded as plus.

If the examiner initially focuses the single line so that it is closest to zero, both the cylinder and the sphere will have the same sign (plus or minus).

In some cases, the examiner may wish to record all prescriptions in terms of plus cylinders. In doing so, it is necessary to first bring the single and then the triple lines in focus. By rotating the axis wheel, the examiner can arrange that the triple lines come into focus when more plus is introduced, thereby ending up with cylinders recorded as plus.

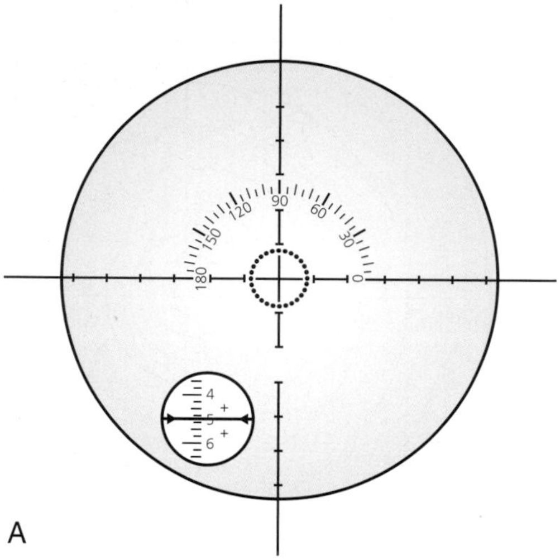

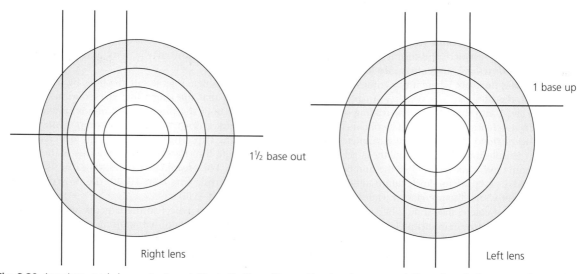

Fig. 8.19 European lensmeter test target. (A) Test target with spherical lens. (B) Test target with spherocylinders.

A

B

1 base up

1½ base out

Right lens

Left lens

Fig. 8.20 American-made lensmeter target. Neutralization of lens with prism incorporated. Note that displacement of target by prism is always recorded in terms of base of prism.

The European dot-type target consists of a circle of dots (or variation thereof) that does not rotate. Instead, a protractor grid rotates in the field of view to determine the cylinder axis. The power of a spherical lens is determined by bringing the dots into sharp focus and then reading the power (see Fig. 8.19).

The power of a toric or cylindric lens is determined as follows:

1. If a lens contains a cylinder, the target will appear as a system of focal lines. These lines focus in two positions, one perpendicular to the other. First, focus the target so that one of these lines is in focus. The reading closest to zero is marked down as the spherical component (e.g., +1.00).

2. Focus the target so that the second set of lines is now perpendicular to the first reading and record the difference in dioptric powers between the first and second readings. This is the cylinder portion. For example, if the first focal point is at +1.00 and the second focal point is at +3.00, then the prescription will be +1.00 +2.00.

3. Adjust the cross line so that it is parallel to the focal lines on this second reading. This is the axis of the cylinder (e.g., +1.00 +2.00, axis 90).

    Note: It is impossible with a very weak cylinder to identify a cylindric lens and its axis when the dots are in focus. (When the user is unfamiliar with this instrument, the most common error is that the axis is off by 90 degrees.) There will be no difficulty with stronger cylinders because the dots will smear into distinct lines and aligning the axis grid offers no problems.

    The technique for neutralizing a lens with a weak cylinder is as follows. First, rock the power-focusing wheel on either side of the target's focus point and note how the individual dots "bloom" or go out of focus. If the blooming is spherical, you have a spherical lens. If the blooming is oval, you have a cylindric lens. While rocking the focusing wheel, rotate the target protractor or reticule to line it up with the direction (axis) of the oval blooming or smearing of the circular dots. After establishing the cylindric axis, determine the spherical and cylindric power.

4. In determining the additions in a reading bifocal lens, move the lens up to the reading segment and then focus again on the lines at the second focal point. The difference between the value of the second focal point in the distance prescription and that found in the reading segment is the reading addition. This is always recorded as plus.

With all lensmeters it is important: (1) to center the lens well before reading the prescription and (2) to measure the prism if present. The lens has a prism if the center of the lens does not coincide with the center of the target. There are circles surrounding the central target of the lensmeter to measure the amount of prism. The distance between each circle represents 1 prism diopter. It is easy to see at a glance how far the optical center of the lens is displaced in prism diopters from the center of the target. Fig. 8.20 illustrates a prism in a lens with the American type of target.

Universal method of using any lensmeter

Many projection instruments make reading of the lens prescription easier. The following method works with any lensmeter, standard or projection type, using any type of target:

1. Place the lens to be measured (in frame or otherwise) in the lensmeter on the table, convex side toward you, with the lens surface firmly against the instrument and with no tilt. Tilting a lens will introduce an error that may result in an inaccurate axis and cylinder power. This is a common error made by the inexperienced user in measuring the bifocal segment. Finding the addition of a fused-glass bifocal requires a special technique, which is covered in detail later.

2. Center the target, then set the power to zero. Move the power wheel from zero to a point well beyond the focus of the target and then back toward zero to the point where the first target meridian or dots come into focus. Take the reading. This is the spherical power.

3. Continue rotating the power wheel in the same direction (do not reverse direction) to bring the second meridian into focus. The algebraic difference is the cylindric power. The sign of the cylinder is opposite that of the sphere. Note the axis of the second meridian. This may be correct or exactly 90 degrees off.

4. Make this check. If the target line or smeared dots are nearly horizontal, the axis is going to be near zero or 180 degrees. If the target line or smeared dots are nearly vertical, the true reading will be near 90 degrees.

This procedure is the same with all makes of lensmeters, and the user actually has a check on a possible cylinder axis error. The user may be in doubt, however, when the axis is near 45 or 135 degrees, in which case another pair of glasses should be tried (or a cylinder from a trial case) to identify which line on the target, or the grid, gives the true axis.

This universal method gives plus cylinder results with minus spheres and minus cylinder results with plus spheres.

Once the user has mastered the instrument, he or she will have no difficulty in modifying the method to work only in plus or only in minus cylinders if this is wished, rather than transposing mathematically from one to the other.

Prism, with the base in any direction, is measured by concentric circles and the displacement of the target. The circles may be in 0.50 or 1.00 prism diopter steps. In addition, some lensmeters have a Risley rotary-type prism as an integral part of the instrument; its secondary use is to center the target for accurate axis reading in a prismatic lens.

Addition

To find the addition of a bifocal lens less than 3.00 diopters, the difference in power between the distance and the reading portions must be found. First, the distance power should be found in the conventional manner, holding the lens being tested in the instrument with the rear surface (usually concave) away from the eye. Second, the reading power should be found, holding the lens in the same position, rear surface away from the eye. If the bifocal is less than 3.00 diopters, the previously mentioned method will produce a correct reading to within 0.06 of a diopter, which is an insignificant error.

For all bifocals greater than 3.00 diopters, the following is the only procedure that gives accurate results:

1. Check the distance portion in the manner indicated previously. This step is identical in checking all lenses and gives an accurate result as to the power of the distance portion.

121

2. The bifocal must now be reversed in the instrument. Hold its front (usually convex) surface away from the eye and check the distance portion at a spot about the same distance above the center as the point at which you will check the reading power is below the center. In the case of aspheric surfaces, measure the distance through its optical center.

3. Note the finding made through the distance portion. Now check the power through the reading, again with the convex surface away from the eye. Subtract the power of the distance portion found from the reading power to determine the addition.

4. When making all readings, the lens must be firmly against the lensmeter stop, its surface at right angles to the axis of the lensmeter. In some lensmeters, it is advisable for the operator to hold the lens in position with his or her fingers and not rely on the lens holder.

Automatic lensmeters

Space-age technology has once again simplified the operator portion of arriving at spectacle measurements. Although costly, this technology will save time and improve accuracy in a busy office. A lens analyzer measures in a single operation the sphere, cylinder, axis, and prism of a lens (Fig. 8.21). The values are digitally displayed and can be recorded, if desired, on a paper tape by the built-in printer. This instrument eliminates the focusing and target alignment tasks,

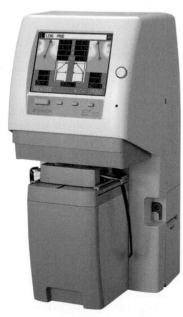

Fig. 8.21 Topcon lens analyzer.

which require a fair amount of skill with a conventional lensmeter. It also does the mathematic tasks of computing cylinder power and of computing the add value of the bifocal segment. The lens analyzer has the unique ability to position spectacle lenses at a given interpupillary distance and then to use prism information collected to compute the net prismatic effect of the spectacle pair. These measurements are made very rapidly. The instrument uses a white light source and a ray trace-type system to make its measurements. It can also measure the amount of ultraviolet lens transmission to let one know exactly how much protection the wearer has.

The minicomputer in the lens analyzer is used to operate a hard copy printer, to make add computations when bifocals are measured, to change the display cylinder convention, to change round-off modes, and to make special tests for errors and improper measurements, in addition to its primary mode of calculating and displaying the basic lens values. When a spectacle pair is measured, the printed copy records the lens values for both lenses labeled "left" and "right" with sphere, cylinder axis, and prism shown, plus the net prism for the pair. This automatic lensmeter operates on a standard electric power source. The newer Lensometer has a communication link with the phoropter for more rapid refraction.

Rodenstock Instruments manufactures a series of lensmeters in their AL Series. These instruments are fully automated with touch screens and built-in printers. Depending on the instrument in the series, they offer simultaneous measurements of lens power and ultraviolet (UV) transmission, automated detection and measurements of progressive lenses, prismatic lens measurements, pupillary distance (PD) measurements, refractive index calculations, precise lens marking, and a contact lens mode.

The Autolensmeter, manufactured by Acuity Systems, similarly is a microprocessor computer that provides ophthalmic and contact lens reading with accuracy. Pressing one button provides a sphere/cylinder and shows both on a display panel and on printed tape. Pressing another button causes horizontal and vertical prisms to be displayed. The "add" button automatically computes the additional power on multifocal lenses. The Autolensmeter also simplifies the measurement of progressive power lenses.

1. Topcon makes a lensmeter that is fast and reliable. It also detects if a bifocal is present in a progressive add. There is a color screen that simplifies readings. The instrument provides a printout and it can be integrated into a computer (Fig. 8.22). All optical parts of the lensmeter, as well as the spectacle lens, should be kept clean with a soft cloth and lens-cleaning solution.

2. In unusual situations, the spherical power may extend beyond the range of the lensmeter scale. If this occurs, it may be necessary to insert neutralizing or

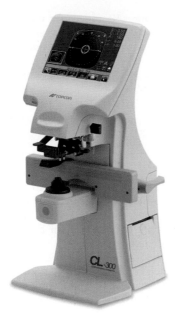

Fig. 8.22 Automated lensmeter from Topcon.

opposite-power lenses in the lensmeter to bring the target into focus. The final figures are approximate only.

3. Prisms may be detected by counting the number of rings from the center crossmark that the optical center of the lens is displaced. The direction of the base of the prism can be read directly. For example, if the optical center of the lens is displaced two rings temporally from the center of the crossmarks, then the amount of prism present in the lens would be 2.00 prism diopters, base out.

4. If the center of the lens cannot be detected in the field of the target, loose prisms may be required to bring the optical center of the lens to fall within the area of the target. Some lensmeters incorporate the variable-adjusting Risley-type prisms (see Ch. 9) for this purpose.

Accommodation

Accommodation is a mechanism by which the eye internally adjusts to changes in the proximity of an object before the eye to maintain a clear image on the retina. This change in the total power of the eye is affected by alterations in the radius of curvature and the thickness of the eye's lens. Increasing the radius of curvature of the anterior face of the lens and increasing its thickness add power to the eye as an optical instrument.

Measurement of amplitude of accommodation

Proximity method

Small print, such as J3 type, is held at a comfortable arm's length and gradually brought closer. The distance at which the patient reports blurring of the letters is measured in centimeters and expressed in diopters. To convert the centimeter measurement into diopters, this measurement should be divided into 100. For example, if the patient detects blurring of the print at 20 cm, the range of available accommodation would be from infinity to 20 cm and the power of accommodation would be 100/20 or 5.00 diopters. It is important that each eye be tested individually and that the patient wear full-distance correction for the test. If the patient is too presbyopic to comfortably hold reading material, an auxiliary lens, such as +2.50, is added to the patient's correction. The amplitude of accommodation is then measured and +2.50 subtracted from the total findings.

Triple line test

In this test, two small vertical lines, as found on the Lebensohn chart, are brought toward the patient. The near point is reached when the patient sees three lines instead of two.

Effect of age

The ability of the eye to make these changes in focusing adjustments is greatest in childhood, when the crystalline lens is softest and most malleable. The range of accommodation declines rather precipitously with age as the lens becomes harder. A 10-year-old child has 14.00 diopters of accommodation and a near point of 7 cm, whereas a 40-year-old adult has only 4.50 diopters of accommodation and a near point that has receded to 22 cm (Table 8.2). This means that a 45-year-old man cannot see fine print closer than 22 cm without the assistance of reading glasses.

Convergence

Convergence is an act by which the eyes are turned toward each other to view an object in the midline plane situated close at hand. It is measured by having the patient look at a small target, such as a pin, letter, or toy (Fig. 8.23). The near point of convergence is that point at which fusion can no longer be maintained and one eye deviates outward.

Table 8.2 Accommodation and near point of the emmetropic eye

Age	Near point in centimeters	Available accommodation in diopters
10	7	14.00
20	9	11.00
30	12	8.00
40	22	4.50
45	28	3.50
50	40	2.50
55	55	1.75
60	100	1.00
65	133	0.75
70	400	0.25
75	Infinity	0

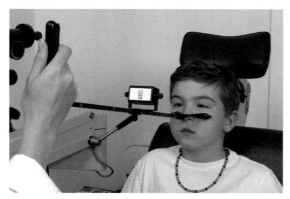

Fig. 8.23 Measuring the near point of convergence.

The patient may report seeing double at the moment one eye begins to drift outward. The near point of convergence (NPC) is measured in centimeters.

The following points should be kept in mind when measuring convergence:

1. It is a voluntary act that requires the cooperation of the patient and the ability to respond to the test with alertness. If the patient is tired or debilitated at the time of testing, the near point may be unusually remote. If the patient is a distractible, uninterested child, again the near point cannot be adequately measured. For these reasons, the near point of convergence is not regarded as a reliable and completely reproducible test in terms of value.

2. This test requires normal fusion; it cannot be performed if one eye is amblyopic.

Color vision

Defects in color vision may be congenital or acquired. Congenital color defects occur in about 8% to 10% of males and in only 0.4% of females. This defect is transmitted through the female and appears predominantly in the male. Acquired color blindness may occur after diseases of the optic nerve or central retina.

Congenital color blindness may be partial or complete. In the completely color-blind patient, visual acuity is reduced and the patient usually has nystagmus. All colors appear as various shades of gray. Fortunately, this form of color blindness is rare. The partial form is a hereditary disorder transmitted through the female, who usually is unaffected. In the majority of patients, the color deficiency is in the red–green area of the spectrum. With the deficiency in red, this color appears less bright than for the normal individual and thus mixtures of colors containing red are often confused with other colors. Deficient color vision of the red–green variety may pose problems for sailors, drivers, pilots, and textile designers. Absence of blue color is very uncommon.

Tests for color blindness are multiple and varied and consist of matching colored balls or yarns, the red–green lantern test and the most popular test, isochromatic plates.

In clinical practice, it is sufficient to test with one of the pseudoisochromatic plates. More scientific approaches to color vision testing (such as the Nagel anomaloscope) are available but are not generally useful for routine clinical practice.

Ishihara test plates

The Ishihara book consists of a series of pseudoisochromatic plates that determine total color blindness and red–green blindness. These plates are viewed by the observer under good illumination. They consist of dotted numbers of one color against a background of another color (Fig. 8.24). If color vision is normal, the dots stand out and the patient can read the appropriate number. A person with normal sight may see one number, whereas the color-blind person viewing the same plate would interpret the dots as forming a completely different number. For patients unable to read numbers, plates are present in the album with colored winding lines that may be traced.

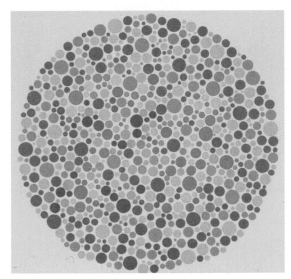

Fig. 8.24 Ishihara's test for color blindness.

Hardy-Rand-Rittler plates

This test is no longer manufactured but may still be found in ophthalmic offices. This series of pseudoisochromatic plates includes plates for yellow–blue color blindness, as well as red–green color deficiency (Fig. 8.25). The background is a neutral gray on which a series of colored circles, crosses, and triangles are superimposed. These geometric designs are present in higher and lower saturations of color to detect the degree of color vision deficiency. Under proper illumination, the observer is required to detect the geometric designs present on each plate. With this color vision test, not only can a graded diagnosis be made (mild, medium, or severe) but also the yellow–blue defects may be differentiated, as well as the red and green.

Although it is possible to memorize the numbers on the round Ishihara plates, this is impossible with the Hardy-Rand-Rittler (H-R-R) test because the patient must identify not only what symbols are seen on each plate but also how many and in what quadrant. To ensure against malingering, the plates may be presented right side up, sideways, and upside down. As a result, the malingering patient will have no clues to guide him or her.

Colormaster

Colormaster is a sophisticated, completely automatic, and programmable computerized form of presenting color sequences of constant hue, saturation, and brightness to an individual. This computer has both clinical and research importance because of its repeatability and reliability.

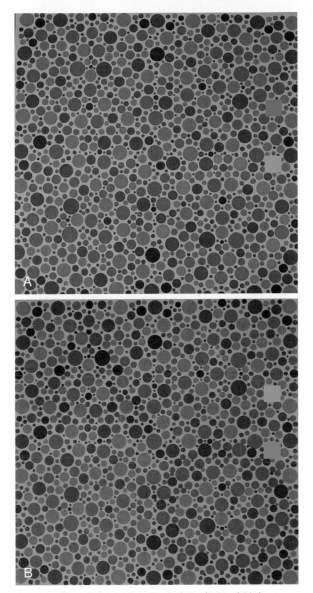

Fig. 8.25 (A and B) American Optical Hardy-Rand-Rittler test for color blindness.

Depth perception

Depth perception is the highest quality of binocular vision because it provides the individual with judgment concerning depth, based on the coordinate use of the two eyes together. A prerequisite for depth perception is good vision in each eye, overlapping visual fields, and normal alignment of the eyes in all positions of gaze. The four main tests available are the fly test, the Wirt stereo test, the Worth four-dot test, and the biopter test.

Fly test

The patient is provided with polaroid lenses and asked to touch the wings of a fly. If the patient has depth perception, the wings will appear to stand out before the picture (Fig. 8.26). This patient will have gross stereopsis of approximately 3600 seconds of arc (when tested at 40 cm).

Wirt stereo test

Animals in three lines are shown to young school-aged children or even to preschoolers who seem able to grasp the idea of the test (see Fig. 8.26). If all three lines of animals are correctly selected, the patient has stereopsis of approximately 100 seconds of arc.

The raised rings in nine frames are shown to older children, adults, or even younger children, if possible, depending on the child's alertness. If all nine groups are correctly selected, it may be assumed that the patient has normal stereopsis of approximately 40 seconds of arc. In this portion of the test, two groups must be missed in succession for the examiner to stop the test. For example, if the patient correctly selects groups 1 through 6 and misses groups 4, 7, and 8, number 6 is counted as the patient's maximum amount of stereopsis.

Worth four-dot test

In the original Worth four-dot test, one white disc, one red disc, and two green discs are presented to the patient, who is wearing spectacles with a red-free green lens before one eye and a green-free red lens before the other eye, thus allowing both the patient's eyes to see the white disc. However, the eye covered with the red lens will see, in addition to the white disc, only the red disc. The eye covered with the green lens will see, in addition to the white disc, only the two green discs. The patient is then asked to report the number of discs seen. If four discs are seen, both eyes are functioning. If three discs are seen, then the eye behind the green lens is seeing (the two green and one white) and the eye behind the red lens is suppressing. If two discs are seen, then the eye behind the red lens is seeing and the one behind the green lens is suppressing. If five discs are seen, then another problem is indicated (the eyes are not fusing and muscular imbalance is suspected) (Fig. 8.27).

Variations on this test include the Project-O-Chart slide, wall-mounted internally illuminated tests or the flashlight form (Fig. 8.28). The symbols shown may be

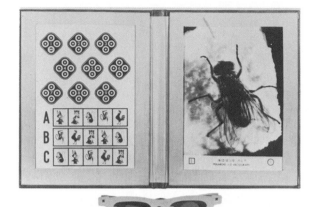

A

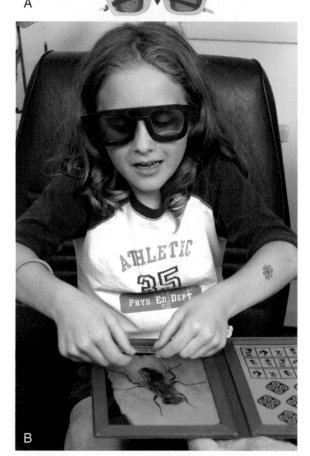

B

Fig. 8.26 (A and B) Wirt and fly tests for depth perception.

four discs set in a diamond pattern or a disc, a cross, a triangle, and a square. For children, a picture presentation in colors of a clown, a seal, and a ball may be used. In all these tests red and green spectacles are worn.

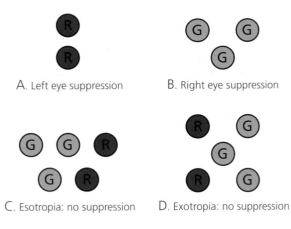

A. Left eye suppression   B. Right eye suppression

C. Esotropia: no suppression   D. Exotropia: no suppression

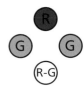

E. Normal 4-dot response:
no suppression

Fig. 8.27 Worth four-dot test. (A and B) The suppressing eye. (C and D) Muscle imbalance and no fusion. (E) Normal four-dot response. *R*, Red lens before right eye; *G*, green lens before left eye.

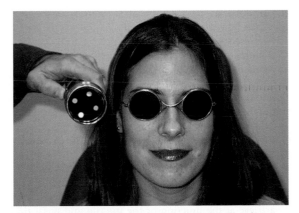

Fig. 8.28 Worth four-dot test to detect suppression. (From Kaiser PK, Friedman N, Pineda II, R. *The Massachusetts Eye and Ear Infirmary Illustrated Manual of Ophthalmology*. 4th ed. Philadelphia: Elsevier/Saunders; 2014.)

Biopter test

This instrument has the fundamentals of a home stereoscopic viewer in which slightly different images are presented to each eye (Fig. 8.29). The sensation of depth is appreciated by the slightly disparate images.

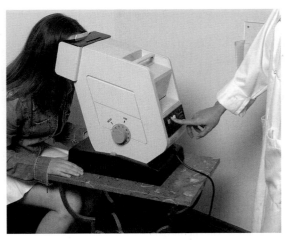

Fig. 8.29 Biopter test for depth perception.

External examination

Although the ophthalmic assistant cannot expect to substitute for the trained eye of the ophthalmologist in recognizing abnormalities of the eye and the eyelid, an awareness of abnormal external features, with documentation of such on the record, will aid the ophthalmologist in the recording of these abnormalities, as well as alerting him or her to problems that are incidental to the main complaint of the patient. This exercise also helps instill an awareness of and interest in unusual eye problems, whether they are abnormal or pathologic.

The ophthalmic assistant should begin the external examination of the eye by systematically noting the symmetry of the orbits, the eyelashes, the lid margins, the conjunctiva, the lacrimal apparatus, the sclera, the cornea, the iris, the anterior chamber, the pupil, and the lens.

Symmetry of orbits

In proptosis (exophthalmos), in which one eye protrudes, the upper lid is often retracted and there is exposed sclera above and below the cornea (Fig. 8.30). Another method of determining the presence of proptosis is to stand behind the patient, draw the upper lids upward, and note which eye appears to bulge more. The ophthalmologist may record the degree of proptosis with an instrument called an exophthalmometer (see Figs. 10.35 and 10.36).

Eyelashes

Cilia, or eyelashes, are hairs on the margins of the lids. They are located in two rows, totaling about 100 to 150 cilia

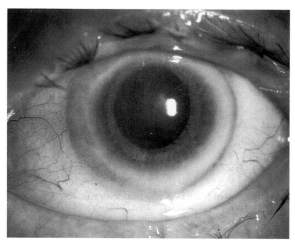

Fig. 8.33 Arcus senilis caused by deposition of cholesterol and lipids in the peripheral cornea. A common aging process. (Reproduced from Spalton D, Hitchings R, Hunter P. *Atlas of Clinical Ophthalmology*. 3rd ed. St Louis: Mosby; 2004, with permission.)

becomes swollen, it loses its shape and transparency so that loss of vision is common. Total corneal swelling occurs with acute glaucoma, and the cornea may develop a ground-glass appearance.

The normal cornea should be smooth, shiny, and free of irregularities. In children, the corneal diameter should not exceed 11 mm. Corneal enlargement 12 mm or greater is strongly indicative of congenital glaucoma. In older adults, a white ring is frequently present near the corneal periphery. This creamy white ring is a result of the deposition of fat and is called the arcus senilis (Fig. 8.33).

The cornea is normally free of blood vessels. The presence of blood vessels indicates a pathologic condition and disease. Blood vessels in the cornea are best seen with a slit-lamp microscope but can be appreciated with strong focal illumination and the magnification of an ophthalmic loupe. Corneal edema often can be seen with the naked eye because of its characteristic ground-glass appearance. Corneal opacities may be detected by oblique illumination with a small flashlight.

Corneal sensation should be tested with a small wisp of cotton directly applied to the cornea. In this test, the patient is instructed to look up. Normally, a blink response should occur if the corneal sensation is intact. It is important that the patient not see the cotton approaching the eye because the visually evoked response of seeing a foreign object approach the eye causes a blink. Because of the wide range in individual response, comparison of the corneal reflexes of the two eyes is most useful. Loss of corneal sensitivity follows herpes simplex virus and brain disease involving the fifth nerve.

Use of fluorescein, rose bengal, and lissamine green stains

Fluorescein is an ocular stain used to show defects and abrasions in the corneal epithelium. The pooling of fluorescein on small corneal defects is best seen by means of ultraviolet or cobalt blue light for illumination. This causes the fluorescein to fluoresce. There is a danger with fluorescein in solution form. It becomes easily contaminated with *Pseudomonas aeruginosa*, which appears to flourish in fluorescein. Sterile dry fluorostrips in which fluorescein has been impregnated are available to prevent this complication. The fluorescein strip should be moistened with a drop of saline and applied to the lower fornix. This will cause liquid fluorescein to replace the tear film. The ulcer or denuded epithelium will be visible as a brilliant green.

Rose bengal is a red dye that has an affinity for degenerated epithelium. Similar to fluorescein, it will stain areas in which the epithelium has been sloughed off. However, unlike fluorescein, intact, nonviable epithelial cells of the conjunctiva or cornea stain brightly with rose bengal. The stain is helpful in diagnosing keratoconjunctivitis sicca or other conditions associated with dryness of the conjunctiva. If the dye stains devitalized epithelium of the nasal bulbar conjunctiva, a diagnosis of keratitis sicca may be made. The technique is to apply at least 10 mL of sterile balanced salt to the test rose bengal strip.

If available, lissamine green can be used as an alternative to rose bengal. It is less irritating.

Iris

The iris is normally clear to inspection. The irides of both eyes are generally the same color. The color depends on the amount of pigment in the stroma and posterior layer of the iris. A heavily pigmented iris appears brown, whereas a lightly pigmented one appears blue. Interestingly enough, there is no blue pigment in the iris. In the blue iris, the light passes through the nonpigmented stroma and strikes the pigmented epithelial cells on the back of the iris so that light of longer wavelength (red) is absorbed and that of shorter wavelength (blue) is reflected.

A difference in the color between the two irides (heterochromia) may be indicative of a congenital abnormality, iris tumor, retained intraocular foreign body (siderosis), or old iritis.

If a light is brought to bear on the iris at close range against the sclera (transillumination), the light may seem to glow in a patchy way in areas where there has been marked pigment loss. This can occur with some forms of glaucoma (pigmentary), after iritis, or with albinism. Freckles on the iris should be noted because iris freckles are frequently associated with intraocular malignant melanomas. Near the root of the iris lies the dilator muscle. When

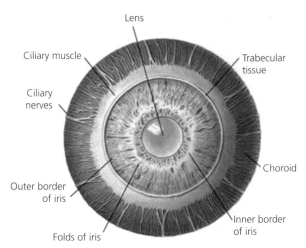

Fig. 8.34 Frontal drawing of the eye showing the iris and pupil (lens). (From Head and Neck Imaging. Mafee, Mahmood F.; Som, Peter M. Published January 1, 2011. © 2011. Modified from Sobotta Atlas of Human Anatomy © Elsevier GmbH, Urban & Fischer, Munich.)

dilation occurs, at a maximum, the pupil may be 9 mm or greater in diameter. When maximally contracted, it may be only 1 mm.

The iris is normally well supported by the underlying lens. Tremulousness of the iris (iridodonesis) usually means the presence of a dislocated or loosely attached lens. Tremulousness of the iris, or undulating movements of the iris structure, is best seen by having the patient look quickly from one point of fixation to another. Near the aperture is a sphincter muscle that constricts the pupil. In the center of the iris, running radially around the pupil and forming a circular web, are the blood vessels of the iris. If the lens is absent (aphakia), the iris loses its support, flattens, and deepens the anterior chamber. It may become tremulous.

A defect in the iris is called a coloboma. A coloboma, which indicates absence of some portion of the iris, may be the result of previous surgery or a congenital abnormality.

Muddiness of the iris is a term used to express the general loss of clarity of the pattern of the iris. It is caused by inflammatory exudates in the anterior chamber or on its surface. Normally, the textured surface of the iris and the white markings of the iris vessels are easily visible (Fig. 8.34).

Anterior chamber

By shining a small penlight from the side, one can make an estimation of the depth of the anterior chamber. If the anterior chamber is shallow, it should be so recorded because the patient may be prone to narrow-angle glaucoma.

Penlight examination for estimating the depth of the anterior chamber

It is important to evaluate the anterior chamber depth in all patients but especially before dilating their pupils.

The depth of the anterior chamber can be estimated by holding a penlight temporal to the eye near the limbus and parallel to the iris plane. Shine the light across the front of the iris and toward the nose of each of the patient's eyes. Observe the degree of shadow formation on the iris between the nasal pupillary border and the nasal limbus. A completely illuminated nasal iris with possibly a small rim of shadow just inside the nasal limbus denotes a deep chamber (Fig. 8.35A). A wide shadow on the nasal portion of the iris (Fig. 8.35B) denotes a shallow chamber. The shadow projected onto the nasal iris denotes that the angle is narrow because the iris is bowed forward and blocks the path of light. Although the oblique penlight test lacks the sensitivity or specificity of a Van Herrick test (a test that uses a slit lamp to create an optic section beam at approximately a 60-degree angle at the limbal cornea that is then compared with the width of the corneal section and the width of the shadow adjacent to it) or gonioscopy, it can be used as a useful tool in detecting a shallow anterior chamber without the use of a slit lamp. An appropriate referral by

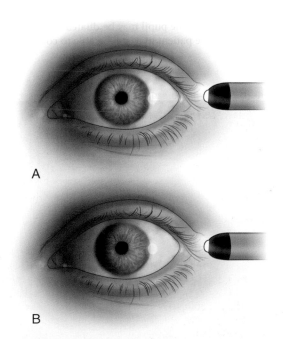

A

B

Fig. 8.35 (A) Fully illuminated iris with little shadow denotes a deep anterior chamber. (B) Partially illuminated iris with a wide shadow denotes a shallow anterior chamber.

Psychic influences, such as surprise, fear, and pain markedly dilate the pupil. Dim light also dilates the pupil, whereas bright light constricts it. At times, the pupil is constantly contracting and dilating; this is called *hippus*.

During sleep the pupil is constricted. This is such a constant finding that it serves as an aid in differentiating true from simulated sleep.

Any irritation of the cornea or conjunctiva, such as an abrasion results in constriction of the pupil.

Shape

The pupil is normally round and regular. Irregularities in the shape of the pupil may result from congenital abnormalities, inflammation of the iris, trauma to the eye, and surgical intervention (Fig. 8.38). Trauma may cause tears of the iris in the form of a wedge-shaped defect, either at the pupillary margin or at its base (iridodialysis). A corneal laceration with prolapse of the iris may result in the drawing up of a segment of the iris to the site of the laceration (adherent leukoma). In severe iritis, the iris may be bound down to the lens by adhesions (posterior synechiae), and irregular changes may occur in the shape of the pupil.

Equality of size

The pupils should be equal in size and react equally to direct light stimulation, consensual light stimulation, and near objects. In the light of an ordinary room, the diameter of the normal adult pupil is between 3 and 5 mm. If the two pupils are unequal in size, the condition is called *anisocoria*. Inequality of size may be caused by a tonic pupil (Adie syndrome). In this condition, which can be mistaken for a partial third nerve palsy, the pupil responds to light stimulation very slowly. Adie syndrome is diagnosed by instilling a low dose (0.125%) of pilocarpine, which can result in the constriction of the tonic pupil caused by cholinergic denervation hypersensitivity, whereas a normal pupil will not constrict with such a low dose of pilocarpine.

Disorders of pupillary function may involve many of the previously mentioned factors together. For example, Argyll Robertson pupils, one of the classic signs of late syphilis, are small, irregularly shaped, and nonreactive to either direct or consensual light stimulation but reactive to near stimulation.

Differential diagnosis of a dilated pupil

A dilated pupil may be caused by third nerve palsy, trauma, Adie's pupil, or acute glaucoma, or it may be drug induced.

Third nerve palsy. If the dilated pupil is fixed, the cause may be third nerve palsy. This condition may be associated with ptosis and a motility disturbance, characterized by the eye being deviated out and down. The pupil responds to constricting drops, such as pilocarpine. This is a neurosurgical emergency, and the possibility of an intracranial mass lesion must be ruled out.

Trauma. Damage to the iris sphincter may result from a blunt or penetrating injury. Iris transillumination defects may be visible with the ophthalmoscope or slit lamp and the pupil may have an irregular shape.

Adie's pupil. In Adie's pupil, the pupil responds better to near stimulation than to light. The condition is thought to

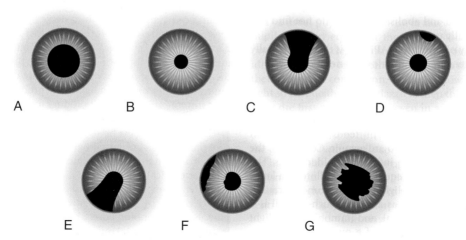

Fig. 8.38 Variations in pupillary size and shape. (A) Dilated or mydriatic pupil. (B) Constricted or miotic pupil. (C) Full or sector iridectomy. (D) Peripheral iridectomy. (E) Congenital coloboma of iris. (F) Iridodialysis. (G) Posterior synechiae.

be related to aberrant innervation of the iris by axons that normally stimulate the ciliary body. Absent knee jerks can be associated.

Acute glaucoma. The patient may complain of pain and/or nausea and vomiting. The eye is red, vision is diminished, intraocular pressure is elevated and the pupil is mid-dilated and poorly reactive.

Drug-induced dilation. Iatrogenic or self-contamination may occur with a variety of dilating drops, such as cyclopentolate hydrochloride (Cyclogyl), tropicamide (Mydriacyl), homatropine, scopolamine, and atropine. The pupil is fixed and dilated and, unlike in third nerve palsy, does not respond to constricting drops.

Differential diagnosis of a constricted pupil

A constricted pupil occurs in Horner syndrome or iritis and may be drug induced.

Horner syndrome. Other signs of Horner syndrome include mild ptosis of the upper lid and elevation of the lower lid. The difference in pupillary size is more notable in dim light because adrenergic innervation to the iris dilator muscle is diminished.

Iritis. Slit-lamp examination shows keratitic precipitates and cells in the anterior chamber and a prominent ciliary flush. The intraocular inflammation stimulates pupillary constriction.

Drug-induced constriction. Iatrogenic or self-induced pupillary constriction may be caused by a variety of drugs, including pilocarpine, carbachol, and echothiophate iodide (Phospholine Iodide).

Lens

The entire lens is normally not visible without the aid of a slit-lamp microscope. However, an advanced cataract may be seen with the naked eye because it causes a gray, opaque appearance in the pupillary aperture.

Blinking

Most people blink 15 times per minute. The duration of a blink is approximately 0.3 to 0.4 second. The average period between blinks is about 2.8 seconds in men and just under 4 seconds in women. Spontaneous blinking does not produce a discontinuity of vision in spite of the fact that vision is interrupted during the blink. Continual squeezing of the eyelids together is called blepharospasm. It occurs as a result of inflammatory diseases of the anterior segment, Parkinson disease, and stress.

Examination of the ocular muscles

The six extraocular muscles in each eye are innervated by a total of three nerves. The action of specific muscles can vary, depending on the position of the eye when it is innervated. Table 8.3 shows the general relationships that apply.

The examiner should determine the range of ocular movements in all gaze positions (Fig. 8.39). Limited

Table 8.3 Extraocular muscle innervation

Innervation	Muscle	Primary action
Third nerve	Superior rectus	Up and in
	Medial rectus	In
	Inferior rectus	Down and in
	Inferior oblique	Up and out
Fourth nerve	Superior oblique	Down and out
Sixth nerve	Lateral rectus	Out

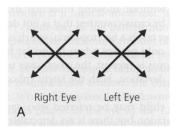
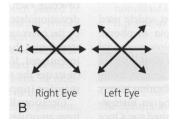
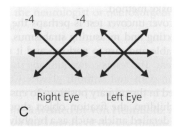

Fig. 8.39 (A) Method for examining and recording ocular motility. (B) Record of sixth nerve palsy of right eye. (C) Record of right orbital blow-out fracture and limited upgaze. (From Stein HA, Slatt BJ, Stein RM. *A Primer in Ophthalmology: A Textbook for Students.* St Louis: Mosby; 1992.)

Answers, notes, and explanations **A**

1. **False**. 6/6 vision in meters is equivalent to 20/20 vision; 6/12 vision in meters is equivalent to 20/40 vision. In Canada and the United States, visual acuity charts are designated in feet, whereas in Europe the metric system is used.

2. **False**. Occlusion nystagmus is a congenital condition in which nystagmus and esotropia may be induced by covering one eye and decreasing vision. The decrease in light sensation is enough to cause the other eye to oscillate. Such children, when given routine vision tests, score poorly because the examiner fails to look for this condition. In these children, the eye that should be occluded can be fogged with a + 10.00 diopter lens to allow proper vision in the other eye.

3. **True**. A pinhole disc before the pupil improves vision to normal limits if the loss of vision is a result of a refractive error. The pinhole test separates refractive visual loss from pathologic visual loss. With disease, a pinhole over the pupil makes vision worse. Shining a light in the other eye causes both pupils to constrict and is a simple way of achieving the pinhole test.

4. **Base**. If the lens has a prism, the center of the lens does not coincide with the center of the target. The displacement measured in circles of expanding radii is a measure of the power of the prism and is recorded as base in, out, up, or down. The distance between each circle represents 1.00 prism diopter. With the new automatic devices, prism power is digitally recorded and the results are instant.

5. **3.50 diopters**. The decline in accommodation is most striking between ages 30 and 40 years when it drops from 8.00 to 4.50 diopters. It is caused by atrophy of ciliary muscle and loss of elasticity of the lens of the eye. Unfortunately, there is no way to halt the process; thus it is inevitable that everyone eventually needs reading glasses, except near-sighted people, who merely take their glasses off.

6. **Boys**. Congenital color defects, red–green being the most common, are transmitted by the female and appear predominantly in the male. In fact, 8% to 10% of males are color deficient. Total color blindness is another matter; it is rare and very disabling and causes blindness and nystagmus in children.

7. **b. The Ishihara test plates**. Ishihara test plates are those most commonly used for the detection of color deficiency. Other devices, such as the Nagel anomaloscope are superior in detection of possible defects and in quantifying them. The Ishihara plates, however, are inexpensive to purchase so they can be used by every industrial or school nurse. They are simple to use, no expertise is required, and the results are reproducible. It is basically a color vision screener and not an analyzer.

8. **d. All of the above**. Most authorities believe that depth perception cannot be acquired. If there is a congenital strabismus and the eyes are straightened at age 3 years, that child will not have depth perception. Having poor depth perception may not be of practical importance because there are so many monocular clues to judge distance. Pilots need it in the rare instances that they have to make a visual landing. Athletes, like baseball or tennis players, are also handicapped without depth perception.

9. **a. Thyroid disease**. Protrusion of the eyes is usually measured with the exophthalmometer. When it occurs in one eye, it frequently indicates a retrobulbar mass, a hemangioma being most common. But when it occurs in both eyes, it means thyroid disease until proved otherwise. Deposits of fat, hyaluronic acid-like material, and inflammatory cells cause the typical bulging of the eyes.

Chapter | 9 |

Visual function and impairment

Bernard R. Blais, Harold A. Stein, and John S. Massare

Introduction

Visual function refers to how well the eye and overall visual system work to produce the ability to objectively observe the outside world. Visual impairment refers to any condition that decreases maximum visual function. It is sometimes considered as vision loss that cannot be corrected by standard means, such as spectacles. There are a whole host of causes of visual impairment (generally considered to be *best corrected* vision below 20/40 or sometimes 20/60). Some of the most common causes of vision loss include cataracts, glaucoma, diabetic retinopathy, macular degeneration, uveitis, amblyopia, retinal detachment, retinitis pigmentosa, and sometimes even stroke.

When considering visual function and impairment, one should consider that there are many ways of looking at anything depending on perspective. Artists all recognize this. Famous ones have unique perspective. Indeed, some even have altered color value in the cones of their retina, for example, yellow-blue blind.

One alters one's perspective when placed in large or small lecture rooms. Magicians can create visual illusions and fool us into seeing things that are not there or making things disappear before our eyes; for example, Houdini made an elephant disappear on stage in front of a large audience and David Copperfield made the Statue of Liberty disappear in front of a large audience.

The eye care doctor's goal is to achieve the best visual function for the individual and to determine if it is possible to minimize any impairments to vision that may be present.

Vision loss

Vision loss can be observed from many different points of view. The most commonly used set of aspects is the International Classification of Impairments, Disabilities, and Handicaps promoted by the World Health Organization (WHO), and the International Classification of Diseases. WHO produced on October 8, 2019 (before World Sight Day on October 10th) a publication entitled "World Report on Vision" (https://www.who.int/news-room/detail/08-10-2019-who-launches-first-world-report-on-vision). The report indicated that more than 2.2 billion have vision impairment or blindness and that "more than 1 billion people worldwide are living with vision impairment because they do not get the care they need for conditions like short and farsightedness, glaucoma, and cataract."

The aspects and ranges of vision loss are also the subject of a recent standard of the International Council of Ophthalmology (www.icoph.org).

Types of vision

The basic structure of the eye is shown in Figs. 1.1 and 1.2. The retina contains receptor cells, rods, and cones, which, when stimulated by light, send signals to the brain (as described in another chapter). These signals are subsequently interpreted as vision.

Most of the receptors are rods, which are found predominantly in the periphery of the retina, whereas the cones are located mostly in the center and near periphery. It is estimated that there are 120 million rod versus 6 million cones in the human eye. There are three types of cone detectors in the human eye roughly corresponding to red, green, and blue detectors.

According to the duplicity theory of vision, the rods are responsible for vision under very dim levels of illumination (scotopic vision) and the cones function at higher illumination levels (photopic vision).

This dual-receptor system allows the human eye to maintain sensitivity over an impressively large range of ambient light levels. Between the limits of maximal photopic vision and minimal scotopic vision, the eye can adapt rather effectively to changes in brightness of as much as 1 billion times. The sensitivity of the eye automatically adjusts to changes in lumination.

Although the human eye can function over a vast range of brightness, the retina is sensitive to damage by light, such as from lasers, bright flashlights (>600 lumens), or unprotected sun gazing or bright computer screens. This potential for light injury exists because the optics of the eye can concentrate light energy on the retina by a factor of 100,000 times.

Both rods and cones function over a wide range of light intensity levels and at the intermediate levels of illumination, they function simultaneously. The transition zone between photopic and scotopic vision where the level of illumination is equivalent to twilight or dusk is called *mesopic vision*. Here is a summary of each type of vision depending upon illumination:

Photopic vision

- Cone photoreceptors/color vision
- Resolves fine detail 20/20 or better: high acuity
- Functions only in good illumination

Mesopic vision

- Both rods and cones function over a wide range of light at simultaneous levels.
- Intermediate levels of chromatic function simultaneously.

- Twilight or dusk occurs in a mixed rod/cone mode.
- Ambient illumination should be from dim to dark.
- No surface (including reflective surfaces) within the subject fields should exact the eye chart luminance. (Standardizing the condition under which visual acuity is measured, that is, chart luminance, is important in determining whether the patient meets required occupational vision standards, as well as being an indicator of any pathologic conditions.)

Scotopic vision

- Uses rod photoreceptors
- Occurs in very low light levels
- Exhibits poorer quality vision
- Is limited by resolution (usually 20/200 or less) for acuity
- Provides ability to discriminate only shades of black and white (confirmed by noting that at dusk different colors of the flowers in a garden become virtually indistinguishable)
- Provides enhanced sensitivity and low detection threshold under marked reduced illumination
- Color vision is absent

The luminance shows typical situations in which the eye would be in each operating mode. The ambient light level created by the sun level is almost independent of position until the sun falls to 5 to 10 degrees above the horizon. The human eye's contrast sensitivity is roughly constant when the sun is much above the horizon. Once the sun is over the horizon, twilight begins and the change from photopic to mesopic and eventually to scotopic vision begins. Pure scotopic operation occurs only when there is no significant light source. Even good moonlight can prevent full scotopic operation.

Adaptation (the response to changing levels of stimulation, which for photoreceptors means light) also differs for rods and cones. Because the cones have three separate "channels," the overall sensitivity is lower and the rods are much more sensitive than cones at lower levels of light. Because of the nature of human visual response, these levels are typically measured in terms of luminance (candela per unit area), but on a logarithmic scale. This means that differences of 1.33:1 or 1:0.75 are the smallest discernible steps, despite the seemingly large changes in the associated luminance values.

Luminance versus illumination

Illumination refers to the amount of light striking a surface. Luminance is a photometric measure of the luminous intensity per unit area of light traveling in a given direction.

It describes the amount of light that passes through or is emitted from a particular area, and falls within a given solid angle. According to the International System of Units (SI), luminance is candela per square meter (cd/m^2). One way to think about this relationship is by considering that illumination times reflectance equals luminance. Luminance may also be considered as the perception of brightness by the human eye, that is, how bright light appears to be that is reflected from a surface.

Luminance is often used to characterize emission or reflection from flat, diffuse surfaces. The luminance indicates how much luminous power will be perceived by an eye looking at the surface from a particular angle of view. Luminous energy in the field of photometry is the perceived energy of light, which is sometimes called "luminous flux," that is, luminous energy per unit time. Luminance is thus an indicator of how bright the surface will appear. In this case, the solid angle of interest is the solid angle subtended by the eye's pupil. Luminance is used in the video industry to characterize the brightness of displays. A typical computer display emits between 50 and $300\,cd/m^2$. The sun has a luminance of about $1.6 \times 10^9\,cd/m^2$ at noon.

It is accepted that luminance is invariant in geometric optics and this means that for an ideal optical system, the luminance at the output is the same as the input luminance and that for real, passive, optical systems, the output luminance may be at most equal to the input. As an example, if you form a demagnified image with a lens, the luminous power is concentrated into a smaller area, meaning that the illuminance is higher at the image. The light at the image plane, however, fills a larger solid angle so the luminance comes out to be the same, assuming there is no loss at the lens. The image can never be "brighter" than the source. (Brightness is the term for the subjective sensation or impression of the objective, actual measured luminance.)

Measurement and assessment of visual loss

When considering visual functioning, we can perceive many different aspects of vision loss, depending on our point of view and the interventions, such as surgery and rehabilitation.

In considering how various causes may result in structural changes, such as scarring, atrophy, or loss, the focus is on the tissue. However, structural changes do not reveal how well the eye functions as a whole. For that we must widen our view from the tissue to the organ, and a clinician is needed to measure aspects of organ function, such as visual acuity, visual field, and contrast sensitivity.

Yet knowing how the eye functions does not disclose how a person functions. Our perspective thus has to expand

even more to encompass the individual level and consider tasks, such as reading, mobility, and face recognition. For this perspective, various vision rehabilitation professionals are needed to work with a patient. Beyond this scope, the person has to be viewed in a societal context and assessed for how all of these changes have an effect on the person's participation in society, such as causing job loss or reducing quality of life. The goal of all of these interventions is to ensure the patient is satisfied with the resulting condition.

Aspects of visual impairment

When organ functions are reduced, we speak of impairments. The most common *ocular visual impairments* are a result of ocular disorders. More recently, increased attention is being given to cerebral disorders, which may cause *cerebral vision impairment*. In infants and children, the cause may be perinatal cerebral ischemia, in adults, it may be traumatic brain injury, and in older adults, it may be a stroke. Cerebral visual impairments may cause abnormal visual functioning, which can be captured under the term *visual dysfunction*.

Visual functions

Ophthalmology has unique tools that can measure *visual function* with great precision. Those with the greatest effect on general functioning are: (1) *visual acuity* and (2) *visual field*, followed by (3) *contrast sensitivity*. Many other functions, such as color vision, stereopsis, light and dark adaptation, and psychophysical and electrophysiologic tests (e.g., electroretinography, visual-evoked potentials) can assess visual function, but they are poor predictors of functional consequence. Because loss of visual acuity has many different causes, it is a good screening test, but adds little to the differential diagnosis. Yet whatever its cause it can help in predicting the effect on activities of daily living (ADLs).

Measurement and assessment of functional aspects

The different functional aspects are measured and assessed in very different ways. Visual functions measure how the eye functions by varying one parameter at a time in a simplified, artificial environment. For example, the visibility of test objects depends on their size, contrast, and illumination. If we vary the size while keeping contrast and illumination constant, we create a *contrast sensitivity* test, like the CV-1200. If we vary the illumination while keeping size and contrast constant, we perform a *dark adaptation* test. Each test provides a threshold value for the measured stimulus parameter. The threshold criterion is generally defined as the response level that is 50% greater than guessing. Threshold measurements are chosen not because threshold performance is the most relevant performance level for ADLs, but because they enable more precise psychophysical calculations (psychophysics deals with the relationship between external physical stimuli and the human reaction/mental response to the stimuli).

For visual functions we measure the variable stimulus needed for a fixed response; for functional vision we measure the variable performance for a fixed task, either objectively (e.g., timing or error rate) or subjectively (questionnaires).

Finally, we must consider the societal context or quality of life. For subjective judgments, such as making and keeping friendships, social skills, and self-confidence, measurement is more difficult. The ultimate goal is satisfaction, which describes the subjective balance between individual achievements and individual expectations.

Parameters of ocular function

1. Macula function
2. Provides binocular vision
3. Visual acuity better than 20/200
4. Central vision less than 10 degrees
5. Stereopsis
6. Color vision

Analysis

Basic visual functions and essential ADL are:

1. Acuity testing for:
   - Monocular (each eye) and binocular (both eyes) vision
   - Both distance and near visual acuity
   - With and without correction (the person's eyeglasses or contact lenses)
2. Stereopsis findings as a baseline; note subsequent changes, if any
3. Color perception, of the three visual hues
4. Visual fields to determine visual acuity from the fovea to the ciliary body
5. Muscle balance (distance and near), also called *binocular balance*. The examination should be for vertical and horizontal phorias
   - General limits of normal functional balance are set for far and near vision when performing the tests.

Ocular (visual screening)

Visual screening (oftentimes called an *eye test* and performed by ancillary personnel rather than an eye doctor)

is an eye examination that quickly attempts to determine if there are any eye disorders or visual problems that needs to be examined further.

Vision screening is especially important in children, including babies, as good vision is critical to the child's development and overall wellbeing. The American Academy of Ophthalmology states that "It is essential to check children's vision when they are first born and again during infancy, preschool and school years" (https://www.aao.org/eye-health/tips-prevention/children-eye-screening). A paper entitled "Vision Screening: Program Models" by Mae Millicent W. Peterseim, MD and Robert W. Arnold, MD (Nov. 10, 2015) reviews in-depth information on the topic of vision screening for children (https://www.aao.org/disease-review/vision-screening-program-models).

Peripheral

1. Visual acuity worse than 20/200
2. Peripheral visual fields more than 10 degrees
3. Scotopic vision—night vision—exclusion area of macula/fovea control

Preventive medicine guidelines, CPT codebook's evaluation/management guidelines, requirements

1. Ocular history, which includes a general overview of the individual's visual history
2. Complete visual (ocular) screening examination
   a. Visual acuity quantitative bilateral tests are measured for far, at infinity (at minimum and especially in pediatrics), for near, and for intermediate distances (based on job description); contrast sensitivity is done periodically; all examinations are performed with and without corrective devices (i.e., glasses, contact lenses).
   b. Color vision
   c. Gross visual fields
   d. Heterophoria/heterotropia (horizontal and vertical) and depth perception
   e. Intraocular tension (e.g., puff tonometers) by separate glaucoma screening

Why perform visual screening

Visual function and visual tasks can analyze anatomic and structural changes caused by disease or injury. Also included here is a discussion of the relationship of these functional changes to the visual requirements of ADL or specific occupational requirements.

The precision and accuracy with which the eye can contrast is exceptional, exceeding many sophisticated cameras. It has unique focusing capabilities, and its ability to work with the brain allows people to undergo special training (e.g., finding specific details or characteristics in a product, such as a flaw in a factory-made part). The eye also can differentiate and distinguish between subtle shades of color and images under conditions of high and low contrast.

Aspects of vision loss and function

Vision loss can be observed from many different perspectives in addition to those of the patient, whether it is the treating physician, a family member, or a caregiver. Each aspect is different, but they all revolve around the same clinical case and reveal something about the patient.

Older adults in North America need to be assessed for the most common sight-threatening conditions they may face, that is, cataract, age-related maculopathy, glaucoma, and diabetic retinopathy. These conditions cause visual sensory impairments, even in early and moderate stages and in later stages, reductions in health-related quality of life, including difficulties in daily tasks and psychosocial problems. Other older adults that may be free from these common conditions, may still experience visual perceptual problems as a result of simple aging relating from changes in the optics of the eye and/or degeneration of visual neural pathways.

Functional vision

Functions describe how the eyes and the visual system function. Functional vision describes how the person functions. When organ functions are reduced, they are referred to as impairments. The most common *ocular visual impairments* are caused by ocular disorders. More recently, increased attention is being given to cerebral disorders, which may cause *cerebral visual impairment*. Cerebral vision impairments may cause abnormal visual functioning, which can be considered under the term *visual dysfunction*.

Another scenario involves screening patients with an identifiable defect during an evaluation required by federal law for entrance into a work position, such as the evaluation that a pilot might undergo. In particular, the Americans with Disabilities Act (ADA) of 1990 requires that an individual be evaluated to determine whether that person is qualified to fulfill the essential tasks of the position, with or without accommodation, without significant increase in risk to self or others.

Binocular vision

Binocular vision (visual perception using two eyes) is normal and confers three benefits: it makes hard-to-see objects easier to detect, it enlarges the total field of view, and it improves a person's capacity to distinguish small differences in depth (allows for more effective depth perception).

The most distinctive benefit of using two eyes derives from the fact that because they are horizontally separated, they do not have exactly the same view of the visual world. The small differences between the images in the two eyes are systematically related to the arrangement of objects in depth, providing information from which the visual system is able to distinguish small differences in the distances at which objects lie. This capability, known as *stereopsis*, is most beneficial for making fine depth judgments, especially when objects are nearby (i.e., within arm's reach).

For all three of these capabilities (enhanced acuity, field of view, and stereopsis), the brain must properly combine information from the two eyes. If the vision in the two eyes differs substantially, the brain may not be able to combine the information in a unified view *(binocular single vision)* or may be unable to use the differences between the images to distinguish small differences in the depth. Binocular vision can be disturbed even though each eye alone is functioning normally. Abnormalities in the brain, or improperly coordinated movements of the eyes, or misalignment of them, can disrupt normal binocular vision. When the brain is unable to combine information of the two eyes, a person may experience double vision *(diplopia)* or *binocular rivalry*, a sometimes haphazard switching of the eyes from one eye to the other. Failure to combine information from the two eyes can lead to a reduced ability to use small differences in depth. Moreover, under some circumstances, vision of the two eyes might conflict, making vision poorer than if one eye alone were used.

Monocular vision

Monocular vision is one-eyed vision. A person with monocular vision usually has one of the following:
- Suppression
- Amblyopia
- Tropia
- Disease
- Trauma

Visual acuity

Visual acuity quantitative bilateral tests are measured for far (or at infinity), for near, and for intermediate distances (based on job description); all examinations are performed with and without corrective devices (i.e., glasses, contact lenses).

A visual acuity test may be an evaluation for those especially who have had cataract implant operations or refractive surgery or are older.

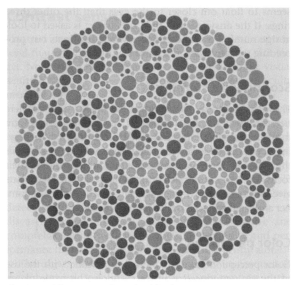

Fig. 9.4 Ishihara's test for color blindness.

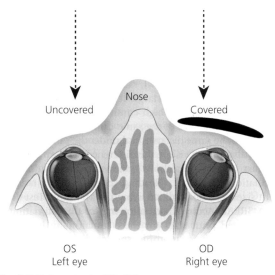

Fig. 9.5 Heterophoria. *OD*, *OS*

plates do not classify as to type of defect. That is determined with follow-up testing using the HRR pseudoisochromatic plate book or the Farnsworth-Munsell 100 Hue Test which will provide a detailed analysis of a person's capacity to accurately perceive colors.

Individuals with low visual acuity (≤20/50) in both eyes may fail color vision testing. The cause of failure in some cases may be low visual acuity rather than faulty color perception. Individuals with low acuity should be identified in the visual acuity section of the vision test series.

Phorias

The term phoria refers to the tendency for an eye to deviate from a straight ahead positioning when covered (i.e., when both eyes are not focusing on the same object).

Heterophoria

Heterophoria is a condition in which both eyes are directed in the same direction except when one eye is covered. The eyes are parallel when both are open but when one eye is covered, the covered eye moves away from the other eye. When an occluder is removed from the eye, the eye then straightens. This is also known as a phoria (Fig. 9.5).

Phorias describe the relative directions of the eyes during binocular fixation on a given object in the absence of an adequate fusion stimulus. With normal binocular vision and with both eyes open, subjects will see a single target in space. Because the phoria indicates a latent deviation of the eyes, dissociation is required to determine the amount and direction of the deviation. The examiner evaluates the subjects' vision under dissociation with the use of a prism to determine whether their lines of sight are parallel or if they diverge or converge.

For an examiner to reveal phoria, the cover–uncover test can be used. Cover one eye of the subject with a card and have the subject look at your fingertip. Move the finger around to break the normal reflex that holds a covered eye in the correct vergence position. Then hold your finger steady and uncover the eye. It may be seen to flick quickly from its correct position. If the uncovered eye moves from outward in, the person has exophoria. If the eye moves from inward out, the person has esophoria. If no movement is detected, the person has orthophoria (Fig. 9.6).

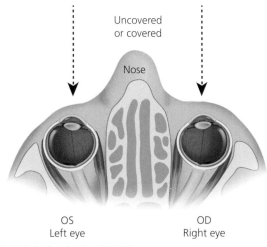

Fig. 9.6 Orthophoria. *OD*, *OS*

It is quite normal for most people to have some amount of exophoria or esophoria.

Heterophoria can be lateral (horizontal) or vertical. A lateral heterophoria can be either an exophoria or esophoria. *Exo* means "turning outward," away from the nose, whereas *eso* means "turning inward," toward the nose. In an exophoria, if the right eye is covered, it will drift outward under the cover. As soon as the right eye is uncovered, it will move back in and fixate on the target again. The same actions occur for esophoria, although the drift is inward.

Lateral phoria

The test for lateral phoria measures, in 0.5 prism diopter steps, the relative posture of the eyes in the horizonal plane when all stimuli to binocular fixation are eliminated.

Vertical phoria

The test for vertical phoria measures, in 0.5 prism diopter steps, the relative posture of the eyes in the vertical plane when all stimuli to binocular fixation are eliminated.

Interventions for rehabilitation

The four aspects of vision loss are not independent but form a loose chain of cause and effect. Rehabilitation, therefore, involves manipulating each of these links to achieve the least possible handicap or the greatest possible participation.

Rehabilitation involves a team of different professionals, and the effects of their interventions must be measured with different yardsticks. Thus it is important that all evaluators not only understand their own responsibilities and the differences in various approaches, but also have a basic familiarity with corresponding issues of the other team members as well.

The decade of the 2020s will see significant advances in vision loss rehabilitation. The confluence of advanced technologies in the coming years including artificial intelligence, quantum computing, biotechnology, human genetics, and nanotechnology, all will play a major role in ameliorating vision loss in the coming decade.

Chapter | 10 |

Understanding ophthalmic equipment

Today, more than ever, the ophthalmologist's clinical acumen is enhanced by the many instruments available that facilitate the determination of refractive errors of the eye, the detection of muscular imbalance, and the magnification and visualization of the interior structures of the eye. This chapter deals with ophthalmic instruments, their purpose and mode of use, and their advantages and limitations.

Equipment used for refraction

Determining the refractive error of an eye permits the ophthalmologist to prescribe lenses that enable the patient to obtain the best possible visual acuity.

Projector and projector slides

The projector provides a means of projecting, on a silver screen, test letters and characters that can be used in assessing visual acuity.

It consists of a housing for a bulb, an opening for introduction of different target slides, and a lens system that can be focused onto a silver screen. The housing for the bulb is made readily accessible for interchange of bulbs when bulbs darken or burn out. Rheostats may be introduced into the power circuits to lengthen the life of the bulb. The lens system and slides should be kept clean and dust free.

Projectors provide a means of illuminating: (1) a horizontal row of test letters or characters, (2) a vertical row of test letters or characters, and (3) a single-test letter or character, and may allow the introduction of red–green to illuminate the letters.

The use of red and green letters is the basis of the duochrome test and a means of fine-tuning the refraction. In this test, half the panel is illuminated in red and half the panel in green. Under the duochrome principle, green is normally focused in front of the retina, whereas red, having a longer wavelength, is focused behind the retina for the emmetrope. Therefore a patient seeing the letters on the green panel more clearly than those on the red panel is hyperopic, requiring more plus to bring the red wavelengths onto the retina. The patient seeing the letters more clearly on the red panel is myopic, requiring more minus to bring the green onto the retina. The emmetrope sees both equally blurred. The duochrome test thus provides a means to arrive at the final correcting lens for the refractive error present.

Available projector slides have a large variety of test targets and specialized tests for refraction. Commonly available slides include:

- Snellen test letters
- Landolt (split circle) rings
- Numbers
- E's
- An astigmatic clock
- A picture chart
- A Worth four-dot test

Projectors may be controlled by remote control units. The use of remote control units is especially important if projectors are installed in inaccessible places or areas that are awkward for the examiner to control.

Trial case and lenses

The trial case is a tray of lenses and accessories used to determine the refractive error of an eye. These lenses are individually marked in the strengths of the dioptric power of each lens, as well as in the direction of axis of the cylindric lenses. The trial case consists of:

- A pair of plus spheres ranging from +0.12 to +20.00 diopters
- A pair of minus spheres ranging from −0.12 to −20.00 diopters
- A pair of plus cylinders ranging from +0.12 to +8.00 diopters
- A pair of minus cylinders ranging from −0.12 to −8.00 diopters
- Accessory lenses
- Trial frame

These lenses are designed to fit a standard trial frame. Each lens is encircled by a metal rim for protection. Handles are provided with spheres for ease of handling and are optional with cylinders. The choice is governed by the type of trial frames used. Cylinders with handles are used with the trial frames illustrated in Fig. 10.1, but not with simple types having no revolving cylinder lens carriers. Handles would interfere with the free rotation of the cylinder in the latter type. The cylinder is marked with reference to its axis and not the meridian. Thus the position on the cylinder, as marked on the lens, is the axis of zero power and indicates the position of the image on the retina.

Accessory lenses available in a trial case are:

- An occluder lens
- A pinhole disc
- A stenopeic slit
- A Maddox rod lens

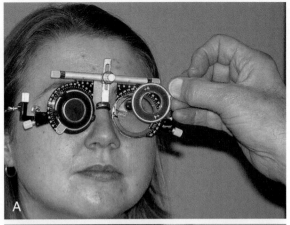
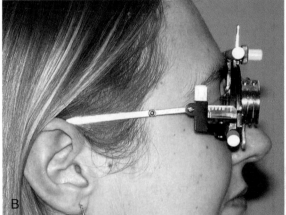

Fig. 10.1 (A) Inserting lenses in a trial frame. (B) Side view of trial frame.

- Prisms ranging from 0.50 to 6.00 prism diopters
- A red glass filter lens

Use of trial lenses

Trial lenses are not used routinely because they have been eclipsed by the *refractor* or *phoropter* (see following text), which offers the ophthalmologist the speed of exchange of lenses in a completely enclosed housing. The trial lens, however, has a place in determining the refractive error of children who are intimidated by the massive bulk of the refractor, or whose narrowly set eyes cannot be positioned properly behind the openings in the refractor (Fig. 10.2). Bifocals are prescribed by use of the trial frame with lenses because the patient can best judge a comfortable working and reading distance with the head bent and the eyes lowered in a natural reading position. Trial lenses are also used in refraction of aphakic and high-myopic eyes because it is

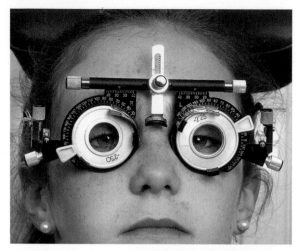

Fig. 10.2 Testing vision with trial frames and lenses.

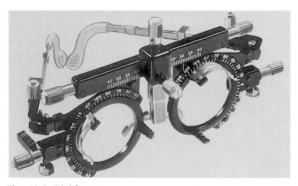

Fig. 10.3 Trial frame.

expedient that the correcting lenses and the spectacles that the patient receives approximate each other with reference to their distance from the eye itself. Trial lenses must be used when low visual aids in the form of high-plus prescription lenses are used.

The trial frame is essentially a frame capable of holding a group of three or four trial lenses for each eye. It has adjustable earpieces and an adjustable bridge that alters the interpupillary distance. Some trial frames have an adjustment for tilting the frames toward the reading position. In high-minus and high-plus prescriptions, the proximity of the lens in the frame to the eye (vertex distance) must be measured. This aids the optician in duplicating the prescription. The calibration scale incorporated on the outer side of the frame can be used for this purpose, but is not really an accurate method of making this measurement. Modern trial frames have a thumbscrew mechanism on the side of the trial frame to rotate the front lens carrier, which is used to house the cylinder. This enables the cylinder to be rotated to the proper axis.

The front surface of the trial frame is marked off in degrees from 0 to 180 (Fig. 10.3). By convention, frames are labeled in a counterclockwise direction beginning on the right-hand side of the horizontal meridian.

Refractor or phoropter

The refractor consists of the entire trial set of lenses mounted on a circular wheel so that each lens can be brought before the aperture of the viewing system by merely turning a dial (Figs. 10.4 and 10.5). In addition to the conventional spheres and cylinders, accessories are available including a polarizing lens, a pinhole, a Maddox rod, and a working lens for retinoscopy. There are many types of refractors on

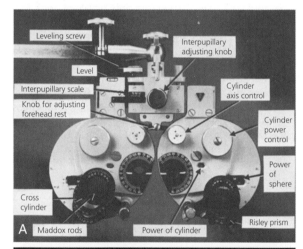

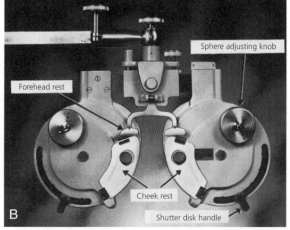

Fig. 10.4 Greens' refractor (older type). (A) Front view. (B) Back view. (Courtesy Bausch & Lomb Co., Rochester, NY.)

154

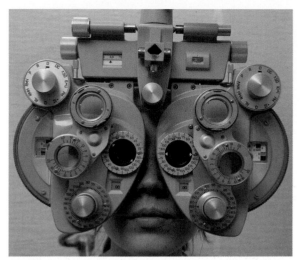

Fig. 10.5 Improved Greens' phoropter II.

the market, varying in the number of accessories available and the mode of housing these accessories. Fundamentally, these refractors are of the same design and purpose.

We shall discuss the Bausch & Lomb Phoropter II (manufactured by Reichert) because it is a typical example of the devices available. (The terms *phoropter* and *refractor* are often used interchangeably.)

Body

The body consists of two disc-like casings that house the lenses. The entire instrument is mounted on a pole or a hydraulic stand. A forehead rest ensures that the patient is correctly positioned and that the eyes are as close to the lens system as possible. The knobs at either end on top of the phoropter adjust the interpupillary distance for the individual patient. If the patient has a head tilt or a vertical muscle imbalance, the phoropter may have to be tilted so that one aperture is higher than the other. Leveling adjustment knobs are adjacent to the interpupillary distance knobs.

Lenses

For each eye, there are large circular discs that contain spheres and cylinders. These lenses may be presented individually or in combination. A large dial on the back surface of the phoropter introduces spheres in units of 3.00 diopters (some older models may be 4.00 diopters). A *side wheel* can be rotated to introduce spheres in small jumps of a quarter of a sphere. The total spherical power is read on the front casing. Plus spheres are recorded in white and minus spheres in red. The range of spherical lenses is from +20.00 to −28.00 diopters.

Phoropters are available in either plus or minus cylinders, but never both. Cylinders are introduced by the top knob on the front surface of the phoropter in units of 0.25 to 2.50. If higher cylinders are required, auxiliary cylinders of 2.50 can be flipped in front of the lens system, extending the range to 5.00. Additional loose auxiliary cylinders may be added to extend the range to 7.50 diopters. Astigmatism may be corrected to 0.12 diopter by introducing an auxiliary cylinder of 0.12 diopter. All cylinders have an axis that is controlled by a small knob, about which the accessories rotate. Markings on the front surface are in degrees, from 0 to 180, with individual axis markings in 5-degree intervals.

Aperture control handle

A small handle on the side of each eye of the phoropter controls the aperture. By moving the handle up or down, one may introduce the following:
1. An occluder to block out one eye
2. A pinhole disc
3. A +0.12 sphere, which can raise the total spherical power of the combination of lenses by 0.12 diopter
4. A retinoscopy lens, which may be custom ordered according to the distance at which retinoscopy is performed (the usual retinoscopy lens ranges from +1.00 to +2.00 spheres and is introduced by the control handle for retinoscopy and removed for subjective testing)
5. Prisms, 6.00 diopters base-up before the right eye and 10.00 diopters base-in before the left eye
6. Maddox rods, vertical and horizontal

From time to time, the complete phoropter should be returned for cleaning of lenses.

Auxiliary lenses

Auxiliary lenses include cylinders of 0.12 and 5.00 diopters for each eye (the phoropter has lenses available in either plus or minus cylinders, but not both), and cross cylinders of 0.25, 0.37, and 0.50 for each eye.

Accessory equipment

Accessory equipment includes Risley's prisms to measure muscle imbalance, a cross-cylinder holder, and a reading-card holder. The *cross-cylinder holder* is geared to follow the cylinder axis control. The cross cylinder is inserted in a double ring of metal, the outer ring being fixed, whereas the inner ring, which holds the cross cylinder, is capable of being flipped or turned to reverse its position. The *reading-card holder*, attached to the front of the phoropter, permits the holding of a reading card at a variable distance from the phoropter. The reading-card holder is a rod, calibrated in inches, centimeters, and diopters, and it is capable of presenting four test cards to the patient.

Aids in care of refractor/phoropter

1. If the lenses are dirty, they should be cleaned with a lint-free swab slightly moistened with either alcohol or ether. Ammonia or ammonia-containing cleansers should not be used. Lenses may be dried with a tissue.
2. Do not put fingers, pens, or pencils in the front aperture to see if a lens is in place because the marks left are extremely difficult to remove. The rear apertures are often protected by a cover glass.
3. The instrument should not be lubricated because the design of the instrument is such that no interior oiling is necessary. It may be helpful at times to oil the bearings on which the cross cylinder and the Maddox rod ride.
4. Cleaning material should not be used on the numbers and workings that indicate lens power. These should be cleaned with a dry, soft cloth.
5. The forehead and cheek rests are removable and should be cleaned periodically with cotton moistened in 70% alcohol solution.
6. The instrument should be covered with a plastic cover when not in use.

Retinoscope

The retinoscope is the most valuable instrument in determining the refractive error of an eye (Figs. 10.6 and 10.7). It is useful in determining the total objective refractive error of an eye and may be the only means of assessing refractive error in infants and small children. It is also useful for the objective estimation of the refractive error in people who cannot read, are learning disabled, are debilitated and

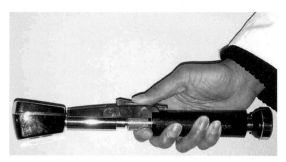

Fig. 10.7 Copeland streak retinoscope.

uncooperative, and have speech loss. There are two basic types: the spot retinoscope and the streak retinoscope.

Spot retinoscope

The spot retinoscope is designed so that the refractionist can look down the center of a slightly diverging beam of light through the pupil of the patient's eye. The modern retinoscope has a light source in the handle of the instrument, shining upward, which strikes a mirror set at 45 degrees. The beam is therefore turned through 90 degrees.

The mirror may be semisilvered or may have a hole through its center through which the refractionist can look. Therefore an area of the patient's retina is illuminated and the refractionist sees this as a red-reflected glow. This is termed a *reflex*.

In the eye with no refractive error, the rays of light come to a focus on a point on the retina and the refractionist sees the whole pupillary area lit with a red glow. This is analogous to an automobile's headlight, in which the whole 6-inch (15-cm) circular diameter of the headlight appears to be illuminated, whereas the source of this illumination is a small filament in the bulb, about 5 mm long, positioned correctly at the point of focus of the optical system of the headlight. Moving the retinoscope away from the pupil extinguishes the red reflex.

If the patient is myopic, the rays of light from the retinoscope will come to a focus in front of the retina, cross at this point, and illuminate a relatively larger area of the retina behind the focal point. If the light source is moved across the pupil, the rays of light from the retinoscope, pivoting on the focal point, will move the illuminated area on the fundus in a direction opposite to that of the retinoscope. This apparent shift of the illuminated area is termed an *against motion*. The refractionist therefore adds minus lenses before the patient's eyes to move the focal point back onto the retina. When he or she has the correct combination of lenses, the movement of the light across the pupil causes no movement of the reflex, it merely turns on and off.

If the patient is hyperopic, the ray of light from the retinoscope, when going through the eye, would focus at a

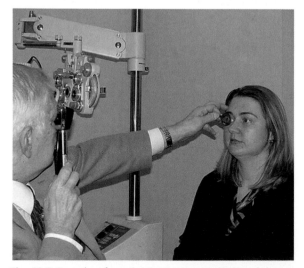

Fig. 10.6 Procedure for retinoscopic examination.

point behind the retina (if the retina does not block the rays of light). Lateral movement of the retinoscope across the pupil causes the area illuminated on the retina (pivoting about the focal point) to move in the same direction as the retinoscope, indicating that the eye is hyperopic or far-sighted. This shift is termed *with motion*. The refractionist then adds plus lenses to bring the focusing point up to the retina until the *on and off* light reflex appears without any apparent movement.

In summary, if a retinoscope beam produces *with motion* of the red reflex, the patient's eye is hyperopic or far-sighted and needs plus lenses to correct the condition. If the retinoscope beam produces *against motion*, the patient is myopic or near-sighted and needs minus lenses to correct the refractive error.

If the eye is astigmatic, it will exhibit two powers on axes at 90 degrees to one another. The retinoscope is then used to correct the power on one axis and then on the other. A cylindric prescription can be obtained in this manner with use of spheres alone, but generally cylinders are added, as well as the spheres, until the *on and off reflex* is observed on all axes.

All the aforementioned theory depends on the patient's relaxed accommodation (i.e., the patient's looking at some object 20 feet [6 m] away) and on parallel rays of light entering the eye and coming to a focus on the retina. The light source of the retinoscope, held about 18 inches (0.5 m) from the patient during retinoscopy, produces diverging, not parallel, rays of light from the retinoscope. Therefore a +2.00 diopter lens (in the refractor, known as the retinoscopy lens) is put in the trial frame so that the divergent rays from the retinoscope are in fact parallel when they enter the pupil. The power of this lens depends on the working distance of the refractionist; for example, if he or she works at 0.5 m (18 inches), this would be a +2.00 diopter lens.

Some refractionists prefer a working distance that requires a +1.50 diopter retinoscopy lens.

The final prescription, taken from the lenses in the trial frame or on the phoropter, is reduced by the working distance power to determine the distance prescription of the patient.

Streak retinoscope (see Fig. 10.7)

The same principles that apply to the spot retinoscope also apply to the streak retinoscope. In the streak retinoscope the light source is a straight-line filament of the bulb. There is a condensing lens between the mirror and the bulb so that the filament itself may be focused onto the patient's eye as a straight line. By means of a movable sleeve that envelops the whole retinoscope, the bulb may be rotated and moved up and down to adjust its focus. Because the light source is a streak of light rather than a cone, if the eye is not emmetropic, the area of the retina illuminated becomes a straight line rather than a spot. If astigmatism is present, it is very easy to determine its axis because the

streak, playing externally across the patient's face and trial frame with its axis graduation, will not be at the same angle as the streak seen on the retina. The retinoscope streak is rotated until it parallels the streak on the retina and the axis is thereby established (see Ch. 12 and Fig. 12.3).

From this point, the procedure is basically the same as with a spot retinoscope and lenses are added until the reflexes on both axes exhibit no with or against motion when the streak is passed across the pupil.

Accessories used in refraction

Cross cylinder

The cross cylinder consists of a plus and a minus cylinder set at right angles to each other, with a handle set midway between the two axes (Fig. 10.8). The axis of the plus cylinder is marked in white and the axis of the minus cylinder marked in red. Cross cylinders are available in dioptric strengths of 0.12, 0.25, 0.50, and 1.00.

The cross cylinder is a refining instrument that determines the exact axis of the astigmatic error and the exact power of the cylinder. The method of use is described in Chapter 12.

Pinhole disc

The pinhole disc is a small disc with a small central opening that eliminates peripheral rays of light, permitting only the central rays to pass through. The pinhole disc permits the examiner to differentiate poor vision caused by refractive errors from poor vision resulting from disease of the eye. In general, vision that can be improved with a pinhole disc usually can be improved by spectacle lenses.

A multiple pinhole disc serves the same purpose as the pinhole disc, but it is an easier device to use because the patient does not have to search for a solitary tiny central hole (Fig. 10.9). The patient is asked to view a small line of print with one eye occluded and with the pinhole disc placed before the other eye. If looking through the pinhole

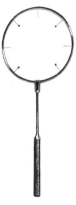

Fig. 10.8 Cross cylinder.

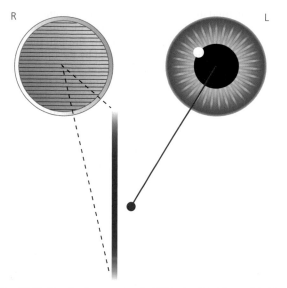

Fig. 10.15 Esophoria or esotropia. With the Maddox rod held horizontally before the right eye, the vertical red line appears on the right side of the point source of light.

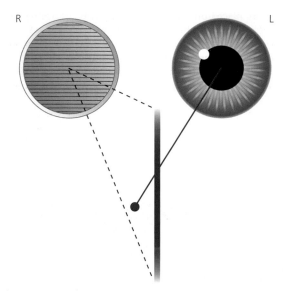

Fig. 10.16 Exophoria or extropia. With the Maddox rod held horizontally before the right eye, the vertical red line appears on the left side of the point source of light.

If the Maddox rod is rotated so that the rods are placed horizontally before the eye, the patient will perceive the red line in the vertical direction. If the Maddox rod is held before the right eye of the patient and the line appears on the right side of the light, then *esophoria* or *esotropia* is present (Fig. 10.15). If the line appears on the left side of the light, then *exophoria* or *exotropia* is said to exist (Fig. 10.16).

The Maddox rod may also be used to detect torsion *cyclophoria* and *cyclotropia*. Torsion is the result of those ocular muscular anomalies that cause the eyes to rotate in a clockwise or counterclockwise fashion. To detect torsion, a red Maddox lens is placed before one eye and a white Maddox lens before the other eye, with the rods of both lenses held in the same direction. If the patient sees that the red line and white line are not parallel, then torsion is present, as well as cyclophoria or cyclotropia.

A prism is needed to measure a phoria or a tropia with a Maddox rod. For example, if the patient has a right hypertropia and reports seeing the red line below the point source of light, base-down prisms are placed before the Maddox rod in increasing strengths until the patient states that the red line runs through the light. The amount of prism required to center the red line on the small light is then a measure of the vertical muscle imbalance in prism diopters.

Prisms

A prism is a triangular, or wedge-shaped, piece of plastic or glass that has the property of displacing a bundle of light toward the base of the prism (Fig. 10.17). If the prism is

placed before an eye, an object viewed in front of the prism will appear to be displaced toward its apex.

Prisms are used in measuring the presence and the amount of any tropias or phorias. The tests most commonly used to measure ocular muscle imbalance with prisms are the Krimsky test, the Maddox rod prism test (discussed previously), and the prism cover test.

In the *Krimsky test*, the observer notes the position of the corneal reflexes when a small light is shone into the eyes. The examiner notes where this reflex is centered in the fixating eye. Prisms are then placed before the deviating eye until the position of the reflex in the pupil of the deviating eye is located in the same position as that of the fixating eye. For example, if the patient's right eye is turned in, the light reflex may be found overlying the temporal margin of the pupil and base-out prisms would be required to displace this reflex to a more central position.

The basis of the *prism cover test* is to displace the image of the deviating eye by the use of prisms so that it falls on the macula of that eye. Thus each eye projects to the same point in space, and covering one eye does not require any movement of the other eye to take up fixation. The amount of prism diopters required to achieve this endpoint is a measure of the deviation (see Fig. 10.17). The mechanics of this test are discussed in Chapter 29.

Types of prisms available are the loose prism, horizontal and vertical prism bars, and Risley's rotary prism.

The *loose* or *individual prism* is made of plastic or glass. These prisms are supplied in low powers in standard trial

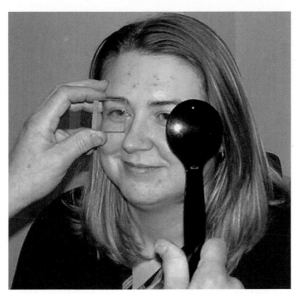

Fig. 10.17 Prism cover test. Handheld prisms are introduced to neutralize a deviation.

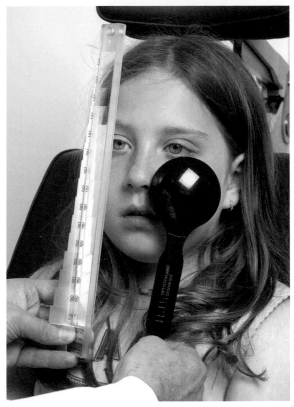

Fig. 10.19 Prism bars used to measure the amplitude or power of fusion.

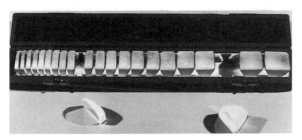

Fig. 10.18 Loose or individual prisms set.

lens sets and in a full range of powers in individual prism boxes (Fig. 10.18).

Horizontal and vertical prism bars (Fig. 10.19) are fused prisms amalgamated into a single bar of gradually increasing strengths. These prisms may be set in a horizontal direction (base in or out) or in a vertical direction (base up or down). The prism bar is principally used to measure the amplitude or power of fusion. It is sometimes used in the cover–uncover test for measuring strabismus in children because it permits rapid examination in a patient whose patience and attention may be limited.

Risley's rotary prism (Fig. 10.20) consists of two counter-rotating prisms mounted in rings, one in front of the other. These rings are easily rotated in opposite directions by a small thumbscrew. When the two bases are rotated so that they lie behind one another, their effective power is additive. When the apex of one prism is rotated so that it lies behind the base of the other, the effective power is zero. Thus Risley's rotating prism provides a rapid and simple increase in prism power strength so that a deviation may be rapidly adjusted and measured without the delay in introducing individual prisms before the eye.

Instruments used to determine power of lenses

Several instruments are available to assist the ophthalmologist and the ophthalmic assistant in accurately determining the strength of the lenses the patient has been wearing.

Lensmeter

The lensmeter (sometimes called *Lensometer* or *Vertometer*) is used to determine: (1) the dioptric vertex power of a lens, (2) the axis, (3) the optical center of a lens, and (4) the

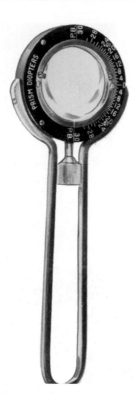

Fig. 10.20 Risley's rotary prism.

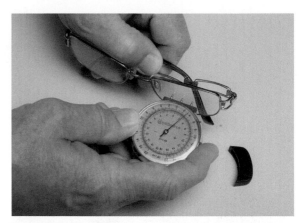

Fig. 10.21 Using a lens clock to measure the curvature of a lens surface to determine the dioptric power of the lens.

presence of a prism and the direction of its base. It consists of an illuminated target, a holder for the glasses to be measured, an adjustable eyepiece, and an optical system designed to focus on an image in the anterior focal plane of the lens to be measured.

To use the lensmeter, see the detailed instructions in Chapter 8.

Geneva lens measure

The Geneva lens measure measures the radius of curvature of the lens surface and records it in diopters. The instrument consists of a dial with a revolving hand and three pins projecting from the instrument. The approximate dioptric power of the lens can be determined by placing the surface of the lens against the pins and then rotating the lens by 90 degrees. If the reading on the scale remains constant, no cylinder is present on that side. The algebraic sum of the readings from the front and back surface of the lens represents the dioptric power of the lens (e.g., −2.00 sphere on one side and +6.00 sphere on the other side is equivalent to a +4.00-sphere lens). If the reading is not uniform over the entire surface of the lens, the difference between the lower and higher readings represents the amount of cylinder present. The disadvantage of the Geneva lens measure

is that the gauges are calibrated for crown glass only and are subject to considerable error in determining the axis of the cylinder. The gauge gives incorrect measurements for hard resin (plastic) lenses, for aspheric surfaces, and for invisible progressive bifocals.

The use of the Geneva lens measure is that occasionally when glasses are made the base curve may have changed considerably so that the patient may develop headaches and eyestrain. The gauge can help in identifying this cause (Fig. 10.21).

Instruments used to examine the interior of the eye

Ophthalmologists enjoy the unique privilege of being able to examine, by direct visualization, the interior of a vital organ. They can study the retina, which is a modification of nervous tissue, the head of the optic nerve (optic disc), and the state of the retinal blood vessels, which to a large degree mirror the state of other blood vessels of the body not visible to inspection. Because many systemic and neurologic diseases first manifest by alterations within the eye, the use of the ophthalmoscope and other such devices has assisted in bringing ophthalmologists into closer contact with their medical colleagues in related fields.

Direct ophthalmoscope

The ophthalmoscope was invented more than 100 years ago by Hermann von Helmholtz. Von Helmholtz's work was based on the observations of Ernest Brücke, a well-known Viennese physiologist, who 4 years earlier had reported noticing a red light in the pupil of a young man standing in the auditorium of the university as the chandelier light reflected from the student's eye in a direction corresponding to that of his own visual axis. With the popularization of the ophthalmoscope, a wealth of blinding diseases could be understood, and investigation of their cause and treatment began.

The ophthalmoscope consists fundamentally of a light source, a viewing device, and a reflecting device to channel light into the patient's eye. The reflecting device can be a mirror or a reflecting prism. If the patient and examiner are both emmetropic, then light from the patient's retina will be in focus for the examiner. If, however, either the patient or the examiner is hyperopic or myopic, the spherical lenses must be used to overcome their refractive error. Because the ophthalmoscope contains no cylindric lenses, astigmatic errors of refraction cannot be compensated for. Thus if a patient has a large amount of astigmatism, a crystal-clear view of the fundus cannot be obtained. The direct ophthalmoscope enables the examiner to use the power of the subject's eye as a magnifying system to see the retina. Although the field of vision is somewhat restricted compared with that seen with the indirect ophthalmoscope, the magnification is greater, being approximately ×15 for the former and ×5 for the latter (Fig. 10.22).

To facilitate pupillary dilation, ophthalmoscopy is best performed in a darkened room. For a better inspection of the fundus, however, the pupils should be dilated with a weak mydriatic agent, such as 2.5% phenylephrine. With heavily pigmented irides, a stronger mydriatic agent, such as 10% phenylephrine, should be used but with *caution*. Because there have been deaths recorded from the application of a single drop, 10% phenylephrine should *not* be routinely used. It should *never* be used with patients who have hypertension or cardiovascular disease. If it is imperative to dilate the pupils of these patients, then cyclopentolate (Cyclogyl) or tropicamide (Mydriacyl) should be used. Pupillary dilation with drops is usually performed in all new patients and in those with extremely small pupils.

The examiner stands directly in front of the patient and examines the patient's right eye with his or her own right eye and the left eye in similar fashion (Fig. 10.23). The first structure in the fundus noted, for purposes of orientation, is the optic disc. The disc is an oval structure and represents the site of entrance of the optic nerve (Fig. 10.24). It is usually pink and may have a central white depression, called the *physiologic cup*. The margins of the disc are sharp and distinct except for the margins of the upper and lower poles, which may be slightly fuzzy. From the disc, the retinal arterioles and veins emerge and bifurcate; they extend toward the four quadrants of the retina. The retinal vein, which is usually found lateral to the retinal artery, is larger and darker red.

Approximately two disc diameters away from the optic disc and slightly below its center is the *macula*. The macula

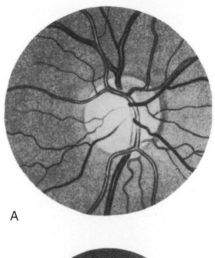

A

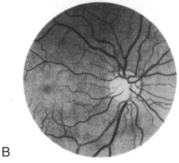

B

Fig. 10.22 (A) Fundus as viewed with the small aperture of the direct ophthalmoscope. Note the magnification obtained but the restrictions in the fields seen. (B) Fundus as viewed with the indirect ophthalmoscope. Note the larger field of view, reduced magnification, and inverted image.

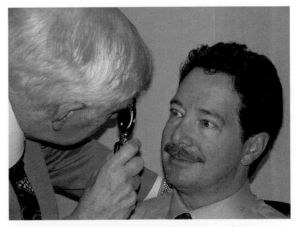

Fig. 10.23 Use of the direct ophthalmoscope to detect pathology in anterior segment and fundus of eye.

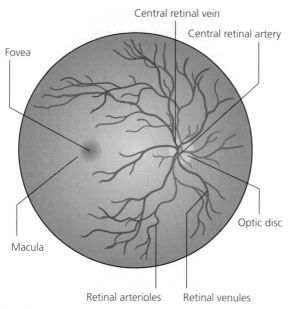

Fig. 10.24 Fundus of eye.

is a small avascular area that appears deeper red than the surrounding fundus. In heavily pigmented individuals, the macula may have a darker hue than the adjacent fundus. In the center of the macula is a glistening oval reflex called the *fovea*. In young people, a second reflex, which appears as a glimmering halo, may surround the entire macular region. Each quadrant of the fundus is examined in turn. To see as much of the peripheral retina as possible, the examiner should ask the patient to look in the direction of the quadrant under study. The color of the fundus is usually an even red hue, but it varies with the general pigmentation of the eye, as well as the individual's pigmentation.

Because the disc of the ophthalmoscope lens permits very close observation of an object, the ophthalmoscope usually examines the lens, the iris, the cornea, and the external eye.

Special devices on the ophthalmoscope

Red-free light

Although a true red-free state cannot be obtained with the yellow-green filters found in many ophthalmoscopes, the filters do serve a purpose. Viewing the fundus with a relatively red-free filter makes the retinal blood vessels appear black and retinal nerve fibers more prominent. The macula stands out against the greenish-gray background of the fundus as a golden-yellow oval patch. The use of red-free light

for examining the fundus is particularly valuable for detecting minute superficial hemorrhages, holes in the retina, and early degenerations of the macula.

Red light

Red filters diminish the contrast between the retinal blood vessels and the retina. However, melanin pigment, which absorbs red rays, contrasts strongly with the surrounding red fundus. Red light illumination is therefore of value in differentiating hemorrhage from pigmented tumors that contain melanin.

Polarized light

Incorporation of two polarizing filters into the optical system, which polarizes the light leaving the ophthalmoscope, minimizes irritating reflections from the patient's cornea. The only problem with the general use of polarized light is that the intensity of the illumination has to be greatly increased to compensate for the filtering effect of the two polarizing filters.

Slit illumination

In the construction of the ophthalmoscope, the insertion of a slit or a diaphragm in the course of the illuminating system simply reduces the illumination. For focal high-intensity illumination, better results are attained when the slit is directed from a slit-lamp microscope and the fundus is viewed with a contact or Hruby lens. The use of a slit lamp is valuable in estimating the level of various areas of the retina.

Aperture discs

Most ophthalmoscopes have two or more aperture discs of different sizes. The smaller apertures are particularly useful for viewing the fundus through a small pupil, such as that found in glaucoma patients under treatment.

Cobalt-blue filters

These are used for fluorescein studies of the fundus.

Many types of ophthalmoscopes are available. Electric-power ophthalmoscopes offer the advantage of illumination that is more controlled and of higher intensity.

Indirect ophthalmoscope

The indirect ophthalmoscope was invented by Dr. C.J.T. Rooter only 1 year after von Helmholtz's invention of the direct ophthalmoscope. The indirect ophthalmoscope permits the examiner to see more of the retina in one

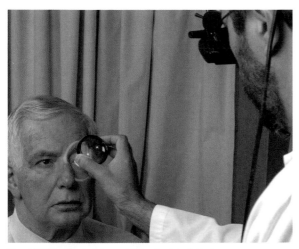

Fig. 10.25 Examination with indirect ophthalmoscope.

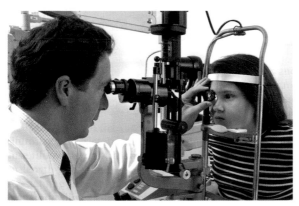

Fig. 10.26 Examination of the fundus with lens.

glance than the direct ophthalmoscope allows. Because of its construction, the instrument also accommodates a larger and brighter light source, which permits the examiner to penetrate moderate cataracts and to see retinal detail. Usually, however, the pupil must be dilated to use this device.

For indirect ophthalmoscopy, the patient's eyes must be fully dilated with a mydriatic agent. The examiner holds a convex lens in front of the patient's eye and through a viewing device attached to the headband of the indirect ophthalmoscope, the examiner sees a real, inverted image at the focal point of the handheld lens (Figs. 10.25 and 10.26). The size of this aerial image varies with the dioptric strength of the lens used. Most commonly used is a +20.00 diopter lens.

The fundus camera is simply an enclosed indirect ophthalmoscope with a camera back.

Relative merits of direct and indirect ophthalmoscopes

The *direct ophthalmoscope* permits a greater magnification (×15), is easier to use with small or undilated pupils, and is mechanically easier to use. The *indirect binocular ophthalmoscope* permits binocular vision and depth perception, permits a wider field of view of a given area, is easier to use in the operating room without contamination, permits indentation of the sclera and thus a better view of the periphery of the fundus, provides more intense illumination, and frees the hand for operative manipulation.

Transilluminator

Transillumination is used when the media are too cloudy to permit inspection of the fundus and the examiner suspects the presence of an intraocular tumor. The transilluminator (also called a muscle light or a Finhoff light) consists of a handle and a small, narrow tip that contains a heat-free or insulated high-intensity light source. The beam of the transilluminator is passed over accessible areas of the sclera and in normal cases, a bright red glow comes from the pupil if there are good transmissions from any point where the light is applied. If the light passes over the site of a solid tumor, the brilliance of the glow in the pupillary space will be diminished and an outline of the tumor revealed. The transilluminator is also useful for providing a bright source of illumination for the inspection of the external eye, the lids, and the iris reflex.

Instruments used to study the anterior segment of the eye

Slit-lamp microscope

Use of slit lamp

This instrument is used to illuminate and examine under magnification the anterior segment of the eye. The slit-lamp microscope enables the observer to view binocularly the conjunctiva, sclera, cornea, iris, anterior chamber, lens, and anterior portion of the vitreous, and it permits the detection of disease in these areas. The slit lamp is the heart of an ophthalmologic examination. The watch glass on a watch appears relatively clear when viewed from the front, yet when a penlight is directed obliquely at the edge of the watch glass, it brings out scratches and smears that are not easily seen in normal lighting. Similarly, the front surface of the eye and the interior of the eye can be seen more clearly when light is placed obliquely and there is backscattering of the light. Allvar Gullstrand of Stockholm, who won the

a manner similar to that for the applanation tonometer. No ophthalmoscope is required. The eye must be anesthetized because the pressure is applied to the cornea rather than to the sclera, as is done with the older types of instruments. After the eye is anesthetized, the slit beam is used to view the optic disc through the microscope while a contact lens exerts increasing pressure on the cornea. The graded pressure dial is turned until the first pulsation of the central retinal artery is obtained. This is the diastolic pressure. The observer then turns the dial until sufficient pressure is exerted to stop all blood flow. This is the systolic pressure. Readings are then taken and recorded. This method provides a greater degree of accuracy and repeatability than others. It is not possible, however, to obtain measurements on the recumbent patient.

Doppler test

The Doppler test has virtually replaced the ophthalmodynamometer as a test of carotid flow. The test measures the flow of the internal and external carotid arteries directly. It is less subject than the ophthalmodynamometer to instrumental and operator errors. If the internal carotid artery of the neck is narrowed by atheromatous plaques, then the flow pattern distal to the obstruction site will be reduced and irregular. The turbulence of flow may be so great that the sound may be audible with a stethoscope placed directly over the internal carotid artery. This sound is called a *bruit*. With transducers in the instrument, however, the precise measurement of flow can provide more accurate information regarding carotid artery patency. This test is used for people with central retinal artery occlusions, transient ischemic attacks, and cerebrovascular accidents.

Automatic refractors

Sophisticated automatic refractors that, in effect, perform retinoscopy and, in most cases, are designed to be operated by the ophthalmic assistant have come onto the market. These instruments do not produce a refraction from which a pair of glasses should be made. The present ones do no more than an automatic retinoscopic or objective refraction. It is essential that the results obtained with these machines be refined by a subjective refraction. In a busy office, however, they save a great deal of time. See Chapter 12 for a more detailed description of autorefractors.

Computerized corneal topography

There has been increased research and growing interest in the field of corneal topography, that is, measurement of the curvature of the anterior corneal surface. With the capabilities of modern computers and software technology, it has become feasible and practical to precisely analyze the radius of curvature (millimeters) and corresponding refractive power (diopters) at thousands of points across the corneal surface.

Computerized corneal topography is a logical advance from the basic principles of keratometry and photokeratoscopy developed during the 20th century. Photokeratoscopy provides the user with only qualitative information about the curvature of the cornea and changes that accompany surgery, contact lens wear, and progressive corneal abnormalities. The keratometer yields quantitative data, but only at four points. These points are located at approximately the 3-mm optic zone along two perpendicular meridians. One pair of points is aligned along the steepest axis of the corneal surface, with the second pair 90 degrees away. Each pair of points is averaged across its respective meridian to yield two *K* values, which approximate the cornea's central refractive power. The keratometer has fundamental limitations in that it is able only to measure points along the annulus of the 3-mm optic zone and it assumes orthogonal symmetry of the flat and steep axis of the cornea.

Topography provides a color-coded representation of the cornea's shape and monitors corneal curvature changes from the apex to the periphery.

See Chapter 41 for more details.

Corneal Tomography

Corneal tomography allows for three-dimensional analysis of the anterior segment, typically using Scheimpflug imaging. In addition, to anterior curvature imaging that is obtained with corneal topography units, the tomography units can evaluate elevation of the anterior and posterior corneal surface, and provide a corneal thickness map. These maps are critical for screening patients before laser vision correction, cataract surgery, and refractive lens exchange. The maps allow for making an early diagnosis of keratoconus, corneal ectasia, or other forms of irregular astigmatism. In addition, there are a wide variety of other clinical situations that tomography maps can be valuable, such as following patients after surgery that have had laser vision correction, corneal transplants, or other corneal conditions.

Visual field equipment, tangent screens, and perimeters

See Chapters 18 and 19 for a discussion of visual fields.

Diagnostic ultrasound: A-scan and B-scan

Ultrasound was first used in World War II; the sound waves were used to locate submarines under water. In a variety

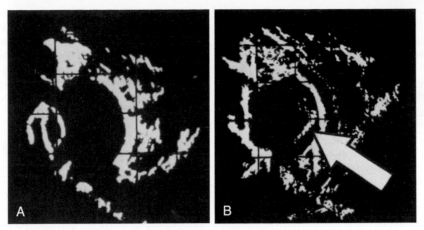

Fig. 10.41 B-echogram. (A) Normal. (B) Showing retinal detachment *(arrow).*

of ophthalmic disorders, diagnostic ultrasound provides information that cannot be obtained in any other way. This is especially true in eyes with opaque media that preclude ophthalmoscopic examination. Intraocular use is stressed because space does not permit a detailed description of the somewhat more difficult field of orbital diagnosis.

Two common types of ultrasound waves are used. The A-wave is a single-beam, linear wave that is directed in a probing manner to detect interference along its pathway. It travels like a beam of light in a straight direction. A B-scan consists of a series of these impulses sent out by a moving transducer that are amalgamated into a two-dimensional image. This not only minimizes possible missed areas but also gives a clearer picture of the underlying pathologic condition. The B-waves are used to detect tumors of the orbit or eye that cannot be identified by any other means. The sound waves, like light waves, pass through certain tissues and are reflected by others. When the sound wave meets firm tissue, such as is found in a tumor mass, the waves are reflected off its surface. The rebounding waves are received by a transducer, which turns the sound energy into electrical impulses that are amplified and displayed on an oscilloscope in a visible pattern called an *ultrasonogram* or *echogram* (Fig. 10.41). Homogeneous tissue, such as normal lens vitreous or aqueous humor, does not reflect ultrasound and produces no echoes. A cataractous lens produces intralenticular echoes. In some centers, ultrasound is used to aid the surgeon in locating a foreign body in the eye.

B-scan ultrasonography also has been effective in diagnosing many ocular tumors, especially choroidal malignant melanomas. Drs. K. Ossoinig and Fred Blodi reported a 95% accuracy using a standard B-scan echogram in a large series of choroidal malignant melanomas.

B-scans differ from A-scans in that they are more complex. An A-scan is a linear echo, and the reflection of this linear ultrasound can indicate the position of the cornea, the lens, and the retina. The B-scan is similar, but it extends above and below the horizontal to sweep the contents of the globe. Both A- and B-scanners are available from several manufacturers as portable devices.

C-scan techniques also are available and are used in diagnosing orbital disease. The C-scan uses a transducer to cover a small aperture. It images soft tissue within the span of a corollary plane that is recorded on polaroid positive–negative film. The corollary plane scans across the axis of the optic nerve. C-scan techniques are used primarily for optic nerve lesions, especially tumors.

A detailed discussion on diagnostic ultrasound can be found in Chapter 43.

Radioactive phosphorus

One test to detect whether an ocular or retroocular tumor is benign or malignant is determination of the radioactive uptake of the tissues. It is known that cancerous tissues proliferate rapidly. Certain highly malignant tumors (especially malignant melanomas) take up and retain certain radioactive elements, particularly radioactive phosphorus (^{32}P), to a greater extent than do normal tissues. In this test the ^{32}P is injected intravenously and the radioactivity is assessed on the surface of the eye by a Geiger counter 24 and 48 hours after the injection. The major difficulty in this test is that the counter has to be directly over the tumor. With tumors at the back of the eye it is difficult to place the tip of the counter accurately. In addition to this mechanical difficulty, some tumors simply do not give a high count. Other tumors, such as retinoblastoma, the most common eye tumor in children, rarely show any alteration in the radioactive uptake of ^{32}P.

A positive ^{32}P test result, then, is of value in providing corroboration for the presence of an actively growing malignant tumor; however, a negative result is of little value because it does not indicate the absence of a tumor.

Electroretinography and electrooculography

Electroretinography (ERG) responses are described as photopic (light adapted) or scotopic (dark adapted). Although the rods outnumber the cones 13 to 1 in the normal human retina, the cones account for 20% to 25% of the ERG response amplitude. The response of the dark-adapted eye to white light breaks down to an early corneal negative A-wave; a corneal positive B-wave; a slower, usually positive C-wave; and, in some mammals, a small D-wave. The resting potential of the normal retinal axis is measured by a silver disc electrode mounted in a scleral contact lens.

An electrical potential exists between the cornea and the retina of the human eye. This potential can be altered by changes in the intensity of light entering the eye, the wavelength of that light, and the state of adaptation of the eye, that is, whether it is light adapted or dark adapted. In some disease states the resting potential is altered and the ability of the electrical potential to be changed by these other factors is abnormal.

There are basically two types of retinal receptors: the rods that serve vision in dim light and the cones that mediate daylight vision and color vision. The electroretinogram reveals disease of either the rod population or the cone population, or both.

For this test, electrodes incorporated into a contact glass are placed directly onto the eye. Eye movements disrupt the values of the test, so the patient must be old enough to fixate on a target, which keeps the eyes still. Because they are unable to cooperate, very young children do not make good subjects for this test.

Total loss of electrical activity can be recorded in siderosis bulbi (caused by retained iron foreign bodies in the eye), in stages of retinitis pigmentosa, and in severe vitamin A deficiency. Selective degeneration of the rods, as manifested by night blindness, also can be detected by this method because the electrical reaction during dark adaptation is faulty. Selective involvement of the cone, as seen in congenital total color blindness, also is revealed by the inability of the eye to electrically respond during conditions of light adaptation.

Electrooculography (EOG) measures the standing potential between the electrically positive cornea and the electrically negative back of the eye. It indicates the activity of the retinal pigment epithelium (RPE) and photoreceptors cells. Diffuse or widespread RPE disease is required to significantly affect the EOG response. The EOG is always abnormal when the ERG is abnormal and therefore provides useful information only when the ERG is normal. One of the current diagnostic uses for the EOG is in Best's vitelliform macular dystrophy.

ERG and EOG are generally performed in university centers. Expert technical knowledge is required to perform these tests and to interpret their results.

Lasers

The laser (covered more completely in Ch. 35) is a device that amplifies light waves. The name itself is taken from the beginning letters of light amplification by stimulated emission of radiation. Intense beams of light have many practical implications, but in the eye, their virtue is that the laser beam may be directed through the pupil to the retinal structures for repairing retinal holes and tears and destroying blood vessels.

The ruby laser emits a beam that creates a heat reaction in the pigment epithelium of the retina, binding the epithelium of the retina to the underlying choroid; it also aids the sealing of retinal holes in a retinal detachment when the retina is adjacent to the choroid. The blue-green light of the argon laser is superior to the red light of the ruby laser in treating certain blood vessel diseases of the eye because it is absorbed by the red blood pigment, which resists the red light of the ruby laser. The argon treatment is a feature in diabetic retinopathy and other retinal conditions, such as Eales disease, in which vessels grow abnormally and bleed easily; sickle cell anemia, which produces sludging of blood in peripheral eye vessels; and several congenital vascular conditions that cause blindness.

It has been well established that argon or neodymium-yttrium aluminum garnet (YAG) laser treatment is a good alternative to the invasive surgery of a peripheral iridectomy in producing a hole in the iris. The former is painless and causes minimal inflammation, which is normally handled by application of steroid drops for about a week. It is most useful in treating angle-closure glaucoma or aphakic pupillary block glaucoma, or in opening an incomplete surgical iridectomy. The Abraham iridectomy lens, a modified Goldmann type of fundus lens, may be valuable in delivering a more intense laser beam to the iris. Blue eyes are more difficult to penetrate than brown eyes because of the lack of the heat-absorbing pigment in blue irides. Laser trabeculoplasty involves using the laser for shrinkage of the trabecular meshwork.

The excimer laser has been developed for two specific uses. First, it enhances vision so that combined myopia and astigmatism, or hyperopia and astigmatism, can be eliminated or refractive errors can be significantly reduced.

Second, it has significant use in removing corneal scars and corneal dystrophies, stopping recurrent corneal erosions and smoothing out corneal surfaces after surgery for conditions, such as pterygium. The current influence of the excimer laser on refractive errors is more thoroughly discussed in Chapter 36.

Summary

The ophthalmic assistant should become knowledgeable about the workings of each instrument in the office. It is important to keep the instruments clean and all lenses free of dust and grease by using a lint-free cloth. The ophthalmic assistant should be able to change bulbs in every instrument inasmuch as the use of the instrument depends on a functioning bulb and an intact power supply. An active inventory of the replacement bulbs in the office should be kept so that bulbs are always available. Another area of expertise that should be developed is calibration of the tonometers. In addition, the ophthalmic assistant should know the purposes of each piece of equipment and what information can be derived from its use. For a more comprehensive look at new imaging equipment (see Ocular imaging).

Questions for review and thought

1. What is the purpose of the red-green test on the projection equipment? Explain the test.
2. Discuss the power and range of the various types of lenses and auxiliary lenses on the lens tray that you have in the office.
3. How can you tell the power of a prism in the standard lens tray?
4. How can you differentiate a cylindrical lens from a spherical lens in the lens tray?
5. What is the purpose of the pinhole disc?
6. What is meant by a retinoscopy lens in a standard refractor? What is its power? Why?
7. What is the difference between phoria and tropia? What instrument is used in detecting these conditions and how?
8. Explain the principle of either the spot or the streak retinoscope.
9. What is meant by vertex distance? How is it measured in a trial frame? In a spectacle? In a refractor?
10. What are the prisms used for?
11. What is the prism cover test?
12. Discuss the relative merits of direct and indirect ophthalmoscopy.
13. What is the purpose of a goniolens?
14. Draw the endpoints of the two half circles from the applanation tonometer as seen when a true reading of the intraocular pressure is to be obtained.
15. What is the value of the ophthalmodynamometer? What does it measure?
16. How can you determine whether a lens is concave or convex without using instruments?
17. What is the exophthalmometer? Describe how either the Luedde or the Hertel exophthalmometer is used.
18. How is ultrasound of value in ophthalmology?
19. Outline the value of automated refractors in clinical ophthalmology.
20. Compare the advantages of automated refractors versus retinoscopy and subjective refraction.
21. Outline the disadvantages of automated refractors versus retinoscopy and conventional subjective refraction.
22. Discuss inherent errors that can occur in the use of an automated refractor.
23. What is instrument myopia?
24. What are the drawbacks to introducing an automated refractor in practice?

Self-evaluation questions   Q

True–false statements

Directions: Indicate whether the statement is true **(T)** or false **(F)**.
1. In the duochrome test, a near-sighted person sees the letters more clearly on the red panel. **T** or **F**
2. Trial frames and lenses are better than the phoropter in determining the refractive status of the aphakic person or a person with high plus or minus lenses. **T** or **F**
3. The Maddox rod is used to dissociate the eyes and prevent them from fusing. **T** or **F**

Self-evaluation questions—Continued Q

4. Manual objective refractors require significant operator skill and time. **T** or **F**
5. Automated objective refractors require significant operator skill and time. **T** or **F**
6. Some automated refractors provide for subjective refinement. **T** or **F**

Missing words

Directions: Write in the missing word(s) in the following sentences:

7. The radius of curvature of any lens can be measured simply by using a _____.
8. Phenylephrine is an excellent mydriatic for dilating pupils. The safest or most commonly used concentration of this drug is _____.
9. The optic disc is best examined with _____.
10. Objective refractors may be used to replace _____.
11. Automated objective refractors still require _____ testing.
12. When an assistant using an automated refractor requires the patient to provide responses to questions, this is considered a _____ refraction step.

Choice-completion questions

Directions: Select the one best answer in each case.

13. If the media are opaque, which of the following tests can be used to determine whether an intraocular tumor is present?
    a. Transillumination
    b. Ultrasound A- or B-scan
    c. ^{32}P
    d. All of the above
    e. None of the above
14. The Hruby lens is:
    a. a −55.00 diopter lens.
    b. a jeweler's loupe.
    c. a lens for detecting the intraocular pressure.
    d. a lens for viewing Schlemm's canal.
    e. none of the above.
15. The results of an automated refractor are least affected by:
    a. large pupils.
    b. cataract.
    c. small pupils.
    d. irregular astigmatism.
    e. corneal scarring.
16. To incorporate an automated refractor in a practice, one usually does not need to:
    a. designate a staff person to be responsible for testing.
    b. provide more housing space.
    c. increase the capital cost.
    d. have a maintenance service agreement.
    e. have a large-volume practice.
17. An accurate automated refraction result usually is found in:
    a. a patient with moderate cataract.
    b. improper alignment of the patient's eyes.
    c. high astigmatism (greater than 7.00 diopters).
    d. macular degeneration.
    e. irregular corneal surface.

Answers, notes, and explanations A

1. **True**. Green normally is focused in front of the retina because of its short wavelength. Therefore a near-sighted person whose entire image is focused in front of the retina would see letters on the red side of the chart more clearly. Red has a longer wavelength and is seen more clearly by the larger eye of the myopic person. The person whose near-sightedness has been overcorrected, however, will see the green letters more clearly. The duochrome test is useful in determining the type and end point of the refractive error.
2. **True**. It is useful that the correcting lenses and spectacle lens that the aphakic patient and all patients with high plus or minus lenses finally wears are similar with respect to the distance of the lens from the eye and its tilt. With four-drop lenses, trial aphakic spectacles are provided so that the margin of error is minimized. Even without minimal effective diameter (MED) lenses or four-drop lenses, trial frames are still the best way of arriving at the aphakic person's, or those with high-plus or high-minus lenses, final prescription inasmuch as the measurement for vertex distance is more reliable. The Halberg clip is an excellent method for determining the true spectacle correction.
3. **True**. This is done by changing the shape and color of the image of one eye. The rod converts a point of light to a linear rod by virtue of cylindric rods that run across it. The red line always runs perpendicular to the axes of the Maddox rod.

Answers, notes, and explanations—Continued | A

4. **True**. To operate manual objective refractions, a person needs skill and time for the alignment and adjustment steps.

5. **False**. Automated objective refractors require little skill by the ophthalmic medical assistant. Skill is required when the patient is not aligned properly or moves during the testing procedure.

6. **True**. Some automated refractors have a subjective component in which the assistant will question the patient as to changes in vision. The instrument can add or subtract both sphere and cylinder to refine the prescription. This is considered a subjective refinement.

7. **Geneva lens measure**. The disadvantage of this instrument is that the gauges are calibrated for crown glass only. Moreover, the axis of the cylinder is not precisely determined.

8. **2.5%**. Recently deaths have been reported with the use of 10% phenylephrine; this concentration should *not* be used for routine dilation. The weaker solution should be used routinely. Phenylephrine should *not* be given to patients with hypertension or active cardiovascular disease. When it is given, care should be taken to occlude the punctum so that minimal drainage into the nose and minimal systemic absorption occur.

9. **The direct ophthalmoscope**. The direct ophthalmoscope permits greater magnification so that the fine details of cupping of the disc are easily observed with this instrument. The indirect ophthalmoscope offers a wider field of vision, but it is not as good for examining disc detail, such as mild cupping, slight pallor, pits or holes, and the growth of delicate new blood vessels off its surface.

10. **Retinoscopy**. The automated refractors can give a beginning prescription for refinement on a subjective basis. This simulates retinoscopy and becomes a starting point for refraction.

11. **Subjective**. Subjective testing is most important after using an automated objective refractor. The refractor provides only the starting point; one must still obtain individual responses to the given refractive finding.

12. **Subjective**. The word *subjective* means that the patient, who is the subject, has input into the final results.

13. **d. All of the above**. Probably, the most widely used test for an intraocular mass when the media are too cloudy to permit direct examination is the B-scan ultrasound. It is precise, easy to perform, and painless. Permanent records can be obtained. The location and type of a retrolental mass often can be detected with this method.

14. **a. A −55.00 diopter lens**. The Hruby lens is a −5.00 diopter lens for viewing the fundus. It is not as good as a fundus contact lens, but it has the advantage that the retina can be examined without placing an instrument on the eye.

15. **a. Large pupils**. Large pupils do not affect the result of the automated refractor. In fact, the opposite is true. Small pupils may yield no information, often because of misalignment.

16. **e. Have a large-volume practice**. Automated refractors can be valuable in any type of practice, whether it is small volume or large volume. They can provide a reference point similar to retinoscopy. The cost effectiveness may have to be questioned if the practice is relatively small, however.

17. **d. Macular degeneration**. Macular degeneration is a dysfunction of the eye's cones. The actual refractive error is not altered, although the vision is markedly reduced centrally. Consequently, the automated refractor usually provides reliable results as far as the refractive finding is concerned.

Chapter | 11 |

Maintenance of ophthalmic equipment and instruments

The maintenance of ophthalmic equipment and instruments often becomes the responsibility of one person in the office. Someone may be more technically adept to take on this responsibility. Simplified instructions on care and maintenance are noted in the following text.

It is important that adequate supplies of replacement bulbs be maintained and that everyone be familiar with the different bulbs required for each of the available pieces of equipment. Lists of the required bulb for each piece of equipment should be made and posted. If batteries are required, a suitable battery supply should also be maintained. If the batteries are the rechargeable type, they should be charged fully the first time. They can be recharged to the same full capacity on each recharging, which should take place on a regular basis. Handles usually contain rechargeable batteries that require nightly recharging in a battery well. All equipment should be kept covered with dust covers supplied by the manufacturer.

Applanation tonometer

Calibration of the applanation tonometer is important, and it should be checked approximately every 2 months or sooner with regular use. Tonometers are always supplied with a calibration bar. The most common applanation tonometer is the Goldmann tonometer. Applanation tonometers may be checked for accuracy by the use of a central weight. For the Goldmann tonometer, a short rod of measured weight is attached to the balancing arm of the tonometer and the rod set at 0, 2, and 6. At each measure, the measuring drum should be placed at the corresponding stop. At each stop, the tonometer head should move only 0.05 to 0.1 g of these settings (Fig. 11.1).

To be specific, follow these guidelines:

1. To check at drum position zero (0), insert the measuring prism at measuring position − 0.05. The zero mark on the measuring drum is set one line width below the index. When the pressure arm, with prism in position, is gently pushed, it should move freely between the two stops and return toward the stop on the examiner's side (Fig. 11.2). At measuring position + 0.05, the zero mark on the measuring drum is set one line width above the index. As this procedure is followed, the pressure arm should move toward the patient's side.

2. Check at drum position 2. For this check the control weight is used. Five circles are engraved on the weight bar. The middle one corresponds to drum position zero, the two immediately to the left and right are position 2, and the outer ones are position 6. One of the marks on the weight corresponding to drum position 2 is set precisely on the index mark of the weight holder. Holder and weight are then fitted over the axis of the tonometer so that the longer part of the weight points toward the examiner (Fig. 11.3).

3. At drum positions 1.95 and 2.05 (graduation mark 2 on measuring drum set one line width below or above the index), the pressure arm should return from the area of free movement to the corresponding stop.

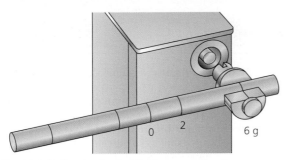

Fig. 11.1 Calibration bar for Goldmann applanation tonometer.

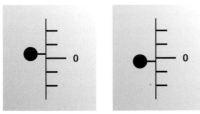

Fig. 11.2 Calibrating Goldmann applanation tonometer at position 2. The tonometer head should move only 0.05 to 0.1 g from zero.

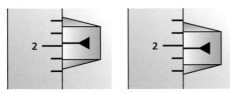

Fig. 11.3 Calibration with larger weight toward the examiner. Balance should show scale variation no greater than zero.

4. The check at drum position 2 is the most important and should be carried out frequently because the measurement of intraocular pressure in this range is of particular importance.
5. Check at drum position 6 in the same manner. The corresponding checking points are 5.9 and 6.1. The graduation mark 6 on the drum is offset by half an interval below or above the index.

The applanation tonometer consists of a plastic prism with a flat anterior surface and a diameter of 7 mm. This prism is brought into contact with a fluorescein-stained tear film of the cornea, which it displaces to the periphery of the contact zone until a surface of known and constant size of 3.06 mm is flattened. The inner border of the ring represents the line of demarcation between the cornea flattened by applanation and the cornea not flattened. The

measuring drum can regulate the tension to produce a force between 0 and 8 g.

Noncontact tonometer

Calibration of the noncontact tonometer is important. The use of the logic circuits in the instrument, which are necessary to measure and record intraocular pressure, enables the operator to check the calibration of the pneumatic-electronic network by the following procedure:

1. Turn the instrument to on (red dot).
2. Remove the objective cap and wait 30 seconds for warm-up.
3. Depress the trigger switch-display at 68.
4. Push the power switch knob and set it at D.
5. Depress the trigger switch-display at 47 + 1.

Triggering is repeated several times 8 to 10 seconds apart. The display must not change more than +1 count. There must be no source light indicator (SLI) light in any of the tests. During the check of calibration, the display number has no quantitative significance; its repeatability must be the concern. The number displayed is a specially selected equivalent to a critical check at approximately 20 mm Hg, with twice the resolution that is used in the actual intraocular pressure (IOP) measurement.

The noncontact tonometer is sturdily constructed and normally requires little care to keep it operationally perfect. Protecting the equipment against dust is important to maintain it in good working order. It is recommended that the supplied dust covers be used.

Bulb replacement

Target illuminator bulb

1. Always disconnect the instrument from its source of electrical power.
   Remove the instrument top by unscrewing two screws with a $\frac{3}{32}$ hex wrench.
   Free the bulb holder by loosening the set screw, marked B, with a $\frac{1}{16}$ hex wrench.
2. Pull out the bulb holder.
3. Remove the bulb by unscrewing the knurled retainer ring.
4. Replace the bulb with a no. 12419 bulb and wipe the bulb clean of fingerprints.
5. To adjust for maximum and even target illumination, view the red-dot target through the objective orifice and adjust the bulb holder on axis with the power on. Tighten the set screw.
6. Replace and secure the instrument cover to protect against dust.

Source light indicator

If replacement is ever necessary, it should be made only by a qualified service technician. An authorized American Optical distributor should be contacted.

Fixation lamp

To replace the fixation bulb, the center joint is separated by pulling apart. The screw base bulb (no. 11583) is exposed for replacement.

Chin rest

The chin rest is easily removed by twisting it 90 degrees, then pulling up. It is made of a durable material that can be sterilized (maximum 250°F [121°C]) or washed in soap and water or alcohol.

Paper chin rests also are available.

Headrest cushions

Headrest cushions are wiped clean with alcohol. They also may be replaced.

Eyepiece and objective

1. The exposed surfaces of the eyepiece and objective should be kept free of dust, fingerprints, and smudges. The lens surfaces should be dusted occasionally with a camelhair brush.
2. The alignment target, as viewed by the operator, may become blurred by accumulation of grease from eyelashes on the annular aperture of the objective. Clean the annulus with a dry cotton-tipped stick.
3. After prolonged service or use in a dusty or humid environment, the inside surface of the objective should be cleaned. Remove the objective by unscrewing it counterclockwise and dust the surface with a brush or, if necessary, wipe it clean with a dampened tissue paper before reassembly.

Lensmeter

The lensmeter requires little maintenance. The eyepiece should always be adjusted for each technician using this instrument. Operators should focus or adjust the eyepiece to their eye.

If the lensmeter has a prism compensator, which is located just under the eyepiece, the compensator should always be set on zero to ensure you obtain the correct reading. (For further details, see Ch. 8.)

Keratometer

We shall use the Bausch & Lomb keratometer as an example.
1. When not in use, or at least overnight, the keratometer should be kept covered with the dust cover supplied with the instrument. Dirt on the daylight-blue filter sometimes causes smudges in the mire imagery. The filter can be removed easily and cleaned by removing the two screws that hold the lamp housing to the body of the instrument.
2. When carbon deposits begin to form on the lamp bulb, the mire imagery will be diminished. If this occurs, a new bulb should be used in the instrument.
3. The lower part of the lamp housing is removed easily for the insertion of a new bulb. To replace the bulb, rotate the instrument by turning the set until the lamp housing is away from the central carriage. The base can be removed by loosening the two screws on the sides of the lamp housing. In replacing the base, one must take care to see that the base rests squarely on the shoulder of the housing; otherwise that part will not clear the carriage when it is rotated back into position.
4. There is also an attachment that can be used for checking keratometer measurements. This attachment comes complete with bracket and three test ball bearings with specific radii. To calibrate, use a spherical test ball of known radius of curvature inserted in a holder. When the correct radius of curvature of the test ball is obtained, the accuracy of the keratometer can be confirmed. If the keratometer is out of alignment, it should be repaired by a trained professional.

Slit-lamp biomicroscope

1. The slit lamp is an important instrument. All personnel who use it should make a habit of keeping it covered with a dust cover when it is not in use. When changing bulbs, be sure the instrument is unplugged. Also, always remember to wipe off all fingerprints on the bulb to extend its life.
2. If the slit lamp will not operate, replace bulbs even if they appear to be in good condition. If the slit lamp does not light when a new main bulb is installed, check contacts on the bulb cap and remove any dirt with a small file or knife. If the instrument still does not operate, check all electrical connections to make sure that all wires are plugged into the transformer and that the main power cord is plugged in. Also check for a faulty fuse in the transformer.

3. The Haag-Streit and copies are the only slit lamps with mirrors that require cleaning. Removal of the mirror is easiest when the microscope and illuminator are well separated and the latter is inclined by approximately 10 degrees or more. Grasp the narrow shank of the long mirror and pull upward. The small mirror, which has no shank, is more difficult to grasp; therefore the point of a pencil should be used to get the mirror started on its way out. The mirror should then be dusted and sprayed with a glass cleaner. Wipe clean with cotton balls or some other material that will not scratch the surface, using a downward stroke. Repeat until dry.

4. If the slit lamp becomes difficult to move with the joystick, clean the joystick pad with a cleaning solution. If slit-lamp movement still continues to be difficult, apply a thin coat of three-in-one oil or sewing machine oil to the pad.

Phoropter (Fig. 11.4)

All personnel should make it a habit to keep the phoropter protected with a dust cover when not in use. Alcohol should not be used on any part of the phoropter.

1. The semipermanent face shields furnished with the phoropter are made of white nylon. This material can be washed with soap and water, soaked in alcohol, or boiled in water.

2. All lenses should be kept clean and free of dust and fingerprints. Do not put a finger in the sight aperture to check lens placement. Fingerprints on the lenses make refraction difficult. Cleaning of dust on enclosed lenses can be done with an ear syringe. The back lenses are the retinoscopy lens, polarizing lens, red lens, and Maddox rod. These are the only lenses that may be cleaned by office personnel; a glass cleaner and cotton-tipped swabs are used. The phoropter should be sent to an authorized repair shop every 2 years for preventive maintenance and lens cleaning.

3. Because the cross cylinder and the rotary prism are not enclosed, it is advisable occasionally to wipe each one carefully with lens tissue to remove dust.

Green's refractor

The Green's refractor (see Ch. 10) should be protected with a dust cover when not in use. Alcohol should not be used on any part of the refractor.

1. Face shields, which can be purchased from a local supplier, should be replaced after each patient use.

2. The only lenses that can be cleaned in the office are the retinoscopy lens and the +0.12 diopter lens. These are

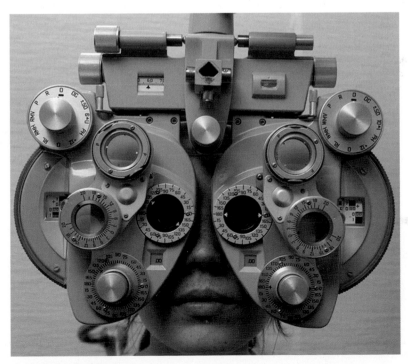

Fig. 11.4 American optical ultramatic phoropter.

located in the shutter disc and may be cleaned with a glass cleaner and cotton-tipped swabs. These two lenses become dirty because they are in the back of the refractor where patients' eyelashes may come into contact.

3. Because the cross cylinder and the rotary prism are not enclosed, it is advisable occasionally to wipe each one carefully with lens tissue to remove dust.

4. Do not put a finger in the sight aperture to check lens placement. Fingerprints on the lenses make refraction difficult.

5. Removing dust from the internal lens may be done by blowing with an ear syringe. It is not recommended, however, for self-cleaning of the internal lens.

6. The Green's refractor should be sent to an authorized repair department for preventive maintenance and lens cleaning every 2 years.

Projector

The vision screen projector requires little care. Occasionally, the glass slides and the lenses in the focusing tube should be wiped with a soft clean cloth. Best results are obtained if the cloth is dry because any moisture can cause streaks that will be projected onto the screen.

1. Do not remove lenses from the objective barrels. The refractor can be easily cleaned because the entire inner lamp house is removable.

2. When it is not in use, switch off the instrument to conserve the life of the lamp and prevent burning it out prematurely. It is desirable to keep several spare bulbs on hand to ensure always having a lamp of correct voltage and proper filament center.

Projection slide

Water or any other substance should not be sprayed on the slide. Wet substances can slip between the lenses and destroy the slide. Only the slide is cleaned by rubbing lightly with a camera lens tissue.

Cleaning the projector screen

The projector screen has a high reflectance characteristic. It is, however, susceptible to damage from abrasive scratches and fingerprints.

1. Periodic cleaning of the screen is advised. Simply use a mild detergent solution, wiping the screen surface gently with dampened absorbent cotton.

2. Fingerprints are normally removed by the recommended cleaning procedure. Scratches, however, cannot be removed and the screen does not lend itself to refinishing.

Replacing the lamp

Warning: Projector must be off for a few minutes before proceeding with lamp replacement!

To replace the lamp, push the small aluminum button on the side of the instrument. This releases the catch and allows the outer lamp house to swing back, exposing the inner lamp house. To remove the inner lamp house, pull the top back until the spring clips have disengaged, then lift out. The lamp is then entirely exposed and can be removed from the socket by a downward pressure, at the same time turning the lamp until it is free of the bayonet slide.

Caution: The lamp socket and reflector are factory-adjusted and should not be disassembled.

Projection front-surface mirrors

Front-surface mirrors have silvering on the first or front surface. They are cleaned by spraying a glass cleaner in small amounts on the mirror, stroking downward with a cotton ball (do not rub back and forth) and disposing of the cotton ball. The process is repeated until the mirror is dry.

Patient viewing mirror

The patient viewing mirror is cleaned like any other mirror (except the front-surface mirror). Most viewing mirrors are not front surface; they are plate glass with rear silvering. A front-surface mirror is identified by touching the mirror surface with an object, such as a pen or pencil. If the end of the object touches the reflection in the mirror, it is front surface.

Refractive errors and how to correct them

Almost all patients who enter an ophthalmologist's office require a determination of the refractive status of their eyes, for either diagnosis or treatment. Only by correcting the patient's refractive error can the ophthalmologist distinguish between visual loss caused by organic disease and that caused by a refractive error. Any visual loss not amenable to correction by lenses is regarded as a pathologic condition. Unexplained visual loss not corrected by glasses must always be investigated.

Many patients, regardless of their problem, be it fatigue with driving or headache, expect to receive a pair of glasses to remedy their complaints. Some patients are methodic about having their glasses changed every year or every 2 years; they believe that glasses, like tires, will wear out in time. Others think that glasses have a therapeutic effect on the eyes, maintaining them in good performance and preserving their integrity. Vision, especially in younger individuals and the presbyopic patient, may deteriorate with time, necessitating a change in correction but the health of the eye is not affected, for better or worse, regardless of changes made in the glasses. There is some evidence, however, that in the young, plus correction may prevent the normal loss of hyperopia and minus correction may exacerbate the development of myopia.

Glasses function to improve visual performance, to relieve the symptoms of refractive errors and muscular imbalance of the eyes, and to prevent suppression of one eye in children younger than 5 years, when the refractive difference between the two eyes is great. This chapter deals with the signs and symptoms of refractive errors and the therapy available for their treatment.

Emmetropia

The emmetropic eye is a normal eye in which all the rays of light from a distantly fixated object are imaged sharply on the retina without the necessity of any accommodative effort. This is a relatively uncommon condition (Fig. 12.1).

Ametropia

There are three basic abnormalities in the refractive state of the eye: hyperopia or hypermetropia, myopia, and astigmatism.

Hyperopia

The hyperopic or far-sighted eye is one that is deficient in refractive power so that rays of light from a distant object come to a focus at a point *behind* the retina with respect

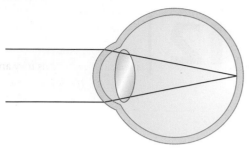

Fig. 12.1 Emmetropic eye. Parallel rays of light come to a focus on the retina.

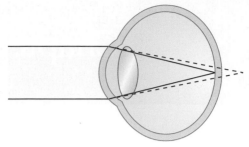

Fig. 12.3 Manifest hyperopia. Accommodation by the lens of the eye brings parallel rays of light to focus on the retina.

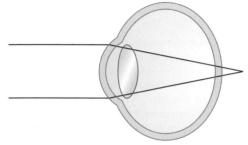

Fig. 12.2 Hyperopic eye. Parallel rays of light come to a focus behind the retina in the unaccommodative eye.

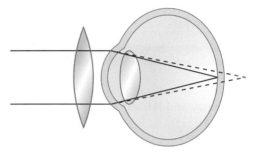

Fig. 12.4 Absolute hyperopia. A convex lens is required to bring rays of light to focus on the retina.

to the unaccommodated eye (Fig. 12.2). Consequently, the image that falls on the retina is blurred and can be brought into focus only by accommodation or by placing a plus, or convex, lens in front of the eye. The convex lens supplies the converging power that the eye is lacking.

Cause

In most cases of hyperopia, the chief cause is a shortening of the anteroposterior axis of the eye. Such an eye is smaller than the normal, or emmetropic, eye. At birth almost all human eyes are hyperopic or shorter than normal, to the extent of 2.00 or 3.00 diopters. With growth, the eye lengthens and approaches the normal length of an adult eye. Each millimeter of shortening of the eye is represented by 3.00 diopters of refractive change. This shortening of the globe results in *axial hyperopia*.

Another cause of hyperopia is found when the front surface of the eye (the cornea or lens) has less curvature than normal so that the image formed is focused at a point behind the normally placed retina. This is called *curvature hyperopia*.

From a practical standpoint, the cause of the hyperopia is not of great importance. What is significant is whether the accommodative system of the eye can supply an additional plus power to correct the hyperopic error. Young people are usually not handicapped by hyperopia because of their excellent range of accommodation.

Types

Hyperopia may be latent, manifest, or absolute. *Latent hyperopia* is the portion of the hyperopic error that is completely corrected by the eye's own accommodation. The compensation is so complete that any attempt to place a plus lens in front of such an eye will merely blur the vision. *Manifest hyperopia (facultative hyperopia)* is the element of the refractive error that can be corrected either by convex lenses or by the patient's own accommodation. In both latent and manifest hyperopia, *the patient has normal visual acuity* (Fig. 12.3). *Absolute hyperopia* is the portion of the refractive error that is not compensated for by accommodation (Fig. 12.4).

To understand the three types, consider the following case. A 32-year-old man is found to have a visual acuity of 20/50. A +1.00 lens is given, which improves his vision to 20/20. This means that the patient has 1.00 diopter of absolute hyperopia. It is found, however, that the patient can still see 20/20 if an additional 1.50 diopters are placed before the absolute correction. Thus the patient is found to have 1.50 diopters of manifest hyperopia. A cycloplegic examination is performed and it is found that the patient requires 3.50 diopters of plus lenses to enable him to see 20/20. Of the 3.50 diopters, 1.00 diopter we know has been accounted for in the form of *absolute hyperopia*, 1.50 diopters were present as *manifest hyperopia*, and 1.00 diopter remains in the form of *latent hyperopia*. Such a patient requires 1.00 diopter, will accept up to 2.50 diopters, but cannot be given the full hyperopic correction of 3.50 diopters.

Role of cycloplegia

Cycloplegic drops paralyze accommodation and thereby prevent the accommodative effort required to compensate for hyperopia. Therefore under cycloplegic examination all of the hyperopia is uncovered. Full correction of hyperopic errors, however, can never be based on cycloplegic findings because correction of the latent factor will only blur distance vision. The findings may be unreliable, however, in the management of accommodating esotropia. Cycloplegic examination indicates the magnitude of the refractive error. Noncycloplegic examination reveals the acceptability of a particular correction.

Symptoms

In the young, the condition may cause no symptoms, because a healthy youngster has an ample reserve of accommodation and, if hyperopic, accommodates for distant and near objects without being conscious of the act. Thus a 5-year-old may have 4.00 diopters of hyperopia and not require any spectacle correction whatsoever. It is usually in older adults that the symptoms of hyperopia become apparent, as educational demands and the time allotted for close work increase and accommodative reserves decrease (Fig. 12.5).

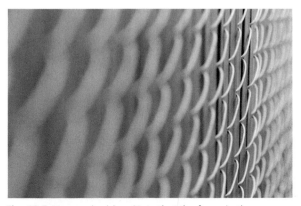

Fig. 12.5 Hyperopic vision. Note that the fence in the foreground is fuzzy, whereas the distance is clear.

The symptoms of eyestrain are many and varied. They include headaches, burning of the eyes, and a pulling sensation of the eyes. These symptoms are generally related to the constant excessive accommodation that is required for close work. In older patients, no symptoms may appear until the power of accommodation has diminished to the extent that the near point is beyond the range of comfortable reading distance, so that close work has to be held farther away than usual to be seen clearly. The greater the degree of hyperopia, the sooner this symptom arises; therefore presbyopia commences at an earlier age than usual in the uncorrected hyperopic eye.

Treatment

The treatment of hyperopia is based on the patient's symptoms, occupation, and ability to compensate for close work. In the very young, the treatment of hyperopia is usually unnecessary. The only exception to this rule occurs with *accommodative strabismus*. In this condition, part or all of the strabismus may be corrected by the use of convex lenses, which decrease the need for accommodation and thus for the associated excessive convergence.

In older adults, hyperopia is always corrected to improve near vision. Some believe the facultative component is never fully corrected unless the patient complains of fatigue and headaches. Whereas a 5-year-old may be oblivious to 4.00 to 5.00 diopters of hyperopia, a young college student may be very distressed by the presence of even 1.00 diopter of hyperopia. Such a patient needs to wear glasses only when the demands on accommodation are the greatest, that is, for performing close work. Some doctors, however, believe that the facultative component should be fully corrected.

In a middle-aged person, reading glasses become a necessity. The decline in accommodative power becomes so great that the patient is totally unable to see at a comfortable reading distance without convex lenses. Moreover, the power of the lenses exceeds the absolute and facultative demands of the hyperopia so that the patient can see comfortably with reading glasses for close work, but the vision is totally blurred when these lenses are used for distance vision.

Older adults, particularly those between 55 and 65 years, find it difficult to accommodate even 1.00 diopter. This type of hyperopic patient usually needs convex lenses for both distance vision and close work.

Myopia

Myopia, or near-sightedness, is that condition in which parallel rays of light come to focus at a point just in front of the retina with respect to the unaccommodated eye (Fig. 12.6). The myopic eye has basically too much plus power for its

c. Cataracts
d. Dirty soft contact lenses
e. Warped corneas from poorly fitting hard contact lenses
f. Lens subluxation
g. Postsurgical corneas.

Streak retinoscope

There are two main types of retinoscopes: the spot retinoscope and the streak retinoscope. The Copeland streak retinoscope has been the most popular. Other streak retinoscopes are the Nikon, the Welsh-Allyn, the Keeler, and the Reichert. The last three retinoscopes work by holding the bar on the handle down, whereas the Copeland and the Nikon work by holding the bar up.

Many ophthalmologists use the streak retinoscope (Fig. 12.13). The streak reflex illuminated in the pupil can be aligned easily with an astigmatic error. Moreover, it can be rotated to any desired meridian. With the streak retinoscope, the point of neutrality sometimes is evidenced by a cleavage in the streak (scissors reflex) so that half the streak moves in one direction and the other half moves in the opposite direction.

The light source for the streak retinoscope has a linear filament. From this source, a divergent collection of light rays strikes the person's pupil. The alignment of the rays from the linear filament is made possible by the adjustable sleeve on the instrument, which provides rotation of the bulb.

Streak retinoscopy is largely plus cylinder retinoscopy, that is, corrected with plus cylinders. A mirror in the instrument bends the path of light at right angles to the vertical orientation of the handle so that light can move across the space between examiner and patient. When the sleeve is up, a planomirror effect is created. The sleeve-down position produces a concave mirror effect. Thus with sleeve up, the most traditional position, diverging rays are emitted (planomirror effect), whereas in the sleeve-down position converging rays are formed (concave mirror effect).

A retinal reflex is found in the pupil when light from the retinoscope is shone into the patient's eye. The movement of this fundus reflex will yield information as to the presence of myopia, hyperopia, or astigmatism. The instrument must be moved to elicit the reflex in the pupil. The movement is perpendicular to the axis of the streak. When the streak is vertical, the movement of the instrument is sideways.

It is important to remember that the light in the patient's pupil is reflected from the retina so that a total picture of the refraction is obtained.

The working distance must be taken into account in retinoscopy. Most refractions use a 22-inch (66-cm) distance, which, translated into diopters, is an added plus

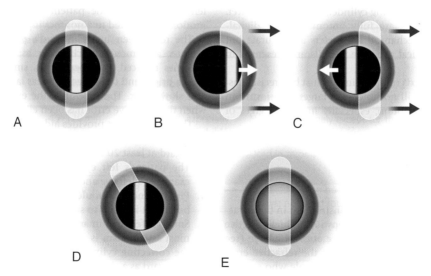

Fig. 12.13 Reflexes produced by the streak retinoscope. (A) Normal. (B) "With" movement. The reflex moves in the same direction as the retinoscope, indicating a hyperopic eye. (C) "Against" movement. The reflex moves in the direction opposite to that of the retinoscope, indicating a myopic eye. (D) Streak is not uniform in size, speed, or brightness over the entire aperture. The band is more prominent in one meridian, indicating astigmatism. (E) Neutralization point. There is no movement of the reflex and the pupil is filled with a red glow.

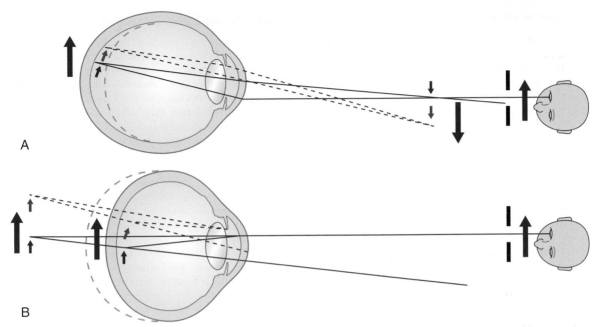

Fig. 12.14 Movement of images on retinoscopy. (A) Myopia: real upside-down image creating "against" motion. (B) Hyperopia: virtual upright image creating "with" motion.

lens of +1.50 diopters. If the person is emmetropic, with this lens no movement will be present in the light reflex of the patient's pupil. The neutralization point can be as much as 0.50 diopter of accuracy. If the patient is hyperopic or far-sighted, the reflex will become a "with" movement (the reflex moves in the same direction with the movement of the retinoscope). If the eye is myopic, there will be an "against" motion from the neutral state (Fig. 12.14).

With a far-sighted eye, plus lenses are added until neutralization occurs. The added plus spheres are then a measure of the total hyperopic refractive error. The same approach occurs with myopia, except that concave lenses are used.

Many practitioners prefer to use the "with" motion because it is easier to see compared with an "against" motion. This can be done by overcorrecting myopic eyes or by reversing the position of the sleeve.

Neutrality of the objective refraction can be determined by the following:
1. **The brightness of the reflex:** the closer one comes to neutralizing the refractive error, the brighter the reflex.
2. **The speed of the light movement:** when the light movement is dull and slow, it means the refractive error is still considerable.
3. **The size of the reflex:** the reflex fills the entire pupil when the neutrality is reached.

A large pupil makes it easier to recognize the motion of the reflex. For this reason, pupillary dilation is helpful in most cases.

With astigmatism, the speed, brilliance, and size of the reflex will be considerably different in one meridian compared with the other principal meridian. Each band of light is neutralized separately and the difference in diopters measures the degree of astigmatism. In all computations, one must reduce the value of the working lens by +1.50 or +2.00 diopters.

Autorefractors

Several refracting instruments have been introduced over the past few years. These include manual objective refractors, automatic infrared retinoscopes, and sophisticated subjective refractors that can modify the results to obtain the optimum visual acuity. Some are quick and easy to use; some take longer and require more operator skill. All of these automated refractors are designed to be managed by the ophthalmic assistant without the need for extensive knowledge of refractometry techniques. Some have subjective components that can refine the readings, some have the capability to assess the patient's vision, and others provide keratometer readings of the cornea.

Historical development

Automated refractors date back more than 100 years, but only recently have some of them become successful. There have been three major problems in obtaining the necessary accuracy. First, many automated refractors have used only small portions of the patient's pupil to make the measurement. Because of the optical irregularity present in many eyes, the refraction obtained through small portions of the pupil may not be valid for the entire pupil. Such optical irregularities are easily visible during retinoscopy, and the automated refractors have no better way to deal with these than does retinoscopic examination. Second, maintaining proper alignment of the automated refractor with the patient's eye was difficult with many of the early instruments. To lessen this problem, automatic tracking capability has been added to some of the newest automated refractors. Third, and most important, most automated refractors have been placed in box-shaped instruments that cause the awareness of near. Patients tend to accommodate when looking into these boxes, even though the visual targets within the boxes may be imaged optically at infinity. Accurate refraction is impossible in the presence of accommodation, and this so-called instrument myopia has been a continuing problem for automated refractors. Various fogging techniques or "free-space" techniques are used to try to overcome the problem of instrument myopia.

Objective refractors

These instruments focus on the ability to determine the corrected refraction that will give the optimum vision. The objective refractor requires minimal cooperation on the part of the patient except to hold still and look straight ahead. The subjective refractors, on the other hand, require responses from the patient, particularly in the final refinement step of the refractive measurement.

Manual objective refractors

In the 1930s several instruments known as *objective optometers* appeared in Europe. The operator focused or aligned a target pattern on the patient's retina to determine the refraction. These manual objective refractors are still used in many parts of the world in preference to retinoscopy. They are less expensive than the other automated refractors, but require more time and more operator skill. Patient cooperation is essential and instrument accommodation is common when cycloplegia is not used. The objective optometers use only small portions of the eye's optics for the measurement and alignment is critical, limiting the accuracy of the findings. One of these refractors, the Topcon, uses infrared light for the alignment and measurement process so that the patient is not dazzled by the bright white-light target pattern used in other models.

Automatic objective refractors

Automatic objective refractors first became available in the 1970s, using infrared light to refract the eye automatically either by retinoscopy or by similar principles. The first instruments in this group were the Safir Ophthalmetron, the 6600 Auto-Refractor, and the Dioptron, now all discontinued. The infrared light refractors give good results in healthy eyes with medium to large pupils, but accuracy decreases in the presence of immature cataracts, corneal haze, or pupils less than 3 mm in diameter.

Operation of autorefractors is extremely simple and the measurement time is rapid, requiring only 1 second or less for most of the instruments. The refractive results obtained, however, must be regarded as only preliminary. Accuracy is good enough to identify "no change" refractions and to monitor postoperative refractions until stable, but the results are not reliable enough to serve as the basis for prescribing glasses or contact lenses. Refinement by subjective techniques is recommended before prescribing.

Combination objective/subjective refractors

Subjective capabilities have been added to several automatic objective refractors. For example, visual acuity can be measured through these instruments both before and after the refraction. Also sphere, cylinder, and axis can be adjusted manually according to the patient's responses to various targets presented. Cross-cylinder testing is incorporated into most of these instruments, with successive views of the two cross-cylinder choices. The objective portion of the refraction with these instruments is the same as with the other automatic objective refractors.

The subjective capabilities of each of the combination refractors may be used, if desired, for refinement of the refraction. Considerable operator skill and knowledge of refracting techniques are necessary for optimal subjective refinement with these instruments and there is still the problem of instrument myopia in patients up to the age of 40 years (Figs. 12.15 and 12.16).

Automated subjective refractors

Two automated refractors with purely subjective capabilities were on the market for about 10 years. The first to appear was the Humphrey Vision Analyzer in the mid-1970s. The Vision Analyzer used a novel optical system to refract the eyes in "free space," using a concave mirror 10 feet (3 m) from the patient. Even the method of refraction was novel, using smeared-out astigmatic line targets in two independent meridians 45 degrees apart to

Because hyperopic patients often accommodated to the plane of the mirror of the Vision Analyzer, overrefraction capabilities were added, creating the Humphrey Overrefraction System. The eyes were refracted while the patient wore glasses, and the results were trigonometrically added to the power of the glasses.

Remote-controlled refractors

Several refractors or phoropters have been motorized in recent years and equipped with remote-controlled keyboards. These are designed to be operated by the skilled refractionist because the techniques of refraction are not automated and still require full knowledge of refractive procedures. These remote-controlled refractors are expensive. Their major advantages are to impress the patient and to ease the practitioner's back strain. Retinoscopy can be performed in the usual manner through these instruments, and accuracy is comparable to that obtained with conventional manual refractors.

Accuracy of measurement

The automatic objective refractors still create problems of irregular refraction in the patient's eye, maintenance of alignment of the instrument with the eye, and instrument myopia. Although accuracy is within 0.25 diopter of the subjective refinement in more than 80% of cases, it is not always obvious which measurements are incorrect, necessitating subjective refinement of most refractions. With a visual acuity check built into some of the objective instruments, valid information can be obtained at least to identify "no change" refractions and to monitor the stability of the refraction after surgery.

The automated subjective refractors were highly accurate but required more operator skill. They also were not free from the problem of instrument myopia, and repeat measurement under cycloplegia was sometimes necessary in younger patients. The patients had to be 8 or 9 years old to respond reliably to the subjective refractors, whereas with the objective instruments, refraction sometimes can be effected in patients as young as 3 or 4 years.

To date, neither a purely objective nor a purely subjective instrument has fully replaced conventional refracting techniques; that is, it is precisely the combination of an objective starting point and subjective refinement that yields the most reliable results throughout the widest range of patients. It is not surprising that automated refractors are evolving into combination objective and subjective instruments, but the subjective portion still requires knowledge of refracting techniques and at least a moderate amount of experience for optimal results. It is likely that more sophisticated methods for subjective refinement will be developed within the next few years, decreasing operator dependence of the present instruments.

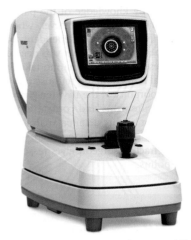

Fig. 12.15 Zeiss VISUREF 100 Auto Refractor and Keratometer. (Courtesy Zeiss, UK, www.zeiss.co.uk.)

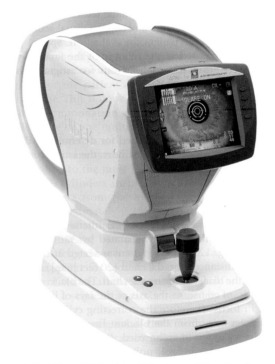

Fig. 12.16 Nidek ARK-1 s Auto Refractor and Keratometer. (Courtesy Marco Ophthalmic, Jacksonville, FL, www.marco.com.)

arrive at the final cylinder and axis. The Vision Analyzer required an entire room, however, and was somewhat complicated to administer. It provided both binocular and near testing capabilities, unique among the automated refractors.

197

one eye and to determine the clarity of the charts with the two positions of the cross cylinder. Additional cylinder or axis shift can be altered until the ultimate endpoint is reached when both lines are equally distinct.

It is immaterial whether one uses a cross cylinder or an astigmatic dial chart for the correction of astigmatism. The results are equally valid with both techniques. The efficiency by which one obtains a good refraction depends more on the skill of the refractionist than on the technique used.

Irregular astigmatism

In irregular astigmatism, the refraction in different meridians is irregular. Usually when irregular astigmatism is found, there is an associated pathologic condition of the cornea. Two of the most common causes of irregular astigmatism are corneal scarring from any cause and the developmental condition called *keratoconus*.

The diagnosis of irregular corneal astigmatism is best facilitated by using Placido's disc. This is a large, flat disc painted with concentric black and white circles (see Fig. 10.37). It is held in front of the eye, and the reflexes are observed through a hole in the center of the disc. The distortion of the circles on the cornea is usually readily visible.

The treatment of irregular astigmatism by conventional cylinders is virtually impossible. The best method of treating either corneal scarring or keratoconus is usually with a contact lens. If the treatment of irregular astigmatism by contact lenses is unsuccessful, often a corneal transplant becomes necessary.

Spherical equivalent

Occasionally in refraction, especially if the patient is an adult who has never worn glasses and requires a large astigmatic correction, the refractionist uses the spherical equivalent. Essentially, the cylinder is reduced, and half of that reduction is added algebraically to the sphere. For example, assume that the patient's correction is a +3.00 sphere combined with a +6.00 diopter cylinder, axis 180. Let us say in this instance that the refractionist decides that this cylindric correction would be too great for the patient to accept at once, and the decision is to reduce the cylinder by 1.50 diopters. Then the refractionist would add +0.75, or half the reduction, to the sphere. The resulting prescription would then read +3.75 sphere combined with +4.50 cylinder at axis 180. If one wishes only to determine the spherical equivalent expressed as spherical, the following examples apply: $-2.00 + 1.00$ at axis $180 = -1.50$ sphere and $+2.00 + 1.00$ at axis $180 = +2.50$ sphere.

Duochrome tests

Duochrome tests are based on the fact that light of longer wavelengths (red) is refracted by optical systems less than light of shorter wavelengths (blue or green). In the *red–green duochrome test*, the projector screen is illuminated through a filter that is red on one side and green on the other. Another form of duochrome test requires the patient to look at a point source of light through a cobalt-blue glass filter. This type of glass is peculiar in that it transmits light in two "bands" of wavelengths that are widely separated: one in the red and the other in the blue.

On one hand, if the red–green test is used and the patient has insufficiently corrected myopia, then the letters on the red side will stand out blacker, clearer, and sharper. They require more minus for the green to be as distinct as the red. On the other hand, if the same myopia is overcorrected and made artificially hyperopic, then the letters against the green background appear blacker, clearer, and sharper. The sphere is adjusted until letters on both sides are of equal quality. In the latter case, they require plus levels for the red to be equally distinct. Similarly, with use of the *cobalt-blue test*, the person with undercorrected myopia perceives a blue circle with a red center, whereas the person with overcorrected myopia perceives a red circle with a blue center. The red–green test is more commonly used than the cobalt-blue test.

Duochrome tests are useful only in refining spherical power, contributing nothing to the determination of cylinder power or axis. Therefore the most appropriate use of a duochrome test is as an endpoint determination in refraction.

Anisometropia

Anisometropia is a condition in which there is a difference in the refractive error of the two eyes. If the difference in the refractive error of the two eyes is slight, binocular vision is easily attained. Each 0.25 diopter difference between the refraction of the two eyes causes 0.5% difference in size between the two retinal images, and a difference of 5% is probably the limit that can be tolerated. Moreover, inasmuch as accommodation is a bilateral act in that it occurs equally in both eyes, there is no internal adjustment that one eye can make to compensate for this difference in refractive error. Because of difference in image size, fusion of images of unequal size becomes impossible. Normally, a 1.50-diopter difference in the refractive errors between the two eyes is quite easily managed with the retention of binocular vision. In large errors, in which the difference amounts to 1.50 to 3.00 diopters, fusion can take place for large and gross objects. With greater differences, some adjustment in binocular vision occurs. For example, the child may learn to alternate his or her vision, that is, to use one eye for distance and one eye for near. This is especially apt to occur when one eye is far-sighted and the other near-sighted.

If the refractive error is negligible in one eye and great in the other eye, the individual tends to suppress the image in the eye with greater refractive error. This is especially true if the eye involved has a large astigmatic error, so that vision for both distance and near is foggy. The constant habit of suppression leads to loss of vision or *amblyopia from disuse*. This condition is preventable because useful vision can be retained if the error in the defective eye is corrected early enough in life, and the use of the eye is encouraged at the time by suitable patching or other exercises.

Aniseikonia

Another problem caused by unequal refractive errors is the development of *aniseikonia*. In this condition, the differences in the size of the retinal image affect the patient's spatial judgments. This is not a common complaint and it is most readily found in people who use spatial judgments at all times in their daily work. People such as carpenters, interior designers, engineers, and artists are most prone to speak of disorders in spatial perception. These patients complain of visual discomfort, fatigue, headaches, distortion of objects, slanting of tables, dipping of surfaces, and so forth. Diagnosis of this condition is made with the patient's history and simple screening tests; for example, the patient reports a rectangular card as trapezoidal. Measurement of aniseikonia can be performed with a special instrument called a *space eikonometer*.

Treatment

When anisometropia occurs in children, especially those younger than 12 years, every attempt should be made to induce them to wear the full correction. For adults, especially when the difference is only between 2.00 and 4.00 diopters, the full correction again should be given, and they should be encouraged to bear with this correction despite symptoms. Often after 3 to 4 weeks of wear, the symptoms of eyestrain disappear and adults become comfortable with their lenses. In older patients, the visual discomfort often becomes intolerable, so that it is frequently advisable to undercorrect the eye with the higher refractive error.

Anisometropia and aniseikonia are treated more successfully today with contact lenses, particularly in the young child who has not yet developed amblyopia. Prisms correct the secondary muscular imbalance; iseikonic glasses are also used to treat this problem.

Aphakia

Aphakia is a condition in which the crystalline lens is absent from the eye. This may be caused by removal of a cataractous lens, or by displacement of the lens from the pupillary space by trauma.

Today implant surgery is performed in most countries, but there are still a dwindling number of patients who have cataract surgery in earlier years without benefit of an implant.

Correction of aphakia is perhaps the most difficult task for the refractionist. The intraocular lens (IOL) today represents the most suitable form of visual rehabilitation after cataract surgery. When indicated, a contact lens may be used. With a contact lens, the magnification is only 7%, compared with 33% for an aphakic spectacle lens. The visual adjustments and distortions with a contact lens are considerably reduced compared with those with spectacles. However, the tendency is toward implants in all new cataract procedures. This is called *pseudophakia*. Fortunately, *accommodating IOLs* permit the aphake to read.

Perhaps one of the most disturbing aspects of aphakic vision is the *jack-in-the-box phenomenon*. In this situation, the aphakic person finds an object through the edge of the spectacles and looks toward it, only to see that it is gone. *Aphakic vision, even though it results in 20/20 vision, requires a complete visual reorientation*. Spatial relationships, distances, and spatial judgments are all altered with this new type of vision.

An aphakic eye can never work together with a normal eye. This is because an aphakic eye essentially is a very far-sighted eye and the anisometropia induced is too great to overcome. Unless one uses a contact lens on the operated eye, it will not coordinate with the unoperated eye.

1. The optical centers must be exact because even a slight error causes a prismatic displacement with a thicker aspheric correction.
2. The distance of the trial lens from the eye and the eventual spectacle glass also must correspond. The distance of the eye from the trial lens (vertex distance) can be measured with a distometer. If this notation is put down on the prescription card, the opticians can make the suitable adjustment in power.
3. The periphery of the lens must be ground off. This type of lens is referred to as a *lenticular aphakac lens*. The lenticular aphakac lens serves to reduce the weight of the glass and abolish the extreme aberrations occurring from the periphery of a normal aphakic spectacle. Newer forms of aspheric spectacles are less curved in the periphery with use of an aspheric front surface instead of a lenticular design.

4. The frames must fit comfortably on the nose and be set straight. Fortunately, the era of aphakia is over because every cataract removal operation is replaced by an intraocular lens.

When to refract after cataract surgery

Historically, it was taught that at least 6 weeks were required after a cataract operation before aphakic lenses could be prescribed. The final prescription was then given when, after a recheck 1 week later, the prescription was still the same. With small-incision cataract surgery, the time has been compressed considerably. Some surgeons use the keratometer as a guide and perform refraction when the *K* readings are stable between two visits.

There has been a marked change in cataract surgery. The phacoemulsification and femtosecond laser method has become accepted and is in widespread use. This method requires only a 1- to 3-mm incision. These patients are mobile almost as soon as the procedure is finished and they can undergo refraction early. Almost all patients today receive lens implants, and the refraction must be performed over the implant. Often glare of the implant can be a problem to the retinoscopist. The surgeon must make the decision as to the timing of a preliminary refraction.

Refractive points specific to the aphakic and pseudophakic person

The aphakic (no lens implant) and pseudophakic person may not have a healthy eye, and the vision may not be refined to 20/20 or 6/6. The eye may have suffered surgical trauma, such as cystoid edema of the macula, or may have macular degeneration. Cataract patients are generally older adults and may have degenerative ocular manifestations, such as glaucoma or optic atrophy. A multiple pinhole may be used to start refraction to assess the potential of the eye.

The use of retinoscopy may be awkward in many ways. The patient who has no accommodation and has hazy vision cannot fixate accurately. The eye may move because of lack of fixation or lack of attention and concentration. If the patient does not hold the eyes steady, erratic and confusing scissor movements of the retinoscopy reflex may occur. Also the axis and the amount of astigmatism will be difficult to gauge.

We have found keratometry an important reference starting point in pseudophakia, particularly when the retinoscopy shadows are poor.

In pseudophakia, with an intraocular lens, the problems are different. The pupil after an implant procedure may be small, and the retinoscopy shadows are more difficult to assess. If the pupil is small, frequently the surgeon will authorize the use of a mydriatic agent for the refraction. An ophthalmic assistant should not even consider dilating the eyes of a patient with an iris-supported intraocular lens without instructions from the surgeon. Fortunately, these lenses are uncommon today. Dilation in older iris-supported implants may be a pivotal step in dislocating the lens. In pseudophakia, retinoscopic examination in the direct visual axis frequently causes disturbing reflections from the intraocular lens surface. These annoying reflections can be avoided by moving side to side until a good reflex is obtained.

Procedure after cataract surgery

After cataract surgery, keratometric reading, which provides the starting point for refraction, can be obtained. Often the glare induced by the intraocular lens implant makes retinoscopic examination difficult. Once the keratometric readings are stable between visits, the final refraction can be considered. The autorefractor, used with dilated pupils, may also provide a good starting point for refraction.

Cataract lens

Aphakic lenses for the person who has had cataract surgery without benefit of an intraocular lens are fast disappearing. Up until the early 1970s, almost all patients underwent this procedure and required cataract glasses. Many cases today have been reversed by *secondary implants* or the benefits of contact lenses, thus eliminating the problems induced by aphakic glasses. Despite these advances, some individuals are still wearing these cataract glasses.

The bull's-eye lenticular lens, a bulbous lens mounted on a plano carrier, has given way to the more cosmetically acceptable, highly aspheric lenses. These lenses are lighter and can be dispensed in a fashion frame. The optical effect is outstanding. The field of clear vision is enlarged and the pincushion distortions are reduced to a minimum.

These lenses commonly have up to a 4.00-diopter drop in power at the periphery of the lens. This aspheric effect creates a marked improvement in the patient's cosmetic and functional rehabilitation.

The patient still has a 30% magnification of image size, but other features of lens scotoma, jack-in-the-box phenomenon, distortion, and field limitation, which are present in regular aphakic lenses, are greatly reduced with the highly aspheric lenses. These lenses are also lighter and more comfortable, with less of a tendency to slide down the nose.

Presbyopic intraocular lenses of various designs are rapidly being developed by several companies, and their success rate in offering the presbyopic patient ability to read at distance and near is becoming predictable.

Presbyopia

Everyone becomes presbyopic with age. The accommodative ability decreases because of loss of the strength of the ciliary muscle and hardening of the lens. However, not everyone who is 45 years or older needs reading glasses. Myopic patients do not because they can simply take off their glasses to read. Those who are near-sighted in one eye may not be aware of this anomaly and may carry on happily without a reading aid indefinitely. Also the needs of people differ. An architect will require reading glasses long before a waiter will. Some people do not read or sew and have little use for a reading assist at any time. Thus the correction of presbyopia is not just optical. The needs of the individual must be kept in mind. What does the person do? What lighting is available? The brighter it is, the better. How much reading is done and at what distance? Does the person need to look up and down to see distance and near for occupational reasons? Are the person's symptoms genuine, or is stress or anxiety making reading difficult?

Symptoms

The primary feature of presbyopia is an inability to do close work. Initially, it manifests as difficulty in seeing the telephone book ("the print is grayer now") or a problem in seeing the menu in dimly lit restaurants. Presbyopic individuals cannot see small print or see without good illumination. They may increase lighting to see clearly. Light adds contrast and constricts the pupil to a pinhole aperture. Some people complain that they have to hold the print farther away, so eventually they are reading with an uncomfortable reach, complaining that their arms have become too short. Other symptoms include fatigue with reading, grittiness of the eyes with prolonged close work, and trouble with threading a needle.

Treatment

Two types of spectacle lenses are available for the treatment of presbyopia: the reading glass and the bifocal (regular, trifocal, or graded). Psychologically, most new presbyopes are much more receptive to the idea of reading glasses. They are referred to as *working glasses, sewing glasses, library glasses*, in other words, by any term that denotes their use rather than the patient's advancing age. Bifocals conjure up a picture of one's grandmother and represent the first step toward declining vigor and old age.

If the patient's distance vision is adequate, reading glasses are usually prescribed first. The patient is, however, warned that the glasses will help only to read at near. They will blur things if they are used for distance work.

The patient also is told that with time the reading glasses now prescribed will no longer suffice as accommodation declines. Many patients think that with time the glasses seem to get stronger, rather than thinking that an intrinsic disorder of the eye is becoming more pronounced. Even if the patient requires glasses for distance, it is often best to give the patient a separate pair of reading glasses for close work. Most patients have several friends or relatives who have had difficult times in adjusting to bifocals, and the patients will relate these stories with great relish. For this reason, and for psychologic considerations, the patient is best left to cope with trying to use two pairs of glasses. Once patients have become sufficiently harried trying to use two pairs they will return, asking for bifocals and will adjust to them quite comfortably. The optician can be of great service in helping patients choose the proper bifocal. For individuals who are conscious of their appearance, no-line bifocals are available *(progressive no-line lenses)*.

Some presbyopes complain that their glasses are too strong. When bifocals are prescribed, the near point of accommodation is measured in each eye with the patient's distance spectacles in place. It is customary to give the weakest possible lens that will enable the patient to see at a comfortable working or reading distance. The stronger the lens given for a bifocal addition, the shorter will be the patient's range of focus. This loss of range can be quite disabling for the executive who must see the corner of the desk or for the typist who has to look away at approximately 30 inches (75 cm) to see the typing. Therefore when lenses are prescribed, it always is advisable to leave some accommodation in reserve. In fact, the rule in prescribing near corrections is to give that correction which will leave half the amplitude of accommodation in reserve.

When strong bifocal additions are required, such as +2.00 to +2.50 or sometimes +3.00, the range of focus is compromised by necessity. For those patients whose occupations demand an intermediate zone—that is, an ability to read at 1 meter—trifocals are used, the trifocal being one-half the strength of the bifocal. Trifocals should not be prescribed with abandon, because to most patients trifocals mean 3 times as much trouble as "regular" glasses. An individual with a +2.50 correction can see clearly only objects located at about 16 inches (40 cm) away. Anything farther than this distance is fuzzy. Progressive or no-line lenses are another option.

Tests for the correct power

The simplest way to test for the correct power is to allow patients to hold a reading chart at their own preferred reading distance and prescribe the lens that gives the needed clarity. A reading add of less than +1.00 diopter does not offer real assistance, and anything greater than +3.00 diopters makes the focal point too close and the reading distance too narrow to work in.

Why not give all patients a +2.50 add when they are 45 years of age and let them grow into that prescription at 65 years of age? This would be a good idea in cost terms, but a doctor could lose his or her entire practice. The stronger the lens, the greater the weight factor, the aberrations, and the distortions and the closer the work distance.

Visual age considerations are as follows:

- At ages 42 to 45 years: a +1.00 to +1.25 is appropriate.
- At ages 45 to 50 years: a +1.50 to +1.75 is a common strength.
- At ages 50 to 65 years: a +2.00 to +2.50 or even +3.00 is common.

The strength of the add varies with the refractive error, being greater with hyperopic people and the presence of pathologic conditions. Cataracts or macular degeneration may demand the higher magnification gained by closer reading distance, and the strength of the add varies with the individual's needs.

Each eye should be tested individually and a record made as 20/20 or J1 and so on. The reading chart is a simple ready test and is desirable because the patient selects the reading distance. A variable light source helps simulate the patient's own illumination at work or home.

Another method is to test the amplitude of accommodation. This is merely the closest focal point at a given print size. For example, if a person's vision begins to blur at 25 cm, the amplitude of accommodation is 4.00 diopters. The patient is given a lens that leaves half the amplitude of accommodation in reserve. If the patient has to work at 33 cm and requires 3.00 diopters of accommodation, then only a +1.00 diopter add is needed. One-half the amplitude of accommodation is 2.00 diopters. To summarize, the need of accommodation is 3.00; thus the added plus strength of the reading aid is +1.00.

The dynamic cross-cylinder test is also useful. A +0.50 cyl/ −0.50 cyl is the one most commonly used. A grid made up of horizontal and vertical lines is the test target. The patient wears the distance correction. If the astigmatism has been properly corrected, the grid lines should be equally clear. The cross cylinder, with minus axis vertical, is added. Plus spheres are added, increasing the power until the vertical lines are clearer. At the same time, spherical power is reduced until the lines are again equally clear. The add is the difference between the total spherical power for near and distance correction.

This test has application for patients in whom the amplitude of accommodation is difficult to measure. It is not a preferred method, however.

Prescription

Patients should be given what they need. A man who works in a factory and walks around with safety glasses requires bifocals. He cannot walk with reading glasses. The same may be said for the musician who must look at the music and see the conductor. This person cannot see in the distance with reading glasses.

Reading glasses should be given in the following circumstances:

1. As a first lens when applicable
2. Whenever one is in doubt about which lens to prescribe
3. For people who spend most of the day reading, writing, or working at a fixed distance

Bifocals should be considered for the following patients:

1. One who requires distance and near vision within moments, for example, a teacher
2. One who already wears distance glasses; two pairs of glasses, one for distance and one for near, are too cumbersome for efficiency
3. One who is disgruntled with reading glasses (no other options are available in a spectacle design and the choice is limited to bifocals or readers)

Do's and don'ts

1. Do not prescribe bifocals for a −1.50 diopter myope. The simplest and cheapest device may be to take off the glasses, which is similar to opening a window; it is always much clearer to look through an open window.
2. Bear in mind that plastic and glass lenses absorb some light transmission.
3. Do not overcorrect the patient's vision. The greatest source of aggravation is with lenses that are too strong.
4. Never prescribe trifocals as an initial lens. A trifocal is used for intermediate range and is half the strength of the bifocal. Usually the bifocal must be a +2.00 diopter in power before a trifocal is valid. The trifocal is +1.00 diopter. This is too complicated and heavy a prescription for a first-time user.
5. Do warn patients of the difficulties and limitations of seamless or no-line bifocals. The no-line or invisible bifocal, often called progressive bifocal, although popular for cosmetic reasons, may induce marked astigmatism when the eyes wander to the sides of the bifocal segment. Some invisible or no-line bifocal lenses have larger clear fields than others, but all contain some limitation of clear, undistorted field in the reading portion. Newer adaptations of these lenses, which go under the trade names of Varilux III (Comfort), Multilux, and Omnifocal, have addressed this problem and have improved the quality of vision, but the fault remains. These lenses are expensive and promise a great deal. Optically, they remove image jump and sharp transitions of focal power. Patients should be informed. This problem is covered in more detail in Chapter 13.
6. Do not change the prescription of a bifocal until the fit has been appraised. The top of the segment on flat-top segment bifocals (used to minimize image jump

in looking from near to far) should be at the level of the lower lid. If the segment is too high, it will cut into the distance segment. If the segment is too low, it will add plus power to the prescription and the patient will in effect have a stronger spectacle. The fit of a bifocal affects the power, the field of vision, the image size, and the distortion factor. Always look at what the patient is wearing before reordering lenses, especially if the complaint regards a new set of spectacles. The flat-top bifocal is conspicuous. If the patient has strong feelings about the symbolic act of moving into bifocals, then respect this attitude. Some people's jobs depend on looking "young"—for example, entertainers, salespeople, and media people—and these individuals frequently prefer a no-line or progressive bifocal.

7. Always check the reading segment monocularly. Sometimes a difference in the prescription between the two eyes indicates a fault in the distance correction. Most people have equal accommodative reserve, and the bifocal addition should usually be the same. If unequal adds are required, an error in distance correction or some pathologic condition should be suspected.

8. Do not prescribe a bifocal if patients can read with their distance glasses. If patients can read through the distance segment, they often never get used to the bifocal segment. It is an intrusion in the field. Besides, they do not need a reading addition.

9. Look at the reading pattern when deciding between bifocals or reading glasses. Bifocals work well for people who drop their eyes to read, because bifocals do not upset any ingrained visual habits. But for those who lower their heads and always look through the center of the lenses, reading glasses should be considered.

Myths to be dispelled

The following myths need to be dispelled:

Myth 1. *Reading glasses ruin powers of accommodation and contribute to the aging of the eye*. In reality, new bifocal wearers quickly become dependent on and enjoy the reading additions. Further loss of accommodation would have occurred anyway.

Myth 2. *Bifocal wearers, in the main, have a difficult time adjusting to bifocals*. In reality, the vast majority (a clinical guestimate is more than 90%) have no difficulty in adapting to bifocals.

Myth 3. *Bifocals are a hazard when a person walks down stairs*. In reality, myopic persons with vision of this power, without glasses, have no difficulty in descending stairs.

Myth 4. *Bifocals should be worn for racquet sports to see the ball close in*. In reality, they should not be worn. Only distance spectacles are needed. Bifocals are not only

unnecessary, but they are a hazard to the game itself and create blind spots.

Myth 5. *Presbyopia is a disease and the eyes become weaker with age*. In reality, presbyopia is a normal change in the refractive error associated with the aging process. It is not a disease. The crystalline lens of the eye loses its ability to accommodate because of changes in the lens fibers. Presbyopic individuals see 20/20 for distance and near and merely require different lenses to accommodate their needs. Presbyopic eyes are healthy.

Complaints: how to anticipate them

Most frames are designed by fashion people in Paris, Italy, or New York and are not particularly practical from an ophthalmic point of view. In the merchandising of lenses, style has become paramount and function downgraded.

A few key points will provide assistance to the patient and prevent much grief at a later date.

1. Jumbo frames are a very poor idea for someone with a large refractive error. People who have worn small frames before and want to move into a high-fashion style should not be encouraged. Large lenses induce large aberrations and increase the weight of the lenses. People will complain of ocular vertigo and blurred vision because of the sliding effect every time they look down.

2. Impact-resistant lenses should always be ordered. In many states and countries this is law, but an ever-present element of neglect or indifference exists and somehow the cheaper lenses occasionally find their way into the market. A lens should be a protection, not a liability. Safety standards for every country are not the same.

3. Bifocals less than +1.25 diopters should not be prescribed. The disadvantages of a new bifocal do not warrant a new device with minimal advantages. Also people tend to like high magnification when being tested and resent the same prescription in their ordinary lives. The ophthalmologist should not overplus a bifocal. When in doubt the rule is, do not change the glasses.

4. Tints should not be prescribed in lenses for indoor use. A tinted lens reduces contrast and makes reading more difficult. A tint, even though slight, makes driving in dim illumination hazardous. Besides, tints can distort colors. A blue tint can make the person more myopic. When driving at night, it enhances the normal night myopia.

5. When a high prescription has been given, it is important to check that the base curve has not been changed. A change of base curve or a change in the tilt of the lens may induce unwanted aberrations.

6. Glasses for older adults should not be changed unless significant visual gains can be made, at least two lines. Frequently, vision of older adults is undercorrected because of slight hardening or sclerosis of the lens of the eye. These patients often like being a little undercorrected for distance and overcorrected at near.

7. Plastic tends to be softer than glass and scratches more easily. This disadvantage is compensated by the lightness. Plastic lenses also do not shatter, a fact of importance when dealing with a high myope who has lenses that are very thin at the center. Plastic frequently results in a thick lens and may not be desirable as a social lens. This consideration can be dealt with by making the lens one-third thinner with flint glasses, which have a higher index of refraction. These lenses should not be used for children or adults working in industry because they are more brittle.

Glasses checks and how to handle them: 12 key points

When a complaint is received from a patient who is unhappy with new glasses, public relations skills are important. Someone may have made a mistake, so it is best to check the total prescription. Arrogance, dismissal, and clichés like "You will get used to your prescription" will drive the patient to obtain a second opinion and jeopardize the doctor's reputation with that family. The following 12 key points should be checked:

1. Poor centration. It is possible that the lenses are not centered properly. The optical centers of the lenses should be checked and aligned with the eyes.

2. Large frames. The frames may be too large compared with the patient's old glasses. If so, the patient will experience new distortions, particularly from the periphery of the lens. It may be necessary to go back to the old size of frames.

3. Incorrect prescription. The lenses should be checked on the lensmeter. They may not be correct. Not only can the doctor make a mistake, but the optician and laboratory are also capable of the same sin.

4. Vertex problem. The distance the present lenses are set from the eyes should be compared with that of the old spectacles. If the vertex distance is not the same as the old lenses, or has not been corrected in the prescription with refractive errors greater than 4.00 diopters, then the power will be wrong.

5. Frame problems. Do the frames slide up and down the nose with head movement in reading? Parallax may be a factor here.

6. Unwanted prism. Because of faulty centration, prisms may be introduced that cause induced phorias, either

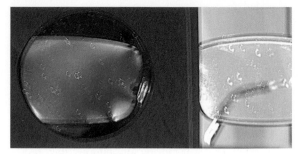

Fig. 12.18 The quality of the spectacle lens viewed against a bright background with Polaroid filters can show crimping in frames, producing distortion in glasses that may cause eyestrain or asthenopia.

vertical or horizontal. This is more common in strong reading glasses.

7. Base curve. Have the new lenses been made up on the same base curve as the old ones? A change may cause difficulty. A Geneva measure may be useful.

8. Stress lines. Are there stress lines in the lenses? Have the lenses been crimped into the frames? Crimping occurs when lenses are inserted in frames under pressure. It downgrades the quality of vision. Perceived through the lenses, crimping can be detected by viewing with a double Polaroid filter (Wilson polarizer) and viewing through the spectacles. If lenses have been crimped in the frames, it will produce distortions in vision (Fig. 12.18).

9. Thick lenses. Are the lenses thicker than they need to be for the power involved, resulting in excessive glass to look through centrally?

10. Tilt. Are the lenses tilted adequately for reading or is the patient reading obliquely through the lenses?

11. Correction of nondominant eye. Has the nondominant eye been corrected so that it has far better vision than the dominant eye? This may result in some difficulties. Check for eye dominance.

12. Segment line of bifocal. Is the lens set too high or too low and interfering with some of the visual pathways, particularly during walking or working? Are the segment heights symmetric?

The prescription should be reviewed. The doctor should rerefract and check the sphere cylinder and axis. An axis change of 10 degrees from previous glasses may not be tolerated even if correct. In higher-cylinder corrections, an axis change of more than 5 degrees may not be tolerated.

If the prescription is wrong, the patient should be told. It is better to admit to an honest mistake and ask the lens company to replace rather than continue a subterfuge.

Cycloplegic drops should not be used for recheck. The prescription may be different with a smaller pupil. Also the smaller the pupil, the greater the depth of focus, a factor that must be taken into consideration.

Summary

Refraction is an art that requires patience, practice, and contact with many people before excellence is attained. Glasses must fill a particular need, and in the final analysis it is the need and not the refractive error that is paramount. The acme of visual efficiency—20/20 or 20/15 vision—is totally unnecessary in a 5-year-old child but may be vital to a young college student. Experience teaches us how to handle the presbyopic mechanic who must lie on his back and look directly at the undersurface of an automobile; the 65-year-old receptionist-typist who must be able to see across the room, type at 26 inches (66 cm), and read at 16 inches (40 cm); and the elderly, illiterate person who comes in for a check-up and neither reads, sews, nor does any close work whatsoever. In addition to knowledge of optics and the method of refraction, the refractionist must be congenial and a little talkative, at least enough to be able to assess the patient in terms of profession or work, hobbies, and special interests.

Acknowledgment

The authors thank David L. Guyton, MD, for his contribution to this section.

Questions for review and thought

1. Illustrate the convergence of parallel rays in an emmetropic eye, a myopic eye, and a hyperopic eye.
2. With full cycloplegia, one measures 3.00 diopters of hyperopia. Will the patient accept this amount in a pair of glasses? Explain.
3. Why does a young person not require as much hyperopic correction as an older person?
4. What is meant by axial myopia?
5. What are some of the causes that have been suggested for myopia? Which are possible?
6. When does myopia usually stop changing?
7. What is with-the-rule astigmatism?
8. Where is the axis of a minus cylinder in with-the-rule astigmatism? Of a plus cylinder?
9. What is irregular astigmatism? How is it treated?
10. Outline the value of automated refractors in clinical ophthalmology.
11. Outline the disadvantages of automated refractors versus retinoscopy and conventional subjective refraction.
12. Explain how the cross cylinder is used.
13. What is Placido's disc? What is its purpose?
14. Outline some of the problems inherent in the correction of aphakia by spectacles.
15. In a strong plus or minus prescription, of what importance is the distance of the spectacles from the eye? Explain.
16. What is the cause of presbyopia?
17. Discuss the shadows seen on retinoscopic examination of a myope.
18. What is the most common problem in the correction of presbyopia?
19. What is the purpose of a cycloplegic refraction?
20. What is a manifest refraction?
21. What is the greatest difference between the refractive errors of two eyes that are compatible with good fusion?
22. What is meant by eyestrain?
23. Outline methods of dealing with a patient who complains of an inability to wear prescribed glasses.

Self-evaluation questions   Q

True–false statements

Directions: Indicate whether the statement is true **(T)** or false **(F)**.
1. The duochrome test is based on the fact that green is refracted behind the retina. **T** or **F**
2. Myopia is largely a hereditary disorder. **T** or **F**
3. Fogging involves discouraging accommodation by blurring the patient's eyes with plus spheres. **T** or **F**

Missing words

Directions: Write in the missing word in the following sentences:
4. Retinoscopy and the correction of astigmatism are best done with a _____ cylinder.
5. Retinoscopy can yield information on an irregular cornea because of _____ reflexes in the pupil.
6. Vertex distance measurements can be avoided by _____.

Self-evaluation questions—Continued

Q

7. Automated objective refractors still require _____ testing.

Choice-completion questions

Directions: Select the one best answer in each case.

8. Aphakic spectacles cause which of the following problems?
   a. Magnification by 10%
   b. Barrel distortion
   c. Jack-in-the-box scotoma
   d. Variable vision
   e. Induced astigmatism
9. Presbyopia should first be corrected by:
   a. reading glasses to prevent it from getting worse.
   b. taking off the glasses if the patient is myopic.
   c. vitamin A.
   d. bifocals if the patient does not need a distance correction.
   e. a decrease in illumination.
10. The results of an automated refractor are least affected by:
   a. large pupils.
   b. cataract.
   c. small pupils.
   d. irregular astigmatism.
   e. corneal scarring.

Answers, notes, and explanations

A

1. **False**. Green is refracted by the optical system of the eye so that a person with normal vision will have green focus in front of the retina and red focus behind the retina. A person who finds the letter on the green side more clearly in focus than that on the red requires plus correction.
2. **True**. Myopia is largely a hereditary disorder, but this is still debatable. Other causes have not been conclusively proved. Other claims of the causes of myopia that are without scientific validity are the following:
   a. Poor illumination
   b. Reading too much, with the eyes too close to the page or without the proper reading posture
   c. Dietary problems, particularly insufficient vitamins
   d. Glasses that have been fully corrected instead of being undercorrected
   e. Wearing glasses (i.e., proper correction) too early in life
   f. A disease that makes the eyes "weak"
   g. A lack of proper eye exercises
3. **True**. It is vitally important in the refraction of the eyes of children or young adults to control accommodation so that this element can be eliminated from the tabulation of a proper prescription. With children, short-acting cycloplegic drops are used. With many adults and in some practices, cycloplegic drops are not routinely used because of practical problems, such as a patient with fully dilated pupils trying to drive an automobile on a bright day. Instead of "dropping" the eyes, fogging may be used to eliminate the accommodative component of the refraction. The pupils are not artificially dilated and a visual hazard is not created. The patient can drive home in safety or return to work or school. In addition, no deleterious side effects occur with fogging. It is a natural way to eliminate or reduce accommodation.
4. **Plus**. Plus cylinders are desirable because a "with" movement is easier to view in the pupil than an "against" movement. Because of this optical effect, the chance of making an error of retinoscopy is least when the reflex is neutralized from the plus side.
5. **Distorted or irregular**. The reflexes in the pupillary aperture should be regular and even. A distorted reflex means the corneal surface is irregular. This could be a result of surgery to the anterior segment, early keratoconus, "warping" of the corneal surface by an ill-fitting contact lens, or inflammation, such as an old herpes scar. Whatever the cause, a proper refraction cannot be performed because there is no valid method of treating irregular astigmatism with regular lenses.
6. **Overrefraction**. There are two ways of handling vertex problems. One method is to make the calculation with a distometer and make the adjustment from distometer tables. A more accurate method is to overrefract over the patient's present spectacles and use the resultant power in a new prescription for the same frame.
7. **Subjective**. Subjective testing is most important after using an automated objective refractor. The refractor provides only the starting point; one must still obtain individual **responses** to the given refractive finding.
8. **c. Jack-in-the-box scotoma**. Aphakic spectacles do cause an increase in magnification of the image size, but it is 30%, not 10%. They also cause distortion but the

Answers, notes, and explanations—Continued

effect of this **distortion** is a pincushion type, with the sides sloping inward. Variable vision does not really occur with proper lenses. However, many aphakic patients receive a poor fit and the lenses may slide down the nose with reading. This slide is strictly caused by the weight of the lens. The newer, lighter lenses control this variability caused by the slide of the frames. Chromatic aberration is a feature of many lenses, not just aphakic ones. Chromatic aberration is the breakup of white light into a spectrum of colors. The jack-in-the-box scotoma does occur with aphakic spectacles, and objects appear to dart suddenly into the peripheral field of the person wearing aphakic spectacles.

9. **b. Taking off the glasses if the patient is myopic**. Presbyopia should be corrected by the simplest device possible. A person who must work and walk around requires bifocals. A presbyope who is in industry requires safety glasses; thus there is no other option but bifocals.

If the patient is near-sighted, an easy solution is to have that person remove the glasses. It is fast and inexpensive and the optical effect is the best if the vision is between -1.00 and -2.50 diopters.

Reading glasses do not make presbyopia better or worse. One practical way to postpone presbyopia is simply to direct more light onto the page. An increase in illumination adds contrast, which is an excellent way to obtain greater clarity. It also makes the pupil smaller, thereby producing more of a pinhole effect.

10. **a. Large pupils**. Large pupils do not affect the result of the automated refractor. In fact, the opposite is true. Small pupils may yield no information, often because of misalignment.

Chapter | 13 |

Facts about glasses

Melvin I. Freeman and Shoshana (Sue) M. Levine*

Virtually every patient who enters an ophthalmologist's or other eye care practitioner's office receives a refraction and most receive a prescription for spectacles. Even if patients plan to use contact lenses as their main corrective device, they should have glasses for backup. Thus the ophthalmic assistant needs some information about the construction and types of spectacle frames and the types of lenses currently used.

Despite an accurate prescription, many patients are unhappy with their glasses because of the design, fit, or prescription. The goal of correcting a refractive error is not only to achieve the best possible vision for each eye, but also to do so with a pair of glasses that match the patient's aesthetics and lifestyle as well. Glasses that make the wearer feel good and look good are more likely to be worn regularly. The purpose of this chapter is to provide a brief résumé of the types of eyeglasses available to the patient, reviewing the advantages and disadvantages of each.

History

The use of spectacles has its origin in ancient history (Fig. 13.1). In the early periods, optical glass was of poor

---

* Chapter revision edited by Katy Murphy, COA.

quality and was made from scarce pebbles of quartz or semiprecious stones. The first primitive spectacles were balanced precariously on the nose, tied to the ears by means of thread or string or held in the hand as one holds a present-day lorgnette. Their use was confined solely to monks and other learned men of the day. By the 17th century, spectacles were in common use and were elaborately fashioned of gold or silver for members of the aristocracy, whereas tortoiseshell frames were used by members of the upper middle class.

Despite the improvements and refinements in the manufacture and dispensing of frames, the final choice of the right set of spectacles is a personal one, derived not by any scientific formula but by the whims, fancies, and needs of the individual.

Today's fashion industry has influenced frame design tremendously. It is common to see fashionable frames with international designer names (e.g., Prada, Tom Ford, and Salvador Ferragamo). The stigma of wearing glasses has transcended into a fashion statement and has exploded into the sunglass arena. Frame selection has evolved from a simple visual necessity to a method of communicating a personal statement, a fashionable tool for displaying an image one wishes to present.

Frames

A frame for every face

As a rule, frames look best when they complement a patient's facial form. Current fashion trends should be taken into account; if the style of the moment is small round frames, public demand will lean in that direction. A knowledgeable assistant will be able to tell whether the trendy look suits a particular patient, and if not, what different styles to offer.

Early History of Glasses

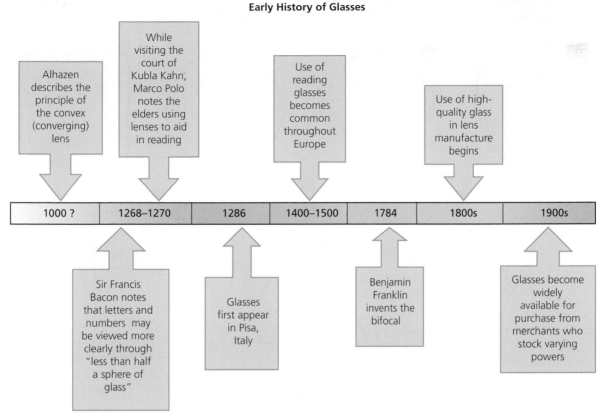

Fig. 13.1 Timeline in the history of spectacles.

Here it is best to refer to classic rules for assistance. The first step is to determine which of the seven basic face shapes the patient has: oval, diamond, round, square, base-down triangle, oblong, and inverted triangle (Fig. 13.2).

The most flattering eyeglass frames are those that are the right depth and width for the face. In general, a flattering frame shape is opposite to the face shape. A round face, for example, looks best with a squared, angular frame, not a rounded shape.

The Vision Council's website (www.eyecessorize.com) devotes an entire section to selecting the correct frame shape. *Oval:* The chin is slightly narrower than the forehead and the cheekbones are high. There appears to be a natural facial balance. *Best options:* Choose frames that are as wide as or wider than the broadest part of the face. Select frames in proportion to the face size. Most frame shapes are good on an oval face.

Diamond: A small forehead and wide temple area gradually narrow to a small chin. Often, cheekbones are high and dramatic. *Best options:* To widen the forehead and jaw and to minimize the cheekbones and wide temple area, select frames that are top-heavy with sides that are straight or angled outward toward the bottom. Frames should be square, rimless, or shaped with a straight top and curved bottom. Avoid frames with decorative temples that make the middle of the face look wider.

Round: Full face with very few angles that appears equal in height and width. *Best options:* To make the face seem longer and thinner, select oval, slightly curved angular frames that feature high or mid-height temples. Clear bridges and color on the temple area flatter this face.

Square: This face has a broad jawline and forehead, with wide angular cheekbones and chin. *Best options:* To lengthen the face, try subtly curved frames, no wider than the widest part of the face. For a high-style look, experiment with stark, geometric shapes that have color concentrated on the outside corners. Square faces can also wear top-heavy frames, oval shapes with temples in the center, and frames with decorative temples hinged above the eye level.

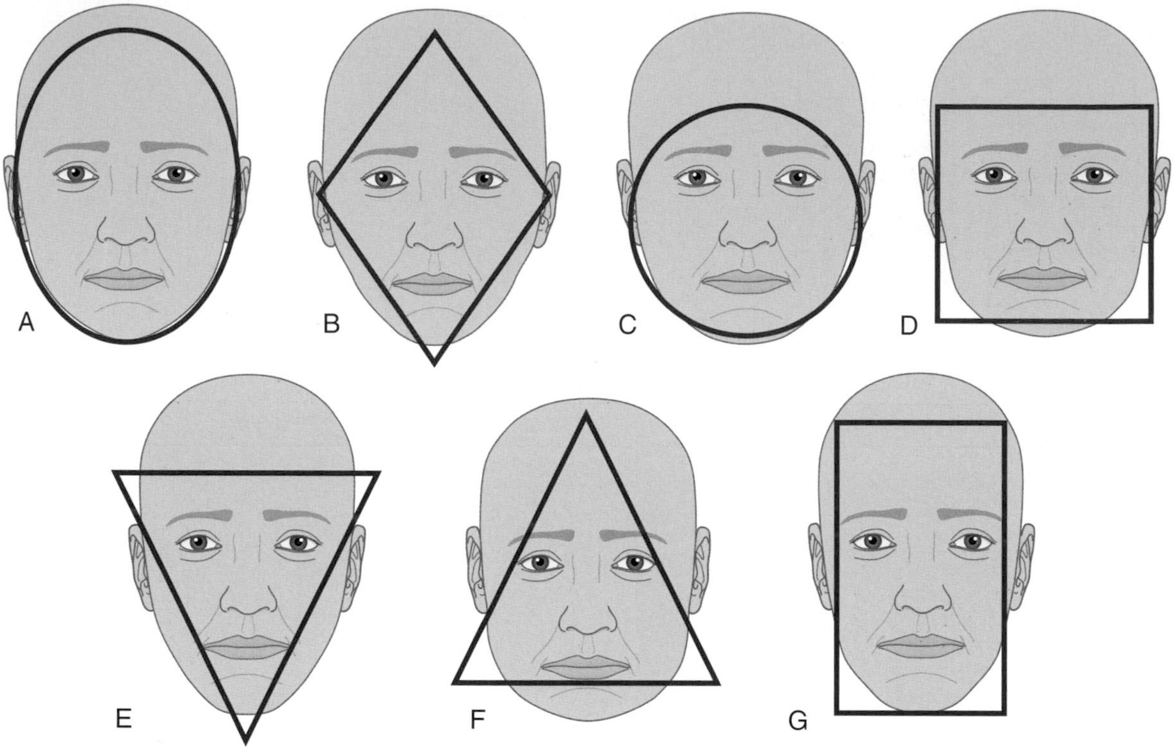

Fig. 13.2 Face shapes. (A) Oval. (B) Diamond. (C) Round. (D) Square. (E) Inverted triangle. (F) Base-down triangle. (G) Oblong. (Modified from photos courtesy of The Vision Council.)

Inverted triangle: Below a wide forehead, this face shape narrows into high cheekbones and a narrow chin. *Best options:* To add width to the chin and cheeks, select frames that angle outward at the bottom but are no wider than the forehead. Low temples, light colors, and rimless styles balance the face. Frames with rounded tops and square bottoms, aviators, and butterfly shapes are other options.

Base-down triangle: A narrow forehead becomes fuller at the cheeks and chin. *Best options:* Frames should add width to the forehead but soften and narrow the jaw, chin, and cheeks. Flattering frames angle outward at the top corners. They should be as wide as or slightly wider than the broadest part of the jaw. Square, aviator, and metal frames with rimless bottoms are flattering selections, or try top-heavy frames with angled bottoms.

Oblong: This face shape is longer than it is wide and the forehead, cheek, and jawline are comparable in width. *Best options:* To shorten and widen the face, select styles that extend beyond the widest part of the face. Choose frames with decorative temples, strong top bars, and round bottom lines. Round, deep, or square shapes shorten and soften an oblong face.

Although fashion is key to frame design, so too are comfort, durability, and thinness. A wide range of frame materials is available; each has its own characteristics.

Spectacles can be defined as an optical appliance composed of lenses and a frame with sides, called *temples*, extending over the ears. The front, main part of the frame holds the actual lenses in front of the eyes, the pads give support on the nose, and the temples hold the front part in the correct position before the eyes. Frames may be made of metal, rubber, wood, plastic, or a combination of metal and plastic.

Fig. 13.3 illustrates the anatomy of frames. Bridge size may be noted as distance between lenses (DBL), which should not be confused with the distance between the (optical) centers (DBC). Temples often are marked with the overall temple length expressed in either inches or millimeters. When two numbers are found on the temple, both overall length and length to the bend are given.

Metal frames

Originally, frames were designed and handmade of silver or solid gold for the aristocracy. These metals have gradually

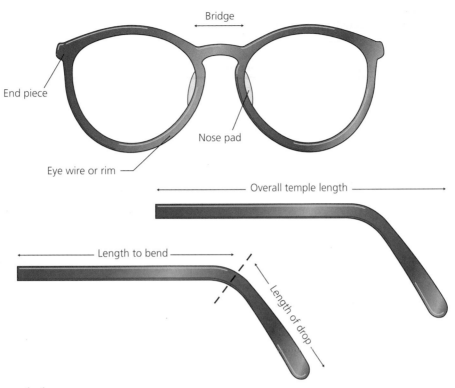

Fig. 13.3 Anatomy of a frame.

been replaced by other metals, such as gold-filled, nickel, aluminum, stainless steel, memory metal such as Flexon, and titanium (Table 13.1).

Plastic and composite frames

There are two types of plastic frames: those molded to shape from *plastic materials* in an injection-molding machine and higher-quality frames cut to shape from a flat piece of plastic, which is then machined and polished to form the finished frame.

Ophthalmic frames made from different types of plastic and composite materials include the following:

Propionate is a spun cast, easy to manufacture lightweight plastic with translucent colors to rival Optyl. It is easily recognizable and needs only a hot-air blower for adjustments. Propionate holds its shape well but, like all plastic, this feature depends on the manufacturing quality.

SPX is stronger and more flexible than propionate, enabling the production of very thin plastic frames. If SPX is overheated, it will shrink and not return to its original size. Thus lenses are mounted while the frame is warm or at room temperature.

Cellulose acetate is a common plastic used today that comes in various colors and patterns. It will burn if a flame is held in contact with the material but is self-extinguishing; when the flame is removed, the plastic will cease to burn. Clear acetate will not change color or yellow with age, and cellulose acetate does not become brittle.

Lucite (Plexiglas, Perspex) is a much tougher plastic and is available in solid colors only (or two-tone or fade-away patterns, produced by laminating two colors). Once the frame is fitted, it retains its shape better than cellulose acetate or nitrate. Lucite does not change color, but manipulation requires much more heat than do other materials.

Nylon (Grilamid, Trogamid) frames are lightweight, hypoallergenic, and relatively unbreakable. They are injection molded and thus of one solid color. Some types are dyed after completion to give the appearance of stock sheet materials also found in cellulose acetate. Nylon requires a high temperature to glaze. Lenses should be cut as close as possible to final size and shape. Because nylon can become dried out, patients should soak the frames in water monthly.

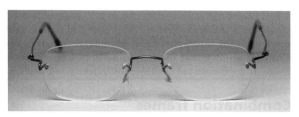

Fig. 13.7 Rimless frame.

frame is viewed from the front the tabs are out of sight behind the top.

Older-model rimless spectacles actually had holes drilled through the lenses and small nuts and bolts placed through these holes to hold the lenses in position (Fig. 13.7). This type of rimless frame was easily shattered when dropped and therefore is now practical only when high-index, polycarbonate, or Trivex lenses are used. Modern-day semirimless spectacles have a pressure mount with a post shim to hold the lenses in place.

Frame measurements

Most frame measurements are based on the box system, whereby the lens is enclosed in a rectangle and the distances between opposite sides are taken as the *eye size*. An imaginary line running through the center of the lenses is called the *datum line*. This is a very important line, because all measurements are taken at this point (Fig. 13.8).

On the back of a frame are a few figures, such as 46×22, which represent the lens size (46) and the bridge size (22). All measurements are in millimeters.

The other measurements are for the temples; they vary according to the use for which the glasses are intended and the consequent shape of the temples.

Temples

The temple is the long strut that extends from the lateral aspect of the eyepiece and rests on the ear. The temple length (e.g., 140 mm) is expressed as the overall length from the hinge end to the end that rests behind the ears. Most plastic temples have a metal core for rigidity and strength.

Several varieties of temples are available. The more commonly used types are:

Cable temples (Fig. 13.9A). Cable temples sometimes are known as *riding bow* temples or *curl side* temples. The cable temple is either metal or plastic, with the ear portion made of a flexible metal that can be shaped to fit the contour behind the ear. Another type of riding bow temple has a much stiffer metal core covered with plastic. A comfortable fit is possible only when this temple is contoured to the back of the ear. This type of temple is ideal for children and active people, for those who are constantly looking down, or for positions in which the spectacles might otherwise slide off the face.

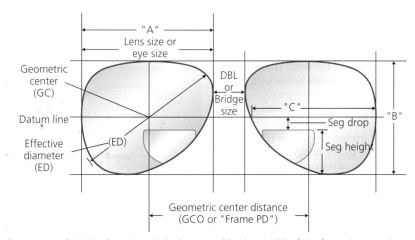

Fig. 13.8 In the boxing system, the "A" dimension is the horizontal boxing width. If the frame is properly marked, the eye size will be equal to the "A" dimension of the frame. The "B" dimension is the vertical boxing length. The "C" dimension is the width of the lens along the horizontal midline. This dimension is seldom used today. The "C" dimension should not be confused with the "C-size" of a lens. The C-size of a lens is the distance around the lens, that is, its circumference. The dispenser uses the C-size to ensure that a lens ordered in isolation (without the frame) will be exactly sized for that frame. *PD*, Pupillary distance; *DBL*, distance between lenses. (Reproduced with permission from Opticians Association of America. *Professional Dispensing for Opticians.* 2nd ed. Philadelphia: Butterworth-Heinemann; 1996.)

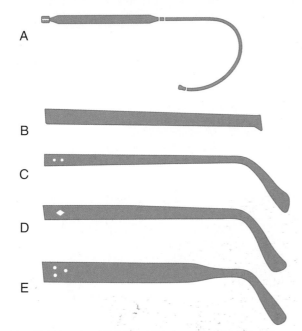

Fig. 13.9 Temples. (A) Cable, riding bow, or curl side temples. (B) Straight or library temples. (C–E) Paddle, skull, or hockey-end.

Straight temples (Fig. 13.9B). Straight temples sometimes are called *library* temples. These are ideal for people who constantly take their glasses off and for those in religious orders whose ears are concealed under a habit, making it difficult to put on or take off glasses that have riding bow or other paddle temples.

Paddle temples (Fig. 13.9C–E). Paddle temples are sometimes called *skull* temples or *hockey-end* temples. These temples are ideal for general use and are the most common type used today.

Specialty frames

Frame manufacturers produce the majority of frames with standard eye sizes and bridge sizes. This leaves a small portion of the population with unusual facial measurements unable to obtain a correct fit with the commercially produced frames. Fortunately, some optical companies will make frames for this group by hand and will produce frames for special vocational or medical requirements. A few of these are mentioned here.

Frames for individuals with low, flat bridges

Because infants and some people have practically no bridge to their noses, the ordinary plastic frame fits too low on the face and is so close to the eyes that the lenses interfere

with the eyelashes. A handmade frame with special nose construction can be made to look like a standard frame yet have the necessary low-set, thickened portion to the bridge so that the spectacles can be properly adjusted in front of the patient's eyes. Before this development, such patients had to be fitted with frames that had adjustable pads to raise the frame and move it away from the face. Today, some manufacturers offer frames which feature a bridge specifically designed to fit this facial shape. These frames are designed with wider pads to move the frame away from the face.

Side shields

There are conditions, such as an anesthetic cornea or a "dry eye," for which it is necessary to enclose the eye between the frame and the face. There are many ways of doing this, but most side-shield constructions are not attractive and usually are bulky, hard, and poor fitting. With the use of a soft, transparent plastic, a shield can be produced and trimmed with a pair of scissors to exactly fit the individual patient. An added bonus is that it is almost invisible and, being soft and pliable, it does not interfere with the glasses being folded up in the standard manner

Ptosis crutch

Although the ideal solution in the case of ptosis is an operation, there may be contraindications to surgery. Frames can be fitted with a ptosis crutch, which is a small piece of wire or plastic affixed to the inside of a spectacle frame. This wire can be adjusted to raise the eyelids of the patient so afflicted.

Dispensing spectacle frames

It is important that spectacles are produced so that the patient, when viewing distance objects, looks through the *optical centers* of both lenses. Consequently, it is essential to know the distance between the visual axes through the pupils of the patient, so that the lenses may be correctly mounted in the spectacle frame at the same interpupillary distance. The term *pupillary distance* is abbreviated PD.

Unfortunately, the visual axis through the human eye does not pass through the center of the pupil, as one might expect, but varies from patient to patient and is on the nasal side of the pupil. Therefore any mechanical device that measures from the center of the pupil of one eye to the center of the pupil of the second eye will give a measurement greater than the actual distance between the visual axes of the two eyes.

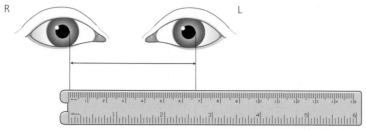

Fig. 13.10 Measurement of pupillary distance. Measurements are made from the nasal edge of one pupil to the temporal edge of the other.

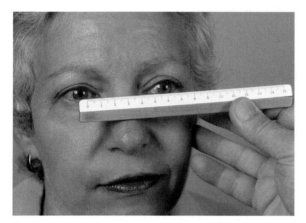

Fig. 13.11 Measuring pupillary distance.

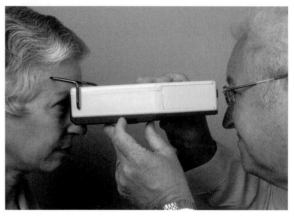

Fig. 13.12 Measuring pupillary distance by pupillary gauge.

This error is of little significance if the prescription is a weak one. However, a few millimeters of error will produce a decidedly uncomfortable pair of glasses for those patients requiring unusually strong (greater than ± 4.00 diopters) prescriptions: binocular aphakes, myopes, hyperopes, or those with large amounts of astigmatism. Because it is difficult to assess the visual axis or the center of the pupil, the practice is to measure (if both pupils are the same size) from the nasal edge of the pupil on the patient's right eye to the temporal side of the pupil on the patient's left eye (Figs. 13.10 and 13.11).

Two PDs are taken, one for distance, where the visual axes are parallel, and one for near, which is the close working distance of the patient.

There is only one accurate method of measuring PD—the *light reflex method*—the result of which gives the distance between the visual axes of the two eyes, rather than the distance between the center of one pupil and the center of the other. The difference between the two methods of measurement may be 2 to 5 mm. There are many optical interpupillary gauges that can give the measurement from pupil to pupil very accurately for distance vision; the PD can then be converted for near vision by means of tables.

One gauge on the market today uses the accurate reflex method (Fig. 13.12).

Special considerations in measuring PD include the following:

1. If the patient has pupils of different size and the standard method with a PD rule is to be used, the measurements should be made from the nasal side of the limbus of the patient's right eye to the temporal side of the limbus on the other, ignoring the measurements from the pupil.
2. If the patient can see from only one eye, the measurement can be taken for the good eye from the center of the bridge of the nose to the center of the pupil, because an inaccuracy of a few millimeters one way or the other has no significance.
3. If the patient has a squint, the measurement can be taken from the inner canthus of one eye to the outer canthus of the opposite eye, giving a reasonably accurate PD. A better way is to occlude the turning eye and measure from the center of the bridge of the nose to the center of the uncovered eye and then repeat with the other eye covered. The sum of the two measurements is the PD.

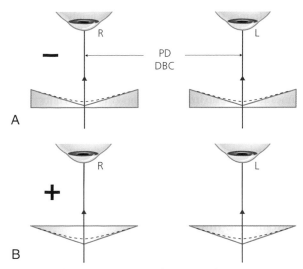

Fig. 13.13 (A) Minus or concave lens. Optical center is at its thinnest part. (B) Plus or convex lens. Optical center is at its thickest part. *PD*, Pupillary distance; *DBC*, distance between centers of lenses.

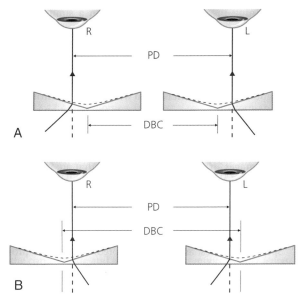

Fig. 13.14 (A) Prism base-out effect is created by inward displacement of the optical centers of two concave lenses. (B) Prism base-in effect is created by outward displacement of the optical centers of two concave lenses. *PD*, Pupillary distance; *DBC*, distance between centers of lenses.

The PD is taken so that the optical centers of the lenses will be directly in front of the visual axes through the pupils (Fig. 13.13). If the optical centers are not so placed, an unwanted prism is incorporated in the glasses.

The *optical center* can be defined as the thinnest part in the center of any minus lens or the thickest part of the center of a plus lens. Only at the optical center do rays of light go through the lens without bending. To make this clearer, a minus lens can be represented by two prisms, bases out, and a plus lens, bases in. When these lenses have their centers in line with the visual axes, they are correctly positioned in front of the patient's eyes (Fig. 13.14).

If the PD is wrong and the lenses are off-center, the vision is bent by the lenses toward the base of the prism in each case and the object would appear to be displaced laterally. The eyes would have to turn in or out to try to correct this, causing discomfort to the patient. If the lenses are high power, plus or minus, so much prism can be introduced that double vision will result. In the case of a lens of +10.00 diopters, if the PD is out 1 mm then 1.00 diopter of prism that has not been prescribed is introduced into the prescription.

Measuring pupillary distance with a ruler and the reflex method

Most times, the PD is measured with a device called a pupillometer. When checking the PD manually, the following equipment is required:

1. Small PD rule, graduated in millimeters

2. Pinpoint of light, such as a bare bulb of an ophthalmoscope battery handle or a penlight

To take a *distance PD*, the procedure is as follows:

1. Sit approximately 16 to 18 inches from the patient to be examined.
2. Hold the light source immediately under your left eye. Place the PD rule across the bridge of the patient's nose so that it will extend to cover the lower half of both pupils.
3. Make sure the patient looks directly at the light bulb.
4. Place the zero mark of the ruler on the pinpoint reflection of the light on the cornea. Use your left eye for this purpose.
5. Without disturbing the PD ruler and without the patient moving the head, move the light to a position underneath your right eye.
6. Make sure the patient is still looking at the light.
7. Note the measurement on the PD rule of the reflection of the light on the cornea of the patient's left eye. (In doing this you will observe that the pinpoint of light is not in the center of the pupil but at some point nasal of center. The measurement is an accurate one of the distance between the visual axes of the two eyes [incorrectly termed the distance PD for want of a better term].)
8. Note the measurement at the center of the nose (this may be useful if the patient's face is grossly asymmetric).

mirror coating can be produced. Popular colors available commercially are green, neutral gray, brown, rose, and transparent (one-way) surfaces.

Color coating of ophthalmic lenses gives an even coloring across the whole surface of the lens, whether it is a strong plus or a strong minus lens. The coating, whether it is antireflection, mirror, or color, may be removed chemically in about 10 seconds, should this be necessary.

Almost all sunglasses are clear lenses coated to the chosen color. However, colored-glass lenses are still available that are perfectly satisfactory for plano or weak prescriptions. If the prescription is a high plus, then the color of the glass is darker at the center than at the edges. Conversely, a high minus lens would have a central light spot. Before the advent of the surface coating process, evenly spread color was obtained by laminating a colored plano lens to a clear prescription lens, an expensive process that is no longer necessary.

Colored plastic lenses are clear lenses dyed the appropriate color. Therefore they have an even color no matter how strong the prescription may be. Gradient tints or even several colors on the same lens can be produced. Plastic lenses can be effective blockers of UV light, but not of infrared light.

A neutral gray tint has been the most popular color for sunglasses in North America for almost half a century. Because of its neutral absorption of all colors of the visible spectrum, light intensity is reduced without color distortion or imbalance, which is a very important factor when proper color perception is essential, for instance, a pilot having to read various colored dials, gauges, or maps; a telephone lineman distinguishing between color-coded telephone wires; a driver who might have difficulties differentiating colors of traffic signals; a participant or spectator at a sporting event where each team is denoted by the color of their uniforms; or a naturalist watching birds, animals, or flowers. In short, gray lenses should be recommended whenever a patient wants protection from intensive light or glare without loss of color differentiation.

The human eye responds to wavelengths of 380 to 780 nm. Shorter or longer wavelengths do not elicit a visual response but may enter the eyes and cause heating or photobiologic damage. Blocking lenses are valuable. The stratospheric ozone layers help protect the eyes, but holes are appearing in the ozone layer owing to manmade chemicals, especially the fully halogenated methanes (chlorofluorocarbons [CFCs]).

A green lens absorbs most of the UV and infrared light and transmission peaks roughly at the same point as the luminous curve of the eye. Naturally, violet, blue, orange, or red colors are less distinguishable. Green lenses are recommended for situations with high amounts of reflected light (which contains large amounts of UV), such as glaciers and open water. They should be recommended for vacations in the tropics and for use during hot weather to protect against (heat) rays. In industry, green lenses of various densities are used for welding and other high light and heat situations. They also have the psychologic effect of "coolness" during hot weather and thus provide comfort to the wearer.

For many years, brown tints were very popular in Europe. Brown-tinted lenses are being dispensed more commonly in North America. Brown lenses absorb almost all of the UV and have a very even progressive curve throughout the visible spectrum. Brown lenses are most useful in moderate to cold climates to protect against UV radiation and excessive radiation, with the added benefit of creating a "warm" visual environment. Three different tints of brown are available in either glass or plastic lenses.

Except for the cobalt-blue lenses used to judge the temperature in a blast furnace, blue lenses are more a whim of fashion than eye protection.

Yellow-tinted lenses are good absorbers of UV, violet, and blue. Suppressing this area of the spectrum enhances contrast in the rest of the visible spectrum. A yellow lens is therefore preferred to increase contrast in marginal light conditions, such as hunting at dawn or dusk or driving in foggy conditions, but should not be worn to protect against excessive light.

Other tints, such as pink, purple, and mauve, are deviants of the aforementioned tints and are used mainly as fashion accents.

Cheap sunglasses, usually in injection-molded plastic frames, are sold widely. These are not ground and polished lenses, although they may appear to be. Some lenses are plastic and can be identified as such by "bending" the lens in the frame. Cheap sunglasses are produced from flat, colored-glass sheets of low quality. Circles are cut from the flat sheet and each circle is placed in a metal concave dish having a curve of about 4.00 diopters. The dish is placed in an oven and left until the glass sags, or "drops," to the shape of the dish. The "lens" now has the shape of a ground lens. Lenses made in this manner are called "dropped lenses," and may be identified as such by: (1) the shallow curve, (2) the distortions of objects *reflected* on the surface of the lens, and (3) usually some unwanted and unprescribed power. A properly ground and polished lens will show no distortions of reflected light and is usually on a base curve of about 6.00 diopters.

A popular type of sunglass on the market is the polarized sunglass. Such lenses usually are made of plastic but are sometimes found in a laminated form, in which the polarizing filter is sandwiched between two sheets of glass. Polarized sunglasses are available in prescription form.

Apart from the color of the lens, the axis of the polarizing material is placed in the frames so that glare coming off a flat horizontal surface is further darkened. The glasses are good for driving into the sun, because a white,

Box 13.1 **Tips on purchasing sunglasses**

1. Ultraviolet (UV) absorption. The most important factor to look for in sunglasses is the indication that they block 100% of UV rays. Check for the manufacturer's label indicating whether the sunglasses are 100% UV absorbent and if they meet the American National Standards Institute (ANSI) guidelines for eyewear.
2. The bigger the lenses, the more coverage and the less damage to the eyes from the sun. Oversized glasses and wraparound-style glasses help decrease UV rays from entering the eyes from the side.
3. The color of the lens and the darkness of the tint are not good indicators of the glasses' ability to filter out UV light. Lens color should cause as little color distortion as possible. Dark gray or dark green tints permit the most normal color vision.
4. The price of a pair of sunglasses is absolutely no indicator of their lenses' ability to absorb UV light.
5. Polarized lenses tend to reduce reflection and glare and are especially effective around water and snow.
6. Photochromic lenses change color in response to sunlight, often preventing the need for two pairs of prescription glasses. Today there is much faster activation and deactivation with new photochromic lenses.
7. Special UV-absorbent coatings are available, which can be applied to everyday glasses. These are often applied to glasses used for skiing, high-altitude flying, and outdoor sports.
8. The US Food and Drug Administration requires that all eyeglass lenses, including sunglasses, be made of impact-resistant glass or plastic. Also the frames must be nonflammable. "Impact-resistant"' does not mean that the lenses are shatterproof, but rather that they can withstand moderately sharp impacts.

(Modified from American Academy of Ophthalmology EyeSmart. How to choose the best sunglasses. 2015. With permission.)

glaring highway will appear dark. People who fish or go boating find that glare off water is reduced considerably when wearing polarized lenses. In rough-surfaced areas, such as grass, they are no improvement over tinted lenses. Brands of polarized lenses include Xperio, KBco, and Drivewear.

The American Academy of Ophthalmology has suggested some guidelines for consumers to follow when purchasing sunglasses (Box 13.1).

Densities

In dispensing tinted lenses, it is important to know the light conditions and environment in which the lenses will be used. Lenses that are too dark will dilate the pupil and visual acuity will be reduced. Should light intensity vary rapidly, such as driving in bright sunlight through shaded areas, vision could be impaired. Therefore very dark lenses may be recommended only for sailors, people who fish, and hikers. Naturally, for driving long distances through prairies and urban areas, a dark shade is most comfortable.

Providing a medium tint with a gradient mirror gives the patient an opportunity to select the density according to the prevailing light conditions. Naturally, in this respect, the photochromic lenses fill a specific void in the eye protection field. Their ability to adapt to the varying light intensities has made them one of the most sought-after lens materials.

Photochromic (indoor–outdoor) glasses

Photochromic lenses have the chameleon-like ability to change from light to dark and back again. In glass photochromic lenses, silver halide microcrystals impart this changeability and never wear out. The halides darken when exposed to UV or the blue end of the spectrum. The more popular technology is plastic photochromic lenses. The range of darkening photosensitive plastic lenses has been developed to the point where a pair of glasses can be perfectly clear lenses indoors and a satisfactory sunglass outdoors. Whereas clear plastic lenses transmit 90% to 92% of light indoors (polycarbonate and CR-39, respectively), advanced technology photochromic lenses (in a 1.50 Refractive Index) transmit 89% of light, which makes them indistinguishable from clear lenses indoors. Indoor transmission can also be enhanced with antireflective coatings. The average pair of sunglasses is designed to filter 70% to 85% of visible light and block 100% of UVA and UVB radiation.

The cycling of the modern photochromic lenses happens quickly. Transition lenses darken to a 70% tint within 35 seconds (Fig. 13.22). During the reverse process, out of UV radiation for just a few minutes, they return to a 70% clarity. All photochromic lenses are affected by temperature. The range of dark to light is greater in cold weather (winter day) than in hot (summer picnic).

UV light boxes are available that allow one to demonstrate the darkening of lenses with UV light. One can place

Questions for review and thought

1. Discuss the manufacture and types of ophthalmic frames.
2. What are the advantages and disadvantages of the different types of ophthalmic frames?
3. How is pupillary distance measured?
4. What is the temple length? What points are measured?
5. What type of glass is commonly used for ophthalmic lenses?
6. What are some of the distortions inherent in lenses?
7. High-power hyperopic lenses usually present a special problem because of their thickness and weight. What type of special lens is available to overcome these problems?
8. Safety glasses are recommended for children, people engaged in sports, and industrial workers. How are they constructed?
9. Sunglasses filter out certain of the color components of white light. Discuss some types of sunglasses that are available.
10. Bifocals are used to provide two focal distances in the same glass. They may be of one-piece or fused construction or even cemented. Draw diagrams to illustrate how fused bifocals are constructed.
11. Special occupations, such as garage mechanics, may require the worker to use a bifocal segment in an uncommon position. Name as many occupations as you can in which the bifocal segment may be required in an unusual position.
12. What are the advantages of the Fresnel prism?
13. Does a large stylish frame size improve or diminish visual acuity in a person with a large refractive error?
14. What lenses would you recommend for night driving?
15. Does a blue lens affect visual acuity?
16. How can thick glasses be made lighter?
17. What types of frames should be avoided because of their flammable potential?
18. What kind of glasses should a welder use?
19. What are the advantages and disadvantages of trifocals?

Self-evaluation questions   Q

True–false statements

Directions: Indicate whether the statement is true (T) or false (F).

1. Cellulose nitrate is the most common plastic used in the fabrication of spectacle frames. T or F
2. The pupillary distance is the distance from the center of the pupil of one eye to the center of the pupil of the other eye. T or F
3. The optical center of a lens is the thinnest part of the lens in a myopic correction and the thickest part of a lens in a hyperopic correction. T or F

Missing words

Directions: Write in the missing word in the following sentences.

4. The primary glass used by opticians is _____ glass.
5. Aphakic lenses tend to distort to a _____ shape.
6. Coating a lens often is referred to as _____ a lens.

Choice-completion questions

Directions: Select the one best answer in each case.

7. The preferred material to be used in children's glasses is:
   a. CR-39.
   b. polycarbonate or Trivex.
   c. high-index glass.
   d. high-index plastic.
   e. none of the above.
8. The invisible bifocal offers:
   a. great vision over the whole lens.
   b. great vision just in a band on either side of the optical center.
   c. great vision nasally where the eyes turn in to read.
   d. best vision in powers greater than +1.50.
   e. none of the above.
9. A Fresnel lens is a press-on lens and:
   a. it can be cut to any shape.
   b. it comes in prisms up to 15.00 diopters, as well as in a range of positive and negative lens powers.
   c. it gets dirty easily, peels off, and has to be replaced often.
   d. it causes a drop of vision because the optics are not sharp.
   e. is all of the above.

Answers, notes, and explanations

A

1. **False**. Cellulose nitrate burns fiercely if a flame is brought to it. Today, the use of such flammable plastics is not allowed in the make-up of spectacles. A lit cigarette near the frames may ignite them. One of the popular plastics used presently is cellulose acetate, which is desirable because it comes in a variety of colors. It can burn if a flame is held to it but it does not ignite and spread on its own.

    Lucite, a much tougher material, is frequently used. For children, nylon and Optyl frames are popular because they are flexible and virtually indestructible. Flexibility allows the frame to fit any face and prevents snapping, which can occur with the more rigid plastics. Nylon is made up in a limited number of colors, but Optyl can be dyed to any color combination.

2. **False**. This distance actually exceeds the true interpupillary distance, which is measured from the visual axis of one eye to the other. The visual axis is a little nasal to the center of the pupil in most instances. Because of the inherent difficulties in measuring visual axis, the PD is normally taken from the nasal edge of the pupil of the patient's right eye to the temporal side of the pupil of the left eye.

    Light reflexes off the pupil can indicate the visual axis of the eye and they are more accurate.

    Two readings should be taken: one for the distance and one for near.

    The PD is an important measurement because many complaints and glass checks stem from a failure of the optician to center the lens to the visual axis of the eye. When this happens, unwanted prism is introduced, and the patient has symptoms.

3. **True**. The optical center of the lens should be marked inasmuch as it does not coincide with the midpoint between the nasal and temporal sides of the frame. Most lensmeters have a marking device to indicate the true optical center of the lens. Some frames are so large and eccentric that the optical centers of the lenses never approximate the visual axes of the eyes. Checking optical centers should be performed on every glass check because centering is the largest source of complaints.

4. **Crown**. Crown glass has been a favorite lens for opticians because it has a lower refractive index and has less of a tendency to color dispersion. However, such lenses are heavy and are particularly cumbersome in higher powers. CR-39, a hard resin plastic lens, accounts for more than 50% of ophthalmic lenses prescribed. The weight of CR-39 is nearly half that of crown glass. Polycarbonate, a thermoplastic resin lens, is used in sport and safety glasses because of its impact resistance.

5. **Pincushion**. A lens that is thick causes distortion because the bending of light at the edge of the lens is not the same as in the middle of the lens. In an aphakic lens, the thickness is in the center of the lens and the lens profile drops off sharply toward the edge. In high myopes, the thickness of the lens is toward the edges, and the distortion created by the thin center moving out to thicken at the periphery causes barrel distortion.

    In aphakic lenses remedies for distortion include: 1) lenticular lenses because they get rid of the lens edge and 2) lenses that are flatter in the periphery because they eliminate the drastic change in power. The four-drop lens does this job well. Basically, these lenses fall into the category of aspheric lenses.

6. **Blooming**. The lenses are coated with magnesium fluoride, which is one-quarter of the wavelength of yellow-green light. The coating imparts a purplish sheen to these lenses, similar to bloom on a ripe plum; hence the name.

    The coating is tough and lasts the lifetime of the lens. The purpose of coating the lens is to eliminate annoying light reflections from lights and bulbs.

    A coated lens allows greater light transmission while depressing the amount of internal reflections.

7. **b. Polycarbonate** or **Trivex**. When dispensing eyewear for children, it is important to address the many safety issues relevant to the child, as well as the concerns of the parents. Infants and toddlers are prone to bumping into objects and falling down; older children who play sports, as well as children of any age engaged in normal child's play, will benefit from the added safety of polycarbonate or Trivex lenses in their eyeglasses. It is for this reason more than any other that polycarbonate or Trivex is the material of choice for all pediatric dispensing. With an impact resistance significantly greater than that of CR-39, high refractive index, and lower specific gravity, there is no more suitable material for children. Still, CR-39 remains an option when polycarbonate's slightly higher cost is an issue. Generally speaking, the use of crown glass in children's eyewear is contraindicated.

8. **b. Great vision just in a band on either side of the optical center**. This lens has become very popular because it eliminates the visible presence of bifocals, which to many people means aging. Optically, it offers some advantages. It eliminates image jump, as the transition between the distance and near portion is not abrupt. It also confers a continuous increase in power looking down so that a longer band of near focal points is available to the wearer. However, this lens does create lateral astigmatism on either side of the central band of the lens. Many people find the distortion disabling for reading. Some of the newer models of this seamless bifocal are better because the diameter of the clear central zone has been expanded.

9. **All of the above**. A Fresnel lens is basically a temporary lens. The advantages of this lens are that it is flexible and lightweight. However, the disadvantages of hazy vision and of lower durability and reliability preclude constant wear.

    It is a good temporary lens for postsurgical cataract cases and for those people with temporary diplopia who require bridge prisms to carry them along until their condition improves.

Chapter | 14 |

Rigid contact lenses: basics

Contact lenses have become a routine part of our armamentarium for visual rehabilitation of the eye. Their use and demand are constantly increasing. More than 20% of the North American population is myopic and many of these people depend on visual correction. Coupled with the increasing use of contact lenses, many myths and fallacies have arisen regarding their indications and contraindications. At the very minimum, the ophthalmic assistant should be able to discuss with the patient the function of a contact lens, its purpose, and its limitations. The ophthalmic assistant can also be of value in some of the technical aspects of contact lens wear, such as method of insertion and removal and, particularly, proper care and storage of the lens itself. This chapter deals with the practical aspects of management of the patient who desires contact lenses, and in particular, rigid contact lenses.

Development

As early as the 16th century, Leonardo da Vinci conceived and sketched prototypes of modern contact lenses. He experimented by neutralizing his own refractive error by placing his face in a container of water. In the following century, René Descartes described and illustrated a glass type of scleral contact lens (Fig. 14.1). However, the first practical type of contact lens was produced in 1887. This lens consisted of a glass capsule containing gelatin that was placed in contact with the cornea, with the glass being molded to correspond to the shape of the eye.

In 1932 the first major advance in the design of the contact lens was made. Investigating impressions made from the human eye, Dr. Joseph Dallos found that no two were identical. From this, he concluded that it was impossible to fit a contact lens manufactured to a preconceived formula. Dallos then developed a technique of making negative casts of the anterior segment of the living eye. However, his lenses could be tolerated for only limited periods of time because of the excessive weight of the glass, and they were difficult to manufacture. In 1938 the first molded scleral contact lens that overlaid the sclera was made from a plastic material called polymethyl methacrylate (PMMA). This lens had many advantages over glass because it was lighter, shatterproof, and easily moldable.

It was not until 1948 that Kevin Tuohy introduced the first fluidless corneal lens, which was designed to rest on the corneal tear layer. These were large, but later smaller microcorneal lenses were introduced, which made possible a great step forward in the successful wearing of contact lenses.

Further developments in rigid lens manufacture came with the introduction of intermediate curves, the practice of refining the edges, and the development of toric lenses. Rigid lens technology made another leap forward

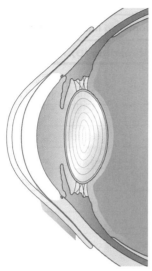

Fig. 14.1 Scleral contact lens. The contact lens fits over the cornea and sclera.

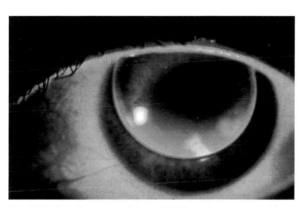

Fig. 14.2 The silicone acrylate contact lens is gas permeable. It may be fitted larger than conventional polymethyl methacrylate rigid lenses. Note that the upper eyelid margin is covering the upper portion of the contact lens.

with the introduction of silicone and fluorocarbon. When combined with PMMA, these materials make the plastic material gas permeable (Fig. 14.2). As a result of these new materials, in most countries today PMMA rigid lenses are rarely used.

Advancement in rigid gas-permeable (RGP, or GP) technology involves improving the biocompatibility of materials to prevent unwanted deposits from tears. Polysulfone has been used in contact lens polymerization. New crosslinking technology stabilizes thin lens designs for comfort and durability. Advancement in manufacturing techniques and new lens material have reintroduced scleral lenses. There

are at least 48 different RGP contact lens materials available by 11 different manufacturers. These manufacturers provide their GP material to labs all across the world that produce numerous GP lens designs.

Optics

The rigid contact lens, for all practical purposes, eliminates the cornea as a major source of refractive error of the eye. The index of refraction of the RGP lenses is slightly greater than the tear layer. The fluid interface between the spherical contact lens and the cornea fills out irregularities in the contours of the anterior corneal surface, converting an astigmatic cornea to a sphere. Thus the fluid may be considered a forward extension of the cornea. If the radius of curvature of the back surface of the contact lens is the same as that of the front surface of the cornea, the fluid lens will be zero. The change in refractive power is produced by altering the curvature of the contact lens, as well as changing the total contact lens power. Change in the contact lens base curve alters the fluid lens power.

How the corneal contact lens works

A contact lens rests on the cornea just as a small fragment of paper adheres to the wet fingertip by just touching it. The natural moisture on the surface of the cornea is sufficient to create a surface tension and permit the lens to adhere quite strongly.

The back surface of the lens is contoured so that it is very similar to the curvature of the cornea. The corneal curvature can be measured by instruments, such as an ophthalmometer (or keratometer) and topographer. It is vital that these measurements be exact because if there is any contact or touch between the cornea and the contact lens, then a scratch, abrasion, or erosion can occur in the superficial layers of the cornea. The contact lens therefore rests on a liquid cushion (tear film) and never on the eye itself. Injury to the cornea is one of the most damaging complications that can result from a poorly fitted contact lens. Not only does it produce a painful red eye that obscures vision, but it also provides a portal of entry for bacteria and other pathogenic organisms to form a corneal ulcer.

The difference between the front surface curvature and the back surface curvature of a contact lens produces the power of the lens.

The edge of an RGP contact lens is thin and polished so that it can gently slide underneath the lid without being dislodged and prevent lid irritation when blinking.

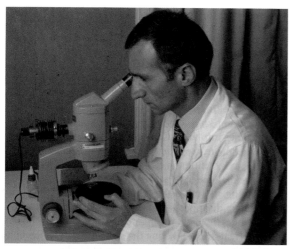

Fig. 14.21 Measuring curvature of a contact lens with the Radiuscope.

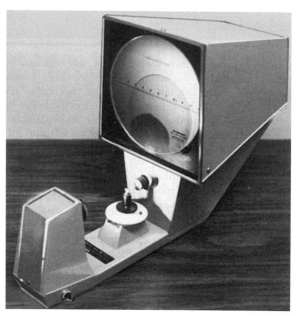

Fig. 14.23 Shadowgraph used to magnify and measure a contact lens.

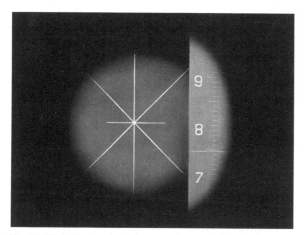

Fig. 14.22 Pattern and inside measuring scale in a Radiuscope. (From Stein HA, Slatt BJ, Stein RM, Freeman MI. *Fitting Guide for Rigid and Soft Contact Lenses: A Practical Approach.* 4th ed. St Louis: Mosby; 2002.)

(2) the width of the peripheral curve, (3) the width of any blending area, and (4) the width of the intermediate curve. The blending zone cannot be seen by the naked eye but can be evaluated only under the large magnification created by the Shadowscope. The Shadowscope is also useful in showing scratches on the optical surface of the contact lens, as well as any cracks or nicks in the edge.

The cross-section view of the contact lens shows up the contour of the edge so the edge thickness can be measured, which should be no thicker than 0.12 mm.

To use the Shadowgraph and Contactoscope, the practitioner places the contact lens on a vertically mounted stage to provide a front view of the lens. The image is focused

on the screen by a lever under the stage. The lens should be scrutinized for scratches, nicks, and cracks. The screen image can be raised or lowered by a knob on the stage so that the lens can be placed against the measuring scale. The diameter of the lens can then be measured on the scale. The peripheral curve width, the blend width, and the intermediate curve width can then be inspected and measured.

To view the lens on the edge, one can either rotate the lens perpendicular to the screen or lay the lens on its convex surface on the stage. The practitioner may need to refocus to get a sharp image of the edge. One can move the stage laterally to project the image of the edge on the reticule scale to measure edge thickness.

Measuring power

The power of a contact lens may be measured on the standard lensmeter. Place the lens concave side down to measure the back vertex power of the contact lens. A small error in the power may arise if the lens is held in place with fingers, particularly with higher-power lenses. To measure the front vertex power, place the lens concave side up on the lensmeter.

Measuring thickness

For measuring thickness, a contact lens is inserted in the thickness gauge, convex side down. The pin of the gauge is allowed to descend slowly until contact is made with the concave surface. The measurement is read from the dial (Fig. 14.24).

Insertion and removal techniques

It is important that the patient be carefully instructed on how to insert, remove, and care for contact lenses.

Insertion

The hands should always be carefully washed and dried before insertion of the lens. The lens is cleaned and wet before inserting, then balanced, concave side up, on the tip of the index finger. The lens is moistened with contact lens solution or methylcellulose. The right hand should be used for the right lens and the left hand for the left lens, although this may vary with patient preference. The patient looks straight down, chin on chest, keeping both eyes open. The upper lid is then held at the lashes with the fingers of the opposite hand pressing up and against the bony margin of the brow. The lower lid should be held at the lash margin with the fourth finger of the hand that is holding the lens pressing down and against the cheek. The lens finger is then brought straight up to the eye until the lens touches the eye (Fig. 14.25). An instant afterward, the lower lid should be released and then slowly the upper lid. It is important to impress on the patient that he or she should not look away at the last moment. The head must always be kept straight and the temptation to turn must be avoided.

In the early stages of learning to insert the lenses, the use of a mirror will help. The patient should learn to insert the lenses without a mirror as soon as possible because one may not be handy at all times.

Some individuals are more successful in placing a lens on the eye when they do not have to look at the lens coming toward the eye. These individuals should look downward, with the upper lid lifted by the forefinger or middle finger.

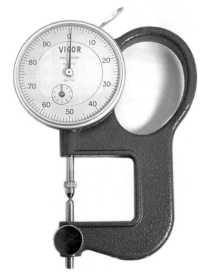

Fig. 14.24 Thickness gauge. Before measuring, thickness gauge must be set to zero. (Courtesy Vigor Optical, Division of Grobet USA, Carlstadt, NJ.)

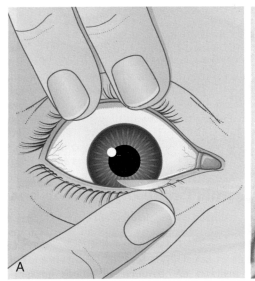
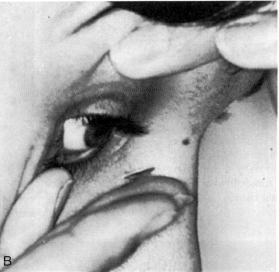

Fig. 14.25 Rigid gas-permeable contact lens insertion by the patient. (A) The upper lid is retracted by grasping the lid near the margin and pulling it. The left hand is used to elevate the right upper lid. The patient's gaze is directed downward and the lens is carried to the eye by the index finger of the right hand. (B) Incorrect method: the upper lid should be grasped near the lid margin and the lens should rest on the tip of the finger.

irritability. The patient has discomfort and even pain when exposed to normal thresholds of light.

3. Spectacle blur. Foggy vision occurs when the contact lens is removed and glasses are worn. The spectacle blur is caused by edema of the central portion of the cornea, which may be a result of inadequate oxygen transport to the cornea, from either inadequate tear transport to the cornea or a material that has insufficient oxygen permeability characteristics.

4. Reflections. Internal reflections may occur from the contact lens itself or from a lens that decenters.

5. Burning sensation. This symptom of corneal irritability may represent corneal edema, corneal erosion, or excessive eyelid contact.

During the adaptation period, because the patient may have tearing, lid irritation, and excessive sensitivity to light, activities that require good visual acuity should be avoided. Until the adaptation period is complete, the patient should avoid driving a car; working on lathes, grinders, and other high-velocity moving equipment; and doing prolonged close work.

Abnormal symptoms

Symptoms may be caused by poor technique on the part of the patient in the insertion or removal of the lenses. A poor insertion method is a common failing of the novice. Among the hazards of incorrect insertion are the tendencies of the person to flinch, move the eye quickly, thrust the lens against the cornea, or squeeze the lids around the lens.

Symptoms caused by low oxygen (hypoxia) to the cornea tend to become more severe and more constant as the lenses are worn. Lenses that prevent adequate tear and oxygen exchange are referred to as "tight" lenses, but symptoms are essentially caused by starvation of oxygen in the cornea. The symptom of corneal hypoxia is a burning sensation that appears after a comfortable induction period of 2 to 3 hours. Such a lens may not lag with eye movement, will not drop when the lids are pulled away, and shows little or no excursion with blinking. However, if the lens is too "loose," it may frequently slip off the cornea or fall out of the eye.

Poor vision may be a result of a variety of conditions. The power of the lens may be in error, the fit of the lens may be poor, the lens may be warped, or it may have been inserted in the wrong eye.

A distinction should be made between foggy vision that occurs on insertion of the lens and that which arises 2 to 3 hours after contact lens wear. The former is usually caused by incorrect cleansing or mucus under the lens. The latter is usually indicative of corneal edema or corneal hypoxia and is a pathologic finding.

Excessive awareness of a contact lens can be a psychologic problem because it is only an extension of the normal conscious feeling of something foreign on the eye. However, the normal contact lens wearer usually has many periods during the day when he or she is free of this sensation. If the patient should suddenly become aware of the contact lens, this symptom may be indicative of roughened and scratched edges of the lens or the presence of dried secretions on its surface.

A burning sensation is generally attributed to a tight lens, to stagnation of tear fluid between the lens and the cornea, to corneal anoxia, or to damage of the corneal epithelium. In the first three cases, the symptom abates on removal of the lens, whereas in the last it does not.

The patient with a foreign body sensation will either harbor a tiny foreign body between the lens and cornea, particularly in dusty areas, or have erosions of the cornea. Any patient who has pathologic symptoms should be told to remove the lenses and be reassessed before wear is resumed.

Abnormal symptoms and signs and the corrections required to eliminate them are discussed further in Chapter 14.

Objective criteria

The fit of a contact lens may be objectively evaluated according to its relationship to the lid margins and its position on the cornea. Ideally, the upper margin of the lens should fit under the upper lid and be free of the lower lid. Blinking action of the lids should raise the lens slightly. The contact lens should be well centered on the cornea and not displaced to either side.

Other objective criteria used to evaluate the fit of a contact lens include: (1) fluorescein patterns, (2) alteration of the blink rate, (3) scratches, chips, and roughened edges of the contact lens, and (4) changes in the cornea.

Fluorescein patterns (Figs. 14.30 and 14.31)

If the size and movement of the lens in the patient's eye appear satisfactory, the fluorescein test should follow. In this test, fluorescein is placed on the superior margin of the cornea. Fluorescein patterns are best seen with an ultraviolet lamp source for illumination and a slit-lamp microscope or handheld magnifier for inspection (Fig. 14.32). The fluorescein dye forms a thin layer between the contact lens and the cornea. The distribution of the dye enables the observer to evaluate the adequacy of the precorneal fluid layer between the contact lens and the cornea.

The patient with a normal corneal contour will have an even and thin layer of dyed tear film centrally surrounded by a slightly deeper ring of fluid peripherally. At the area of marginal touch at the extreme periphery of the lens, the depth of the tear film is minimal. A flat lens, which is a lens with a flatter posterior curvature than the anterior central surface of the cornea, tends to rest on the optic cap of the cornea and touch it (Fig. 14.33). At the area of contact there is an absence of the green fluorescein dye (Fig. 14.34). A steep lens has a steeper posterior curvature than the cornea and bridges it, making contact at its margin with the

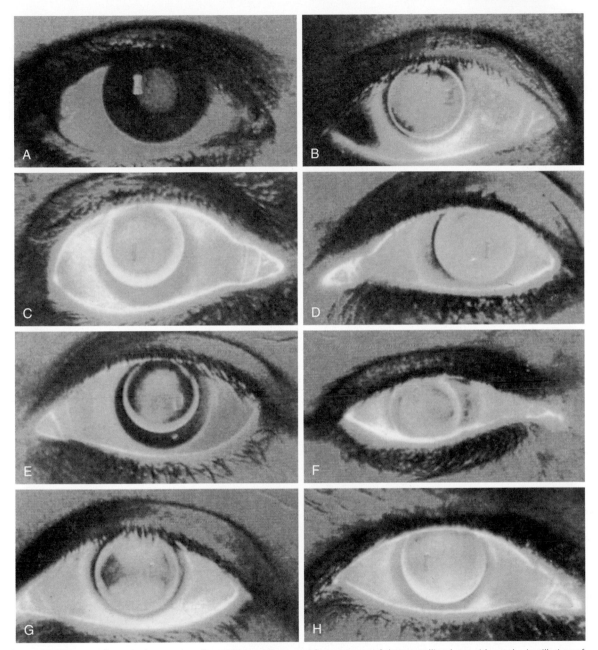

Fig. 14.30 Common fluorescein patterns. Corneal lens. (A) Normal fluorescence of the crystalline lens without the instillation of fluorescein. This is a source of confusion to the novice in assessing the fit. (B) Minimal apex-clear fitting in a corectopic patient with the pupil at the limbus at the 12 o'clock position. Note that a more apex-clear lens would show a broader dark band of contact adjacent to the peripheral curve. (C) The apex-clear pattern in the normal eye. Note the fluorescence of the crystalline lens within the pupil. (D) Flat-fitting lens. There is touch at the apex of the lens. (E) Flat-fitting lens. A pool of fluorescein with a curved lower limit is seen above the central touch. (F) Flat-fitting lens. A pool of fluorescein with a curved upper limit is seen below the central touch. (G) Flat astigmatic picture. The other eye of the patient with corectopia is seen in (B). (H) Apex-clear astigmatic pattern in a normal eye. (A–H, Reproduced with permission from Duke-Elder S, Abrams D, editors. *System of Ophthalmology, Vol 5: Ophthalmic Optics and Refraction*. St Louis: Mosby; 1970.)

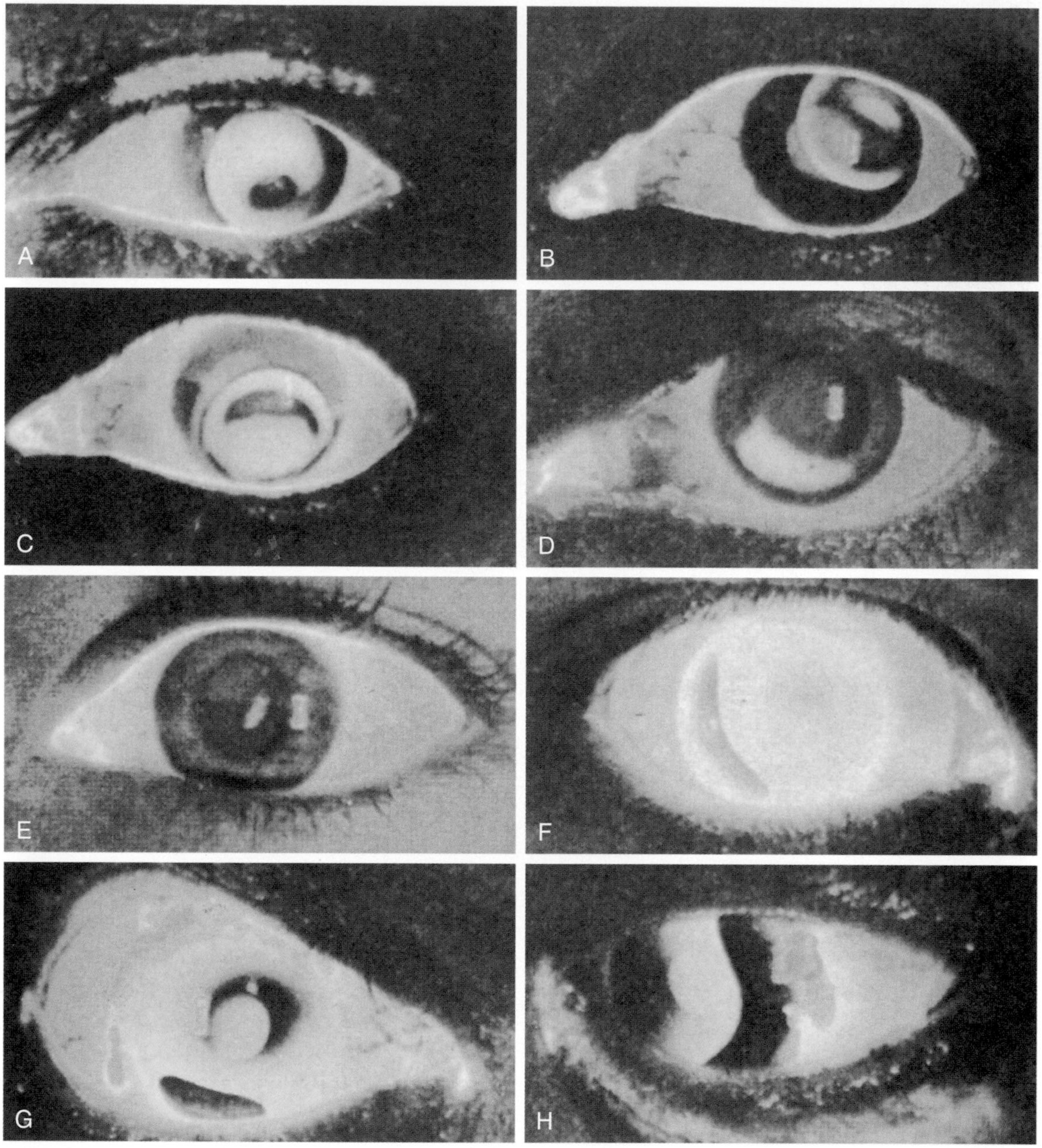

Fig. 14.31 Corneal lens. (A) Keratoconus. A hard touch in the area of the cone, lifting off the lens in other areas. (B) Keratoconus, a thin, small lens fitted to the flattest keratometry reading. This lens proved satisfactory. (C) Same case as in (B) with the lens in a lower position, showing a completely different fluorescein pattern. (D) Asymptomatic corneal stain of a superficial punctate type, 6 days after cessation of corneal lens wear. (E) Transient crescentic staining of a granular of punctate type with a corneal lens, differing from that resulting from central corneal edema and not giving rise to any serious complications. Scleral lens. (F) Normal eye, scleral lens. There is a light corneal touch with adequate limbal clearance and a sausage-shaped bubble associated with the fenestration. (G) Central corneal touch. Poor limbal clearance. (H) Nasal corneal touch and enlargement of the bubble on adduction. (A–H, Reproduced with permission from Duke-Elder S, Abrams D, eds. *System of Ophthalmology, Vol 5: Ophthalmic Optics and Refraction*. St Louis: Mosby; 1970.)

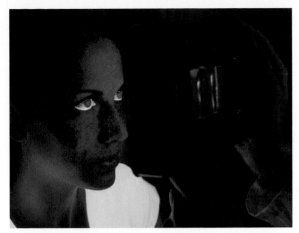

Fig. 14.32 Burton lamp used to evaluate fit of contact lens.

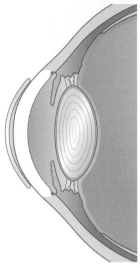

Fig. 14.35 Tight lens: base curve is too steep. (From Stein HA, Slatt BJ, Stein RM, Freeman MI. *Fitting Guide for Rigid and Soft Contact Lenses: A Practical Approach*. 4th ed. St Louis: Mosby; 2002.)

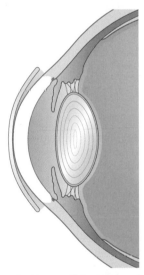

Fig. 14.33 Flat contact lens resting on apex of cornea.

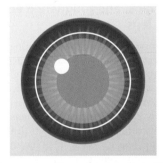

Fig. 14.36 Fluorescein pattern of a steep lens. Note absence of dye at the periphery as a result of marginal touch.

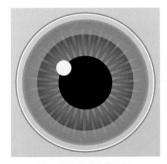

Fig. 14.34 Fluorescein pattern of a flat lens. Note absence of dye centrally.

peripheral portion of the cornea (Fig. 14.35). Peripheral contact tends to cause central pooling of the dye, with a ring of touch marginally (Fig. 14.36).

Alteration of the blink rate

Blinking properly is an important factor in the successful wearing of a contact lens. With blinking there is an interchange of tears between the contact lens and the cornea, thereby bringing fresh oxygen and nutrients to the cornea. As tears are produced, they form a small ring around the lid margins. When the lids close, as occurs in blinking, they act like a windshield wiper and sweep the tears over the cornea. When a contact lens is worn, the lids move the lens and a new precorneal tear film is produced, which interchanges with the existing tear film.

A patient whose lenses fit comfortably blinks normally, is free of squinting, and shifts gaze in a normal manner. If excessive blinking develops, it is usually in response to a lens that has excessive movement. Normally the lens makes a small, quick excursion upward with the blink and then gently falls. A loose lens is generally indicative of a flat lens–cornea relationship. A loose lens slides more easily off center and the patient begins to blink excessively trying to recenter the lens.

If the blink rate is reduced and the patient is given to staring, the contact lens may be irritating the eyelid. By opening the eyes wide and controlling the blink rate, the patient avoids the unpleasant contact of the superior margin of the contact lens and the upper lid. The nonblinker may show a reduction in the blink rate from the normal of 12 times a minute, or once every 3 or 4 seconds, to 3 or 4 times a minute.

Changes in the blink rate often occur because of awareness of the contact lens and persist despite a perfect contact lens fit. To avoid this habit, many fitters advocate blinking exercises. The patient is asked to fixate on a distant object and perform voluntary closures of the lid until the lid awareness diminishes in intensity.

Scratches, chips, and roughened edges of the contact lens

Scratches may occur from incorrect handling of the contact lens. If the scratches are central and numerous, they can cause scattering of light and a diminution of visual acuity. Chips and roughened edges may cause erosion of the corneal epithelium by scratching it. Roughened edges may be caused by incorrect cleansing of the lens if the normal secretions and sediment are allowed to collect and dry at the margin of the lens. A contact lens should be examined under magnification to ensure that the lens is free of surface defects and adherent deposits.

Changes in the cornea

Alteration of the surface of the cornea occurs either in the form of diffuse or localized corneal edema or in the form of erosion of the epithelium. Corneal edema results if the contact lens fits so tightly against the cornea that the surface epithelium cannot breathe or become oxygenated. Depriving the cornea of oxygen interferes with its metabolism, which in turn causes the formation of edema. The factors that cause corneal edema are: (1) a flat lens, which causes compression of the apex of the cornea; (2) a steep lens, which causes stagnation of tears; (3) a poorly centered lens, which causes pressure in one area; (4) incorrect blinking; and (5) incorrect cleansing of the lens.

Patients complaining of spectacle blur or photophobia that persists beyond the first week or two should be examined for edema. On retroillumination, the edema will

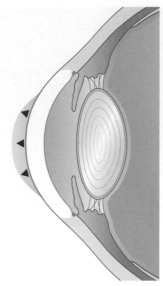

Fig. 14.37 The rigid lens produces a discrete type of corneal edema, confined to the corneal cap, which does cause spectacle blur because it produces a radical steepening of the corneal curvature. (From Stein HA, Slatt BJ, Stein RM, Freeman MI. *Fitting Guide for Rigid and Soft Contact Lenses: A Practical Approach*. 4th ed. St Louis: Mosby; 2002.)

appear as a smoky area in the center third of the cornea. Another method of detecting edema is by keratometry (follow-up K readings). Edema often produces K readings higher than those originally found (Fig. 14.37).

During the adaptation period, edema is almost inevitable. It should not, however, be present after 2 or 3 weeks. If edema persists, it will be accompanied by subjective complaints of photophobia, burning smokiness, and spectacle blur. The usual cause of edema is a tight lens resulting from too steep a base curve. However, the peripheral curve may be too shallow or poorly blended, or the lens may be too large.

Erosions of the corneal epithelium may occur because of the incarceration of tiny foreign bodies between cornea and lens. They are visible as slightly depressed spots that tend to take up the fluorescein stain (Fig. 14.38). Other causes of corneal erosions, or punctate staining, of the cornea are: (1) a chipped or roughened edge, (2) flat peripheral curves, (3) a flat lens, (4) incorrect recentering of a lens, (5) poor insertion and removal techniques, (6) dust or other particles under the lens, and (7) overwearing of lenses.

Corneal edema has become much rarer owing to the development of high-DK GP materials. A patient with corneal edema will complain of blurred vision or veiled vision. In punctate staining, the most common symptom is a foreign body sensation of the eyes either during contact

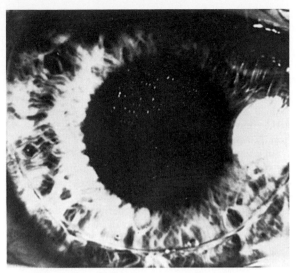

Fig. 14.38 Punctate staining of the cornea. (Courtesy Dr. J. Dixon.)

lens wear or after the lens has been removed. If a patient continues to wear contact lenses despite signs and symptoms of a punctate keratitis, he or she can easily develop a corneal scratch or abrasion or, eventually, a corneal ulcer. The occurrence of corneal erosions requires immediate removal of the contact lens and reevaluation of the fit.

Adjustments

The most common problems with contact lenses are that they are either too loose or too tight. If the lens is too loose, it may be redesigned to provide greater adherence to the cornea by:

1. Increasing the optic zone diameter
2. Increasing the overall diameter of the lens
3. Decreasing the radius of the optic zone (mm)
4. Decreasing the radius of the intermediate or peripheral curve (mm)

All modifications that produce a tighter-fitting lens require the manufacture of a new lens. A lens can always be adjusted to fit more loosely, but never more tightly. Note that some newer materials do not allow for in-office adjustment.

Problems associated with overwearing contact lenses

Moderate to severe pain, lid edema, lacrimation, and marked photophobia can occur if contact lenses are worn for too long. These symptoms usually occur if the patient has been too ambitious in the early adaptive period in trying to prolong the wearing time. They may occur as a result of carelessness, as typified by the person who falls asleep while wearing contact lenses. The pain usually occurs 2 to 3 hours after the lenses have been removed and is intense. The patient is usually very agitated and in such distress that examination of the cornea can be made only after local anesthetic drops have been instilled in the eye. The cornea shows diffuse erosions over its apex and stains intensely with fluorescein. This condition usually responds to patching of the eye. Within 24 hours the surface of the cornea is usually clear.

Acute hypoxia of the cornea was a common event with PMMA lenses, but is a rare occurrence with any of the GP lenses. Most of the hazards of insufficient oxygen to the cornea, whether acute or chronic, have been eliminated with GP lenses and, with the newer type of these lenses, extended wear for varying periods is a reality. The oxygenation of the cornea under the closed lid is sufficient to sustain metabolism despite the presence of a contact lens.

Uses

The popular thought regarding the use of contact lenses is that they are of value only for cosmetic purposes. It is true that many patients experience a tremendous psychologic emancipation when freed from the burden of heavy, thick, and unsightly glasses, but this is not their primary function. Contact lenses are a wonderful visual aid that can provide vision unobtainable by any other means. They are of particular value to a patient with high myopia. Myopes constitute the largest group of contact lens wearers, probably because of their high degree of motivation.

Contact lenses offer a more normal image size because they are closer to the eye. Just as high-plus cataract spectacles magnify the image on the retina by virtue of lying in front of the eye with an air interspace, high-minus spectacles tend to minify the retinal image. When contact lenses are used for myopia, the retinal image is more normal, enlarging about 10% for a −6.00 diopter lens and much more for a higher-minus lens. Therefore contact lenses result in a retinal image of more normal size and better visual acuity. They allow an unrestricted field of view because the lenses move with the eyes and the appearance is like that of unaided vision.

RGP contact lenses also treat irregular astigmatism caused by corneal scarring.

Hyperopic patients form a small portion of those desiring contact lenses because a far-sighted person needs a comparatively low-powered lens and can usually obtain satisfactory distance vision without glasses.

The patient who has had cataracts removed suffers the same visual disabilities as the high myope and therefore enjoys the same advantages with contact lenses, such as freedom from the weight of heavy glasses, a wider range of field of vision, and a more natural-appearing image. For the aphakic or postcataract patient, spectacles enlarge the image by 33%. With contact lenses, there is a restoration to a more normal image size because the contact lens reduces the magnification to only 7%. In addition, the aphakic individual suffers from many aberrations while looking through the periphery of the spectacle lens. With contact lenses, distortion never occurs because the lens moves with the eye and vision is always obtained through the central portion of the lens.

Nowadays, intraocular lenses are inserted after all cataract removal operations. For patients who had the procedure performed before the advent of intraocular lenses, contact lenses offer restored normal vision. Contacts may make the image size approximately the same size as the image seen by the fellow eye, or at the very least only slightly larger.

Contact lenses have also been used for children who have undergone surgery for congenital or traumatic cataract.

Keratoconus is a developmental anomaly of the cornea, which is characterized by progressive thinning and an apical bulge of the central portion of the cornea (Fig. 14.39). This condition results in irregular myopic astigmatism that cannot be corrected by glasses. Contact lenses mask the corneal irregularity, flattens, and possibly stabilize the condition, and, by virtue of the fluid interface between the contact lens and the cornea, eliminate irregular astigmatism and permit clear vision.

For repeat laser treatment the cornea may be too thin. Following laser surgery, a condition of keractesia may have developed and the only option may be glasses or a contact lens. This condition is an excellent indication for contact lenses. Keractesia is an induced form of thinning of the cornea may be too thin for crosslinking. The only option may be glasses or an RGP contact lens.

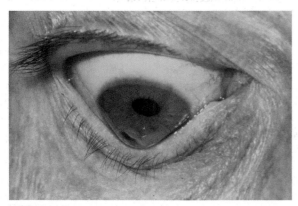

Fig. 14.39 An advanced case of keratoconus.

Besides correcting refractive errors, contact lenses may be used to cover unsightly eyes. In these cases, the contact lens is colored to disguise disfiguring features of the eye.

Contact lenses also have been useful in treating patients with nystagmus. In these cases, vision is improved because the correcting lens moves with the eye. Another use for contact lenses is for a patient with congenital albinism. A small pupillary opening is provided and a collarette of darkly tinted soft lens is produced to protect the patient from excessive glare.

An interesting field of research is under way to investigate the potential of GP lenses for reducing myopia progression (peripheral blur hypothesis). If these studies result in valid scientific evidence, the use of such lenses in young people may become standard practice, in particular in those Asian countries that have a very high rate of myopia.

In orthokeratology, RGP lenses with flat base curve are used overnight to reshape the cornea. The reshaped flat cornea remains during most of the day and therefore 3 to 4 diopter of myopia is corrected temporarily. In this method a series of two to three pairs lenses over a period of time are used until the desired flat corneal shape is maintained. This vision treatment will be maintained by constant overnight use of the lenses.

Many professional people, including actors, politicians, and public speakers, wear contact lenses to improve their appearance before the public. Professional athletes, such as hockey players and football players can participate in competitive sports only by being free of the encumbrance and hazard of spectacles. Among athletes, however, soft contact lenses may be the wiser choice because they are less likely to be lost than are rigid lenses.

Summary

One of the major concerns with contact lenses is education of the contact lens patient. Each patient should be instructed about the symptoms that can be expected and tolerated and those that are danger signals and indicate immediate consultation. Also each patient should be shown the methods of handling the lenses, their insertion and removal, and their storage and hygiene.

Each phase in the adaptation period should be clearly outlined to the patient. The patient must be given an orderly schedule to follow and a routine to perform.

The patient also should be told the function that the contact lens will perform. This function may be optical, therapeutic, or cosmetic. The wearing of contact lenses demands the payment of a price, in attention, care, and finances. The patient should know the benefits and be aware of the hazards.

Questions for review and thought

1. Name factors that contraindicate the wearing of rigid contact lenses.
2. List the advantages and disadvantages of corneal rigid contact lenses.
3. What holds a contact lens in place?
4. What are the characteristics of the plastic used in rigid lens manufacture?
5. Outline a method of evaluating a patient before prescribing contact lenses.
6. The keratometer is an important instrument in evaluating the anterior corneal curvature. Outline a method of performing keratometry.
7. How can you verify the diameter of a contact lens? The radius?
8. Given a patient with $-2.75 + 0.75 \times 90$ and K readings of $43.50 \times 44.50 \times 90$, with normal lid and pupillary opening, how would you compute a possible type of rigid lens for initial trial?
9. What effect would contact lenses have on the visual field of a patient with a -6.00 diopter lens?
10. Describe spectacle blur and its causes.
11. Describe how you would instruct a patient to clean and insert contact lenses.
12. Describe three methods of instructing the patient in lens removal.
13. What is the value of a wetting solution? Name several that are available.
14. What is the value of a lens cleaner? Name several that are available.
15. What are the advantages of using a trial set in contact lens fitting?
16. What is the importance of blinking?
17. What causes corneal edema after wearing of contact lenses?
18. How can a lens be adjusted that is too tight? Too loose?
19. Contact lenses are frequently used for cosmetic or refractive purposes. However, after cataract surgery they aid considerably in overall vision. Why?
20. What is your routine wearing schedule for rigid lenses?
21. What symptoms may be attributed to a loose lens and to a tight lens?
22. List the features of a contact lens that can be modified without making a new lens.

Self-evaluation questions **Q**

True–false statements

Directions: Indicate whether the statement is true **(T)** or false **(F)**.

1. The keratometer is an instrument that is used to measure the radius of curvature of the front surface of the cornea. **T** or **F**
2. If the keratometer measurements show a difference in dioptric power from one meridian to the opposite meridian, then irregular astigmatism exists. **T** or **F**
3. With fluorescein staining, if a dark area appears centrally, then the corneal lens is considered too steep. **T** or **F**

Missing words

Directions: Write in the missing word in the following sentences:

4. With-the-rule astigmatism is present when the horizontal meridian is _____ than the vertical meridian.
5. The optic cap is the _____ zone of the cornea.
6. The power of a rigid contact lens may be measured by an instrument called the _____.

Choice-completion questions

Directions: Select the one best answer in each case.

7. Defects in lens material or edge design may be identified by which piece of equipment?
   a. Radiuscope
   b. Shadowgraph
   c. Lensmeter
   d. Keratometer
   e. Profile analyzer
8. A rigid lens that is too loose may result in:
   a. spectacle blur.
   b. burning sensation.
   c. blurring of vision after blinking.
   d. night blindness.
   e. pain after lens removal.
9. Fluorescein patterns may be most helpful in identifying a poorly fitting lens. A lens that shows a large dark central area with an absence of fluorescein is indicative of:
   a. a normal fit.
   b. a steep lens.
   c. a flat lens.
   d. incorrect fenestration of the lens.
   e. none of the above.

Answers, notes, and explanations

A

1. **True**. The keratometer measures the front surface of the cornea, which acts as a convex mirror reflecting the mires or images of the keratometer. The keratometer measures only a very limited circular area of the cornea, approximately 2 to 4 mm apart, depending on the manufacturer of the keratometer. The keratometer makes an assumption as to the index of refraction of the cornea.

2. **False**. If the dioptric power from one meridian to the opposite meridian is different, then regular astigmatism is said to exist and the difference in diopters between the two meridians indicates the amount of corneal astigmatism present. When irregular astigmatism exists, the mires are distorted and it is difficult to obtain satisfactory reflecting images from the cornea. Such conditions as keratoconus and scars of the cornea produce irregular astigmatism.

3. **False**. The dark area indicates that there is no fluorescein pattern centrally, which signifies that the lens is touching the central portion of the cornea. This exists when the lens base curve is flatter than the curvature of the cornea so that the central portion of the lens rests on the central portion of the cornea and prevents the dye from entering the center and pooling centrally.

4. **Flatter**. The eye is shaped in some ways like a football whose long axis is positioned horizontally in the palpebral fissures so that the steeper meridian is vertical and the flatter meridian is horizontal. This is known as with-the-rule astigmatism. When this occurs in the opposite direction, it is considered against-the-rule astigmatism.

5. **Central**. The optic cap lies in the central 5 to 7 mm of the cornea, which involves the visual axis of the cornea. This is the area that should be measured with the keratometer in determining the central corneal radius of curvature. This is the area that becomes involved when a rigid contact lens is overworn and edema results, causing fogginess of vision.

6. **Lensmeter**. By holding a rigid contact lens between the thumb and forefinger or letting it rest concave side down, the examiner may measure the back vertex power of a contact lens. The lens should always be placed so that the concavity of the lens lies toward the instrument so that the back power is measured. This is of minor significance in low powers, but in high minus or high plus powers, it may become significant.

7. **b. Shadowgraph**. The Shadowgraph is a type of magnifier and projector that permits the examiner to check the details of the lens material and edge design for chips, roughness, or sharpness. Important features such as sharpness or roughness of a rigid lens may be fundamental to the comfortable wearing of rigid contact lenses. It is the edge design, which must ride against and under the eyelid, that tends to produce the lid awareness of a contact lens. The surface quality of the lens, as well as defects in material can be identified with the magnification of the Shadowgraph instrument.

8. **c. Blurring of vision after blinking**. A loose lens will often decenter after a person blinks and will ride either to the side or low, resulting in poor vision and fluctuating vision. Burning sensations are a result of hypoxia that develops from stagnation brought on by the accumulation of metabolites centrally from a steep lens that does not permit adequate venting and exchange of tear film. This is a tight lens symptom. Spectacle blur is a result of hypoxia with edema that develops in the central portion of the cornea and is usually a result of either overwear of a contact lens or a tight lens that does not permit adequate tear exchange. Pain following lens removal is also a symptom that there has been corneal hypoxia or complete anoxia brought on by incorrect venting or tear exchange and indicates a tight lens rather than a loose lens.

9. **c. A flat lens**. The absence of fluorescein is indicative that the lens is touching the apex of the cornea so that fluorescein does not intervene between the lens and the cornea. This central touch may cause warpage of the cornea with compression changes on the surface of the cornea. If the lens is too flat, it may rock and usually decenters. Also there may be a flattening of the cornea and an undesirable type of reduction of myopia at the expense of possible permanent structural changes in the cornea. The principle of orthokeratology is to provide very slight changes by central touch so that small degrees of astigmatism can be reduced on a regular basis in this manner. This, however, may result in irregular flattening of the cornea by compression, with resulting induced irregular astigmatism.

Chapter | 15 |

Soft contact lenses

There are approximately 90 million contact wearers worldwide. In the United States alone, data indicate that approximately 13% of the population (>36 million) use contact lenses for vision correction and it is estimated that the United States represents approximately 40% of the number of wearers worldwide. Most contact lens wearers also own a pair or two of spectacles. Data indicate that in 2015, the number of spectacle units (number of eyeglasses manufactured) worldwide was approximately 3.5 billion.

The soft lenses rival rigid lenses in their quality of vision and surpass them in the realm of comfort and ease of adaptation (Fig. 15.1). The two basic types of soft lenses are the hydrogel (hydrophilic) lens, which owes its softness to its ability to absorb and bind water to its structure, and the silicone hydrogel lens, which owes its softness to the intrinsic property of the rubbery material.

History of hydrophilic lenses

In 1960 two young New York lawyers established a company with the unique function of promoting patent exchanges among corporations. Their specialty was combing through the dusty corporate files for idle patents and setting up licensing agreements with other companies interested in putting the dormant ideas to use. In 1965 the men who had established the National Patent Development Corporation suddenly dissolved their patent law business. They had uncovered a patent with so many exciting possibilities that they decided to pick up a license themselves. In effect, they became their own client, eliminating their role as middlemen.

The new material was a plastic that they called hydron. It was developed by Dr. Otto Wichterle, head of the Institute of Macromolecular Chemistry of the Czechoslovakian National Academy of Science and a leading expert on polymer chemistry, and by Dr. Drahoslav Lim. The new material appeared to be like other plastics in that it was a hard transparent substance that could be cut, ground, or molded into a variety of shapes. When placed in water or an aqueous solution, however, the tough, rigid plastic became soft and pliable. In this wet form, it could be bent between the fingers until the edges met or could be turned easily inside

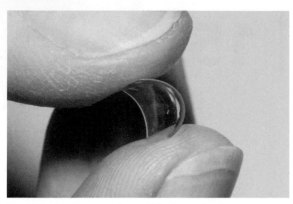

Fig. 15.1 A soft contact lens will fold completely.

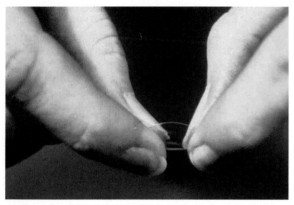

Fig. 15.2 The soft lens is sturdy despite its flexible quality. It can be stretched, dried, or crumpled and still retain its integrity.

out, yet it would snap back into its original shape quickly. When allowed to dry, the supple waterlogged material became as dry as a cornflake and crushed to a powdery dust if smashed. The substance was subjected to rigorous biologic tests and was found to be inert and fully compatible with human tissue. One of its properties was that although highly elastic when wet, it remained strong and able to hold its shape (Fig. 15.2).

The plastic is hydroxyethyl methacrylate (HEMA), a plastic polymer with the remarkable ability to absorb water molecules. Chemically, the polymer consists of a three-dimensional network of HEMA chains crosslinked with ethylene glycol dimethacrylate molecules about once every 200 monomer units. As the water is introduced to the plastic, it swells into a soft mass with surprisingly good mechanical strength, complete transparency (97%), and the ability to retain its shape and dimensions.

Five vigorous years of improvements and clinical trials were conducted on the soft lens before the U.S. Food and Drug Administration (FDA; which considered the lens a drug) approved the lens as a safe prosthetic device of good optical quality. The FDA's caution, after the thalidomide tragedies in which a drug produced severe deformities in the babies of pregnant women, was understandable. Both the public and the practitioner needed protection. In the first phase of research, the soft lens was tested with laboratory animals to ensure that it was nontoxic; later it was given to selected practitioners and independent research workers for clinical trials on human beings.

It soon became apparent that the soft lens was an innovation of major importance, with widespread application not only as an instrument for treating diseased corneas, but also as a superior contact lens. In the early stages, however, the therapeutic possibilities of soft lenses overshadowed any other consideration because it appeared that these lenses would replace many conventional treatments of external diseases of the eye.

As the number of contact lens companies throughout the world expanded, a search for newer and better lens plastics and lens designs developed. Many modifications were made as new monomers were discovered and crosslinked to create differing polymers; polyvinyl pyrrolidone (PVP) was added to increase oxygen permeability, and methyl methacrylate (MMA) to create more stiffness to aid in handling ease. Non-HEMA hydrogel polymers were introduced.

Research activity was also directed toward lens designs to correct astigmatism, bifocal corrections, and tinted lenses for cosmetic appearance, as well as therapeutic application. Ultrathin and higher-water-content lenses have opened up significant new areas in contact lens development, with increased success rates. In the manufacturing arena, the emphasis is on automated computer-driven systems and advanced molding processes.

The most recent developments have been the addition of ultraviolet-screening agents to soft polymers and the amplification of the concept of biomimesis. *Biomimesis* is defined as the ability to create or mimic biologic surfaces. Various approaches have been tried to improve the biocompatibility of materials for use in the human body. The surface properties of foreign materials play a critical role in triggering a biologic response and initiate undesirable and unwanted interactions with proteins and other biomolecules at the material surface. The formation of blood clots on surface materials, dental plaque buildup, and contact lens deposits are examples of the same phenomenon. A synthesized phosphorylcholine added to soft lens material to promote biocompatibility has produced the Proclear lens from CooperVision. Current soft lens research aims to produce a contact lens that replicates the tears in the human eye. Materials with water content as high as 92% are under investigation.

With the proliferation of soft materials, it became necessary to classify lenses in several ways. Classification by water content means that the soft lens contains that percentage of water, for example, low water content (37.5%–45%), medium water content (46%–58%), and high water content (59%–92%). The FDA classifies lenses into four basic groups based on water content and ionicity for the purpose of evaluating disinfecting systems with different lens material groups. With the development of new high-DK materials, a fifth classification group is being considered. The process used to manufacture a soft lens is another method of classification. Lenses may be spin cast, lathe cut, or cast molded; 90% of soft lens production in the world today uses the cast-molded method. Finally, soft contact lenses may be classified by design or function (e.g., daily wear, flexible wear, extended wear, or continuous wear).

Silicone hydrogel lenses with higher oxygen permeabilities are the latest development in soft contact lens material (Boxes 15.1 and 15.2).

Advantages

The advantages of hydrophilic contact lenses are as follows:
1. Comfort
2. Rapid adaptation
3. Lack of spectacle blur
4. Disposability
5. Minimal lens loss
6. Minimal overwear reaction
7. Lack of glare and photophobia
8. Difficulty in dislodging
9. Protection of entire cornea
10. Attractive alternative for rigid lens dropouts
11. No serious corneal abrasion on insertion

Comfort

These lenses are exceptionally comfortable from the initial period. It is impressive to witness the rapid tolerance of the cornea to the presence of the contact lens. The lack of awareness of a soft lens is caused partly by the flaccidity, water content, and thin edges of the lens, which mold to the white of the eye (the sclera). Therefore there is almost no interference from the upper lids during normal blinking. The lens hugs the eye so closely that the advancing surface of the eyelid just glides over it (Fig. 15.3). Its supple quality when wet also contributes to the easy acceptance of the soft lens. Being hydrophilic, or water-loving, it forms a cushioned fluid buffer between itself and the cornea. It also contours itself to the unique shape of the individual cornea. With no hard edges to irritate the eyelid edge and no rigid structure to compress delicate living tissue, there are minimal frictional erosions. Because of its soft qualities,

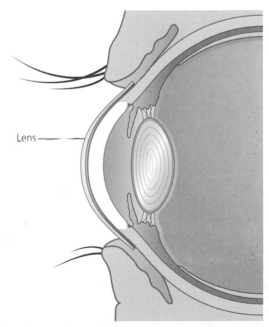

Lens

Fig. 15.3 The soft lens fits under the eyelid margins and the advancing lid edge just glides over its surface. This accounts for part of its comfort factor. (From Stein HA, Slatt BJ, Stein RM, et al. *Fitting Guide for Rigid and Soft Contact Lenses: A Practical Approach.* 4th ed. St Louis: Mosby; 2002.)

a normal tear exchange takes place by diffusion through the lens matrix and under the lens.

A rigid lens has to be fitted according to the precise shape of the cornea. If the fit is poor, or if the laboratory does not make the lens according to exact specifications, a rigid lens will irritate the eye. A soft lens is more flexible on the eye. A wide latitude is possible without corneal injury and less exacting measurements are required.

Rapid adaptation

Tolerance is extremely high compared with that of the rigid lens. The lenses are frequently comfortable to a new patient within 30 minutes. Wearing schedules can be easily increased to full-time day wear within 10 days.

Lack of spectacle blur

Removal of the lenses permits patients to switch directly to their glasses within 5 to 10 minutes without the spectacle blur that occurs with edema induced by polymethyl methacrylate (PMMA) rigid lenses. Spectacle blur is uncommon because of the diffuse nature of any edema, which spreads evenly over the cornea and does not alter its radius (Fig. 15.4).

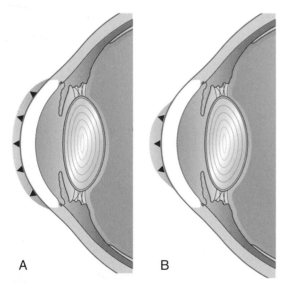

A   B

Fig. 15.4 (A) The soft lens produces a diffuse area of corneal edema that does not alter the radius of curvature of the cornea and does not cause spectacle blur. (B) A low-DK hard lens produces a discrete type of corneal edema, confined to the corneal cap, which does cause spectacle blur because it produces a radical steepening of the corneal curvature. (From Stein HA, Slatt BJ, Stein RM, et al. *Fitting Guide for Rigid and Soft Contact Lenses: A Practical Approach*. 4th ed. St Louis: Mosby; 2002.)

Disposability

Soft lenses may be replaced on a disposable regimen, for example, replaced daily, weekly, or biweekly, reducing patient discomfort and risk of infection. Soft lenses replaced on a disposable regimen are ideal for occasional or intermittent wear.

Minimal lens loss

With new patients, rigid lenses are sometimes lost in the first 3 months, when handling is still somewhat clumsy. Rigid lenses also dislodge with aggressive sports activities. The technique for removal of a soft lens is such that loss is less frequent than with a rigid lens. The larger size of the soft lens, coupled with the firm adherence of the lens to the cornea with minimal sliding effect, reduces the loss factor considerably. It is rare for a patient to report the loss of a soft lens (Fig. 15.5). The lenses do not fall out.

Minimal overwear reaction

Every ophthalmologist remembers cases of the overwear syndrome experienced by the old PMMA rigid lens wearer, who appeared at the hospital emergency room in the middle of the night with excruciating pain, having worn these lenses longer than the normal time limit. This problem is virtually eliminated with the soft lens. In older low-DK soft lens material, 2% of patients reported slight corneal edema with halos about lights and a burning sensation of their eyes. At the end of the day, no serious disabling disorder has occurred. The edema effect was further reduced by the advent of materials with greater oxygen permeability.

Oxygen is carried to the cornea through the tear film and is replenished through the circulation of tears under the lens and diffusion through the lens. This is the same method by which the cornea receives its oxygen supply under a rigid lens. The evidence of a good tear layer between the soft lens and the cornea has been demonstrated by a French ophthalmologist, Dr. Paul Cochet, who showed spherical particles 1 to 3 μm in diameter passing underneath the lens. When the tear layer has been stained, it has been shown to ripple with the blinking motions of the lids. The respiration of the cornea is provided by tear exchange during blinking.

Lack of glare and photophobia

Glare and light sensitivity are seen almost routinely in the early weeks of rigid lens wear. These symptoms are virtually absent with the soft lens, making it the ideal lens for outdoor athletes, such as golfers and tennis players. Also

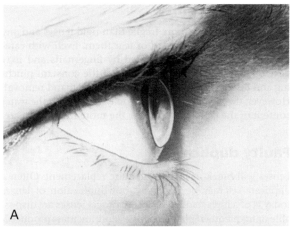

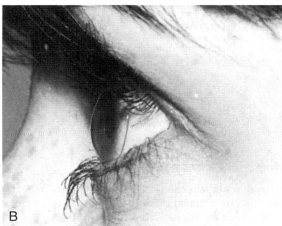

Fig. 15.5 Comparison of hard and soft lenses. (A) The hard lens is smaller than the cornea and can be easily dislodged with the edge of the lid. (B) The soft lens is larger than the cornea, hugs the eye tightly, and seldom is displaced even during body contact sports.

the generous size of the optic zone means that the pupil is always covered; this minimizes glare.

Difficulty in dislodging

The firm adherence of the soft lens to the eye permits it to be used in body contact sports and reduces embarrassment associated with dislodgment (Fig. 15.6).

Protection of entire cornea

Hydrophilic lenses cover the entire cornea. They can be used to reduce corneal exposure for such conditions as facial paralysis and corneal insensitivity (Fig. 15.7). In this sense, these lenses are used as bandage lenses for entropion, trichiasis, dry eye, and corneal dystrophies.

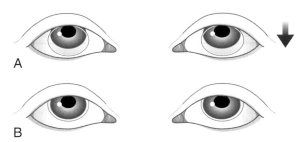

Fig. 15.6 (A) With rigid lenses, the lenses drop when the tennis player moves his eye up to hit the ball. (B) Soft lenses move with the eye and show only minimal lag; thus they are an ideal sports lens. (From Stein HA, Slatt BJ, Stein RM, et al. *Fitting Guide for Rigid and Soft Contact Lenses: A Practical Approach.* 4th ed. St Louis: Mosby; 2002.)

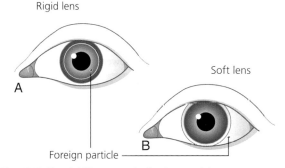

Fig. 15.7 The rigid lens permits foreign particles to enter under the lens, whereas the soft lens tends to prevent the entry of foreign bodies under it by its scleral impingement and minimal movement. (A) Foreign body under rigid gas-permeable (RGP) lens. (B) Soft lens prevents foreign bodies from getting under. (From Stein HA, Slatt BJ, Stein RM, et al. *Fitting Guide for Rigid and Soft Contact Lenses: A Practical Approach.* 4th ed. St Louis: Mosby; 2002.)

Attractive alternative for rigid lens drop-outs

A significant percentage of rigid lens patients are unable to persist in wearing their lenses. This intolerance may be the result of dryness as a result of pregnancy, birth control pills, allergies, or a change of environment. Most of these patients readily accept soft lenses and are able to wear them comfortably.

No serious corneal abrasion on insertion

In the rigid lens, incorrect insertion can cause an abrasion of the cornea. This does not occur with the soft lens because of its soft nature.

Cosmetic lenses

Colored and opaque hydrogel lenses to enhance or change eye color have been available since the 1980s.

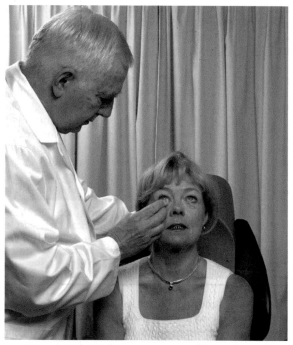

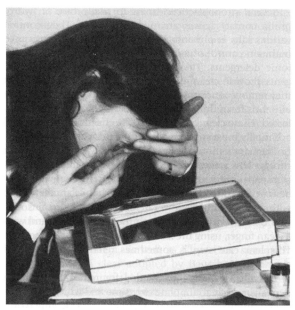

Fig. 15.23 A large mirror is a helpful adjunct in inserting a lens. (From Stein HA, Slatt BJ, Stein RM, et al. *Fitting Guide for Rigid and Soft Contact Lenses: A Practical Approach*. 4th ed. St Louis: Mosby; 2002.)

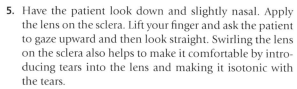

Fig. 15.22 Insertion of contact lens by the practitioner. The middle finger retracts the lower lid while the contact lens is gently rolled into the lower conjunctiva.

5. Have the patient look down and slightly nasal. Apply the lens on the sclera. Lift your finger and ask the patient to gaze upward and then look straight. Swirling the lens on the sclera also helps to make it comfortable by introducing tears into the lens and making it isotonic with the tears.
6. Have the patient close the eyes and lightly massage the lid to help center the lens.
7. Repeat the same procedure for the left lens.

Removal by the fitter

The following technique is used for lens removal by the fitter:
1. Wash the hands before removal, as was done for insertion.
2. Be sure the lens is on the cornea and freely moving before attempting removal.
3. Have the patient look up. Place the middle finger on the lower lid and touch the edge of the lens with the forefinger.
4. While the patient is looking up, slide the lens down onto the white of the eye. Bring the thumb over and compress the lens lightly between the thumb and index finger so that the lens folds and comes off easily.

Insertion by the patient

Careful patient instruction in the care and handling of soft contact lenses is frequently left to the ophthalmic assistant. It is important that the patient understand the procedure and care system and comply with it. Failure to comply with instruction is the greatest single cause of difficulties with well-fitted soft contact lenses.

The following technique is used for lens insertion by the patient. For beginners, a large mirror is helpful (Fig. 15.23).
1. Keep the nails short and carefully wash and dry the hands.
2. Take the right lens out of the vial either with forceps or by pouring the contents of the vial into the palm of the hand.
3. Rinse the lens with normal saline solution.
4. Place the lens on the tip of the index finger of the dominant hand. With thin lenses, permit the lens to dehydrate for 1 to 2 minutes in air and dry finger.
5. Look at the mirror, retract the lower eyelid with the middle finger, apply the lens on the eyeball.
6. Express any air, remove the index finger, and then slowly release the lower lid.
7. Close the eyes and gently massage the lids to help center the lens (Fig. 15.24).

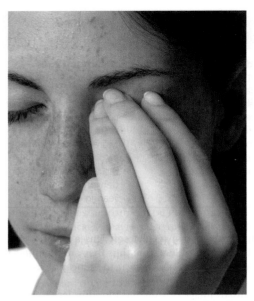

Fig. 15.24 Centering the lens through the closed eyelid.

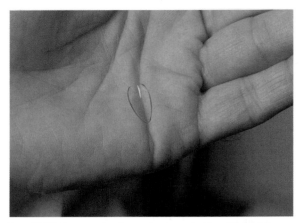

Fig. 15.25 Taco test to determine correct side of the lens.

the correct position. If the edge appears to fold back in the fingers, the lens is everted and must be reversed. For new ultrathin lenses the taco test may not be valid, however.

Removal by the patient

The following technique is used for lens removal by the patient:

1. Check vision in each eye separately to be sure the lens is in place on the cornea.
2. Wash hands and rinse thoroughly.
3. Look upward. Retract the lower lid with the middle finger and place the index fingertip on the lower edge of the lens.
4. Slide the lens down to the white of the eye.
5. Compress the lens between the thumb and index finger so that air breaks the suction under the lens. Remove the lens from the eye.
6. Prepare the lens for cleaning and sterilizing according to the recommendations of the manufacturer and the practitioner.
7. An alternative method of removal is to look nasally and slide the lens to the outermost portion of the eye before removal.

Taco test

If there is any question of whether the lens is inside out, the "taco test" should be performed (Fig. 15.25). In this test, the lens is flexed between the forefinger and thumb. If the edges are erect and point inward like a taco, the lens is in

Precautions for wear

1. Do not insert lenses if eyes are red or irritated.
2. Do not use tap water, distilled water, or spring water directly in the eye; always use commercially manufactured saline solution.
3. Do not use any solutions with contact lenses other than those specifically recommended.
4. If the lens becomes uncomfortable when first inserted or while wearing, or if vision becomes blurred, foreign material may be present on the inside surface of the lens. The lens should be immediately removed, cleaned, rinsed, and reinserted.
5. Lenses should not be worn in the presence of irritating fumes or vapors.
6. Lenses should not be worn overnight unless specifically advised.
7. If the lens is difficult to remove or difficult to slide down, place a comfort drop (lubricating drop) or two on the eye or a few drops of commercially manufactured normal saline solution. The lens should soon once again move freely and be easily removable.
8. If vision is blurred while wearing the lens, consider the possibility that the lens may be inside out, off center, or not clean, or that the right and left lenses have been switched.
9. If the lens is left exposed to air, it will dry out and become hard and brittle. Should this occur, handle it gently and place it in saline solution and it will again become soft and flexible.

lens. Thus each patient must have a trial fitting with a set of trial lenses, with markings that identify the position of the soft lens at all times. By using a soft lens as a diagnostic lens, the practitioner can incorporate correcting values to arrive at the final lens for incorporation of the cylindric power and axis.

Medical uses

A revolution has occurred in the treatment of corneal diseases by judicious use of soft contact lenses. A large number of patients who could not previously be helped can now use the soft contact lens, which can act as a bandage. It is not a panacea for all diseases but, if well fitted and used wisely with well-selected patients, contact lenses can be of inestimable value to promote healing and epithelial regeneration.

The soft lens acts by delicately covering the cornea and thereby protecting it. Its water-absorbing qualities keep the surface of the cornea moist and well lubricated under the agreeable protective shell. Soft lenses best used as a bandage are those that are extremely thin or those that have a high water content.

Bandage lenses can be used in a variety of medical and surgical situations. These include: (1) corneal dystrophies (e.g., bullous keratopathy); (2) corneal erosions (e.g., dry eye, trichiasis, entropion); and (3) after surgery (e.g., corneal graft, and postlaser photorefractive keratotomy [PRK]).

Blisters of cornea (bullous keratopathy)

Bullous keratopathy in its late stages is characterized by blind and excruciatingly painful eyes. In this condition, the cornea becomes swollen and the superficial layer of the epithelium is raised into convex mounds. Some of these corneal blisters rupture and, when they do so, there is a raw, burning feeling and often pain in the eyes, along with a marked reduction in visual acuity. The attendant scarring and irregularity of the cornea that follow the rupture of these blisters can, on a cumulative basis, cause permanent loss of vision. This condition is brought on not by lack of oxygen to the epithelium but by damage to the inside layer of the cornea, the endothelium, so that aqueous humor from the anterior chamber can percolate through the cornea.

The introduction of the soft therapeutic contact lens and its popularization by Dr. Herbert E. Kaufman revolutionized the treatment of the disease. A bandage lens is a safe, simple, nonsurgical method of relieving both the pain and the profound visual loss. It can be inserted in the office rather than an operating room. Its application does not require sophisticated surgical expertise and can therefore be performed by virtually every ophthalmologist or ophthalmic technician in any part of the world. Numerous reports in the ophthalmologic literature confirm that these lenses are well tolerated and can be worn continuously for prolonged periods on diseased corneas without adverse effects. In each case, the patient is comfortable and may experience improvement in vision as long as the lenses remain in place. For terribly scarred corneas, the only improvement is freedom from pain. Some patients become so frightened of possible reactivation of discomfort that they wear their soft contact lenses 24 hours a day for months without removal.

Fitting of the soft lens for bullous keratopathy is more challenging than fitting for refractive errors. A trial lens may be used. In many cases, it may be possible to use an inexpensive soft lens. A properly fitted lens has both central and peripheral contact so that it does not flex in the center with each blink. It may be necessary to fit the lens with minimal or no movement. Extra movement is painful because it erodes tissue under the lens. Because patients with bullous keratopathy wear soft lenses continuously, 24 hours per day, dehydration of the lenses is a concern. Daily lubricating drops are advised. Regular (monthly) replacement gives the best results and keeps the lens comfortable.

For aphakia, one can use a planolens to achieve the corneal change; once the cornea improves, however, the refractive power needs to be considered. In some cases, it is necessary to use medication, such as hypertonic saline 5%, along with the lens.

Corneal ulcers

An ulcer is a large defect in the tissues and its appearance on the cornea is viewed with alarm. If a corneal ulcer increases in size and grows deep, it can cause perforation of the cornea and a loss of the structures inside the eye, which can herniate through the defect. This usually means loss of the eye. The likelihood of such a contingency is quite real. Pressure within the eye itself can cause a perforation if there is a weakness of the coats of the eye, such as a thinning of the cornea or sclera. Furthermore, because the cornea is devoid of any blood vessels (a factor that aids in its transparency but prevents the successful mobilization of the body's resources to a damaged site), it is an extremely vulnerable organ. The cases in which soft lenses have been tried have been those in which antibiotics and pressure dressings have failed and the surgeon has had to perform corneal transplantation. The major cause of infection and corneal ulcers is poor hygiene. Dirty hands, nails, and contact lens cases are often most responsible. Contaminated distilled water is also a common cause.

Recurrent corneal erosion

Many people have had a piece of grit fly into the eye and have required professional help to remove it. Once the eye is patched for 24 hours, the cornea repairs itself and the mishap is forgotten, relegated to the domain of unpleasant minor memories. If, however, the eye is injured by anything organic, such as a fingernail, the cornea may heal but break down again weeks or months later.

The entire sequence of the initial accident is relived and the person suffers pain, sensitivity to light, watering eyes, redness of the eye, and marked blurring of vision. The event may seem unreal because there is no antecedent injury the second or third time. Soft lenses may prevent this recurrent breakdown.

Dry eyes

The primary disturbance in keratitis sicca is a result of a gross deficiency of tears, which parches the cornea and causes dryness of its surface so that it develops pits and erosions. Patients with dry eyes complain of a terrible burning sensation that is much worse when indoors. They are constant visitors to drugstores and will buy anything that comes out of a dropper, provided it is wet.

Again, the mechanism by which soft lenses achieve these clinical results is not clear. They do act as a protective bandage and their tendency to retain water probably accounts for their successful lubricant value. In patients affected with this condition, improvement in their general corneal status gives symptomatic relief and improves their vision, in some instances in a spectacular fashion. These lenses are often effective if used in conjunction with artificial tears and local antibiotics that do not contain preservatives. In some cases, however, soft lenses fail to be of help.

Contact lens wearers as well as laser-assisted in situ keratomileusis (LASIK) patients experience dry eye syndrome. In addition, there are many dry eye conditions, such as Sjögren syndrome that can contribute to this dry eye feeling. Anywhere from 15% to 25% of the average population has dry eyes. A Japanese study pointed out that 82% of contact lens wearers had dry eyes. In late stages of dry eyes, the cornea often becomes desiccated and ulcerated and eventually scar formation occurs. Symptoms of dry eyes are listed in Box 15.6.

Medical specialist situations that can lead to dry eyes include:
- Keratoconjunctivitis sicca or Sjögren syndrome
- Thyroid
- Chemical burns
- Post-LASIK

In the contact lens wearer, there is often blurred vision as a result of lens dehydration. The thinner the lens, the more the dehydration occurs. After LASIK, dry eyes can occur in

---

Box 15.6 Symptoms of dry eye

Scratchiness
Intermittent blurring
Dryness
No tears on crying
Mucoid discharge
Relief with tear substitutes
Discomfort or pain
Occasional burning and itching

80% because of the severance of the corneal nerves at the limbus and by the compression of the microkeratome.
- The function of the tear film is to hydrate and protect the ocular surface
- Reduce friction on blinking
- Enhance oxygen to the cornea
- Remove waste and cellular debris
- Protect against infection
  A dry eye workup consists of:
- A history
- Schirmer's test
- BUT (break-up time of tears)
- Tear meniscus height
- Rose bengal test for staining of the conjunctiva
- Evidence of lag ophthalmos

The more sophisticated tests, such as the lactopheron test and tear osmolarity are rarely used in clinical practice.

The management of dry eyes consists essentially of:
- Copious drops
- Humidifier in bedroom and at work
- Flaxseed or fish oil capsules 1000 mg, 2 to 4 times daily
- Swim goggles
- Bedtime patching
- Punctal plugs

Many artificial tears are available for use. If one is using them in any copious amount, the ones that are preservative free are better. Punctal plugs are easily inserted. There are numerous types available on a temporary or a permanent basis.

Two developments are of interest. Cyclosporine (also, ciclosporin) drops in dilute 0.05% solution (Restasis) correct the inflammatory process that occurs on the conjunctiva and that may give rise to a blockage of the reflux from the conjunctiva to the brain and to the lacrimal gland. Testosterone 3% has also been used in a transdermal patch.

Hormones are said to increase meibomian secretions. Lid hygiene is important and there are surfactant gels that can be applied to reduce the inflammation around the meibomian glands. Of benefit has been the development of a goggle-style sunglass, the Panoptx/7-Eye Orbital Seal, which seals to the skin and protects the eye (Fig. 15.30).

3. Patients should be educated about the need for hygiene procedures with respect to wearing of lenses.
4. Lenses should be worn preferably on a flexible-wear basis and disinfected at least once weekly.
5. The lenses should not be worn longer than 1 week continuously.
6. Follow-up examinations are essential. Patients should be seen at least twice a year by the ophthalmologist.
7. Any complications, such as a red eye or pain in the eye, should be reported immediately.
8. We advocate a hydrogen peroxide disinfecting and cleaning system for most extended-wear patients. This has been shown to kill the AIDS virus. Hydrogen peroxide needs long exposure to kill *Acanthamoeba*. This parasite requires heat or ultraviolet exposure to kill it.
9. It is recommended that any patient wearing extended-wear lenses be offered a form of disposable lenses or planned replacement lenses for added cleanliness.

With long-term use of extended-wear lenses or daily wear soft lenses, vacuoles and microcysts may occur in the epithelium of at least 40% of patients. This condition probably occurs because of prolonged low levels of cell death by hypoxia. It usually clears up after lens use is discontinued.

The sucked-on lens syndrome, reported by Wilson and others, involves a tight, unmovable lens that is associated with red eye. Its cause is still controversial but it may result from chemical changes that alter the steepness of the lens. It may be relieved by the use of alkaline drops, such as balanced salts in solution.

Silicone hydrogel lenses (continuous wear)

Patients still want the convenience of safe vision around the clock and for extended periods. Extended wear lenses fit in with busy and unpredictable schedules and eliminate the daily hassle of inserting, removing, and cleaning contact lenses, enabling wearers to lead a more normal life. Research has shown that approximately 38% of contact lens wearers worldwide are interested in lenses that they can sleep with without removal. These lenses:

- Have a high oxygen transmission
- Have a biocompatible lens surface
- Have a low incidence of complications
- Can be worn safely for up to 30 days with overnight wear

It is recommended to remove these lenses weekly, and clean, disinfect, and reinsert them the next day. These lenses are promoted as a safe and reliable alternative to LASIK surgery and provide at least 6 times more oxygen than ordinary soft lenses. Patients want safety, good vision, comfort, affordability, and convenience. The practitioner, on the other hand, is interested in ocular health and the newer technology that is available. The fluorosilicone hydrogel material partially resists deposits and bacterial adhesions

---

> **Box 15.7 Characteristics of Air Optix Focus Night and Day Lens (CIBA Vision) lenses**
>
> Base curve: 8.4 and 8.6 mm
> Total diameter: 13.8 mm
> Power range: + 6.00 diopters (D) to − 10.00 D
> Central thickness: 0.08 mm @ − 3.00 D (varies with power)
> Oxygen permeability: 140×10^{-11} (cm^2/s) (mL O_2/mL × mm Hg), measured at 35°C (95°F) (intrinsic *DK* – coulometric method)

to the surface. A well-fitted lens does not show any edge lift and mucin balls are not created.

Available today are 30-day silicone hydrogel extended-wear (continuous-wear) lenses manufactured by Alcon (Night and Day lens; Box 15.7) and by Bausch & Lomb (PureVision). Silicone hydrogel material has a high *DK* value and can be worn night and day on a continuous basis for up to 30 days. This eliminates care systems for storing lenses as well as possible hand contamination. These lenses meet the standards required for minimizing corneal edema in the morning.

The following is taken from the package insert for the Night and Day contact lens:

> *"Night and Day and Air Optix 'Night and Day'® Aqua (lotrafilcon A) soft contact lenses are made from a lens material that is approximately 24% water and 76% lotrafilcon A, a fluorosilicone containing hydrogel which is surface treated. Lenses may contain the color additive copper phthalocyanine, a light blue handling tint, which makes them easier to see when handling."*

The following is taken from the package insert for the Bausch & Lomb PureVision lens:

> *"The Bausch & Lomb PureVision® (balafilcon A) Visibility Tinted Contact Lens is a soft hydrophilic contact lens which is available as a spherical lens. The lens material, balafilcon A, is a copolymer of a silicone vinyl carbamate, N-vinyl-pyrrolidone, a siloxane crosslinker and a vinyl alanine wetting monomer, and is 36% water by weight when immersed in a sterile borate buffered saline solution. This lens is tinted blue with up to 300 ppm of Reactive Blue Dye 246."*

Vistakon (Johnson & Johnson) has developed a silicone hydrogel (Acuvue Oasys), with hydraclear plus, which has a *DK/t* value of 147. An advantage of this soft flexible material is its low *modulus*, which is a material's stress divided by its strain. It also has an ultraviolet (UV) blocker incorporated. It is recommended to be replaced on a 2-week basis and worn on a daily wear regimen. The following was taken from the instruction guide for the Acuvue Advance lens:

"The lenses are made of a silicone hydrogel material containing an internal wetting agent with visibility tinted UV absorbing monomer. The AcuvueOasys with hydraclear® Contact Lenses Visibility Tinted with UV Blocker are tinted blue using Reactive Blue Dye #4 to make the lens more visible for handling. A benzotriazole UV-absorbing monomer is used to block UV radiation. The transmittance characteristics are less than 1% in the UVB range of 280 nm to 315 nm and less than 10% in the UVA range of 316 nm to 380 nm for the entire power range."

This lens is also available in a toric design for astigmatism.

Table 15.2 compares the features of various silicone hydrogel lenses. The silicone hydrogel lenses are available in single vision, toric, and bifocal design.

Conclusion

The search for a lens that can be worn for prolonged periods was risky and adventurous. Today, new plastics and better manufacturing techniques are available, although risk factors still are present with extended-wear lenses.

The fitting of the young myopic person with extended-wear lenses is much easier and more successful than that of the aphakic person because of the thinner lens centers, the healthier corneas, and the better tear film often found in the myopic individual. As a result of advances in cataract surgery and intraocular lenses, fitting aphakes with contact lenses is becoming a thing of the past.

Disposable lenses

Lens technology has continued to advance so that disposable replacement regimens are available. This replacement modality is being recommended for 80% of fittings. These disposable lenses may be thrown away and replaced on a daily, weekly, or biweekly basis. With regard to the wear regimen (to differentiate from the replacement regimen) for our own patients, about 20% wear disposable replacement lenses on an extended-wear overnight basis, whereas 80% wear them on a daily wear basis.

The development of disposable replacement contact lenses has ushered in a new era in contact lens safety. Many brands are available on a disposable replacement basis with varying wear regimens from 1 day, 1 week, 2 weeks, to 1 month. Consult a high-quality summary guide for a complete listing of these various brands with their different replacements and regimens.

Disposable replacement of lenses is a practical choice. A person can purchase disposable lenses and discard them frequently.

Disposable lenses have the following advantages:

1. Clearer vision is obtained because clean lenses are introduced regularly.
2. The cost of lens-care solutions is greatly reduced.
3. There is minimal deposit formation.
4. Better compliance occurs because daily wear disposable lenses require minimal care compared with the cleaning routines necessary for regular soft lenses.

Table 15.2 Hydrogel silicone lens comparison

	Acuvue Oasys (J&J)	PureVision (B&L)	Air Optix Night and Day
Material	Galyfilcon A	Bafilcon A	Lotrafilcon A
Power range	+ 8.00 diopters (D) to −12.00 D	+ 6.00 D to −12.00 D	+ 8.00 D to −10.00 D
Diameter	14 mm	14 mm	13.8 mm
Base curve	8.4 and 8.8 mm	8.3[a] and 8.6 mm	8.4 and 8.6 mm
Center thickness	0.07 mm	0.07 mm	0.08 mm
Water content	38%	36%	24%
Oxygen transmissibility *DK/t*	147	110	175
Visibility tint	Yes	Yes	Yes
Ultraviolet (UV) blocking	Yes	No	No
Recommended replacement	2 weeks	30 days	30 days

[a]Low minus powers only.
B&L, Bausch & Lomb; *J&J*, Johnson & Johnson.

Loss or removal of the lenses

Loss of a lens is a common occurrence, particularly with rigid lenses.

1. Lenses can become lost during activity in certain occupations or sports.
2. Cigarette and pipe smoke can force the wearer to remove contact lenses.
3. In case of fire, smoke and toxic gases may become trapped behind the contact lens and irritate the eye, making removal necessary.
4. Foreign particles underneath a contact lens may scratch and irritate the eye, requiring removal of the lens.
5. Soft lenses dehydrate relatively quickly in low-humidity environments, such as aircraft, which may necessitate their removal because of discomfort.

Problems with contact lenses

1. Contrast sensitivity in the everyday world is often reduced with contact lenses. In critical areas of visual function, this may become a hazard.
2. Scratches may occur on hard and soft contact lenses, which necessitates replacement of the lens to improve vision.
3. Debris may accumulate on the surface of the contact lenses as a result of mixtures of lipids and proteins. This can make the eye uncomfortable and impair vision.
4. Poor fitting can result in complications.

Common questions and answers

1. Should a contact lens be removed before evaluation with use of the air tonometer?
   Yes. The practitioner does not obtain reliable results of pressure unless the contact lens is removed before this measurement.
2. Should lenses be removed before a field test?
   No. The best visual acuity is required to perform a field test. If the lenses provide this, then the lenses may remain in the eyes.
3. How long should a contact lens be removed before an eye examination?
   If the examination does not involve a refraction, the contact lens need not necessarily be removed. The lens must be removed during the tonometric examination, however.
4. How long should a contact lens be removed before refraction?
   To obtain a suitable refraction, a contact lens should be removed at least 24 to 48 hours before examination. This permits the corneal epithelium to regain its full corneal curvature and thus provide a suitable refraction. Sometimes epithelial edema is present, which clouds the refraction and produces an error in the refractive surface.
5. Can patients who wear contact lenses be considered for implant surgery?
   Yes. The correct lenses provide no impairment to implant surgery. The use of biometry provides a new measurement for an intraocular lens that often will eliminate contact lenses.
6. Can contact lenses be used after refractive surgery?
   Yes. The keratometer readings often are misleading. These patients should be fitted according to their original *K* readings. Soft lenses, if worn for any extended basis, provide some vascularization at the knee of the depression. Consequently, the patient should receive instructions for daily wear and minimal wearing times. Hard lenses are probably more suitable and will reduce any corneal toricity that may be present.
7. Can soft or rigid lenses be worn after implant surgery?
   Yes. Usually, however, these are not required. On the other hand, in cases of higher astigmatism or residual refractive error, they may provide a very useful form of visual rehabilitation.
8. What are the major problems in care of contact lenses?
   The most common problems are those caused by lack of compliance; that is, the patient does not follow the regimen given by the instructor. Because patients often become haphazard about lens care, care must be emphasized at almost every repeat visit. Reduced vision, discomfort, red eye, infections, and allergic responses are the problems that occur most frequently.

Role of the ophthalmic assistant

A high percentage of the tasks in an efficient contact lens practice may be delegated to the ophthalmic assistant. Supplies and inventory of lenses add a dimension of expense to a practice that must be supervised and continually looked after. Unlike rigid lenses, soft lenses spoil and deteriorate once the vial has been opened unless cleaning and sterilizing routines are applied to trial sets and unopened vials. The ophthalmic assistant in a clinical contact lens practice is often responsible for maintaining inventory and helping in cost efficiency.

The following list indicates some of the duties of the ophthalmic assistant in a busy contact lens practice:
1. Maintain inventory and cost efficiency.
2. Handle insurance programs.
3. Provide instruction on lens care and handling.
4. Schedule appointments.
5. Make follow-up calls for drop-outs, particularly those prescribed extended-wear lenses.

6. Handle telephone calls.
7. Understand adaptive and abnormal symptoms.
8. Perform office cleaning of lenses.
9. Perform collections.
10. Order replacement lenses.

The assistant must become familiar with telephone communication with patients and in particular must be able to distinguish purely adaptive symptoms for both rigid and soft lenses from abnormal symptoms. Abnormal symptoms, such as persistent red eyes, blurring of vision, excessive glare, and unusual discomfort require an emergency appointment with the ophthalmologist. When in doubt, assistants should exercise caution, turn the call over to someone more experienced, or schedule the patient for an examination. They should not assume responsibility for diagnosis on the telephone.

Questions for review and thought

1. Why is a soft lens so comfortable?
2. Describe a method of teaching a patient insertion and removal of a soft lens.
3. What are the advantages of soft hydrogel lenses compared with rigid lenses?
4. Review the fitting method of one type of soft lens.
5. How are soft lenses sterilized?
6. How are soft lenses cleaned?
7. How can you inspect and evaluate a soft lens returned by the patient?
8. Name some medical uses for the soft contact lens.
9. If the diameter of a lens is increased, is the lens made flatter or steeper?
10. How can you determine whether a soft lens is inside out?
11. Can fluorescein be used with a soft lens? Explain.
12. Which candidates are not suitable for soft lenses?
13. If the water content of a soft lens is increased, is its durability increased or decreased?

Self-evaluation questions Q

True–false statements
Directions: Indicate whether the statement is true **(T)** or false **(F)**.
1. Soft lenses are better than rigid lenses in reducing glare and photophobia. **T** or **F**
2. Measurement of a soft lens is labeled in the fully hydrated state. **T** or **F**
3. Thin soft lenses are better for occasional wear, such as sporting activities. **T** or **F**

Missing words
Directions: Write in the missing word in the following sentences:
4. Circumlimbal compression and injection are characteristic of a soft lens that has been fitted too _____.
5. Ultrathin lenses have _____ oxygen transmission compared with lenses of standard thickness.
6. Soft lenses worn in a dry environment should not be thin but be of _____ thickness to reduce dehydration.

Choice-completion questions
Directions: Select the one best answer in each case:

7. Soft lenses can be of great therapeutic value as a bandage lens. Which of the following conditions could benefit from a bandage soft lens?
   a. Bullous keratopathy
   b. Recurrent corneal erosion
   c. Keratitis sicca
   d. All of the above
   e. None of the above
8. Which of the following is true for present-day conventional extended-wear lenses for myopia?
   a. Difficult-to-handle lenses
   b. Loss factor common
   c. Deposit formation common
   d. Infection common
   e. Neovascularization
9. To maintain corneal integrity and proper cornea–lens relationship, the fit should exhibit:
   a. central touch.
   b. no movement.
   c. apical vaulting.
   d. three-point touch.
   e. slight edge lifting.

Answers, notes, and explanations | A

1. **True**. Soft lenses reduce foreign body sensation and thus reduce the incidence of lens-induced photophobia. Also the large optic zone eliminates the glare that can be experienced when light passes through the peripheral curves of a rigid lens or when the pupil dilates.

2. **True**. All soft lenses contain some percentage of water. The expressed parameters are measurements when the lens is fully hydrated. A lens tends to shrink and steepen as it dehydrates. In the manufacturing process of a soft lens, the measurements usually are made initially for the manufacture of the soft lens while it is still in the hard state. An allowance factor for the constant swelling of the material in the hydrated state is taken into consideration to arrive at the final dimensions of the required hydrated lens. The soft lenses are then measured in the fully hydrated state.

3. **True**. Thin and ultrathin lenses show better oxygen transmission and may be fitted larger and tighter and thus track with rapid movements of the eye. This reduces loss and prevents particles from getting under the lenses. This can be a most useful feature in the stability of vision required for most sports.

4. **Tightly or steeply**. A lens that is too tight will show minimal or no movement and cause inadequate tear exchange under the lens, along with compression of the vessels at the limbus.

5. **Higher**. Oxygen permeability is a function of the material, whereas oxygen transmission also takes into account the thickness of the material. When any material thickness is reduced by 50%, the transmission of oxygen is doubled. Thus the thinner the lenses, the better is oxygen transmission through to the cornea.

6. **Standard**. In a dry environment the standard-thickness lenses perform better because they carry more water and permit greater evaporation before they become depleted of their water reservoir.

7. **d. All of the above**. These are but a few of a long list of indicators for the soft lens as a medical device in the therapeutic armamentarium against corneal disease processes.

8. **c. Deposit formation common**. Buildup of minerals, protein, and lipids is still the single main feature of contact lenses that are not cleaned on a daily basis. Although weekly or semimonthly cleaning routines are recommended for most patients with conventional extended-wear lenses, those who fail to follow this regimen often allow deposits to build up and cause spoilage of their soft lenses.

9. **d. Three-point touch**. The proper cornea–lens relationship for a soft lens involves slight central touch with touch of the lens at the periphery. For the smaller-diameter soft lenses, this peripheral touch may be at the limbus, whereas for the larger lenses this may be on the sclera. With each blink, there is some movement of the lens and a small amount of tear exchange under the lens.

Chapter | 16 |

Advanced techniques in soft and rigid contact lens fitting

Many ophthalmic assistants play an expanded role in contact lens delivery and thus require detailed knowledge of contact lenses. Although the changing and ordering of lenses may be beyond the scope of the ophthalmic assistant, an understanding of how to modify lenses and a review of abnormal symptoms and signs are not. This chapter highlights only some of the problems encountered; further information may be obtained from our textbook, *Fitting Guide for Rigid and Soft Contact Lenses: A Practical Approach*. 4th ed. St Louis: Mosby; 2002.

Abnormal symptoms and signs

It is important to recognize purely adaptive symptoms and differentiate them from pathologic symptoms that could result in corneal damage. The ophthalmic assistant may be the first to hear of these symptoms and should alert the ophthalmologist to patients' complaints that might lead to serious corneal damage.

Flare or streaming of lights or glare from oncoming headlights may occur when the lens or the optical portion of the lens (optic zone) is too small. This symptom occurs because the pupil of the eye dilates at night or in a darkened room and the patient begins to have interference in his or her vision from the edge of the optic zone or the edge of the lens. It can be corrected by making the lens larger or by increasing the size of the optic zone.

Blurring of vision in daytime through the normal pupil may be a result of the lens riding too high or gravitating too low after each blink. This can be observed directly by watching the patient view a vision chart or distant object. The patient may respond by producing streaming opposite to the displacement of the lens (Fig. 16.1). Lenses may ride high because of a high minus power and edge thickness that cause the lens to be lifted up by the upper lid. A small lens under a tight lid will also ride high. A lens that rides low may be too heavy because of thickness or because of high plus power or there may be insufficient edge thickness that will not permit the upper lid to grasp the lens and lift it. Redesigning the edge to provide proper compensation will permit the lens to center better. If this fails, smaller lenses may be required. Occasionally, the lens will slide nasally or temporally because of an abnormally centered cornea. These lenses should be replaced with lenses of larger diameter or a larger optic zone.

Central corneal edema (Fig. 16.2) with consequent blurring of vision occurs when there is insufficient oxygenation of the cornea brought about by poor tear exchange. The edematous area appears hazy on the slit-lamp microscope, particularly if the light is shone off to the side of the area to be viewed so the area is illuminated from behind rather than directly. When the epithelial edema advances, some cells may die, causing central stippling, which will stain with fluorescein dye. The stippling may represent only a

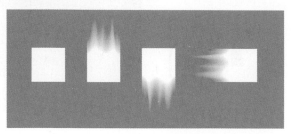

Fig. 16.1 Flare. The zone of streaming is always opposite to the displacement of the lens. Such a lens requires recentering. Uniform flare indicates that the optic zone of the lens is too small. (From Stein HA, Slatt BJ, Stein RM. *Fitting Guide for Rigid and Soft Contact Lenses: A Practical Approach*. 4th ed. St Louis: Mosby; 2002.)

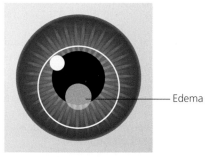

Edema

Fig. 16.2 Corneal edema created by a contact lens. (From Rosenthal P. Corneal contact lenses and corneal edema. *Int Ophthalmol Clin*. 1968;8:611.)

few small, discrete spots at the beginning, but the spots may increase in number as the condition progresses. If the condition progresses, *punctate staining* is said to occur. Patients who develop these objective signs will often complain of spectacle blur for some time after the lenses are removed. To correct this situation, the tear exchange must be improved. This can be done in the original rigid lens by:

- Blending the junctions of the curve better
- Flattening the peripheral curve
- Reducing the total diameter
- Reducing the diameter of the optic zone by increasing the width of the peripheral curve
- Fenestrating the lens

Corneal abrasion (Fig. 16.3) may follow corneal edema caused by lack of oxygen, but may also result from too flat a lens rubbing on a portion of the cornea. Evaluation of the fit of the lens to indicate that the abraded area lies just under the touch area of the contact lens will determine whether the lens is rubbing the cornea and is too flat, too loose, or both. The excessive movement adds to the friction of the cornea and can be corrected with a new lens by:

- Increasing the rigid lens diameter
- Increasing the optic zone diameter
- Reducing the edge thickness
- Steepening the lens case curve
- Steepening the peripheral curve

Three o'clock and *nine o'clock staining* (see Fig. 16.3) of the cornea with fluorescein refers to erosions at the 3 and 9 o'clock positions in the exposed portion of the palpebral fissure. It is usually believed to be a result of dryness because of inadequate blinking while wearing the contact lens so that the small exposed portion of the cornea on each side of the lens becomes dry. This symptom is not usually seen with smaller and thinner lenses. Various methods, such as a smaller, thinner lens; blinking exercises; or artificial tears may help eliminate this problem.

Insertion abrasions may result from improper or clumsy insertion. Abrasion causes either immediate pain or pain after removal of the lens. Further practice in insertion should be undertaken under observation of the instructor.

Foreign bodies trapped under the lens will show varying types of zigzag scratch marks on the cornea, which will stain with fluorescein. Common substances, such as mascara and cosmetics may be the offending agents and should be used with caution.

Arc staining may occur either from poor insertion technique or most commonly from a sharp junction line between the central posterior curve and the intermediate or peripheral posterior curve. A proper blend is required.

Bubbles with staining occur when the lens is steep and there is too much sagittal depth to the lens so that air is trapped under the central curve. A flatter lens is required.

Blurring after reading may occur in the myope nearing the age of 40 years. The introduction of contact lenses requires a further accommodative effort and convergence that the patient cannot compensate for. Reading glasses may be required.

If the blur in the nonpresbyope occurs soon after insertion, it may be caused by the lower lid pushing the lens upward, thus causing poor centering of the lens in the reading position. This may be corrected by making the lens smaller.

If blurring occurs after prolonged reading, it may be the result of inadequate tear exchange and corneal anoxia. Concentrated reading reduces the blink reflex, induces staring, and consequently permits less tear exchange. A smaller lens, a flatter peripheral curve, or a material with a higher *DK* may alleviate this problem. For individuals who require prolonged reading activity, blinking exercises can be recommended.

Corneal warpage or induced astigmatism, both regular and irregular, can occur, resulting either from poorly fitting lenses that alter the corneal curvature or from chronic hypoxia of the cornea from overwearing the contact lenses. A complete reassessment of the fit is called for and possibly refitting in a more permeable material.

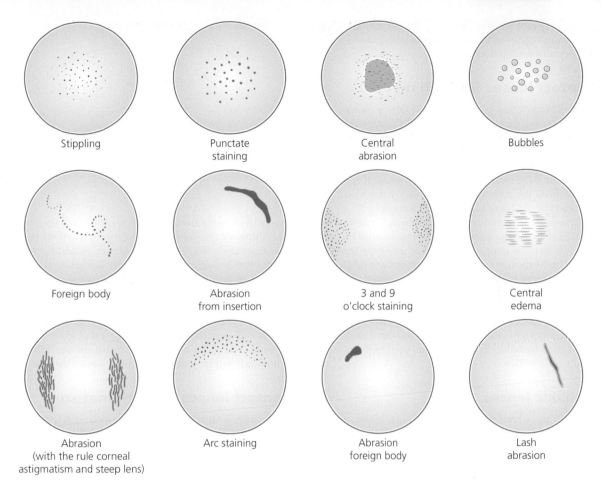

Stippling

Punctate
staining

Central
abrasion

Bubbles

Foreign body

Abrasion
from insertion

3 and 9
o'clock staining

Central
edema

Abrasion
(with the rule corneal
astigmatism and steep lens)

Arc staining

Abrasion
foreign body

Lash
abrasion

Fig. 16.3 Abnormal staining patterns.

Follow-up keratometry

By performing keratometry on repeat visits, one can detect any molding or distortion of the cornea or induced astigmatism. One should record the difference in the K readings at subsequent visits. A notation, such as $K + 1.25 + 0.50$, indicates that the cornea has steepened by this amount in each meridian. Any changes over 1.00 diopter indicate that the wearing time should be reduced or the lens adjusted. Distortion of the mires also indicates that a change is needed.

Special lenses

The methods of contact lens fitting for correction of the most common defects of the eye were described in Chapter 14.

The techniques and devices available have proved highly successful for the majority of cases. However, as with other natural systems, variations in the anatomy and physiology of the eye are broad. Thus for those defects associated with more extreme variations, corrective devices and methods must be custom-built to a highly sophisticated level. For example, patients with extremely high myopia (−6.00 diopters or greater) or aphakic patients (+8.00 diopters or greater) require modifications of the normal lens design because of an extrathick (myopic) or extrathin (hyperopic) peripheral edge of the corneal contact lens. Similarly, extreme cases of keratoconus require bicurvature lenses for effective apposition to the eye, whereas highly astigmatic cases require an asymmetric (nonspherical), nonrotating lens design. Special rigid lenses have been developed for a steepened apical characteristic of the cone in keratoconus. Many eye patients older than 40 years require bifocal lenses, and special lens systems with bifocal lens characteristics

307

can be prepared for their accommodation. Certain pathologic cases requiring telescopic lenses also present a need for specially designed lenses.

Contact lenses for high myopia

Myopia is the most common reason why a patient seeks contact lenses. Contact lenses for high myopia have not only the added feature of cosmetic enhancement by replacing glasses but also increased optical benefit because the contact lens rests on the eye, and thus the retinal image is larger and more normal than it would be with spectacles. In addition, the high myope no longer has a visual field restricted by the edges of glasses and frames.

However, as the minus power of a contact lens increases, so does the edge thickness. This increase in edge thickness creates a base-up wedge effect, which causes the lens to be pulled up by the upper lid and consequently to ride high so that the patient fails to look through the center of the lens. To reduce the thickness of the edge, it must be shaved off to prevent the upper lid from tugging upward on the lens. This in effect results in a lenticular-designed lens for high minus powers. The higher the minus power, the more the anterior edge has to be reduced. Aspheric lens designs have thinner peripheral profiles.

Aphakic lenses

With the more common use of intraocular lenses, aphakic lenses have declined in use. Aphakic contact lenses are primarily used when an intraocular lens is not appropriate, or for an older-generation patient when intracapsular cataract procedure was the surgery of choice. It is obvious why intraocular lenses are preferred: they generally offer better vision and freedom from the daily handling of contact lenses. For an older adult who may have a hand tremor, lax eyelids, or a tear deficiency, this freedom from the hazards of contact lens wear is important. Yet not all cataract extractions are treated with intraocular lenses. Implants **may not be inserted** if any of the following occurs:

• Angle-closure glaucoma
• Recurrent iridocyclitis
• Any surgical contingency that makes the insertion of an intraocular lens hazardous

Thus knowledge of aphakic contact lenses should be acquired despite a definite downgrading of their importance in the management of a cataract patient.

Aphakic individuals require strong plus lenses. As the power of a plus lens increases, so too does its central thickness. This increase in central thickness creates a base-down wedge effect at the upper edge of the lens, thus the upper lid forces the lens downward. The high-plus lens is also heavy, which causes it to gravitate downward. One way of reducing the thickness and thus the weight of a high-plus

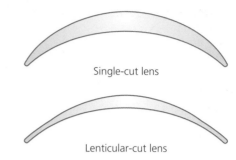

Fig. 16.4 Single-cut and lenticular-cut lenses.

lens is to keep the overall diameter of the lens very small. Unfortunately, this does not solve the problem if the patient has large pupils or keyhole iridectomies, in which case the patient may be looking through the lens edge. A more practical way of fitting a high-plus lens with a reduction in the thickness and weight is to add a lenticular design on the lens (Fig. 16.4). It is important that the lenticular optic portion of the lens completely covers the pupil, otherwise the patient will complain of blurry vision and glare. Another solution is to put a myopic edge finish on any high-plus lens, which will help the upper eyelid elevate the lens.

Contact lenses for astigmatism

Residual astigmatism occurs when a contact lens is placed on an eye and an astigmatic refractive error still results. Several conditions may contribute to this residual astigmatism, but it is most commonly induced by the crystalline lens of the eye (so-called *lenticular astigmatism*). If the amount is small, it will not significantly interfere with vision. If the amount of astigmatism is large, however, vision will be substandard unless one can compensate for this with the contact lens. Although this requires a complex type of lens, essentially a toric surface is ground on the front or back of the lens to prevent the lens from rotating, so that the toric surface is lined up with the axis of astigmatism. One must stop rotation of the lens by introducing a weight, such as a prism ballast to the lens at the correct position.

Nonrotating lenses

Patients with a moderate or high degree of astigmatism will experience difficulties in wearing spherical contact lenses. Symptoms of blurred vision, excessive awareness of lens edge, and slipping of the lens off the cornea or even completely out of the eye will be encountered because of the rocking effect of the lens over the flatter meridian. Residual astigmatism, in which the cornea is spherical but the patient has a cylindric spectacle prescription, is another indication for nonrotating lenses. In these cases, the astigmatism comes from the lens of the eye and it is necessary to add prism to the lens to stop lens rotation and to properly orient the cylinder over the correct optical axis.

Several types of nonrotating lenses have been designed.

Noncircular shapes

A *truncated* lens is really a circular lens in which the bottom or top portion, or both (double-truncated lens), has been cut off. The corners at the edge of the truncation are smoothed off. A double-truncated lens, although infrequently used, will tend to stabilize so that the flat portion lies adjacent to the upper and lower lid edges. If the edges are rounded off more, the lens assumes an oval shape, but this type of lens rotates frequently and thus negates the use for which it was intended. Rectangular and triangular lenses have been designed, but they have shown little practical value.

Toric curve lens

A lens may be cut so that it is not spherical on its back surface. It is called a *toric back curve lens* when it has two meridians of curvature on its back surface that are designed to conform somewhat to the two meridians of curvature of the front surface of the cornea. This lens is used to correct a high degree of astigmatism. When the lens is placed in the eye, it tends to align its curvature with that of the cornea. However, an optical problem of astigmatism may exist that may require the grinding of a toric surface on the front of the lens, the so-called *front surface toric lens*. These are used primarily to treat residual astigmatism in patients with spherical corneas. In some instances, toric surfaces may be ground on both the front and back surfaces, the so-called *bitoric contact lens*.

Prism ballast lenses

When a prism is ground into a contact lens, the heavier base of the prism swings the lens around so that the heavier base rides low, attracted by gravity, and thus further rotation of the lens is eliminated (Fig. 16.5). One can incorporate up to 3.00 diopters of prism in a lens to provide sufficient weight. In addition to preventing rotation, a prism may be used to create weight in a lens that tends to ride high or to reduce excessive lens movements. The weight of prism ballast lenses and the thinner superior edge of the lens, which fits under the upper lid, provide stability and prevent rotation of the lens.

Correction of high astigmatism

Astigmatism may result from corneal surfaces of different radii or from changes in the lens of the eye. The latter is

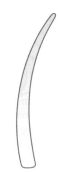

Fig. 16.5 Prism ballast to provide weight and stop rotation of a lens.

less common, but nevertheless does occur and accounts for residual astigmatism when corneal astigmatism has been fully corrected. It may also account for a very irregular corneal surface. Corneal topography is an excellent way of analyzing the corneal surface.

Keratometer readings provide a good index of the amount of corneal astigmatism present. Most spherical-based lenses are the first choice for fitting eyes with corneal astigmatism. Tear fluid readily fills in the interface and provides a good optical result in most cases. However, in some cases, these lenses will not provide adequate tear interchange, rocking occurs, or poor staining is found. A back surface toric lens will be required that will conform to the corneal toricity. Diagnostic trial lenses may be a valuable adjunct. Frequently, changing the back surface to a toric surface causes induced or residual astigmatism; this must be corrected by grinding a toric surface on the front of the lens. This constitutes the so-called *bitoric lens*.

Toric soft contact lenses

A wide variety of toric soft contact lenses are on the market, and fitters must familiarize themselves with what is available on a lens-by-lens basis. Specific lenses are not discussed here because there are excellent fitting guides available from the manufacturers. Before choosing a specific lens, the fitter must make sure that the lens is available in parameters that match the patient's refractive error.

Some "off-the-shelf" toric lenses are available in a limited range of cylinders and axes. Manufacturers make lenses in the most commonly requested power ranges and these are available immediately. Most soft toric lenses are available in powers from − 8.00 to + 4.00 diopters, with cylinder powers of − 0.75 to − 2.50 diopters. Daily disposable toric lenses are available in limited cylinder power and axis. A diagnostic lens of the selected toric design must be evaluated on the patient's eye for fit and position of axis.

For "custom" work, a fitting set must also be used. The fitting lenses are spherical designs with the diameters and excessively flat eventually cause corneal abrasions. Minimal apical clearance of the cone has been advocated but this point of view does not represent the majority. Gaspermeable (GP) materials are the best choice for better maintenance of corneal integrity.

The majority of early to moderate cones exhibit a manifestation of the irregularity at or below the midline of the cornea. Because keratometric readings can be misleading, it is important to remember that the superior portion of the cornea may be relatively normal or much flatter than the K readings suggest. These early to moderate and some more advanced oval cones can be effectively fitted using spherical and aspherical designs that will align with the superior cornea. Diagnostic fitting and fluorescein evaluation are required to accurately fit rigid contact lenses over an irregular corneal surface. The fitter should not be alarmed at the slight to moderate inferior edge lift of the lens if it aligns well superiorly. The upper lid especially aids in holding the lens in position. It is not uncommon to fit an oval cone with irregular K readings in the 50.00-diopter range with a lens, such as the Boston Envision, or Fluoroperm 90 with a base curve of 7.5 to 7.3 (45.00–46.25 diopters).

For more classic nipple-type cones, the Soper keratoconus lens can be of value. In our experience, the Soper keratoconus trial lenses (Fig. 16.11), combined with fluorescein assessment of their fit, have been a necessity in fitting these lenses. These trial lenses have a steep central base curve to permit the bulging of the cone and a much flatter peripheral curve. Ten lenses make up the trial set, extending from a central curve of 48.00 to 60.00 diopters, with increasing sagittal depth to accommodate an increasingly projecting cone (Table 16.3). There is a range of dioptric powers in the set to approximate normalcy for the average keratoconus patient. From the trial set, a lens is selected that has either a slight central touch or a slight vaulting at the apex.

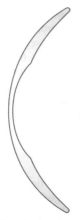

Fig. 16.11 Soper cone lens for keratoconus.

Newer versions of the Soper design keratoconus lens with small modifications are available. The most current lens design is the Rose "K" design by Dr. Paul Rose of New Zealand. The design provides a smaller central optic area to fit over the cone with rapid flattening of the midperipheral curvature. The peripheral lens design consists of a series of computer-controlled curves to form an aspheric edge.

A global licensing agreement with UK-based UltraVision CLPL to market and sell KeraSoft soft contact lenses throughout the world, through the network of Bausch & Lomb laboratory channel partners, was announced in 2011. KeraSoft lenses, which have been awarded the UK's Queen's Award for Enterprise and Innovation, are a patented combination of the latest technologies in soft and silicone hydrogel materials using geometries from complex mathematics to offer comfortable wear and excellent vision. KeraSoft patented technology allows for custom-made contact lenses for irregular corneas and keratoconus.

The Boston Foundation for Sight can work with practitioners on difficult or advanced keratoconus cases and offers its prosthetic replacement of the ocular surface ecosystem (PROSE), which uses U.S. Food and Drug Administration (FDA)-approved custom-made prosthetic devices to replace or support impaired ocular surface system functions that protect and enable vision. Information on PROSE is available on the Boston Foundation for Sight website (bostonsight.org).

Trial lens fitting

In the early phase of keratoconus, K readings are a guide to selecting a lens. As the condition develops, the mire image becomes irregular and the cone becomes steeper than 50.00 diopters so that the radius of curvature cannot be determined by ordinary keratometry. The only alternative is to fit the patient by diagnostic trial lens and fluorescein assessment.

The range of the keratometer can be extended to 61.00 diopters with an auxiliary +1.25 diopter lens. However, because of the disordered mires, problems in fixation and optic defects in the system, the results merely serve as a guide to trial lens selection. Fixation can be improved by using the viewing light of the topogometer; however, topography of the cornea provides the best making of the cornea to aid in keratoconus fitting.

A good fit should have a central touch of 2 to 3 mm centrally with a thin band of touch at the lens periphery, as determined by the fluorescein test. The three-point touch adds to the stability of the lens on the cornea and distributes the weight of the lens not only over the apex but also over other bearing areas. The peripheral touch area corresponds to the zone of the intermediate curve. The initial lens selected, using the K readings as a guide, should have a base curve flatter than K. Then, by using the fluorescein

Table 16.3 Soper cone diagnostic lens set

Sagittal depth (mm)	CPC	Power	Lens diameter (mm)	Thickness (mm)	Diameter of CPC (mm)
0.68	48/45	−4.50	7.5	0.10	6.0
0.73	52/45	−8.50	7.5	0.10	6.0
0.80	56/45	−12.50	7.5	0.10	6.0
0.87	60/45	−16.50	7.5	0.10	6.0
1.00	52/45	−8.50	8.5	0.10	7.0
1.12	56/45	−12.50	8.5	0.10	7.0
1.22	60.45	−16.50	8.5	0.10	7.0
1.37	52/45	−8.50	9.5	0.10	8.0
1.52	56/45	−12.50	9.5	0.10	8.0
1.67	60.45	−16.50	9.5	0.10	8.0
(Optional)	52/43	−8.50	8.5	0.10	7.0
	64/45	−20.00	8.5	0.10	7.0

CPC, Central posterior curve.

test, the examiner exchanges the lens until one is found that results in slight apical touch of 2 to 3 mm or 1 to 4 mm flatter than *K*. A light apical touch is desirable so that the lens can function as a pressure bandage on the thin, central, corneal apex (Fig. 16.12). Overrefraction is then performed to arrive at the correct power.

Role of corneal topography

Contact lens fitting may be improved with the use of corneal topography. Corneal topography is covered in more depth in Chapter 41.

Piggyback and hybrid lenses

Piggyback lenses were introduced by Dr. Joseph Baldone for patients with irregular corneal astigmatism or keratoconus who could not tolerate a rigid lens. They consist of a soft lens carrier for comfort, with a rigid lens riding in the soft lens to add definition. The soft lenses have been modified to provide a donut groove. The diameter and wall height of the groove can be varied according to the needs of the patient. The following rules for fitting are simple:

1. Always evaluate the piggyback lens with the rigid lens in place.
2. Use the same disinfectant and storage solutions for both lenses.
3. The groove diameter when available should be 0.2 mm larger than the diameter of the rigid lens being used.

The Softperm lens was a successor to the Saturn II lens. It had a base curve of 7.1 to 8.1 mm. The lens was 14.3 mm in diameter and ranges from +6 to −13. This is used in contact lens management of keratoconus. The Softperm lens consisted of a hard styrene lens core or central button supported by a soft hydrogel lens skirt. The rigid lens button provides a clear, regular optical surface to yield good vision, and the soft lens flange gives the patient stability and comfort. With a keratoconus patient, in whom the shape and position of the cone button are unpredictable, stability of the lens fit is vital and use of the Softperm and Saturn II lenses has been discontinued. Clearkone Synerge hybrid lenses series are now produced. These lenses have higher *DK* values, have wider range or power availability, and have variety in the skirt curvature design. A broader range of irregular corneas are fitted with the SynergEyes lenses.

Thick-set lenses

For early to moderate keratoconus patients, Softk and Softk toric lenses have proven to be effective in correcting corneal irregularity. They are available in B-C 7.30 to 8.20 mm, with a diameter of 14.2 mm and water content of 67% with xylofilcon A material.

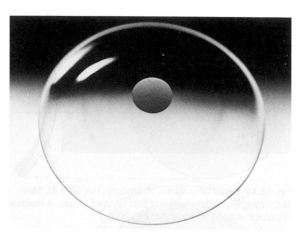

Fig. 16.17 Central add bifocal contact lens.

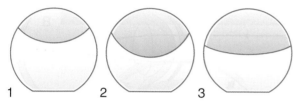

Fig. 16.18 Variations in design of one-piece bifocal lens. 1, Standard lens design; 2, concave lens design: this lens affords greater side-to-side viewing for a near object; 3, flat lens design: this lens affords a wider sweep for distance vision. (From Stein HA, Slatt BJ, Stein RM. *Fitting Guide for Rigid and Soft Contact Lenses: A Practical Approach.* 4th ed. St Louis: Mosby; 2002.)

truncation to weight the lenses and prevent rotation. The segments on these bifocal contact lenses may be either fused or in one piece (Fig. 16.18).

Of recent origin is a type of aspheric one-piece contact lens that provides a distance correction at the center, a reading correction off center, and an intermediate correction at midway points. This is available in both a soft lens and a rigid lens (variable focal lens [VFL]) design (Fig. 16.19).

The other soft lenses of multifocal designs are the reverse type of aspheric lenses such as the PS 45 and Unilens. These designs combine the maximum prescription in the center of the lens with progressively more minus as you move away from the center. This helps to eliminate peripheral distortion at a distance, especially under low illumination.

All bifocal lenses are affected by ambient light. The most affected are those with either a central distance optical zone surrounded by a collarette of reading prescription or the opposite type in which the reading portion is central

(Fig. 16.20). Success in fitting a presbyope depends on the following conditions:

1. Suitable patient screening
2. Understanding of the strengths of each type of lens
3. Using the strengths of each lens to the best advantage for a particular patient
4. Good patient education and motivation
5. Enthusiasm of the fitter
6. An increased rate of success with the experience of the fitter

With well-motivated patients and knowledgeable, experienced, and enthusiastic fitters, the rate of success can be as high as 90%. It is recommended to carefully follow the manufacturer's fitting guide for their specific bifocal contact lens. Many companies provide fitting consultation services that can be very helpful to the practitioner.

Research since 1990 has been directed toward the aging baby-boomer population. The result is an explosion of bifocals, both soft and rigid, addressing this age group. Progressive-add designs are available with increased reading power. The Essential rigid bifocal from Blanchard (Fig. 16.21) is an example, although most companies have their own version. The bifocal lenses of today have high success rates. With more designs on the way, fitting will be easier for both patient and practitioner. Bifocal contact lenses are available in a disposable replacement modality from a number of manufacturers including Bausch & Lomb (Soflens Multifocal, Pervasion multifocal), Johnson & Johnson Vision Care (Acuvue Oasys for presbyopia), and Alcon (Air optic multifocal). Toric multifocal soft contact lenses are manufactured by numerous companies. With changes in the field occurring quickly, practitioners are advised to review often a quality manufacturer's reference guide as a resource to available designs and materials. Some of these lenses are Essential soft toric multifocal by Blanchard, and Proclear topic multifocal by CooperVision.

Magnification with contact lenses

Patients with low visual acuity may benefit from contact lenses for two reasons. First, many visual defects may be a result of small corneal scars, which produce areas of irregular astigmatism. Rigid contact lenses overcome these surface irregularities of the cornea by providing a smooth tear film interface, which eliminates irregularities and can significantly improve vision. Second, visual improvement may be achieved by a telescopic system devised by a combination of a minus contact lens with high-plus glasses, which produces a magnified retinal image. This is the same system found in standard opera glasses, which magnify 4, 5, 6, and even 7 times. The greater the magnification, however, the narrower is the field of vision, as can be appreciated when one looks through strong field glasses.

Contact lens combination with spectacles, such as a −30.00 diopter contact lens and a +20.00 diopter

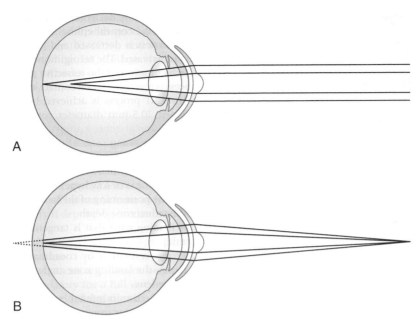

Fig. 16.19 (A) Central add bifocal contact lens. Light from distant objects focuses on the retina; light from near objects is ignored. (B) Light from near objects focuses on the retina; light from distant objects is ignored.

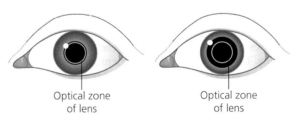

Optical zone of lens   Optical zone of lens

Fig. 16.20 Ambient lighting affects the size of the pupil. A large dilated pupil may result in ghosting.

spectacle lens, provides a magnification of ×1.5 when there is 17-mm separation between the contact lens and spectacles. Often this magnification is a great help to the patient with markedly reduced vision. It certainly is a more pleasant and cosmetically better method than wearing only thick telescopic lenses. It is optically advantageous as well because in addition to the limited field of vision resulting from telescopic lenses, each time the patient turns his or her head, there is a rapid movement of the visual field in the opposite direction. Also many of the other disadvantages of magnification that appear with the use of thick telescopic lenses (such as making objects appear closer than they actually are) are removed or diminished through the use of contact lenses in combination with spectacles.

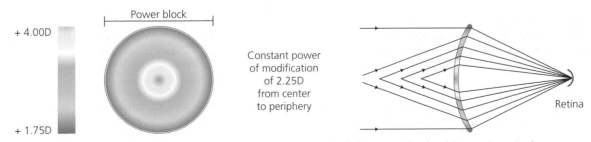

+ 4.00D

Power block

Constant power of modification of 2.25D from center to periphery

+ 1.75D

Retina

Fig. 16.21 Essential rigid gas-permeable bifocal contact lens from Blanchard. (Courtesy Blanchard Contact Lens, Inc.)

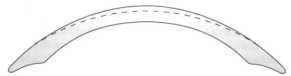

Fig. 16.24 Adding minus power. (From Stein HA, Slatt BJ, Stein RM. *Fitting Guide for Rigid and Soft Contact Lenses: A Practical Approach.* 4th ed. St Louis: Mosby; 2002.)

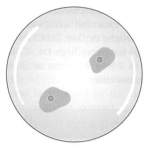

Fig. 16.25 Fenestrations reduce corneal edema in a 1- or 2-mm zone around the aperture. (From Stein HA, Slatt BJ, Stein RM. *Fitting Guide for Rigid and Soft Contact Lenses: A Practical Approach.* 4th ed. St Louis: Mosby; 2002.)

of a brass lens holder or suction cup. To add plus power, the lens is held so that its convex surface is against the velveteen and is exactly centered on the tool. To add minus power, the lens is held so that the convex surface is against the velveteen at the outer edge of the tool. In either case, the lens is rotated once or twice a full 360 degrees against the rotation of the tool (Fig. 16.24).

Peripheral curve

A peripheral curve can be applied by the use of a tool having a radius of curvature of 12.25, 11.5, 10.5, or 9.5 mm. The lens is carefully mounted on the lens block so that it is not at an angle, or it is fixed by means of double-sided tape. The block is held perpendicular to the tool, concave side down, by a sharp-pointed pencil acting as a spindle. The polishing agent (such as X-Pal) is then applied to the surface of the radius tool. The lens is held so that the concave surface rests lightly against the tool, revolving at about 1500 revolutions per minute; the entire edge of the lens must touch the tool at the same time. Equal pressure should be exerted on all meridians of the lens.

Fenestration of rigid lenses

Small holes drilled through a contact lens permit better tear exchange and consequently better oxygenation of the cornea. This is also a remedy for moderately tight contact lenses. Practitioners vary as to whether one or several holes should be used or whether the lens should be completely redesigned. In any event, these holes should be no larger than 0.5 mm and the interior walls must be highly polished to prevent clogging with secretions and irritation to the cornea. The fenestrations, although they do not interfere optically, do have a tendency to allow warpage of a lens and to weaken its structure. They should lie over the area of corneal edema because they provide only a small amount of increased respiration to a very limited underlying area of the cornea (Fig. 16.25).

Removing scratches

Care must be exercised when removing scratches from a rigid contact lens so as not to ruin its optics. In many cases, a new lens is preferred to trying to remove scratches. When scratches are removed from the front surface of a lens, the lens is held with a suction cup or spindle against the velveteen-covered drum while the drum is rotated. As in other modifications of contact lenses, X-Pal is the polishing compound used.

Removing scratches from the inside (base curve) of a lens can be done by use of a convex-shaped tool and X-Pal as the polishing compound. The best method is to use a sponge tool to polish the concave side of the lens.

Gas-permeable lenses

The GP polymer is a huge step forward in lens technology. The contact lens industry has not witnessed such an upheaval because the soft hydrogel lens was introduced.

GP lenses are made from materials that permit oxygen and carbon dioxide to diffuse through the plastic. These materials also wet more easily than the ordinary rigid lens and thus permit the tears to flow better under them.

GP lenses have become well established in clinical practice. They have replaced the conventional polymethyl methacrylate (PMMA) lenses because they offer all the advantages of a rigid lens but have fewer complications. GP lenses are also safer and more comfortable than rigid lenses.

The scope of GP materials is widening. The materials available to date include the following:
1. Cellulose acetate butyrate (CAB)
2. Silicone
3. Combinations of various materials, which include:
   - silicone-PMMA (silicone acrylates)
   - PMMA-silicone-CAB
   - combinations of fluorocarbon-PMMA-silicone
4. Polystyrene

The attractive feature of these lenses is their oxygen permeability, expressed as *DK*.

$$\text{Oxygen transmissibility} = DK/T$$

where:

D = the diffusion coefficient for oxygen movement in any substance
K = the solubility constant for oxygen in that substance
T = the thickness of the center of the lens
(Sometimes the letter L is used for thickness: DK/L.)

The oxygen permeability varies from lens to lens and according to the method used for measuring this factor. The silicone combinations, mixed with PMMA, have a high rating. The lenses with the highest oxygen permeability are those made of pure fluorocarbon or combinations of fluorocarbon and other proven contact lens materials.

The lens thickness of any given material must also be considered. The thicker the lens, the less permeable it is. Thus a lens that is made 0.1 mm thick has much greater permeability than one that is made for aphakia and is 0.5 mm thick.

Rigid lenses have been developed with a DK value of 140 and greater. This means greater freedom from the complications of corneal hypoxia, which permits the application of such high-DK lenses for extended wear. High-DK lenses

Table 16.4 Silicone-acrylate and fluorosilicone-acrylate data for rigid gas-permeable lenses

Lens name	Material	DK	Wetting angle
Boston II	Itafocon A (SA)	18.0	20
Boston IV	Itafocon B (SA)	26.0	17
Boston 7	Satafocon A (FSA)	73.0	33
Boston ES	Enflufocon A (FSA)	36.0	52
Boston EO	Enflufocon B (FSA)	82.0	49
Boston RXD	Itabisfluorofocon A	45.0	39
Boston Equalens	Itafluorofocon A (FSA)	71.0	26
Boston XO	Hexafocon A (FSA)	140.0	49
Boston EO Envision	Enflufocon B (FSA)	82.0	33
Boston Multivision	Enflufocon A (FSA)	31.0	n/a
Paragon HDS	Paflufocon B (FSA)	58.0	14.7
Paragon Thin	Paflufocon C (FSA)	29.0	12.8
Fluoroperm 30	Paflufocon C	30.0	12.8
Fluoroperm 60	Paflufocon B	60.0	14.7
Fluoroperm 92	Paflufocon A	92.0	16
Fluoroperm 151	Paflufocon A	151.0	42.0
Fluorex 700	Fluisifocon A	70.0	15.3
Latitude Multifocal	Telefocon B	43.5	n/a
Optacryl 60	Kolfolcon A	18.0	<25.0
Optimum Extra	Roflufocon C	100.0	<23.0
SGP II	Telefocon B	43.5	<30
Tyro-97	Hofocon A	97.0	23
PMMA		0.0	n/a

DK, Diffusion coefficient for oxygen movement in lens material and the solubility coefficient of oxygen in the material; FSA, fluorosilicone acrylate; PMMA, polymethyl methacrylate; SA, silicone acrylate.

Visual fields

When determining the visual field, the perimetrist attempts to make a two-dimensional map of a patient's entire area of vision. Normally in everyday living, we do not place much importance on the width of our vision, the emphasis being directed on seeing clearly straight ahead. However, those people who have lost much of their peripheral field are just as incapacitated functionally as those who have lost much of their central field. Try rolling up two sheets of paper and placing them before your eyes so that you are basically looking through two large-diameter straws. Although you can see directly ahead clearly, it is very difficult to walk through a room without bumping into the furniture.

The circumference of the visual field depends on many factors. Obviously, the field of vision needed for seeing a mosquito flying about would be different than for seeing a jumbo jet. Thus the size of an object is important in referring to the dimensions of the seeing area. Also the ability to perceive at the sides is not as great when the visibility is poor, as opposed to when it is clear; therefore illumination is an important factor in mapping the field of vision. The state of adaptation of the eye, whether light-adapted or dark-adapted, although not a critical factor, influences the measurable size of the visual field area.

These factors are objective and can in all instances be controlled by the perimetrist. The difficulty in qualitative or quantitative perimetry is not in assessing the factors of size, illumination, and adaptation but in assessing the patient. Perimetry depends entirely on obtaining an accurate and rapid subjective response. How does one compare the replies of a 72-year-old belligerent, slightly confused patient who has recently had a stroke to those of an intelligent 25-year-old woman with no cerebral disease? Because it is difficult to evaluate such factors as reaction time, fatigue, and general health, what is done and noted in every case is a simple evaluation (good, fair, or poor) of the patient's cooperation and reliability.

Although perimetry is not an exact science because it is entirely dependent on the subjective replies of the patient, the visual field for a given reliable patient should be reproducible. Many methods have been devised for estimating visual fields. We discuss only those methods that have survived the tests of time and their applications and limitations.

Preliminary procedures

A general statement should be recorded about the patient's visual behavior. If it is noted that the patient tends to bump into objects located on either the right or left, a right- or left-sided total loss of visual field (homonymous hemianopia) may be present.

Visual acuity, with and without glasses, should be noted before taking a visual field. As a rule, it can be stated that the poorer the patient's visual acuity, the larger is the test object that must be used to plot an accurate visual field. The manner in which the patient responds to visual acuity testing should be recorded. If the patient appears to see only the last three letters of all the lines on the chart, a loss of one-half of the visual field may be present.

Color vision should be checked, especially if colored test objects are going to be used.

The purpose of the visual field examination should be noted so emphasis can be given to specific areas. Such instruction must come from the ophthalmologist, who has made a complete ocular examination and a tentative diagnosis. For instance, for a patient with papilledema, the tangent screen might be thoroughly explored, with particular attention paid to the state of the blind spots, as opposed to the patient with retinitis pigmentosa, in whom a ring scotoma might be anticipated.

Facilities for field testing

Ideally, every office or clinic should have a visual field room that is quiet and out of the way of the normal practice traffic. This room should be of simple design so that distraction is kept to a minimum. Approximately 7 footcandles of illumination (see Ch. 3) are necessary for adequate visual field tests if the test apparatus does not contain its own light source.

Realistically, most offices do not have special visual field quarters because of the cost involved and lack of available space. Similarly, the equipment used varies from place to place. Although it is helpful to have the best ophthalmic equipment, the room and equipment always take a subordinate position to the skill and ingenuity of a competent perimetrist. If the patient understands what is expected and has rapport with the examiner, adequate perimetry can be performed.

Confrontation test

Of all methods of perimetry, the confrontation test is the most widely used because it requires no special facilities or equipment and can be performed in the home, on bedridden patients, and in hospitals. This is essentially a screening test. Any pathologic condition discovered requires a more sophisticated test when possible to determine the exact nature of the visual defect.

In this test, the examiner compares the range of the patient's field with his or her own, which is presumed to be normal. The examiner stands facing the patient at a distance of approximately 2 feet (60 cm). Opposite eyes are occluded; that is, the patient's left eye is covered while the examiner closes his or her right eye. Each of them then fixes the exposed eye of the other. The examiner moves a finger or a white test object, such as a small hatpin mounted

on a handle, from the extreme periphery midway between examiner and patient and notes when it comes into the field of view; the patient and examiner should see it simultaneously (Fig. 18.1). The test is best performed while the patient's back is to the light and the background behind the examiner is uniform and dark.

All four quadrants of the visual field should be tested and two different approaches should be used in each quadrant. If any defect is indicated or suspected, the field should be accurately mapped and recorded with the perimeter and tangent screen. When vision is extremely poor, a small penlight may be used for a rough test.

A modification of this test is to have the patient count fingers. While one eye is occluded, the examiner brings in from the periphery one, two, or three fingers and asks the patient to count the number of fingers brought in from each quadrant.

The confrontation test is an excellent method of screening patients and, if used skillfully, can be surprisingly accurate. It may be the only method of examining children, people who cannot read, and the cognitively challenged. With children, a small article of interest, such as a brightly colored plastic toy may be used as a test object. The preservation of a field in a particular area is indicated when the child makes a quick glance at the object of interest detected in the peripheral field. Finally, when fixation is lost or essential vision is grossly impaired, this method may be more valuable than a more refined technique. For example, in a patient with a cataract, the accurate perception and projection of light or a hand in all four quadrants may be the only method of determining retinal function.

However, this should be regarded only as a rough test, and failure to demonstrate a field defect does not imply a normal field. Defects of large size may easily be missed by this method.

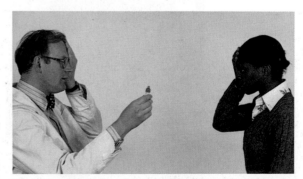

Fig. 18.1 Confrontation test. A test object is brought in from the periphery to the seeing area. (Reproduced from Spalton D, Hitchings R, Hunter P. *Atlas of Clinical Ophthalmology*. 3rd ed. St Louis: Mosby; 2004; with permission.)

Perimeters

Many perimeters are constructed in such a manner that the eye is at the center of rotation of a hemisphere that has a radius of curvature of 33 cm. Some perimeters consist of an arc of a circle that is rotated, and the test object is moved either manually or mechanically along this arc from the periphery toward the center. The more elaborate perimeters, such as the Goldmann perimeter, are constructed from a half shell, in which the test object is projected (Fig. 18.2). In this type of perimeter, the intensity of the illumination of the test object can be controlled and the patient's fixation can be continually checked by a viewing device behind the perimeter.

Before use, the Goldmann perimeter should be aligned and calibrated as follows:

1. Level the instrument so that the projector arm will swing back automatically into the protected position on the sphere when the instrument is not being used. Insert the chart paper and position the vertical and horizontal lines with the V-notch on the frame. If a fixation light projector is used, the chart is positioned 5 degrees from the center line.

2. Use the 15-degree position to the right and left for examination when the central scotoma device is indicated.

3. Adjust the telescope so that the reticule and the patient's eye are clear and in plain focus. Proper adjustment of the light within the sphere and of the projected target is most important. Position the recording arm at the 70-degree mark on the chart. This allows you to lock the projector arm in the proper position by pushing the centering pin on the operator's side into the socket on the upper left side of the instrument. When the arm is locked in, light from the projector will fall onto the light meter.

4. Position the size and brightness control levers to the far right. Turn the instrument on and the room lights off. Turn the appropriate control knob and adjust to a reading of 1000 apostilbs on the light meter.

5. Set the gray filter level to the 0.0315 position. This produces an illumination of 31.5 apostilbs.

6. Interpose the white photometer shade between the projected light and the light meter.

7. At this point, look at the photometer screen through the cut-out on the opposite side of the sphere. Match the sphere's brightness to the brightness on the photometer shade or screen by moving the diaphragm up or down.

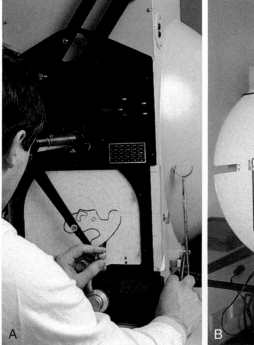
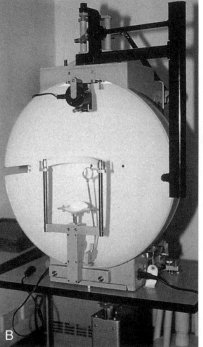

Fig. 18.2 (A, B) Goldmann spherical projection perimeter, an excellent apparatus for both peripheral and central fields. (Reproduced from Spalton D, Hitchings R, Hunter P. *Atlas of Clinical Ophthalmology*. 3rd ed. St Louis: Mosby; 2004; with permission.)

To achieve reliable and accurate fields, calibration of the instrument should be performed before each examination, but from a practical standpoint once monthly is adequate. You are now ready to proceed with the visual field test.

When the visual field has been mapped out on a perimeter, the following notations should be made: (1) the size of the test object, which can vary from 1 to 25 mm, (2) the test distance, which is always 330 mm in a perimeter, (3) the color of the test object, and (4) the cooperation and reliability of the patient.

Measuring a field on the perimeter

Just before the actual perimetric examination, the patient should be told in detail what is expected during this test. It is essential that the patient be comfortable, relaxed, and alert. Glasses are not required. The patient is brought to the perimeter and his or her chin is set on the chin rest. The chin should be placed comfortably on the rest so that the patient's face is held vertically and not tilted to one side. One eye is covered. The other eye, situated in the center of the arc, fixes on the white fixation target at the center of the perimeter around which the arc revolves.

The size of the test object chosen depends on the accuracy of the patient's fixation and reaction time. If the patient is young and alert and has 20/20 vision, the examination is begun with a 1- or 2-mm white target (I-2-e or I-3-e on the Goldmann perimeter). However, if the patient is confused and suffers with early stages of dementia, or has dementia, and has vision no better than 20/200, it would probably be best to use a 10 mm, 20 mm, or even larger test object (III-4-e) as the initial stimulus. The test object is always brought in from the periphery toward the center (from the nonseeing to the seeing area). The test object should be brought in slowly so that the time lag from the patient's response to the mark of the examiner will not be great. In many instances, the ophthalmologist will request a perimetric examination to be performed with certain test targets. These different targets show characteristically larger fields with the larger target. In follow-up visits, it is important to reuse the same targets to show any regression or progression of the field changes. The different targets show a different-sized field at a common illumination and distance; each of these completed mappings of a single target size and brightness is called an *isopter*. The ophthalmologist will inform the ophthalmic assistant which isopters are desired.

The patient should be taught to buzz or tap when the stimulus is seen. Conversation during the test should be kept to a minimum because it only serves to distract the patient and cause head movement.

Ideally, 24 meridians should be tested. The normal physiologic response to an object in the peripheral field is to turn the eyes toward it. When the field of vision is charted, this normal response has to be suppressed because fixation by the patient must be rigidly maintained on the central target. Therefore it is imperative to observe the patient's fixation at all times. In some of the more elaborate perimeters, a viewing system at the back of the shell enables the examiner to constantly watch the patient's eyes during the entire examination.

Field testing is taxing. Accuracy depends on the subject's accurate and quick response. It should not be laborious because prolonged visual field testing will tire a patient and cause erroneous results. Drooping eyelids or eyeglass frames interfering with a clear view of the test object can cause these erroneous results.

Errors in field testing can occur on the part of either the patient or the examiner. Errors attributable to the patient may include following the test object rather than maintaining proper fixation, tilting the head or moving the chin off the chin rest, not understanding the test or being generally uncooperative, responding slowly, most often done by mentally challenged patients with low visual acuity or obvious field defects, and physical, mental, or psychologic handicaps. Errors attributable to the examiner may include poor patient instruction, too-rapid movement of the test object, incorrect monitoring of the patient's fixation, poor or inaccurate marking of the chart, and poor or incorrect adjustment of the perimeter.

Charts

The visual field chart is merely a permanent record of the patient's responses at tangent screen and perimeter examinations. The best type of tangent screen chart is that in which both fields are represented on a small pad that can be fastened to the patient's record so that the whole picture of the patient's visual status can be seen at a glance. The right eye and left eye should be indicated and the chart should be as the patient sees the visual field; that is, the field for the right eye is on the right side of the chart. A notation should be made of the patient's name, the date, and the examiner's name. In addition, the size and color of target used, the corrected visual acuity, the pupillary size, and the patient's cooperation and reliability should be noted.

An isopter is the map of the circumference of a visual field determined by a test object of a certain size, with the patient at a certain distance from the tangent screen or perimeter. The isopter, as indicated on the visual field chart, should be noted as a fraction, the numerator indicating the size of the test object used in millimeters, and the denominator indicating the distance of the patient from the field chart in millimeters. Thus the fraction 5/1000 indicates to anyone what test object was used and at what distance in millimeters.

Special perimetric techniques

Visual field screening

Visual field screening is a good method for rapidly determining the presence or absence of a field defect. It is useful as a preliminary procedure in offices or in testing large groups, such as military personnel or students.

Automated visual fields

The automated perimeter or visual field plotter is a quick, randomized test to determine field defects (Fig. 18.3). A complete discussion of automated visual field equipment is found in Chapter 18.

Indications of a field defect include the following:

1. Two or more adjacent test spots that were missed at a single test intensity
2. A single spot missed at two or more stimulus intensities
3. Marked contraction of the visual field

The automated suprathreshold screener is extremely useful for preliminary visual field testing because it does not take up the amount of time required for the Goldmann perimeter (Figs. 18.4 and 18.5). Those patients examined in the office whose responses to the Amsler grid (see following text) are questionable or who reveal constriction during finger confrontation tests should be examined by the automated screener. If results are normal, generally no further testing is required. If defects are found during the automated screener test, however, then more detailed visual field examination must be done, with particular attention paid to the areas having defects as noted on the automated screener.

There are other models of visual field screeners, all using these principles.

Amsler grid

The Amsler grid was devised to detect abnormalities in the central 20 degrees in the field of vision. This chart consists essentially of vertical and horizontal lines with a central white fixation dot. The squares on the grid are 5 mm in size and subtend an angle of 1 degree at 30 cm. The Amsler chart is of greatest value in detecting small areas of macular or perimacular edema in which visual distortion is a prominent sign (Fig. 18.6).

To use the Amsler grid, one looks at the central black dot one eye at a time while covering the other eye. The illumination should be good and the patient should wear reading glasses if required. Any areas that appear blurred, missing a grid pattern, or wavy lines should be noted. Home Amsler

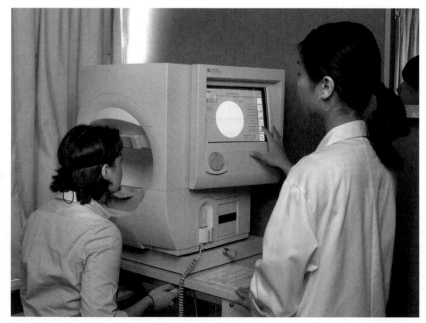

Fig. 18.3 Assessing fields with the Humphrey Visual Field Analyzer.

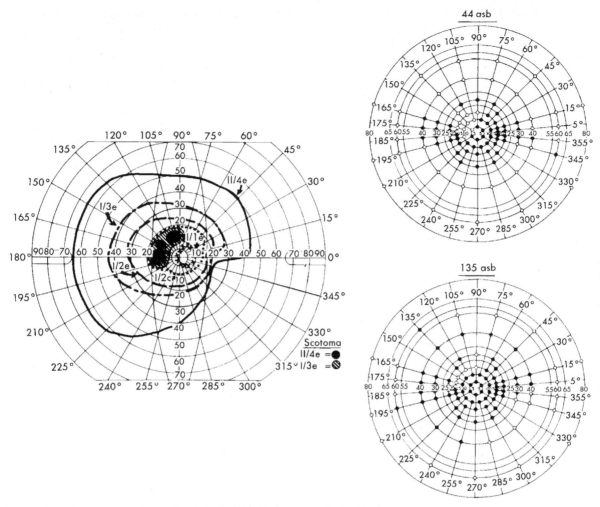

Fig. 18.4 Goldmann *(left)* and suprathreshold *(right)* field plots in a patient with glaucoma.

grids are available. One can rotate the grid card 90 degrees to capture more of the horizontal periphery.

The following series of questions should be asked while the patient is viewing the central white spot:

1. Is the center spot visible? If not, a central scotoma may be present.
2. While viewing the center, can you see all four sides? If not, an arcuate scotoma or a cecocentral scotoma may be present.
3. Do you see the entire grid? Are there any defects? If any areas are absent, then a paracentral scotoma may be present.
4. Are the horizontal and vertical lines straight and parallel? If not, then metamorphopsia is present. The parallel lines may bend inward, indicating micropsia, or bend outward, indicating macropsia.

Normal visual field

The normal visual field is determined by the size of the test object and the distance at which the test was made. With a 3-mm white target on a perimeter of a 330-degree radius, the average peripheral limit is about 95 degrees outward, 75 degrees downward, 60 degrees inward, and 60 degrees upward (Fig. 18.7). If the size of the target is increased, the temporal limit can be pushed outward to about 110 degrees. In many cases, allowances have to be made for the contours of the face. Especially to be considered during field testing is the loss of field caused by the projection of the brow and nose. If the visual field is taken without making allowances for these contours, the field is called a relative visual field.

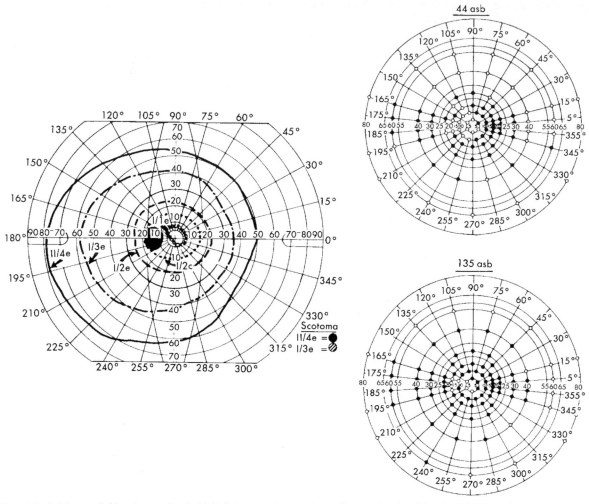

Fig. 18.5 Goldmann *(left)* and suprathreshold *(right)* screens in a patient with nutritional amblyopia and a central scotoma.

The absolute field is obtained by rotating the eye and the head to escape these limitations.

The blind spot marks a physiologic blind area of the retina. It corresponds with the entrance of the optic nerve to the posterior pole of the eye. This blind spot is located about 12 to 15 degrees to the outside of the fixation point and about 1.5 degrees below the horizontal meridian. It measures approximately 7.5 degrees high and 5.5 degrees wide.

Pathologic defects in the visual field

Pathologic field defects resulting from derangement within the optic nerve or its extensions to the occipital lobe of the brain cause a loss of vision but not a sensation of blackness.

Only field defects that arise from disturbances in front of the retina, such as those caused by a vitreous or macular hemorrhage, result in awareness of something black before the eyes. The distinction between the two is subtle. In disorders of the brain, the patient complains of the effects of the field loss but not of any particular sensation associated with this loss. With retinal disease, the patient will complain of both types.

Field defects are classified according to those that emanate from the periphery of the field and those that originate from within the confines of the field itself.

Scotoma

The scotoma is an area of partial or complete blindness within the confines of a normal or relatively normal visual field. Within a scotoma, the vision is more depressed than in the area of visual field surrounding it. When the depressed area of a scotoma expands into the periphery of the field, it is said to have "broken through."

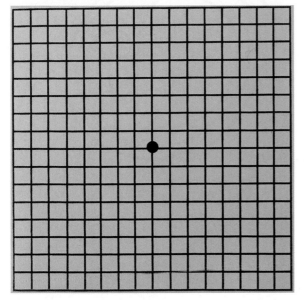

Fig. 18.6 Amsler chart used to detect small central visual field defects and distortions of the central visual field.

Scotomas may be divided into the following types:
1. *Central*, which involves the fixation area and is always associated with a loss of visual acuity (Fig. 18.8).
2. *Pericentral*, in which the fixation area is relatively clear and the field immediately surrounding it is deficient.
3. *Paracentral*, in which the area of depressed visual field is to one side of fixation (Fig. 18.9A). These scotomas also may be denoted as to their position: whether they are nasal or temporal to the fixation point.
4. *Cecal*, which involves the area of the normal blind spot (Fig. 18.9B).
5. *Nerve fiber bundle scotoma*. This is also referred to as an arcuate, Bjerrum, or comet type of scotoma (Fig. 18.9C). This type of lesion extends around the fixation point from the blind spot in an arc and ends typically on the nasal field with a sharply demarcated border. It can occur either above or below the blind spot. In some instances, it is not even attached to the blind spot, but seems to issue from it (Fig. 18.10).

The intensity of a scotoma varies from absolute blindness to a minimum detectable loss of visual acuity. If there is complete blindness to test objects of all sizes, the scotoma is absolute. If the area involves loss of only the smaller test objects, it is referred to as a relative scotoma.

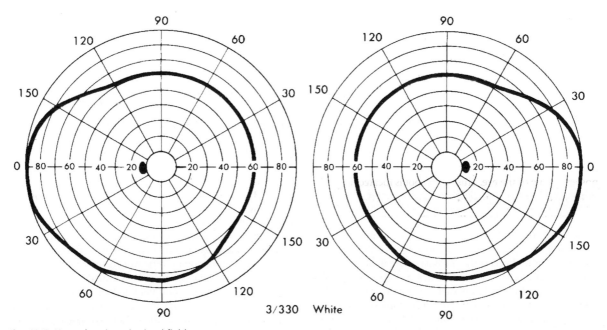

Fig. 18.7 Normal perimetric visual field.

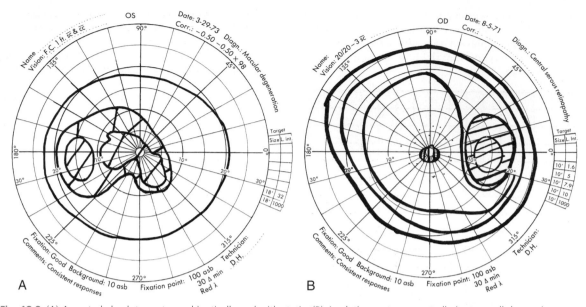

Fig. 18.8 (A) A central absolute scotoma, kinetically and with static. (B) A relative scotoma centrally (note small depression on static).

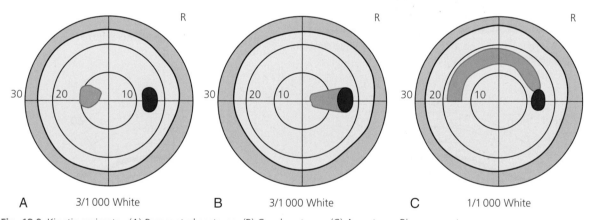

| A | 3/1 000 White | B | 3/1 000 White | C | 1/1 000 White |

Fig. 18.9 Kinetic perimetry. (A) Paracentral scotoma. (B) Cecal scotoma. (C) Arcuate, or Bjerrum, scotoma.

Contraction of the visual field

Contraction usually occurs as an area of blindness emanating from the periphery of the field toward the center. If the contraction affects only one part of the field, it often is referred to as a *sector defect*. Sector defects bounded by vertical diameters of the field are hemianopic defects. The term *hemianopic* is used to indicate a defect occupying half of the visual field; invariably it is a bilateral defect. A hemianopic defect is homonymous right or left when the corresponding half of both eyes is affected (Fig. 18.11). In this instance, there is total blindness in the temporal field of one eye and the nasal field of the other eye. The vertical dividing line between the seeing and the nonseeing portion of the field is midline. When a quadrant of each field is affected, a quadrant hemianopia or quadrantanopia is present (Fig. 18.12). A bitemporal hemianopia is a visual field defect in which part or all of each temporal field is depressed (Fig. 18.13). The defect may vary from the slightest depression of the upper temporal portion of the field to complete blindness in each temporal field.

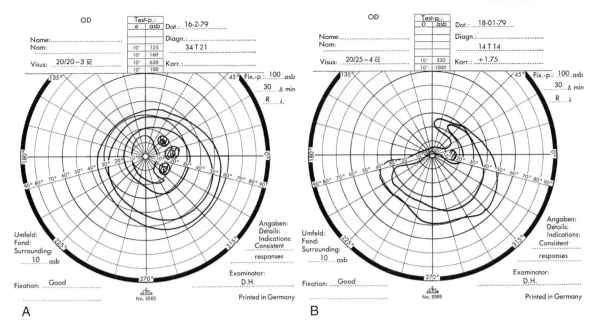

Fig. 18.10 Glaucoma field. (A) Early. (B) Late.

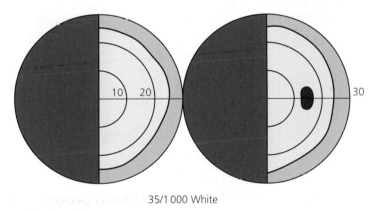

35/1 000 White

Fig. 18.11 Left homonymous hemianopia.

A congruous homonymous hemianopic defect is one in which the defect in the two fields is superimposable; that is, completely identical. In this instance, when the examiner maps the visual field of one eye, its margin will be identical to the visual field of the other (Fig. 18.14).

Hysterical visual field

In some instances, defects of the visual field are functional rather than organic; that is, they are caused by disturbance of the patient's emotional status or malingering rather than by disease of the retina or its visual pathways. In this instance, the most common field of vision seems to be narrowed down to only 10 to 20 degrees in diameter. If the patient is free of any organic disease, a tubular defect should indicate, or at least give rise to suspicion, that the patient has hysterical or malingering fields (Fig. 18.15).

The presence of such a functional defect can easily be checked by moving the patient back another meter from the tangent screen and doubling the size of the test object. By doing this, the visual angle of the field remains the same, but the diameter of the field on the tangent screen should

345

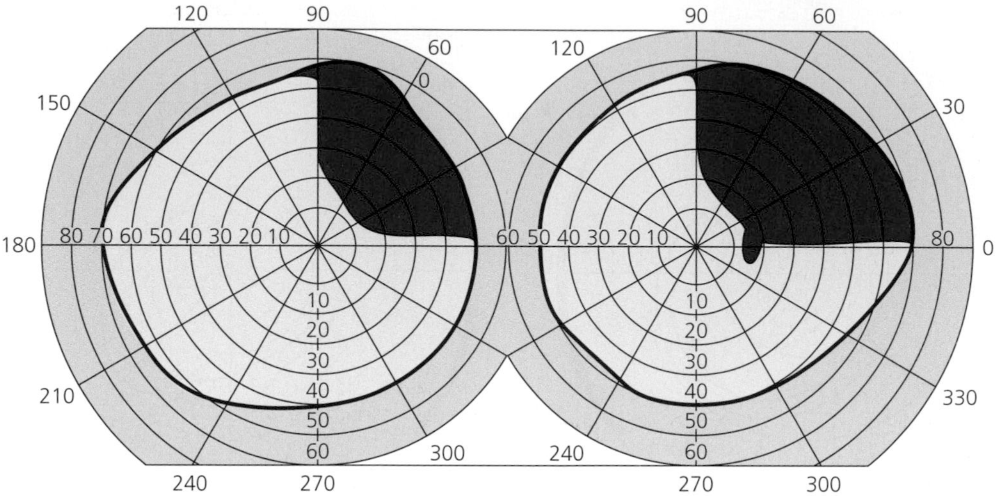

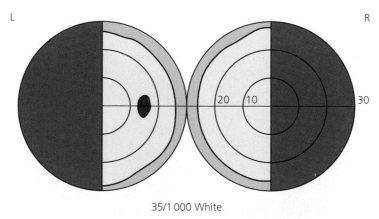

Fig. 18.12 Right incongruous homonymous superior quadrantanopia.

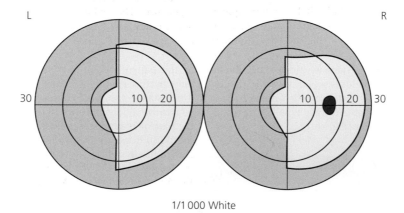

35/1 000 White

Fig. 18.13 Bitemporal hemianopia.

1/1 000 White

Fig. 18.14 Left congruous homonymous hemianopia.

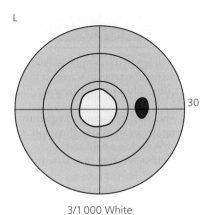

L

30

3/1 000 White

Fig. 18.15 Tubular, or hysterical, field. The size of the field remains unchanged when testing at 1 or 2 m.

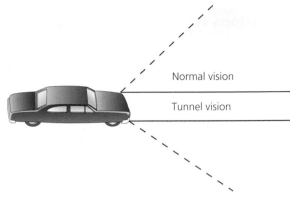

Normal vision

Tunnel vision

Fig. 18.16 Tunnel vision, with gross construction of the visual field as is found in retinitis pigmentosa. Driving is hazardous.

double in size. If the diameter remains the same at 1 and 2 meters, a nonorganic cause should be strongly suspected.

If the diameter of the visual field increases as it should, organic visual loss must be considered. In this case, the differential diagnosis of tubular fields includes vitamin deficiency, retinitis pigmentosa, and glaucoma.

With hysterical or malingering patients, the size and shape of the field defect can be suggested by the examiner. Other field defects frequently noted with this type of situation are the spiraling field and the star-shaped field. With retinitis pigmentosa, the patient has true tunnel vision. Driving a car with this type of field restriction is hazardous (Fig. 18.16).

Summary

The assessment of the visual field is vital to any complete ocular examination. It is of paramount importance in diagnosing lesions of the visual pathway, retinal lesions, and glaucoma. It is the mainstay of deciding whether glaucoma therapy has been adequate for an individual patient, because the entire principle of glaucoma therapy is to prevent loss of visual field. Its importance cannot be emphasized strongly enough. Many professionals believe that visual field testing is so important that it should be performed only by a trained visual field technician. We are in total agreement with this principle. We do believe, however, that the ophthalmic assistant, if properly trained to do a meticulous examination, can perform a valuable service in visual field testing as a preliminary examination. The final interpretation of the visual field must always be done by an ophthalmologist because only the physician can correlate the results of the visual field test with the patient's problem and the signs obtained on physical examination.

Instruction in visual field examination is best done by demonstration. Competence in visual field testing requires experience. The ophthalmic assistant should take every opportunity to perform routine normal visual field examinations to become familiar with the best techniques of visual field testing.

Chapter | 19 |

Automated visual field testing

Richard P. Mills and Joanne C. Wen

Visual field testing has continued to evolve because of advances in technology. In the past, the standard of excellence revolved around the manual Goldmann perimeter and the perimetrist. The visual field was plotted (Fig. 19.1A) after a lengthy examination during which both kinetic (moving) targets and static (stationary) targets were presented in random fashion. Technicians required extensive training and, perhaps more important, considerable patience to perform this task accurately. Kinetic testing has been almost exclusively replaced by static techniques (Fig. 19.1B) because the latter are more easily automated. Infrared and mosaic video cameras now monitor fixation. Patient consistency is constantly evaluated during the test by catch trials designed to elicit false-positive and false-negative responses. Improved testing algorithms have decreased the total test time.

In spite of these advances, perimetry remains a subjective test. The entire process depends on the patient's ability to concentrate and respond to the test stimulus. The key person interfacing between the patient and the computer is the technician. It is his or her responsibility to ensure that the patient understands the test and that the testing process runs smoothly. It is also the responsibility of the technician to ensure that fixation remains aligned, that the patient is given a break, and that he or she is reinstructed if fatigue is observed. No automated perimeter available today has eliminated the need for a technician to administer the test and monitor its quality in real time. In this chapter, the basics of perimetry are reviewed, the technician's duties are outlined and, when appropriate, suggestions are given to make the task easier and more relevant to the patient's needs.

Understanding the principles of perimetry

There are two types of perimeters: kinetic and static. Both kinetic and static perimetry ultimately perform the same function: they test the field of vision, but they do so in different ways. Kinetic devices highlight moving targets to map out the visual field (see Fig. 19.1A) and spend less time exploring the field with stationary or static techniques, whereas static devices depend on static techniques almost exclusively (see Fig. 19.1B).

The analogy of the visual field to an island of vision sitting amid a sea of blindness is a useful one (Fig. 19.2). The highest point near the center of the island corresponds to the area of greatest visual sensitivity (for the fovea of the retina). As a person moves toward the water's edge, the sensitivity falls to zero. In other words, the farther away from the area of greatest visual sensitivity a person is, the brighter a light target must be to be seen. At the water's edge, in the analogy, not even the brightest target can be seen.

The task of perimetry is to map the island of vision. The problem is that the island is enshrouded in a fog bank (Fig. 19.3), and indirect methods of mapping it are required.

Kinetic testing can be likened to airplanes flying toward the visual island at different altitudes (Fig. 19.4). If we know the altitude at which the planes fly and if we record the coordinates of each "crash site" of many planes flying

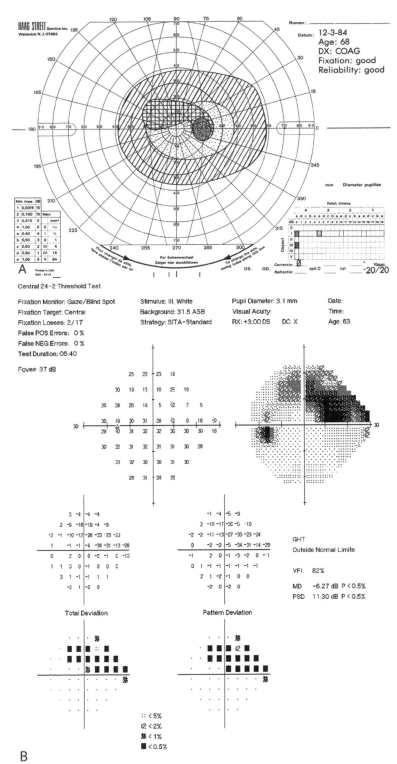

Fig. 19.1 (A) Example of a Goldmann kinetic visual field. (B) Example of a Humphrey visual field of a similar visual field defect.

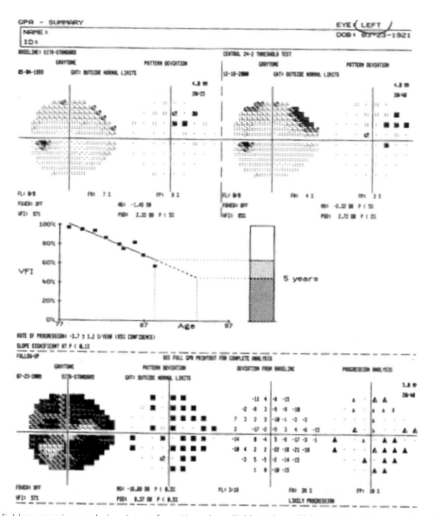

Fig. 19.14 Visual field progression analysis printout from Humphrey Field Analyzer (Zeiss Meditec). (See text for description.)

Summary

The role of the perimetrist is continuing to evolve as the automated perimeter eases many aspects of testing. As this occurs, the attention of the technician is now directed toward other areas. In particular, the perimetrist has more time for guiding and encouraging the patient through the testing procedure. Perimetry is essential in the management of many ophthalmic conditions, and the key component is not the computer or sophisticated software programs; rather, the key component to excellent perimetry continues to be the technician.

Chapter | 20 |

Computers in ophthalmic practice

Michael L. Gilbert, Michael J. Gilbert, and Gerald E. Meltzer

Computer technology is relatively young, the first digital computer as we know it having been built in 1937. However, the computerization of the world has had an enormous effect on nearly every aspect of contemporary daily life and a major effect on the way ophthalmology is practiced. It is estimated that more than 95% of all ophthalmic offices use computers for such tasks as insurance billing, practice management reporting, payroll, sending recall notices, or even calling patients automatically to remind them of missed appointments or to notify them that their contact lenses have arrived. Beyond the myriad practice-centered uses of desktop, laptop, and tablet or handheld computers, computerization not only controls data acquisition but also aids in interpreting the results of many of the instruments commonly used in direct patient care, including the lensometer, keratometer, phoropter, perimeter, ocular coherence tomography, ultrasound, and optical biometry, as well as non-ophthalmic but otherwise critical tools, such as Internet-based telephone (Voice Over Internet Protocol [VOIP]), digital copy machines, and the cell phone. Thus computers increasingly contribute to better patient care as well as increased office productivity.

The effect of computers in the field of ophthalmology is a reflection of an accelerating trend towards office automation. Universal acceptance of computer technology by worldwide industries, coupled with markedly decreasing costs and widespread availability of increasingly sophisticated computer hardware and software programs, has defined a new era in computer-assisted medical care. Well-used computerization is a boon to quality patient care, staff efficiency, and practice success at all levels. This chapter is designed to expand the ophthalmic assistant's knowledge base about computers, how they work, and what they can do for an ophthalmic office and its personnel.

Computer basics

A computer is a device capable of accepting, storing, retrieving, and manipulating or processing information automatically at high speeds by applying a sequence of logical arithmetic or textual operations. In simpler terms, a computer is able to execute a series of instructions that allow the user to ask questions as simple as "What does Fred Smith owe on his account?" The ability to instantly and invisibly respond to sequential instructions at ever increasing speeds allows computerization to aid in more sophisticated tasks, such as the analysis of complex data generated by the automated lensometer, autorefraction, retinal tomography, or corneal topography. With mounting hardware speed, complexity, and capability, computers can even make some complex decisions and predictions through the use of artificial intelligence. By comparing new patient data with stored historical databases of comparable results from normal patients, computers are able to aid in the interpretation of visual fields, corneal topography, intraocular lens (IOL) calculations, or optic nerve analysis. This ongoing evaluation process not only aids in the initial diagnosis of disease but also helps track clinically

Optical coherence biometry

Microprocessor-controlled laser-based diagnostic equipment can be used to determine the axial length of the eye for intraocular lens calculations. This technology offers advantages and disadvantages over ultrasound biometry. Both ultrasound-based and optical coherence–based biometry products generally offer integrated software to calculate intraocular lens powers. They also typically include database software to track outcomes and create surgeon factors intended to enhance future precision and predictability of surgical results.

Wavefront analysis aberrometry

Computer-based wavefront analysis is finding increasing application in ophthalmic practice through laser-assisted in situ keratomileusis (LASIK), IOL advances, and applications in glasses and contacts. These devices analyze light rays that emerge or are reflected from the retina and pass through the optical system of the eye. Light rays are projected into the eye onto the macula. Rays that emerge from a single point in the fovea and pass through the optical system of the eye are analyzed. One such technology uses multiple tiny lenslets located in front of the eye that isolate a narrow beam of light emerging through different parts of the pupil. A digital camera registers the true position of each ray and compares it with the calculated expected position of such a ray for a perfect optical model of the eye without aberrations. This difference enables sophisticated computer-based calculations of the aberrations or distortions of the total true optical system of the individual eye.

Wavefront analysis offers useful information for disease detection and management and selecting surgical parameters, and holds the potential to revolutionize the optical correction of refractive errors.

Fundus photography

Classic film-based narrow angle images have been used for decades in imaging the retina. These cameras are now often computerized as well, taking pictures that are digitized and uploaded into databases for review and analysis by the doctor. More recently, technologic advances have allowed for wider fields of view of the fundus, such as ultrawide field laser-based imaging of the retina that may not even require dilation of the patient. These imaging techniques have enabled tremendous advantages in fields, such as diabetic retinopathy where telemedicine programs and, more recently, artificial intelligence algorithms can analyze these images to determine a patient's risk of vision loss.

Emerging and future computerized technologies

It is almost certain that any new technology adopted in ophthalmic practice will be computer-based. Likely it will use computerization and even artificial intelligence to perform tasks more quickly and to compare individual patient results with a database of normal patients, as well as with that patient's previous results. Increasingly, such applications will use networking and central databases to allow integration of complementary technologies throughout the practice into the EHR. Such integration will, by definition, improve clinical efficiency, data utility, and analysis, while almost certainly promoting improved quality of patient care.

Special ophthalmic applications

Online databases and Internet resources

It is difficult to overestimate the vast effect that Internet resources have had on society in general and on ophthalmic medical practice in particular. Email and messaging are important tools for near-instant communication within the office or around the globe. Such communication can have a powerful effect on patient care and office efficiencies.

Patient engagement is promoted with the use of patient portals. Physicians can exchange information and laboratory results with patients and patients can now readily communicate with their physician using secure messaging. Direct mail allows physicians to coordinate patient care by exchanging sensitive information securely with other physicians.

The Internet itself is seemingly a diffuse, endless resource. Importantly, there are now hundreds of medical databases with an enormous range of information from important primary resources, such as state and federal government, specialty medical societies and journals, commercial researchers, such as the pharmaceutical industry, the National Institutes of Health, the National Library of Medicine, and the Centers for Disease Control and Prevention, to name just a few. Any of these databases can be accessed instantly by computer from the office, from the home office, or while on the move through any Internet connection. The ability for such databases to be kept precisely up to the minute with the latest research makes them powerful resources indeed, lending their power and authority to the latest options in medical care choices.

Health Insurance Portability and Accountability Act and patient privacy

The Health Insurance Portability and Accountability Act (HIPAA) was enacted in 1996 to ensure that employees who changed jobs would not lose their health insurance. However, since that time, the law has been modified so that sensitive patient information is protected from being disclosed without the patient's consent or knowledge thus giving patients greater control over their medical information.

HIPAA demands that safeguards be implemented to ensure the confidentiality, integrity and availability of protected health information (PHI). In addition, the law places limits on the usage and disclosure of PHI. Finally, the law requires that patients be notified if the privacy or security of their PHI is compromised. The Health and Human Services Office of Civil Rights is responsible for enforcing HIPAA. Any violations of the provisions of the law could result in a fine or even criminal prosecution.

What is PHI? Any individually identifiable health information is considered protected under federal law and cannot be disclosed except under certain instances only as authorized by law without a patient's permission. Examples of protected health information include:

1. Information in a patient's medical record
2. Discussions about a patient's medical care
3. Patient's billing information
4. Any information that could be used to link a patient with his or her medical condition, such as a medical record number, a phone number, an address, birthdate, test results or even a license plate number.

Healthcare providers are required to give patients a clear written explanation telling them how the healthcare provider will use their personal information, to whom it may be disclosed, as well as how it will be protected. Information may not be released other than to other healthcare providers who may be involved in the patient's care without consent. Violating these rules may result in significant financial penalties, as well as federal criminal penalties.

1. Remember, all healthcare information is private. Be careful not to display any medical information, such as might be found in a chart or a photograph or on a computer screen so that a patient or nonstaff member could read it.
2. When discussing a patient be mindful of your surroundings so that other patients cannot overhear your discussions.
3. Do not leave patient information in plain sight
4. Do not share your login information with other employees.
5. Do not take files or documents containing PHI out of the clinic or office.
6. Fax transmittals should always include a cover sheet.
7. Never leave PHI on a voice mail message.
8. Call the patient using only phone numbers that have been approved by the patient.
9. Do not discuss PHI with any family member or friend without the patient's written consent.
10. Do not include PHI in an email, whether to a patient or other healthcare provider.
11. All mobile devices or laptops that contain PHI MUST be protected (encrypted) so if lost or stolen, unauthorized individuals would not have access to any protected health information contained on them.

Summary

The incredible effect of computerization on the ophthalmic practice is impossible to overstate. Increasingly, computers are finding their way into every aspect of ophthalmic practice and patient care. Much of medical care involves gathering information, processing selected information, storing data for future reference, and decision-making based on available data. Computer technologies and management resources—available through office-based and networked computers, computerized diagnostic technologies, increasingly sophisticated analysis and tracking software with artificial intelligence, and instant access to a universe of the latest research—define new levels of patient care. With each advance in sophistication facilitated by greater affordability, new horizons in practice efficiencies and enhancements of patient care are opened before us.

Chapter | 21 |

Ocular injuries

Harold A. Stein and Sara M. AlShaker

The ophthalmic assistant and associated allied personnel in ophthalmology should have knowledge about the prevention of eye accidents and the first-aid therapy of trauma in industry, as well as at home. Reports from the National Society for the Prevention of Blindness reveal that ocular injury is responsible for 5% of all blindness in children of school and preschool age. Many athletic activities, including racquet sports, boxing, and hockey, carry the risk of visual casualties. Industrial eye injuries are virtually a daily occurrence in every ophthalmologist's office and in every emergency center of a hospital.

The escalation of traumatic eye injuries is partly attributable to the progress achieved in the field of transportation, to the development of potentially dangerous consumer home products and children's toys, and to advancements in industrial mechanization, without corresponding advances in personal safety devices. Only in large industrial plants have safety programs been inaugurated to detect visual disabilities and to prevent eye accidents. Prevent Blindness America, formerly known as the National Society to Prevent Blindness, launched Wise Owl Club in 1948, an industrial and school eye safety incentive program. The program recognized over 85,000 cases who have had one or both eyes saved from a serious injury by the use of protective lenses. Guidelines for preventing eye injuries are published on their website https://www.preventblindness.org/preventing-eye-injuries.

Despite rigid precautionary safety measures, however, eye accidents will continue to occur because of carelessness, chance, and the tendency of people to ignore the safety measures provided for them.

This chapter deals with first-aid therapy of eye injuries and preventive measures to help reduce the loss of vision from trauma.

Diagnosis of ocular injury

The diagnosis of an eye injury can be made by a careful history of the injury in relation to the time and type of injury. A history of discomfort and reduction in vision may indicate the severity of injury. Objective signs require careful external examination that includes comparison with the unaffected eye. Pressure should never be exerted in separating the eyelids, but the upper lid should be pushed up against the bone under the eyebrow and the lower lid depressed with pressure only on the bone of the cheek below. All injuries to the globe, until proved otherwise, should be examined as if the globe has been ruptured. If magnification is required, a × 2 loupe or slit-lamp microscope can detect areas of damage not otherwise discovered.

Conjunctival and corneal foreign bodies

Despite the many anatomic and physiologic protective factors around the eye, nearly everyone at one time or another has had a foreign body in the eye. In most instances, the ensuing tearing and blinking of the lids have been sufficient to dislodge the irritant. It is when these natural mechanisms fail to remove a foreign body that one has to have it located and removed (Figs. 21.1 and 21.2).

When a foreign body has lodged in the cornea, examination should always begin by determining the patient's best-corrected visual acuity of the injured eye with glasses on or with the addition of a pinhole disc if the vision is reduced. In this way, any preexisting visual impairment will not be attributed to the trauma and removal of the foreign body. In taking the history, the examiner should attempt to ascertain the source of the fragment because the type of foreign body will influence the amount of tissue destruction and rate of repair. Particles of copper and brass are notoriously more irritating to the eye than are iron and steel. High-velocity foreign bodies—that is, those catapulted by hammering, chiseling, or lathing—are prone to penetrate the cornea deeply, or even to perforate it, as opposed to the wind-blown particle that embeds itself in the superficial corneal epithelium.

It usually is expedient to place two or three drops of a local anesthetic, such as proparacaine hydrochloride 0.5%

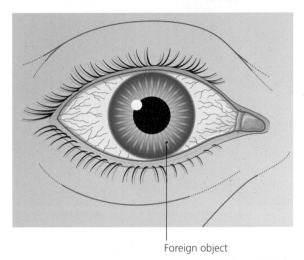

Foreign object

Fig. 21.2 Redness, foreign body sensation, and photophobia occur in the presence of a corneal foreign body. (From Stein HA, Slatt BJ, Stein RM. *A Primer in Ophthalmology: A Textbook for Students*. St Louis: Mosby; 1992.)

(Alcaine) or tetracaine hydrochloride 0.5% (Altacaine), into the lower conjunctival sac to facilitate surface anesthesia. This makes the patient more comfortable and allows the examiner to scrutinize the injured eye with ease. The best instrument for examining the cornea is the slit-lamp microscope because it offers simultaneously high magnification and strong focal illumination. If a foreign body cannot be seen, a strip of fluorescein paper can be placed in the eye to stain the surface of the cornea because foreign bodies become visible when surrounded by the stain. If the foreign body has become dislodged by the patient's blinking and tearing, the fluorescein will stain the resultant corneal defect. In many cases, the cornea will show many surface scratches and the foreign body will be located on the undersurface of the upper or lower lid. Routinely, an examination of the palpebral conjunctiva lining both the upper and lower lids should be performed. Inspection of the conjunctiva lining the lower lid is carried out simply by depressing the lower lid. The undersurface of the upper lid is examined by everting it. The patient is asked to look down while the eyelashes are grasped and pulled over a glass rod, toothpick, or cotton tip applicator (Fig. 21.3). Alternatively, this examination can be accomplished by everting the upper lid over a transilluminator or muscle light. The foreign body is usually revealed as an opaque speck in the red glow of the lid tissue.

The treatment of corneal foreign bodies is total removal. A superficial foreign body can sometimes be dislodged by a gentle stream of saline solution delivered from an irrigator, or it can be wiped off by moist cotton tip applicator.

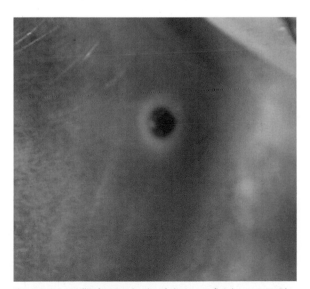

Fig. 21.1 Metallic foreign body of the superficial cornea with surrounding cellular infiltration. (From Kanski J, Bowling B. *Clinical Ophthalmology—A Systematic Approach*. 7th ed. Edinburgh: Saunders; 2011.)

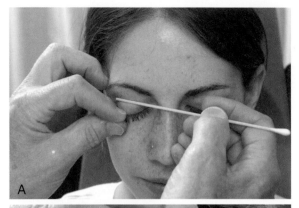

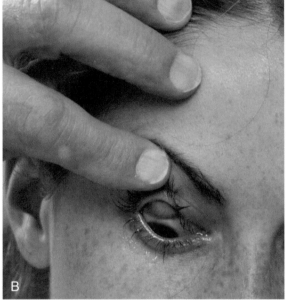

Fig. 21.3 (A) Eversion of the upper eyelid over an applicator. (B) Identification of foreign body on underside of eyelid.

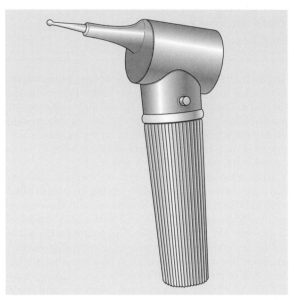

Fig. 21.4 Rotating burr for removal of rust rings.

If these measures fail, a nonpenetrating superficial foreign body can be carefully dislodged using the tip of a 27- or 25-gauge needle or it can be lifted from its base by the use of a sterile jeweler's forceps. The upper and lower eyelids must be immobilized using a speculum or by gently holding them in place. After 6 to 8 hours, a metallic foreign body may form a brownish-orange rust ring in the corneal tissue. This rust spot can be difficult to remove because it becomes adherent to the surrounding corneal stroma. It can be lifted with a needle, jeweler's forceps or it can be smoothened out by a corneal spud or burr (Fig. 21.4), under magnification by a slit-lamp microscope (Fig. 21.5). In such cases, it can help to have a corneal burr on hand to remove the rust ring. Small dental drills make excellent corneal burrs. The

tenacity of the rust is so great that often the corneal spud will only fragment the rusted spot. The goal is to remove as much of the rust ring as possible without causing too much tissue disruption or corneal perforation.

After the removal of a foreign body, the patient is cautioned about the discomfort caused by the epithelial defect from the foreign body and the removal process. Broad-spectrum topical antibiotics are prescribed and the patient is seen the next day. Rarely, in the case of severe discomfort, a bandage contact lens can be used with the precaution that this can promote an infective process; antibiotics and next day follow-up are essential if this is done. A short-acting topical cycloplegic drop can be used to alleviate any pain resulting from iris spasm. A pressure patch can be used cautiously but is not usually necessary. A corneal foreign body should be treated as an ocular emergency. It is desirable, but not mandatory, that the foreign body be removed as soon after the mishap as possible. If there are extenuating circumstances, however, such as the ophthalmologists being involved in surgery, the injured eye should receive some antibiotic drops until the patient is seen. It is imperative, however, to relieve the patient's symptoms. The discomfort of a corneal foreign body can be intense. Some relief of pain can be obtained with over-the-counter medications, such as acetaminophen (Tylenol) or ibuprofen (Advil). The patient should never be given a local anesthetic ointment or drops to take home because local anesthetics only interfere with wound healing and mask complications.

If the foreign body becomes dislodged by forceful and frequent blinking and the profusion of tears, the patient

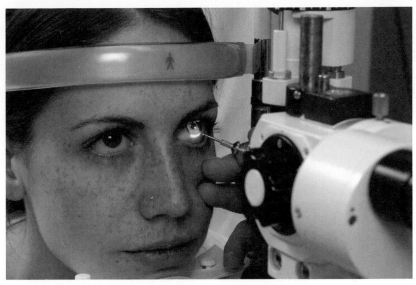

Fig. 21.5 Removal of foreign body under magnification of the slit-lamp microscope.

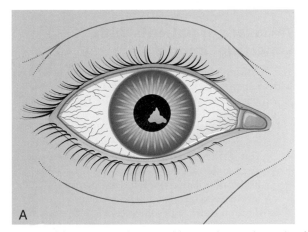

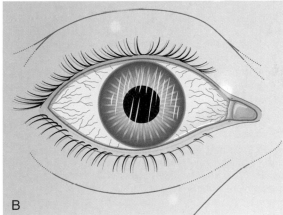

A

B

Fig. 21.6 (A) Deep corneal erosion. (B) Vertical corneal scratches from foreign body under upper lid.

may still feel that something is in the eye. This is because injury to the cornea, whether it is caused by inflammation, a foreign body, or an abrasion, yields the same symptom: a foreign body sensation.

Conjunctival foreign bodies do not, as a rule, give rise to pain or discomfort in the eye. If they lodge in the bulbar conjunctiva, they usually are easily visible because of the white background of the underlying sclera. Exceptions that are not visible are chips of glass and plastic from a broken contact lens. Superficial conjunctival foreign bodies are removed either by the application of a moistened cotton-tipped applicator or by gentle irrigation with saline solution. Occasionally, forceps may be required if there is blood around the foreign body; the ophthalmic assistant should be aware that penetration of the eye may have occurred.

Corneal abrasions

Corneal abrasions are superficial scratches and erosions of the cornea (Figs. 21.6 and 21.7). They are found after corneal foreign bodies have been removed, either spontaneously or with treatment. They are most commonly found after injuries caused by paper, fingernails, wires, and so

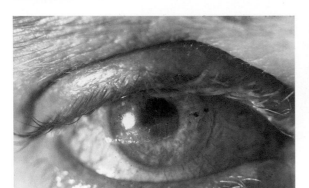

Fig. 21.7 Corneal abrasion as a result of thermal burn from hair curler.

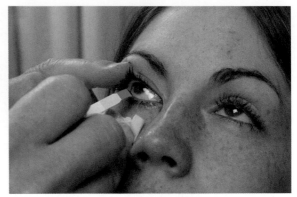

Fig. 21.9 Application of moistened fluorescein paper strip. Some practitioners find the lower cul-de-sac easier to use.

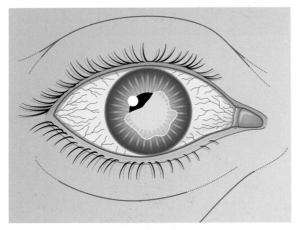

Fig. 21.8 Corneal abrasion is characterized by ciliary injection and an epithelial defect (which stains with fluorescein). (From Stein HA, Slatt BJ, Stein RM. *A Primer in Ophthalmology: A Textbook for Students*. St Louis: Mosby; 1992.)

forth. A corneal abrasion, unless it is large, cannot be seen with the naked eye. Patients with a corneal abrasion complain of a foreign body sensation of the eye. Often these patients are seen by a nurse or a friend and told that there is nothing in their eye and as a result they suffer until they are finally seen by the ophthalmologist. Any patient who complains of a foreign body sensation of the eye should be seen. Fluorescein strips should be placed in the eye (Figs. 21.8 and 21.9) to stain the area of the corneal defect. Careful assessment of the eye with eversion of eyelids, as mentioned before, is necessary. A dilated fundus examination is essential in the case of a history suggestive of a penetrating foreign body.

Most corneal abrasions heal spontaneously. Some ophthalmologists choose to prescribe broad-spectrum topical antibiotics as a prophylactic measure. The larger the abrasion, the more time it takes to heal. Follow-up is usually to ensure no infection has occurred and the cornea has healed well. The same principles mentioned earlier apply with regards to the use of a bandage contact lens.

Aftercare of patients with superficial injuries

The following points summarize the aftercare of a patient with a superficial corneal and conjunctival injury:
1. Arrangements should be made to have the patient driven home.

    The patient should be warned that discomfort in the eye may occur an hour or two after office treatment. This is the length of time that the local anesthetic given in the office usually remains effective. If a feeling of irritation continues, the patient should be instructed to take a pain-relieving drug.
2. Medication other than some general analgesics should not be given. The patient also should be told that it is best to return home and rest.
3. The rate of healing depends on the area of the tissue injured, the amount of tissue devitalized, the presence or absence of infection, and the nature of the injuring agent.
4. The patient should be instructed to return to their follow-up as planned or earlier if there is significant worsening in vision, pain, or discharge.

Intraocular foreign bodies

Intraocular foreign bodies constitute a surgical emergency. Often the site of penetration is not visible externally

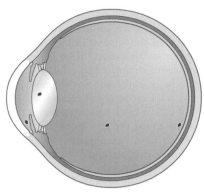

Fig. 21.10 Intraocular foreign bodies can be found in a variety of sites: in the anterior chamber, lens, vitreous, or retina. (From Stein HA, Slatt BJ, Stein RM. *A Primer in Ophthalmology: A Textbook for Students.* St Louis: Mosby; 1992.)

(Fig. 21.10). The ophthalmic assistant should not make a judgment on the gravity of a foreign body injury on the basis of the eye's external appearance.

Because the severity of the intraocular damage depends on the size, shape, and composition of the foreign body, the assistant should attempt to obtain an accurate description of the nature of the type of metal embedded. Often, it is possible to ascertain the source of the fragment. This is very important because the success of the operative procedure depends to a large extent on whether the fragment is magnetic. The patient should be reassured that everything possible will be done, but should not be promised a full recovery of the eye because eyes injured by foreign bodies, particularly those lodged in the posterior pole (i.e., in the retina or vitreous), often do poorly.

One can serve the patient best by making sure that this type of injury is seen by the attending ophthalmologist immediately. Relatives should be notified and the hospital, particularly the operating room personnel, should be informed of the emergency. Transportation to the hospital should be arranged so that the patient is not kept waiting in the office. A protective shield should be placed over the patient, primarily to prevent from causing further damage to the eye by rubbing it or by cleaning it with a dirty handkerchief.

The ophthalmic assistant should always be aware of the possibility of the presence of an intraocular foreign body. Intraocular foreign bodies usually are high-velocity small missiles and should be suspected in accidents in which striking, grinding, or cutting force is applied to metal. Fast-moving particles may penetrate the eye without producing any pain, discomfort, or gross visible signs and yet still may cause severe damage to the eye. Fig. 21.11 shows an air pellet in the eye that passed through the upper eyelid.

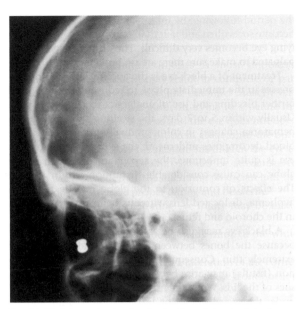

Fig. 21.11 Intraocular foreign body. Air pellet entry into the globe.

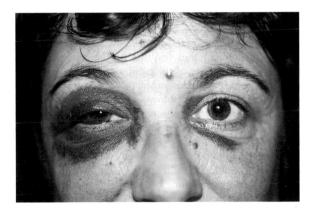

Fig. 21.12 Contusions of the eyelids with ecchymosis. (From Kanski J. *Clinical Ophthalmology.* 8th ed. Oxford: Elsevier/Mosby; 2015.)

Contusion of the eyelids: black eye

A black eye is the result of an injury to the orbital margin or eyelids from a blunt object, such as a fist (Fig. 21.12). The appearance of a black eye is quite alarming to the patient because of the large extravasation of blood underneath the skin. A patient with this type of injury should be seen immediately because examination of the globe is easiest in the game. Since that time, certified face protectors attached to a certified helmet have become mandatory for most minor hockey players in Canada and the United States and are voluntary for professional hockey players. In Canada, ocular trauma decreased by 90% after certified full-face protectors attached to the headgear were made mandatory in organized amateur hockey.

Annually in the United States, there are more than 600,000 eye injuries related to sports and recreational activities; 40,000 of these require emergency department visits. Most injuries occurring in school-aged children are sports-related, and eye injuries are the leading cause of blindness in children. Water and pool activities are the leading causes of sports-related eye injuries in children 14 years and younger, and basketball is the leading cause in youths 15 years and older. A listing of sports-related eye injuries by age is shown in Table 21.1. More than 90% of eye injuries can be prevented by the use of appropriative protective eyewear. Protective eyewear includes safety glasses and goggles, safety shields, and eye guards designed for a particular sport. Polycarbonate lenses with appropriate sports-formulated frames provide the best eye protection for many sports, are 10 times more impact-resistant than other plastic lenses, and do not adversely affect vision. Ordinary prescription glasses and "street wear" frames, contact lenses, and sunglasses do not protect against eye injuries. Safety goggles need to be worn over them. BB guns should be avoided and darts should be played with safety goggles.

Injuries caused by radiant energy

Ultraviolet radiation: photokeratitis

The most common radiation injury encountered results from the absorption of ultraviolet by the cornea. The ultraviolet light of the sun is absorbed mainly by the atmosphere. Except in high altitudes or on exceptionally clear days, the ultraviolet content of the sun seldom exceeds 1% or 2%. Sunlight reflected from the sea, snow, or bright sand, however, may contain 4% to 6% ultraviolet light, and such reflections constitute a greater ultraviolet light hazard than the sun itself. Industrial and domestic sources of ultraviolet rays include the carbon arc lamp, the arc used in welding, and sunlamps used for tanning. The ultraviolet rays from these sources may be reflected and that reflection, as well as direct viewing, may be a source of injury.

With ultraviolet burns to the cornea there are no immediate symptoms, but a few hours later, the recipient's eyes begin to water and feel gritty. Later, as the symptoms

Table 21.1 Sports-related eye injuries by age

Activity	Estimated injuries[a]	Ages 0–14 years	Ages 15+ (years)
Pool & water sports	4675	2795	1880
Basketball	4507	1412	3095
Nonpowder guns, darts, arrows, slingshots	3669	2026	1644
Baseball/softball	1998	1452	546
Exercise, weight-lifting	1871	295	1577
Soccer	1519	473	1046
Other sports & recreational activities	1476	464	1014
Playground equipment	1130	947	183
Bicycle & accessories	1115	295	820
Football	1106	506	600
Boxing, martial arts, wrestling	863	37	826
All-terrain vehicles (4 wheels)	705	18	687
Fishing	640	157	483
Misc. Ball games	617	111	506
Racquet sports	590	191	399
Ball sports, unspecified/other	580	335	245
Volleyball	408	178	231
Trampolines	295	239	55
Golf	270	92	178
Sports & recreational activity, not elsewhere classified	155	116	39
Winter sports	87	6	81

Continued

Table 21.1 Sports-related eye injuries by age—cont'd			
Activity	**Estimated injuries[a]**	**Ages 0–14 years**	**Ages 15+ (years)**
Scooters, Skateboards, Skating, Go Carts	55	34	21
Totals Top 22 Categories	**28,332**	**12,179**	**16,154**

[a]Totals may not equal because injuries are not mutually exclusive. Based on statistics provided by the U.S. Consumer Product Safety Commission, Directorate for Epidemiology; National Injury Information Clearinghouse; National Electronic Injury Surveillance System (NEISS). Product Summary Report—Eye Injuries Only—Calendar Year 2018.
Prevent Blindness. Reproduced by permission of Prevent Blindness.

progress, the foreign body sensation becomes extreme and the patient is in a great deal of pain. Tearing, congestion of the globe, and marked photophobia (inability to tolerate light) occur. Staining of the cornea with fluorescein reveals slight pitting of its surface, which is caused by erosion of the superficial epithelium.

Before commencing therapy, the ophthalmic assistant should attempt to record the patient's visual acuity. The ocular examination is facilitated by placing an anesthetic agent in the patient's eyes, which relieves the distress and enables the patient to cooperate for the ensuing eye examination. Management is mainly supportive and similar to that of a corneal abrasion. Healing occurs within 24 to 72 hours. However, during that time, the patient may experience a great deal of discomfort. Artificial tears, ointments and a topical antibiotic ointment to prevent secondary infection can be used. One hour or so after leaving the ophthalmologist's office, the patient may have a recurrence of symptoms because the local anesthetic wears off. The patient should be warned that a scratching sensation and pain may occur at home. Most ophthalmologists provide the patient with pain-relieving medication. The patient is best advised to rest as much as possible.

The patient should be told that some blurring of vision and sensitivity to light may remain for a week or so after the accident. The patient also should be advised to wear protective lenses against ultraviolet radiation in the future.

Infrared rays

The most common infrared calamity to the eye is an eclipse burn to the retina. This follows direct observation of a total eclipse of the sun. The effect of this injury to the retina is a reduction in visual acuity that may be permanent. Ordinary protective devices, such as tinted glass, Polaroid lenses, and the usual filters are of no value in protecting against this hazard. Direct viewing of eclipses should be avoided.

X-rays

X-rays are of very short wavelength, shorter than ultraviolet radiation and considerably shorter than the visible violet end of the spectrum (see Fig. 3.4). Exposure to x-rays can produce many ocular complications, including glaucoma, cataracts, necrosis of the skin, loss of lashes, and iritis. Great care has consequently been taken, in the clinical use of x-ray exposure about the eye, to protect the patient from excessive dosage and the hospital staff from unnecessary exposure to dangerous radiation. As a result, the incident rate of eye complications among x-ray and radium workers is extremely low.

Prevention of traumatic injuries to the eye

Prevention in industry

At present, the only effective area where safety measures have significantly reduced the number of ocular injuries is in industry. Most industrial safety programs revolve around four categories:

1. The detection of ocular disabilities before placement of workers in specific jobs
2. The wearing of protective goggles, visors, or masks
3. The education of workers in eye safety
4. The correct diagnosis and early treatment of eye injuries

The use of safety glasses has been of greatest importance inasmuch as the glass itself becomes a protective shield for the eye. Although ordinary glasses for street wear and industrial glasses may look alike, the similarity ends there. The difference between the two types of lenses and frames is vast.

Regular street glasses, for example, can shatter easily into the eye. In contrast, industrial safety lenses are thicker and hardened so that they resist, without shattering, the impact of a standard steel ball dropped onto their surface (see Fig. 13.20). The best safety glasses are made of polycarbonate plastic. The frames of safety glasses are also of different construction. In addition to being flame-resistant, they are designed to retain the safety lenses under heavy impact.

Contact lens wear may be hazardous in the fume- and chemical-laden environments of some industries. Contact lens wear, however, should not be considered a deterrent to employment in most industries. In some industries, contact lens wearers must wear protective goggles, as well as a protection against flying missiles.

The urgent case

The decision as to whether a patient requires an immediate examination is important and it rests heavily on the shoulders of the ophthalmic assistant. Without previous medical training and amid the noisy clatter of the outer office or clinic, the assistant must be prepared to screen the incoming calls and decide in a period of 30 seconds or less which patient has a complaint or symptom that can be an ocular emergency.

With industrial or traumatic injuries, this decision can be discharged rapidly and with authority. Obviously, a patient who has suffered a flash burn of the cornea or a laceration of the eyelid cannot be kept waiting until there is an open appointment. On the other hand, each patient who calls to make an appointment has some ocular problem that is causing some real or functional derangement of vision. The high myope with lost glasses is just as incapacitated as is the individual who has suffered an episode of acute chorioretinitis. Both patients cannot see. The only difference between the two situations is that the myope has a static problem that can be solved the moment spectacles or contact lenses are received, whereas chorioretinitis is a progressive problem that must be stopped before serious damage has occurred.

When patients are screened, a system of priority must be established that can be exercised rapidly and efficiently. In this section, instead of merely cataloging the diseases that constitute an immediate threat to an eye, we discuss their symptoms and signs and attempt to assemble them into a meaningful classification. As with all classifications, the purpose is to provide an orderly way of thinking about a particular symptom or disease. It is impossible to cover all situations. Professionals cannot blame patients for not presenting "textbook" problems, but with some flexibility they can realize that exceptions will occur. We favor, in cases of doubt, erring on the side of caution and providing an appointment rather than letting the single "functional patient" with a flashing-lights symptom silently extend a retinal hole or tears to a full retinal detachment while patiently awaiting that cherished appointment 3 months hence.

Ocular emergencies

True emergencies (therapy should be instituted within the hour)

1. Sudden loss of vision
2. Central retinal artery occlusion (Figs. 22.1–22.3)
3. Chemical injuries of the eye
4. Penetrating injuries of the eye (Fig. 22.4)

Urgent situations (patients should be seen the same day)

1. Acute narrow-angle glaucoma (Fig. 22.5)
2. Corneal ulcer (Fig. 22.6)
3. Corneal foreign body
4. Corneal abrasion
5. Acute iritis (Figs. 22.7 and 22.8)
6. Retinal detachment
7. Hyphema (hemorrhage in the eye)
8. Lid laceration
9. Blow-out fracture of the orbit
10. Temporal arteritis

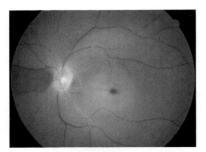

Fig. 22.1 Recent central retinal artery occlusion with a cherry-red spot at the macula. (From Kanski J, Bowling B. *Clinical Ophthalmology—a Systematic Approach*. 7th ed. Edinburgh: Saunders; 2011.)

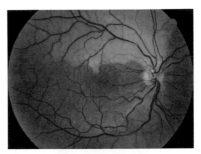

Fig. 22.2 Superior branch retinal artery occlusion caused by an embolus at the disc with ischemic whitening of the superiotemporal retina. (From Kanski J, Bowling B. *Clinical Ophthalmology—a Systematic Approach*. 7th ed. Edinburgh: Saunders; 2011.)

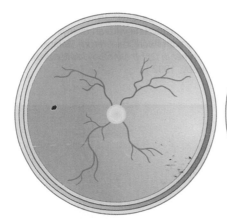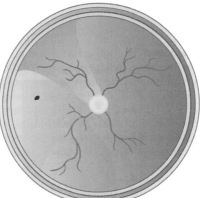

Fig. 22.3 Ischemic whitening of the retina is indicative of a central retinal artery occlusion *(left)* or a branch retinal artery occlusion *(right)*. (Modified from Stein RM, Stein HA. *Management of Ocular Emergencies*. 5th ed. Montreal: Mediconcept; 2010.)

Semiurgent situations (patients should be seen within days)

1. Optic neuritis
2. Ocular tumors
3. Protrusion of an eye
4. Previously undiagnosed glaucoma
5. Old retinal detachment.

Urgent case: to be seen within the hour

Sudden loss of vision in one eye without pain

This symptom in an adult usually means a central retinal artery occlusion, a central retinal vein occlusion, a vitreous

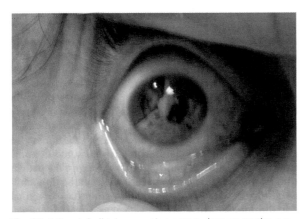

Fig. 22.4 Tennis ball injury causing severe damage to the eye.

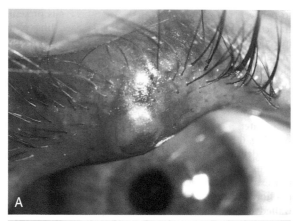

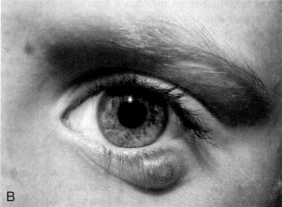

Fig. 22.15 A meibomian cyst (chalazion) develops from a blockage of one of the meibomian glands in the tarsal plate. Clinically, it presents in the acute stage as a red, tender swelling within the tarsal plate of the upper or lower eyelid (A). This either resolves completely or leaves a firm nodule (B). (Reproduced from Spalton D, Hitchings R, Hunter P. *Atlas of Clinical Ophthalmology.* 3rd ed. St Louis: Mosby; 2004, with permission.)

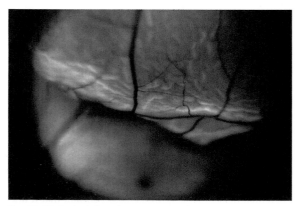

Fig. 22.16 Retinal detachment superiorly.

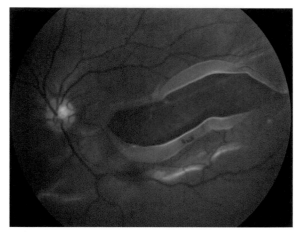

Fig. 22.17 Large retinal tear with associated retinal detachment. (From Kanski J, Bowling B. *Clinical Ophthalmology—a Systematic Approach.* 7th ed. Edinburgh: Saunders; 2011.)

Patients with this symptom in one eye should undergo wide dilation to permit a complete examination of the retina for a retinal tear and associated retinal detachment (Fig. 22.17).

Double vision or lid droop

Any person aged older than 5 years will see double if a single extraocular muscle becomes weak or paralyzed. The eye may be turned in (*esotropia:* Fig. 22.18) if a lateral rectus muscle is paralyzed, or turned out (*exotropia:* Fig. 22.19) if a medial rectus muscle is paralyzed. *Hypertropia* occurs if there is paralysis or weakness of any of the muscles that move the eye up or down (Fig. 22.20). The symptom of double vision is of grave importance because it occurs as a result of disease within the brain itself, the nerves going to the extraocular muscles, or the muscles themselves. Among the more serious conditions that produce double vision are brain tumors, aneurysms, myasthenia gravis, and strokes.

The lid is primarily held open by the action of the levator palpebrae superioris, which is innervated by the same nerve that supplies many of the extraocular muscles of the eye. Weakness of the levator muscle results in lid droop, or *ptosis*. The significance of an acquired lid droop has the same gravity as the onset of double vision.

Temporal arteritis

Temporal arteritis (also called giant cell arteritis or cranial arteritis) is a condition caused by chronic inflammation of the large and medium arteries of the head that can result

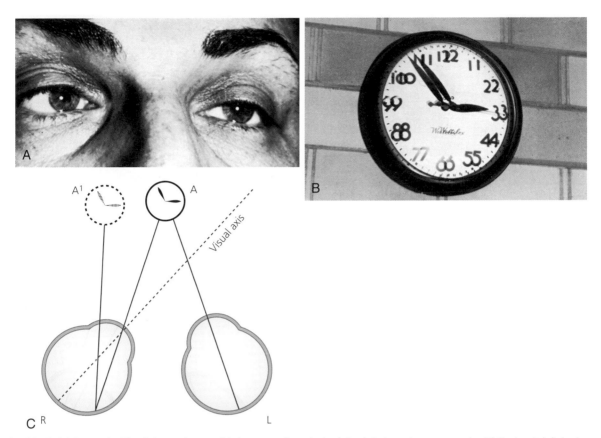

Fig. 22.18 (A) Esotropia. The right eye is turned in because of paralysis of the right lateral rectus muscle. (B) Horizontal diplopia. The patient sees two clocks side by side. (C) Image of the clock falls on the macula of the left eye and a point on the retina nasal to the macula of the right eye. The projection of the image of the clock is displaced horizontally to A^1 and is on the same side as the turned eye.

in an inadequate supply of oxygen to areas of the head and brain. It is an autoimmune disorder in which the body's immune system mistakenly attacks normal healthy cells and tissues causing inflammation. Temporal arteritis often affects the temporal arteries of the head, but can also affect other arteries throughout the body. Temporal arteritis can cause a wide variety of symptoms that can affect the eyes, head, face, and the body in general. Although a relatively uncommon disorder, it is the most frequent cause of inflammation of the blood vessels. It is more common in people aged older than age 50 years, and it affects women more often than men.

Symptoms of temporal arteritis can include blurred vision; reduced vision; double vision or sudden permanent loss of vision in one eye; throbbing headache, especially on one side of the head (usually in the temple) or back of the head; tenderness in the scalp and temple areas; facial pain; jaw pain with chewing; fatigue; weakness; and a general ill feeling.

The diagnosis of temporal arteritis includes a physical examination with emphasis on the head to determine whether there is any tenderness of the arteries. Examination of the pupils and a positive relative afferent pupillary defect can help with the diagnosis. While speaking to the patient who has a suspicious history, be sure to show the ophthalmologist the pupils before dilating the patient. In addition, certain blood tests can be useful in the diagnosis. These tests include a hemoglobin and hematocrit, platelets, erythrocyte sedimentation rate (ESR), C-reactive protein, and a liver function test. A high sedimentation rate and high C-reactive protein are often diagnostic. To make a definitive diagnosis, a biopsy of the artery that the ophthalmologist suspects is affected needs to be performed. This can be done as an outpatient procedure after treatment is initiated. Other tests that may be used in making a diagnosis include a computed tomography (CT) scan and magnetic resonance imaging (MRI).

refractive errors or disturbances in oculomotor balance. For example, such a patient often has decided to finish a university degree at night, been promoted to a desk job, or returned to the workforce. Part of the discomfort may be visual, but the factors of anxiety in doing unfamiliar activities, in forced concentration, and in learning can be of significance as well.

The types of headache that should be included in the category of the priority case are nonocular because they may be indicative of serious neurologic or systemic disorder. Headaches not related to the eyes may:

- Occur at any time and be so severe as to awaken the patient during the night
- Be associated with other systemic symptoms, such as nausea, vomiting, fainting spells, drowsiness, or stiffness of the neck
- Be preceded by an aura of flickering lights and jagged lightning flashes lasting 15 to 20 minutes (an aura often precedes a migraine headache)
- Be throbbing in nature and occur in clusters
- Be aggravated by the position of the head or movements of the body.

In practice, one should be aware that a headache may be a serious symptom and give the patient with consequential associated findings priority treatment. (Many brain tumors are first noticed in ocular assessment.)

Lost or broken spectacles

Although lost or broken spectacles appear to be a minor problem, this can be a disabling event to the patient. A myope of −3.00 to −4.00 diopters without correction may not be able to see better than 20/200 and legally may be considered blind. The patient with a considerable refractive error who has lost his or her spectacles can be totally incapacitated. The high myope cannot drive a car, the presbyope cannot read, and the patient with high astigmatism cannot do either activity. For these patients, improving vision with glasses can be as dramatic, satisfying, and rehabilitating as any other form of therapy involving drops or surgery.

Gradual loss of sight in quiet eyes

Gradual loss of vision occurs in conditions in which a progressive deterioration develops without obvious external signs of ocular disease. In children, this symptom is generally caused by uncorrected refractive errors. Once the child receives spectacles, the difficulty with vision is improved for a time. As the child grows, the refractive status constantly changes until physical maturity is reached. These changes are particularly prone to occur in myopia. Once the age of 19 or 20 years is reached, the growth of the eye is complete and changes in vision are less likely to be caused by errors of refraction. A quiescent period supervenes for about 20 to 25 years, and then most people find that focusing at near becomes difficult and the era of the presbyope is ushered in. Again, a reduction in the ability to see, this time at near, occurs and the presbyopic patient's reading glasses must be strengthened from time to time.

Apart from uncorrected refractive errors, the most common pathologic causes of painless progressive loss of vision are cataracts and macular degeneration. They occur most commonly in older adults, but are by no means restricted to this group. The patient with a cataract sees as though looking through a frosted window or gazing at something through a piece of paper. Objects appear hazy because of irregular refraction of light and are dim because some of the light is reflected by the opacities in the lens and does not reach the interior of the eye. Often, the cataract patient complains of photophobia or sensitivity to light because the retina cannot adequately adapt to the vagaries of illumination coming through a semiopaque lens. Most cataracts are bilateral, but their development may be asymmetric, so that a patient may have a moderate reduction of vision in one eye and a severe visual loss in the other. It is only when the cataract becomes mature or totally opaque that vision drops to the point of mere light perception and projection. Most people who have access to a medical center have their cataracts removed before the cataracts become mature. In areas where medical facilities are not available, cataracts are a leading cause of blindness.

The patient with macular disease has difficulty seeing clearly straight ahead because of destruction of this most vital region of the retina. Macular disease may be slow or acute in onset. Often it is bilateral, but rarely do both eyes become involved simultaneously. Central vision is lost and the patient usually cannot see looking straight ahead. Side vision or peripheral vision, however, is intact so that patients afflicted with this problem can still navigate through a room without bumping into things even though their visual acuity is 20/200 or less. To envision what a patient with macular disease sees, close one eye, place your thumb close to your open eye in your line of vision and look at a framed picture hanging on the wall. You will find that all you can see is the frame on the surrounding wall; the picture is blotted out.

Summary

The task of screening or triaging patients on the telephone is difficult and a heavy responsibility for the ophthalmic assistant. It would be impossible even for a well-trained ophthalmologist to adequately screen large numbers of patients through a conversation that lasts only minutes. The only method of solving this problem is to make errors of inclusion rather than exclusion. Far better to reward the functional patient with a bit of eye time than to turn away the patient with a serious but treatable organic problem.

Every patient who calls an eye doctor's office believes he or she has an important, serious problem that requires immediate attention. Even though all complaints do not fall under the category of urgency or priority, they should not be minimized and dismissed as trivial. Patience and understanding are required in the handling of all patients. Discretion must be used to ferret out the urgent patient.

Questions for review and thought

1. A patient telephones, complaining of sudden loss of vision in one eye. What are the possible causes? When should the patient be seen?
2. Severe pain in an eye, accompanied by nausea and vomiting, is often an indication of what condition? How should the telephone receptionist handle such a call?
3. When a patient calls complaining of redness of one or both eyes, what is the common differential diagnosis? What are the common characteristics that differentiate types of red eyes?

4. What is the significance of flashes of light?
5. What is the significance of sudden onset of double vision?
6. Compose a list of possible causes of headaches.
7. A patient calls in and says that her baby scratched her eye. What advice would you give her?
8. What advice would you give an ophthalmic assistant who gives medical advice over the telephone?
9. A patient has been hit by a fist and has a simple black eye. Should that patient be seen the same day? Why?
10. A high myope loses his glasses. Is the problem urgent?

Self-evaluation questions   Q

True–false statements

Directions: Indicate whether the statement is true (**T**) or false (**F**).
1. A central retinal artery occlusion can be salvaged if seen within 2 hours. **T** or **F**
2. Pain in the eye represents a severe corneal malady. **T** or **F**
3. A chalazion of the upper lid can cause a loss of vision. **T** or **F**

Missing words

Directions: Write in the missing word(s) in the following sentences:
4. A person who has an esotropia has the displaced image on the _____ side.
5. A headache that is preceded by flashing lights for 15 minutes is invariably a _____ headache.
6. The most common cause of halos around lights is _____.

Choice-completion questions

Directions: Select the one best answer in each case.

7. Patients with cataracts:
   a. have better distance vision than near vision.
   b. develop better near vision than distance vision.
   c. have variable vision depending on the time of day.
   d. see better at night.
   e. see better with miotics.
8. The most common cause of headaches is:
   a. eyestrain.
   b. sinusitis.
   c. migraine.
   d. stress-anxiety-depression (SAD).
   e. hypertension.
9. Flashes of light can indicate:
   a. syneresis of vitreous.
   b. migraine.
   c. retinal detachment.
   d. a blow to the back of the head.
   e. all of the above.

Answers, notes, and explanations | A

1. **False**. A true central retinal artery occlusion rarely can be salvaged. Usually 20 minutes is all that the retina can take without oxygen before permanent damage sets in. It is unusual for the diagnosis and treatment to be done that fast once the incident occurs. Sometimes the occlusive plug fragments and lodges in a branch so that the entire retina is not destroyed. The typical fundus picture is that of a retina drained of blood; thus the retinal arteries are narrow and the macula appears red because of the choroidal blush. The glowing epithet, cherry-red spot, applied to the condition of the macula does not really do justice to this blinding event.

2. **False**. Pain in the eye is commonly corneal and can be caused by anything from a foreign body in the cornea to herpes simplex keratitis. The pain of iritis, and especially of acute glaucoma, however, is far more severe than corneal pain.

   Naturally, everyone with pain in the eye should be seen right away. If the eye is fiercely red and the vision is hazy, the worst should be suspected. If the patient states that the pain occurred suddenly and reveals that the pupil is dilated, the assistant can almost start booking the hospital for an acute glaucoma admission.

3. **True**. Any mass, nodule, or lump on the upper lid can cause a slight ptosis of the lid and a flexure of the cornea by compression. It is like pressing on a balloon: the top goes in and the sides go out. The eye is not as flexible as a balloon, but alteration in the corneal curvature does occur. The radius of curvature becomes steeper and more toric in shape. Visual loss of one to three lines on the Snellen chart is common.

4. **Same**. Because the eye is turned in, the nasal side of the retina is exposed to the object of regard. The projection is straight ahead and the false second image is beside the real one and located on the same side as the paralyzed muscle.

5. **Migraine**. Migraine is characterized by the following:
   - A family history of headaches
   - An aura lasting 15 to 20 minutes consisting of light flashes, off-and-on signals, and loss of visual field
   - Precipitation of the headache by stress, drugs, birth control or diet pills, or trauma
   - A tense, commonly compulsive personality
   - Onset in young adults, although it can occur in childhood

6. **Mucous deposits on the cornea**. A halo is caused by the presence of water droplets breaking up white light into its colored components. Its most sinister cause is acute glaucoma, in which episodes of corneal edema occur. Other causes of corneal edema, however, can produce halos.

   The most common causes are mucus droplets on the cornea in association with chronic conjunctivitis, atopic conjunctival allergies, and ocular irritations. Cigarette smoke, pollution, and dry office buildings are a common source of ocular irritation, mucus production, and halo formation. Thus the assistant should not panic over halos.

7. **b. Develop better near vision than distance vision**. Patients with cataracts often see poorly in the distance but still manage to read. This occurs because the hardening of the lens of the eye increases the index of refraction of the eye. This is the reason why the elderly get "second sight."

8. **d. Stress-anxiety-depression (SAD)**. Problems of living are the most common cause of headaches. It is the so-called tension headache that is so endemic. Eyestrain rarely causes a headache. Further, the eye is a sensory organ, a fact that cannot be overlooked. Anybody with persistent headaches should have a physical examination to rule out hypertension, sinusitis, or a neurologic disorder.

9. **e. All of the above**. Flashes of light are a dangerous symptom for the patient to report. The most urgent condition that it might indicate is a retinal detachment, which requires immediate surgery. Other symptoms to be worried about in association with flashes of light include a veil over the affected eye, a shower of spots before one eye, and loss of vision or distortion of vision in the same eye.

   Migraine is sometimes a puzzle. On occasion, patients have the flashes of light for 15 minutes but no headache.

   Syneresis of vitreous is a result of the liquefaction of a part of the vitreous. The remaining gel-like vitreous bumps into the retina whenever the eyes move. The impact of the vitreous against the retina causes flashes of light.

Chapter | 23 |

Common eye disorders

Perhaps the most interesting part of an ophthalmologist's professional life is the challenge presented in diagnosing diseases of the eye. It is toward this end that his or her training has been directed, first as a medical doctor, then as a specialist. Although refraction will often occupy much of an ophthalmologist's time, it is merely a step in the process of defining disease.

For the ophthalmic assistant, the study of disease processes can aid in making the examination of the eye more rewarding. Despite the assistant's limitations in training and instrumentation, there are many common eye disorders seen daily that should be appreciated. The function of this chapter is not to make diagnosticians out of ophthalmic assistants, but to enrich their career through the study of the various disorders that are commonly seen.

Conjunctiva

The conjunctiva commences at the lid margin, lines the inner surface of the lids, forms a cul-de-sac, and then lines the surface of the eye itself, becoming circumferentially attached to the cornea at the limbus. It is translucent, moist, and membranous; has a rich vasculature; and is kept supple by the tear film.

Hyperemia

Hyperemia, or redness, of the conjunctiva is perhaps the most common condition seen. Everyone gets red eyes at one time or another. The redness is caused by dilation of the normal vascular channels in the conjunctiva. It can result from such transitory and innocuous events as exposure to dust, wind or air pollutants, fatigue, excessive reading, exposure to strong light or heat, poor ventilation, excessive dryness, and even the moderate consumption of alcoholic beverages. Many people equate red eyes with infection or inflammation and become alarmed. It is for this reason that proprietary medications "to get the red out" are so successful with their in-depth media advertising. Many people think that by getting the red out they are nipping a disease process in the bud, as well as removing a socially unacceptable disorder.

Transitory redness of the eyes requires no treatment because it is not a disease. People who find some relief with the use of eyewashes or astringent drops get only a temporary abatement of their symptoms and become addicted to eye-whitening drops for the rest of their lives. When the medication wears off, the conjunctival vessels have a tendency to dilate again so that the redness becomes more prominent than before: the so-called rebound reaction.

Subconjunctival hemorrhage

Subconjunctival hemorrhage is caused by a ruptured conjunctival blood vessel. It usually produces an irregular red patch because of pooling of blood under the conjunctiva (Fig. 23.1). Its appearance is particularly gruesome and alarming because it is accentuated by the white of the sclera (Fig. 23.2). Invariably, a collection of blood, like any other bruise under the skin, spreads and seems to enlarge as the blood is disseminated. Eventually, the blood pigment breaks down to its component parts until it is absorbed. This process can take anywhere from 7 days to 3 weeks, depending on the size of the hemorrhage.

Subconjunctival hemorrhage occurs most often in older adult patients with diabetes or hypertension, but commonly

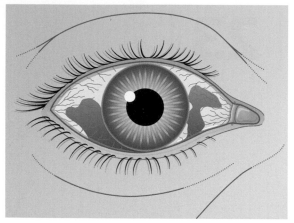

Fig. 23.1 A ruptured vessel with blood accumulation in the subconjunctival space is diagnosed as a subconjunctival hemorrhage. (From Stein HA, Slatt BJ, Stein RM. *A Primer in Ophthalmology: A Textbook for Students*. St Louis: Mosby; 1992.)

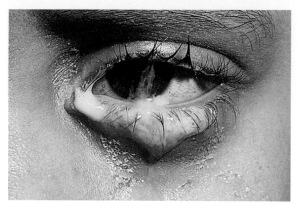

Fig. 23.3 Purulent conjunctivitis.

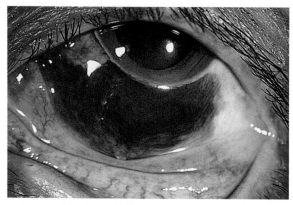

Fig. 23.2 Subconjunctival hemorrhage.

no cause can be found. A predisposing cause appears to be events that produce a sudden rise in venous pressure, such as coughing, straining, lifting, sneezing, or vomiting. There is no required treatment for this condition, which is entirely innocuous, other than reassurance. Occasionally, a subconjunctival hemorrhage is part of a general bleeding disorder, but it must be emphasized that such an event is rare. If there is a history of recurrent hemorrhages, patients should be sent to their family doctor to rule out high blood pressure, diabetes, or blood disorder. Cold compresses on the first day followed by warm compresses may speed up recovery.

Conjunctivitis

Conjunctivitis is an inflammation of the conjunctiva characterized by redness of the conjunctiva, swelling, a discharge that can be watery or purulent, and congestion of the tissues (Fig. 23.3). The patient commonly complains of a burning or grittiness of the eyes. Characteristically, the discharge accumulates during sleep, and its resultant drying on the lashes makes the lids difficult to open in the morning. Usually the lids have to be bathed to open the eyes.

Conjunctivitis may have an *infectious, allergic, or toxic* cause. The most common infectious agents are viruses, bacteria, and chlamydial organisms. A virus is the most common cause of conjunctivitis. Unlike bacterial or chlamydial conjunctivitis, the discharge is characteristically watery. Adenovirus is the most common viral conjunctivitis. Certain serotypes of this infectious agent may be responsible for epidemic keratoconjunctivitis (EKC) or pharyngoconjunctival fever (PCF). EKC is highly contagious and is often associated with epidemic outbreaks in a localized area. This disease is characterized by conjunctival and corneal involvement. PCF differs from EKC in that patients usually exhibit symptoms of a sore throat just preceding or at the time of their ocular symptoms.

Staphylococcus aureus is the most common cause of *bacterial conjunctivitis*. The organism is also responsible for such common conditions as boils or impetigo of the skin. Gonococcal conjunctivitis can be a severe infection resulting in blindness if appropriate treatment is delayed. The disease can be seen in newborns, who contact the organism while traveling through the birth canal. The sequelae of neonatal conjunctivitis can be so devastating that it is mandatory in most countries for either antibacterial drops or ointment, or 1% silver nitrate to be placed into the lower conjunctival sac of all newborns immediately after birth. Gonococcal conjunctivitis also can be seen in adults and is characterized by a significant purulent discharge. These patients and their sexual contacts need to be evaluated for a venereal disease that was probably the source of the conjunctivitis.

Haemophilus influenzae, another bacterial organism, can cause pinkeye, especially in children.

Chlamydial conjunctivitis can be caused by inclusion conjunctivitis or trachoma. The disease is characterized by a red eye and often a mucoid discharge. Inclusion conjunctivitis is the more prevalent of the two in North America and occurs in newborns and young adults. Trachoma is a more severe disease that can give rise to extensive scarring of the lids, conjunctiva, and cornea. It is an epidemic in some parts of the world, such as North Africa, the Middle East, and South Asia, where poor hygiene, poor sanitation, deficient diets, and crowding are the norm. It is a major cause of blindness in the world.

The features that distinguish acute conjunctivitis, acute iritis, and acute glaucoma are shown in Fig. 23.4 and Table 23.1. In cases of acute conjunctivitis, a swab for a smear and culture may be required in selected cases, especially in patients with *ophthalmia neonatorum* (conjunctivitis of the newborn), membranous conjunctivitis (diphtheria), and purulent conjunctivitis (gonococcal).

Allergic conjunctivitis is basically a hypersensitivity reaction (Fig. 23.5). It may occur as a component of hay fever or as an independent ocular allergy. There may be large formations of papules or cobblestones under the eyelid. At times, the conjunctivitis may be an allergic response to an invading organism, such as tuberculosis, protein, or staphylococcal bacillus. Contact allergies to drugs are a common occurrence and one of the main reasons why an inflammation can progress despite copious applications of medication. Neomycin and sulfur preparations are particularly sensitizing. Many pharmaceutical agents are available to bring relief. Agents such as cromolyn, lodoxamide, olopatadine, naphazoline/antazoline, and a corticosteroid may be helpful.

Chemical conjunctivitis is often seen in the summer and is caused by irritation from chlorine in swimming pools. It may also occur in industrial workers after exposure to irritating fumes.

Evidently, the treatment of conjunctivitis depends on identifying its cause and applying the appropriate therapy. Local antibiotic drops that are effective for a bacterial conjunctivitis would obviously be of no value for a viral infection.

In most offices, the diagnosis of conjunctivitis is made largely on clinical grounds and, if serious enough, enhanced with laboratory studies. For example, in a membranous conjunctivitis caused by diphtheria, swabs are taken from the discharge for a smear preparation, and samples are cultured for growth identification and drug sensitivity. Routine cultures and sensitivity tests are rarely done because the time lag in obtaining the results of such investigation does not warrant the delay in treatment. When the conjunctivitis is potentially serious, the ophthalmologist will do appropriate laboratory investigations but will institute therapy first. If the trial of therapy does not work, it can later be altered when the precise etiologic agent has

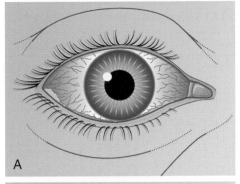

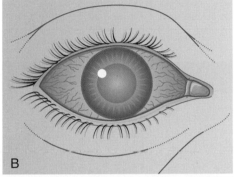

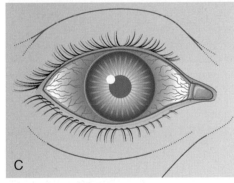

Fig. 23.4 (A) Acute conjunctivitis, characterized by discharge, injection greater in the fornix, clear cornea, and pupil normal in size. (B) Acute glaucoma, characterized by tearing, extreme injection of entire eye, hazy cornea, and pupil that is dilated, oval, and fixed to light. (C) Iritis, characterized by absent discharge, circumcorneal injection, clear to slightly hazy cornea, and small pupil.

been identified and the exact drug to which it is sensitive has been determined.

Episcleritis

Episcleritis is characterized by a salmon-pink hue of the superficial layer of the eye, with involvement of the

Table 23.1 Differential diagnosis of common eye disorders

Factor	Acute conjunctivitis	Acute iritis	Acute glaucoma
Pain	None to grittiness or foreign body sensation	Moderate to severe	Severe
Discharge	Watery or purulent	None	Tearing only
Sensitivity to light (photophobia)	Mild	Severe	Moderate
Cornea	Bright and clear	Clear or hazy	Hazy
Pupil	Normal	Constricted or small	Dilated, oval, fixed to light
Intraocular pressure	Normal	Usually normal	Elevated

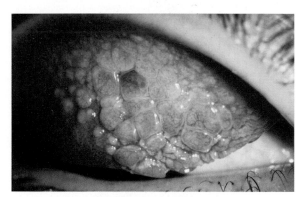

Fig. 23.5 Vernal conjunctivitis. Note cobblestone formation of upper tarsus when lid is everted.

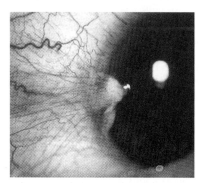

Fig. 23.7 Pterygium actively invading the cornea.

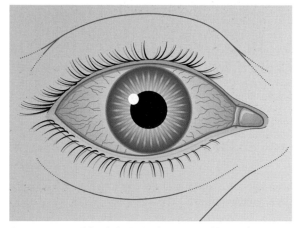

Fig. 23.6 Sectorial episcleritis is characterized by a salmon-pink color of the conjunctival and episcleral tissues. (From Stein HA, Slatt BJ, Stein RM. *A Primer in Ophthalmology: A Textbook for Students*. St Louis: Mosby; 1992.)

conjunctiva and episclera (Fig. 23.6). At least one-third of the lesions are tender to touch. Simple episcleritis may be sectorial in 70% or generalized in 30% of patients. In nodular episcleritis, the nodules that form are movable with a cotton-tipped swab, unlike nodular scleritis.

Pinguecula/pterygium

A *pinguecula* is a triangular, wedge-shaped thickening of the conjunctiva, usually found encroaching on the nasal limbus. If it invades the cornea, it is then referred to as a *pterygium* (Fig. 23.7). These lesions appear as yellowish or white vascularized masses. They are common in tropical climates where people spend a great deal of time outdoors and are exposed to sunlight and the harmful effects of ultraviolet light. Pingueculae usually do not cause symptoms. Occasionally, they may cause some irritation, or may be a cosmetic blemish. Treatment with artificial tears, vasoconstrictors, or, rarely, surgical excision may be indicated. Pterygia can occasionally extend across the cornea and eventually encroach on the visual axis and cause loss of vision. If there is documented evidence of growth, if the lesion is close to the visual axis, or is of cosmetic concern, then surgical excision is indicated. Unfortunately, there is a high incidence of recurrence with a simple excision, and therefore surgical removal is commonly combined with mitomycin C application or beta-radiation. Amniotic membranes or conjunctival grafts have been grafted in place and introduced to reduce recurrence.

Conjunctival nevus

A *nevus* is a benign neoplasm that appears on the conjunctiva at birth or in early childhood. The most common appearance is that of a flat, slightly elevated brown spot that is occasionally cystic. It usually becomes pigmented late in childhood or adolescence. It is uncommon for a nevus to become malignant. This condition should be differentiated from the acquired pigmented lesion that can occur by the age of 40 to 50 years and that can, with growth, turn into a malignant melanoma.

Cornea

The cornea, which forms the anterior one-sixth of the globe and functionally is the main refracting surface of the eye, is the structure most vulnerable to injury or inflammation. It is almost completely exposed so that it receives the brunt of chemical injuries to the eye, foreign bodies, particulate matter, and organisms that can invade it from such contiguous sources as the conjunctiva and the lacrimal sac. It is avascular tissue, which means that it is robbed of the defense mechanisms that normally are marshaled against any inflammatory insult elsewhere in the body. The corneal epithelium provides a strong barrier against bacterial invasion. The integrity of this surface is best appreciated by applying fluorescein to its surface and noting any defects in the integrity of this layer by staining and the accumulation of fluorescein pools.

Keratoconus

Keratoconus is an abnormality in which the cornea progressively becomes thinned and bulges forward in a conical fashion (Fig. 23.8). It is bilateral in 90% of patients and occasionally can be inherited. Keratoconus is often found more frequently in patients who have hay fever, atopic dermatitis, and eczema. Frequent eye rubbing has been recognized as a cause of keratoconus.

The disease results in irregular corneal astigmatism that defies correction by ordinary spectacles. Rigid contact lenses, and sometimes a piggyback of soft and rigid lenses (see Ch. 16), have been used to correct the visual defect.

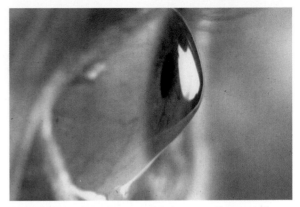

Fig. 23.8 Keratoconus cornea showing cone-like protrusion. (From Levin L, Albert D. *Ocular Disease: Mechanisms and Management.* Philadelphia: Saunders/Elsevier; 2010.)

If the patient is unable to be fitted properly with contact lenses because of high irregular astigmatism, keratoplasty is necessary to restore vision.

Keratoconus in the very late stages is recognized by *Munson's sign.* This is observed when the examiner has the patient look down and notes from above the indentation of the lower lid by the cone of the cornea. The diagnosis may be made by slit-lamp examination showing Vogt's striae or stress lines of the cornea; by the keratometer or retinoscope, which shows the presence of irregular corneal astigmatism; or by use of computerized videokeratography or tomography, which may show corneal irregularity of the anterior surface, elevation of both the anterior and or posterior surfaces, and abnormal steepening. Computerized topography and tomography (see Ch. 41) are now the most popular method to detect keratoconus.

Corneal cross-linking has become a popular technique in the treatment of keratoconus. Cross-linking with ultraviolet light and riboflavin drops often arrests the progress of keratoconus and keractesia. (For more information see Ch. 37.)

Herpes simplex keratitis

Herpes simplex keratitis is a common corneal inflammatory disorder created by the herpes simplex virus, which is the offending agent of the common cold sore. The first exposure to herpes simplex virus in 90% of cases results in subclinical, usually mild, disease. Characteristically, the young child is infected by salivary contamination from an adult who has labial herpes. The incubation period is 3 to 9 days. The clinical features of herpes simplex are both ocular and nonocular. The symptoms are relatively mild and consist of an irritating foreign body sensation, mild tearing with no frank pus or purulent discharge, and some haziness of vision accompanied by sensitivity to light. The classic herpes lesion is the dendritic figure, which, when stained with fluorescein, reveals a branchlike erosion of the cornea, as a single lesion or as multiple disturbances (Fig. 23.9).

The virus will remain dormant in the sensory nerves to the face, where it can be aroused by a variety of precipitating factors, including emotional stress, trauma, menstruation, sunlight, or the use of either local or systemic steroid drugs. When aroused, the virus will travel down the sensory nerves to the face, lids, conjunctiva, and cornea to produce a recurrence of the disease. These recurrences may be frequent, adding insult to each previous episode, so that reduction of vision over the years is a common complication. If only the epithelium is involved, no scarring occurs. However, the inflammatory process commonly extends deep down toward the stroma, which heals with vascular proliferation from the limbus and results in corneal scarring.

This condition can be a diagnostic danger because it appears to be a simple conjunctivitis. Many patients treat themselves or are treated by their family physician with antibiotics for several days before arriving in the ophthalmologist's office. Local antibiotics are of no value in this condition because it is caused by a virus. In many instances, self-medication severely aggravates the condition because many antibiotic preparations are coupled with steroids, which cause the virus to proliferate even more, thus ensuring the spread of the ulcer and further necrosis of tissue.

The treatment of herpes keratitis is instillation of trifluridine (Viroptic) drops and or oral antiviral agents like Acyclovir. The cornea heals in 7 to 14 days in approximately 85% of cases. Some ophthalmologists prefer to remove the offending virus by scraping off the diseased epithelium. This can be done at the slit lamp with a dull blade.

Other forms of the disease include the following:
1. *Gingivostomatitis.* Symptoms are fever, malaise, and lymphadenopathy, along with sore throat.
2. *Pharyngitis.* Often pharyngitis occurs with vesicles on the tonsils.

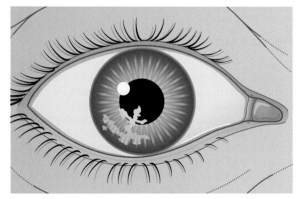

Fig. 23.9 Dendritic figure, typical of herpes simplex keratitis.

3. *Cutaneous disease.* This usually manifests as type I, which occurs above the waist, or type II, below the waist. The disease is seen in wrestlers and rugby players.
4. *General infection.* Type II infection, which is more common than type I, is characterized by fever, myalgia, extensive vesicular lesions, and inguinal and pelvic lymphadenopathy.

Recurrent herpes simplex

The virus develops a symbiosis with human beings. Any of the previously mentioned precipitating factors (trauma, fever, etc.), which provoke viral shedding and the immunologic functions, may be causative factors in episodes of recurrence. The trigeminal ganglion is a reservoir for the type I disease. The virus has a 50% recurrence rate over 5 years and may be highly localized in the lymph nodes, chin, eyes, and genitals. Cultures are usually unnecessary because this is chiefly a clinical diagnosis.

Superficial punctate keratitis

Superficial punctate keratitis consists of fine erosions in the corneal epithelium that can be diagnosed by means of the slit lamp and fluorescein staining. These lesions are common and can be seen in dry eye conditions, infections, such as adenovirus and herpes simplex, and chemical injuries. Treatment varies, depending on the cause of the superficial punctate keratitis.

Herpes zoster ophthalmicus

Herpes zoster ophthalmicus (HZO) is caused by the varicella virus, which causes chickenpox in children. In the adult, it is ushered in by a severe neuralgic type of pain, which usually includes the upper lid and extends upward beyond the brow to envelop the forehead through the scalp almost to the vertex of the head. After the pain, a vesicular eruption of the skin usually occurs and the skin surface becomes swollen, red, and heavily blistered (Fig. 23.10). The severe pain and vesicular phase last approximately 2 weeks. With healing, the skin is often pockmarked with deep, pitted scars and sensitivity to normal sensation is depressed. The incidence of HZO is 10% of all herpes zoster infections. HZO is frequently seen by an ophthalmologist first.

The virus has a predilection for dermatomes T3–L3, but the most common site is the trigeminal nerve. Cutaneous lesions of herpes zoster are histopathologically identical to varicella but have a greater inflammatory reaction, which can cause scarring. The dermatome pattern of herpes zoster may occur in three sites supplied by branches of the trige-minal nerve:
- The ophthalmic nerve distribution (V_1), where it occurs 20 times more frequently than at the V_2 or

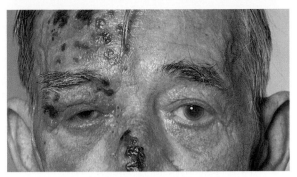

Fig. 23.10 Herpes zoster ophthalmicus. (Reproduced from Spalton D, Hitchings R, Hunter P. *Atlas of Clinical Ophthalmology*. 3rd ed. St Louis: Mosby; 2004, with permission.)

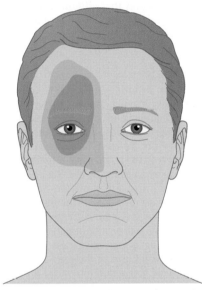

Fig. 23.11 Herpes zoster ophthalmicus is characterized by vesicular skin eruptions in the distribution of any of the branches of the trigeminal nerve. (From Stein HA, Slatt BJ, Stein RM. *A Primer in Ophthalmology: A Textbook for Students*. St Louis: Mosby; 1992.)

V_3 sites. Frontal involvement is the most common, including the upper lid, forehead, and superior conjunctiva, which are supplied by the supraorbital and supratrochlear branches (Fig. 23.11). Alternatively, herpes zoster may spread to the lacrimal and nasociliary area, which supplies the cornea, iris, ciliary body, and tip of the nose.

- The maxillary nerve distribution (V_2)
- The mandibular nerve distribution (V_3)

The virus may affect none, any, or all of these branches.

If the tip of the nose has a vesicular eruption, it usually means that the nasociliary nerve has been affected and that the underlying eye will also be affected by the herpes zoster virus. This occurs in about 50% of patients. Ocular disturbances include superficial and deep corneal ulcers, iritis, secondary glaucoma, and even paralysis of an extraocular muscle in the minority of instances.

Treatment may include the use of systemic steroids to decrease the scarring and pain that are so common after the inflammation has subsided. Ocular treatment may include topical steroids to decrease the inflammation and a cycloplegic agent to make the patient more comfortable. The antiviral agents acyclovir sodium (Zovirax), famciclovir (Famvir), and valacyclovir (Valtrex), administered in an oral form, have been shown to be effective in shortening the course of disease in herpes zoster.

The use of the herpes zoster vaccine (Zostavax) is becoming popular. Almost all adults older than 50 years may be susceptible to the virus. The vaccination has been shown to reduce not only the disease but also the postherpetic neurology that follows.

Marginal corneal ulcers

Marginal corneal ulcers are usually secondary to inflammation caused by the toxin of *S. aureus* combined with cells and other mediators involved in the body's immunologic response. Ulcers are extremely painful, and most patients believe that they have a large foreign body in their eye. There is marked redness around the eye, and usually a white infiltrate extends from the limbus into the substance of the cornea for 2 to 4 mm. At times, the cornea is ulcerated over the surface, but the epithelium may also be intact. The discharge is scant and usually watery.

Because this condition has an immunologic basis, it responds well to antibiotic-steroid medication. Other less common causes of marginal ulcers include nonimmunologic bacterial infections, herpes simplex, and inflammation secondary to a variety of systemic diseases, such as rheumatoid arthritis.

Recurrent corneal erosion

The typical history of recurrent corneal erosion is abrasion of the cornea by a fingernail, a branch of a tree, the edge of a piece of paper or cardboard, or any other organic agent. The actual injury heals temporarily, but a few days, weeks, or even months later the person experiences a complete recurrence of signs and symptoms of the original injury; however, the patient does not have any recollection of having reinjured the eye. Invariably, the symptoms occur in the morning and are thought to be caused by opening the eyes or by the trauma of rubbing the eyes, which removes the area of freshly healed epithelium on the cornea. The disorder is disabling because of the recurrent pain and is somewhat baffling because the features of the disorder are not evident between attacks. The symptoms may last anywhere from 30 minutes to several hours or several days.

The use of hypertonic drops during the day and ointment at night is helpful in dehydrating the corneal epithelium, which makes it less likely to slough off. If this is unsuccessful, a therapeutic soft contact lens can be tried. Another treatment modality is the technique of anterior stromal puncture, in which a fine needle is used to make multiple puncture marks in the anterior third of the cornea. This technique decreases the recurrence rate by forming stronger bonds between the epithelium and the underlying tissue. Another option is to debride the corneal epithelium in the local area and use a diamond burr polisher to roughen Bowman's layer, which promotes stronger epithelial attachments.

Eyelids

Certain anatomic features of the lids affect the manner of lid response. For instance, the skin of the lid, unlike that in the rest of the face, is extremely thin, loosely attached, and devoid of thick connective tissue and a fatty layer. Therefore any inflammatory swelling may cause the skin of the lid to balloon out and look puffy, whereas the weight of the collection of fluid is commonly sufficient to cause ptosis. The lid margins contain the openings of the meibomian glands (oil-secreting glands), as well as small sweat glands (Moll's glands). It is easy to understand why people who put eyeliner on their lid margins get recurrent cysts. They do so by obstructing the orifices of these tiny glands with cosmetic pigments.

The cilia or eyelashes are strong, short, curved hairs arranged in two or more closely set rows. They are longer and more numerous on the upper lid than the lower. They have a protective effect, eliminating debris from the eye except when they themselves are caked by debris of a heavy mascara brush.

Chronic inflammation of the lid margins results in thickened, heavily vascularized lids. At times, lashes fall out and, even worse, grow aberrantly. Instead of curving out, they turn in to rub against the sensitive cornea, creating erosions and even ulcerations.

Normally, the upper lid just covers the upper millimeter or so of the cornea, whereas the lower lid skirts at its lower level. If the sclera is visible either above or below the cornea, it suggests either retraction of the lids or protrusion of the eye, which might be seen in hyperthyroidism, orbital inflammation, or a tumor.

If the lid droops more than 1 to 2 mm over the cornea, the eye seems smaller by virtue of narrowing the palpebral fissure. This condition, called *ptosis*, is caused by the weakness of the muscles that elevate the upper lid (Müller's smooth muscle or the levator palpebrae superioris muscle).

Epicanthus

Epicanthus is a common congenital variation in young white children. A vertical fold extends from the upper lid over the medial angle of the eye and the caruncle (Fig. 23.12). Epicanthus makes the eyes seem closely set together, and many parents and general practitioners mistake this condition for strabismus. Invariably, the condition is self-correcting with the growth of the root of the nose and the face. In Asians, this variation persists throughout adult life. Surgical procedures that eliminate this fold to make the eyes look rounder or more like those of Westerners are popular in Japan.

Entropion

An *entropion* is an in-turning of the lids, and usually one of the lower lids is affected. The spastic type is more common in old age than in youth. Its major disability is created by irritation of the cornea by in-turned lashes (Fig. 23.13). The inversion of the lid margin is caused by a spasm of the orbicularis oculi, the washer-like muscle under the skin of the lid. The spasm closes the eye. This muscle spasm is often induced by ocular inflammation or irritation. In an older adult, it is easy for a spastic muscle to turn in on an atonic lid. A more severe form of entropion is caused by scarring, which can follow inflammation of the conjunctiva, such as in ocular pemphigus, trachoma, lacerations of the lid, and chemical burns of the eye with attendant scarring. Again, surgery is required to remedy the condition.

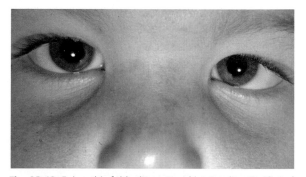

Fig. 23.12 Epicanthic folds. (From Kanski J, Bowling B. *Clinical Ophthalmology—a Systematic Approach*. 7th ed. Edinburgh: Saunders; 2011.)

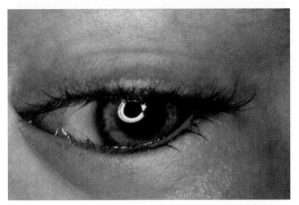

Fig. 23.13 Congenital entropion. (From Kanski J, Bowling B. *Clinical Ophthalmology—a Systematic Approach*. 7th ed. Edinburgh: Saunders; 2011.)

The treatment of entropion is generally surgical, although temporary relief can be obtained by drawing the skin of the lower lid down toward the cheeks by means of adhesive tape. The surgery is safe, simple, and effective and is usually performed with the patient under local anesthesia.

Ectropion

In *ectropion*, the lid suffers a loss of tone and flops away from the eye (Fig. 23.14) so that the conjunctiva lining the inner surface of the lid becomes exposed, irritated, and thickened. It occurs primarily in older adults and is aggravated by attendant tearing as a result of aversion or stenosis of the punctum. The wiping away of tears from the lower lid makes the lower lid droop further, setting up a vicious cycle of tearing and progressive ectropion. Exposure of the conjunctiva causes burning and irritation and predisposes the eye to secondary inflammation. Again, the most common type is a result of senile atrophy of the lid structures, which causes the lids to stray outward. Scarring can also produce the same defect and is caused by the same conditions that create *cicatricial entropion*. This type of entropion is a mechanical defect of the lids that can be remedied only by surgery.

Ptosis

In unilateral ptosis, there is a conspicuous droop of the upper lid and the opening of one eye seems smaller than the other (Fig. 23.15). Commonly, the lid fold is absent or smooth on the affected side. It is evident when the individual has to look up, because the lid on the affected side does not move upward with the globe compared with the opposite normal side. If both lids are involved, a child will develop a characteristic head posture with the head thrown

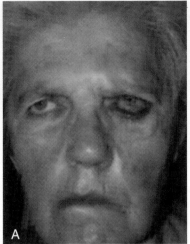

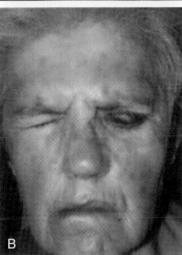

Fig. 23.14 Paralytic ectropion. (A) Left facial palsy and severe ectropion. (B) Lagophthalmos. (From Kanski J, Bowling B. *Clinical Ophthalmology—a Systematic Approach*. 7th ed. Edinburgh: Saunders; 2011.)

back and the upper lids elevated as a compensatory mechanism to raise the drooped eyelids.

Treatment of the condition is invariably surgical. It is directed toward shortening the levator palpebrae superioris muscle, the primary elevator of the lid. Resection of a section of this muscle and advancement of its insertion strengthen it and increase its leverage.

In congenital ptosis it is often bilateral.

Exaggerated blink activity

Exaggerated blink activity is a common condition seen especially in children. The sole feature is the presence

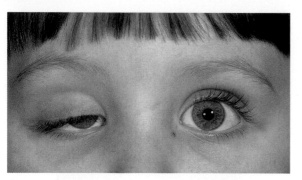

Fig. 23.15 Simple unilateral congenital ptosis. (From Hoyt C, Taylor D. *Pediatric Ophthalmology and Strabismus*. 4th ed. Philadelphia: Elsevier/Saunders; 2013.)

of conspicuous, repetitive blinking motions of the lids, called *myokymia*. Invariably, the ocular examination reveals the presence of normal eyes. The rapid reflex blinking is thought to be the mechanism by which anxiety and restless motor activity are released in a young child. It clears up on its own, so parents are best advised to ignore this self-limiting condition, which disappears more rapidly if it is ignored. Constant attention to these repetitive blinking motions only increases the child's anxiety.

A corollary to reflex blinking in the adult is tremor of the orbicularis oculi muscle. Many adults complain of a fine lid flutter that is like a current going through the lower lid. Other than the annoying spontaneous twitch, it does not cause any other symptoms. The condition is usually caused by a mixture of tension and fatigue and disappears on its own. Rarely, however, it can be caused by serious conditions, such as Parkinson disease, multiple sclerosis, and hyperthyroidism.

Blepharochalasis and dermatochalasis

Blepharochalasis is a condition that often drives middle-aged individuals to the plastic surgeon. It is caused by recurrent swelling of the upper lids and appears most prominently in the morning. The continuous stretching of the skin of the upper lids and the accumulation of edema cause the skin to lose its tone and hang lifelessly as a redundant fold or curtain over the upper lids. One disability is that it interferes with the application of eye make-up to the lids. In extreme cases, it can even weigh on the lashes, creating a sensation of heaviness and ocular fatigue. It may cause restriction of the upper field of vision. At times, this condition is accompanied by the protrusion of fat from behind the eye through the orbital septum just under the skin. These fat pads most prominently appear on the medial side of the upper lids and on the lower lids as rather large, unattractive mounds.

This condition is mainly, but not entirely, cosmetic and can be remedied surgically by removing the excess skin and the fat and repairing the septum so that further protrusion of the retroorbital fat cannot occur.

Although blepharochalasis is largely innocuous, occasionally, it is a manifestation of thyroid disease, kidney disorder, severe allergic reaction, or angioneurotic edema. This condition should be differentiated from dermatochalasis, which is predominantly an involutional aging change. Dermatochalasis is a result not of recurrent edema, but of loss of elastic tissue and relaxation of the fascial bands that connect the skin and underlying orbicularis muscle.

Trichiasis

In *trichiasis*, instead of being directed outward, the lashes turn in toward the eye, causing irritation and sometimes erosion and ulceration of the cornea. Often, there are irregular rows of lashes. Trichiasis may be a result of scarring of the lid, which can be caused by previous injury, chemical burns of the lids, and severe lid inflammations. Simple epilation of the offending cilia is really a palliative measure because the lashes tend to regrow aberrantly. If only a few lashes are irritating, their base can be cauterized by electrolysis. In more severe cases, a freezing technique applied to the base of the cilia, referred to as *cryosurgery*, or surgical reconstruction of the lid margin may be necessary to remove the aberrant lashes that rub against the conjunctiva or cornea and cause the irritation.

Blepharitis

Blepharitis is a common chronic inflammation of the lid margin. Patients usually complain of a sandy or itchy feeling of their eyes, especially in the morning. There is usually redness, as well as a thickening and irregularity of the lid margins. The disease may occur at any age. The two most common types of chronic inflammation of the lids are *staphylococcal blepharitis* and *seborrheic blepharitis*. Seborrhea is a common cause of dandruff. Telltale diagnostic patches of seborrheic involvement in such patients are commonly seen in the medial aspect of the brows, the forehead, and sometimes behind the skin of the ear or on the nose. The base of the eyelash is usually caked with a greasy type of scale that comes off easily, leaving an intact lid margin.

At times, blepharitis can be infective in origin; when this is the case, it is invariably a result of *S. aureus*. The lid margins become ulcerated and congested and adhesive exudate forms on the base of the follicles and on the lid margin.

When the scale is removed, it always reveals an ulcerative defect on the lid margin. The ulcerative type of blepharitis is more serious because if the inflammation reaches down to the base of the follicles it can cause permanent scarring, with either loss of lashes or misdirection of lash and regrowth with accompanying trichiasis. Also the cosmetic consequences are undesirable because the lids become thickened, heavily vascularized, and unattractive.

An uncommon pathogen is the *Demodex* mite. Demodex increases with age and is fairly common after age 60 years. Once the mite lodges in the skin, it moves to the eyelashes and can be seen with the slit-lamp microscope. Once demodex gets out of control, blepharitis follows. The adult version of demodex folliculorum is the most resistant to treatment. Lid hygiene is most important.

Essential blepharospasm

Essential blepharospasm is a condition in which the individual is severely handicapped by spastic closure of the eyes along with severe sensitivity (photophobia) to light. Closing the eyes every few seconds renders the individual virtually blind. By being closed a great deal of a patient's waking hours, the patient is seriously handicapped. Remedies range from special tinted glasses (fl-41), sedatives, and mild tranquilizers to botulinum toxin (Botox) injections. The last is used to paralyze the orbicularis oculi muscle that surrounds the eye and reduce the spasm. If this does not relieve the spasm, then surgical myomectomy of the orbicularis may be performed.

External hordeolum (stye) and internal hordeolum

A *stye* or *external hordeolum* is an acute suppurative inflammation of small sebaceous glands on the lid margin, the *glands of Zeis*, which empty their secretion into the hair follicles of the cilia. An internal hordeolum is an acute inflammation of the sebaceous glands that reside in the tarsal plates: the meibomian glands. In the early stages of the inflammation, the affected gland becomes swollen and the lid becomes red and edematous. An abscess forms with a small collection of pus, which usually points at the apex of one of these glands. Unless the suppuration is opened, the discomfort can be considerable. The inflammation generally results from invasion by bacterial *S. aureus*. It is a common affliction of young adults, but it can occur at all ages, especially in patients with blepharitis.

Treatment consists primarily of hot compresses to reduce inflammation and promote drainage. If this is unsuccessful, the ophthalmologist can incise and drain the hordeolum or inject local steroids into the lesion in the hope of bringing about its resolution.

Chalazion

A *chalazion* is a chronic inflammatory granuloma of the large meibomian glands embedded in the tarsus of the lid. Multiple chalazia can occur in the upper or lower lids. Unlike the infectious causes of the internal and external hordeolum, chalazia are the result of a sterile process. Initially, the orifice of the meibomian gland becomes occluded by a small inflammatory swelling and the accumulated sebum ruptures the gland, creating a granulomatous type of inflammatory reaction in the lid itself. The lid becomes swollen, painful, and inflamed until eventually, the inflammatory reaction is walled off and a cyst forms (Fig. 23.16). If the cyst is large and thickly walled, it must be opened surgically and evacuated with a curet and blunt dissection.

Occasionally, the injection of localized steroids into the lesion may obviate the need for surgical drainage. Sometimes, in the early stages, hot compresses may reduce inflammation, open the meibomian duct to promote drainage. Many times, the patient comes to the ophthalmologist with a nonpainful, localized swelling of the lid after the inflammation has subsided. The lesion may be surgically excised.

One must differentiate from other benign and malignant growths as listed in the following text. Traditional medical treatments include warm compresses, lid massage, lid scrubs, and topical steroids.

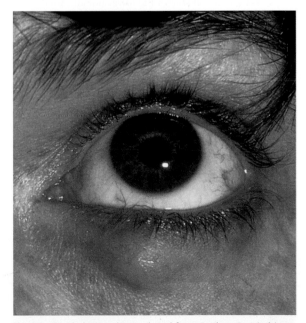

Fig. 23.16 Chalazion. (Reproduced from Spalton D, Hitchings R, Hunter P. *Atlas of Clinical Ophthalmology*. 3rd ed. St Louis: Mosby; 2004, with permission.)

Tumors of the lid

Milia

Milia are small, white, slightly elevated cysts of the skin with a pedunculated apex. They can create a cosmetic blemish when they appear in crops.

Xanthelasma

Xanthelasma are yellowish fatty deposits, or plaques, that occur in the upper and lower lids on the medial side. The condition is largely cosmetic, but it may indicate a more serious lipid disorder because it represents a deposit of circulating cholesterol or other lipids. The deposits can be destroyed or removed by trichloroacetic acid, carbon dioxide snow, or surgery. The purpose of removing xanthelasma is strictly cosmetic.

Carcinoma

Eyelid tumors account for 5% to 10% of skin cancers. The most common malignant growth of the lid is the *basal cell carcinoma* (BCC) (Fig. 23.17). This carcinoma accounts for 90% of cancers of the eyelid. Exposure to ultraviolet radiation is the main cause, although there is a hereditary component. It rarely metastasizes, but can recur. Eyelid reconstruction or grafts are uncommon unless the tumor is very large.

It usually appears on the lower lid near the inner canthus or on the lateral side of the lower lid, and finally and least commonly on the upper lids. The tumor typically has a raised ulcerated surface. Its margin is pearly white and, despite the appearance of tissue destruction, it rarely causes any symptoms. If it is treated early with either radiotherapy or surgery, a complete cure can be effected. The tumor is invasive if it is not treated and tends to spread directly to the tissues surrounding it.

Squamous cell carcinoma (SCC) is more malignant and can spread throughout the body. It must be entirely

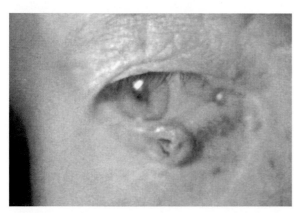

Fig. 23.17 Basal cell carcinoma of eyelid.

removed. Excisional biopsy is sometimes the only way to differentiate BCC from SCC.

Seborrheic keratosis (senile verruca)

This is one of the most common lesions involving the eyelid skin. It appears as a well-defined, small, elevated, brown to brownish-black lesion on the eyelid, much like a button flush on the skin surface. It is benign but may be surgically removed for cosmetic reasons.

Keratoacanthoma

This is a benign lesion but, because of its rapid growth, it is often mistaken for a malignancy. It grows rapidly but reaches maximum size in 6 to 8 weeks. There may be spontaneous regression, but it is usually excised.

Molluscum contagiosum

These are waxy, raised nodules, often with an umbilicated center. The lesions are caused by a member of the pox virus group. Toxic debris released from the lesion into the tears may give rise to a chronic conjunctivitis. The lesion usually has to be surgically excised. Other treatments include cauterization, cryotherapy, and laser.

Lacrimal apparatus

Acute dacryoadenitis

Acute dacryoadenitis is an inflammation of the lacrimal gland that causes pain and discomfort in the upper outer portion of the orbit and swelling of the lid laterally. Eversion of the upper lid reveals a swollen, reddened gland on its lateral surface. Mumps and infectious mononucleosis are the usual systemic causes of this condition.

Lacrimal gland enlargement

Mass lesions of the lacrimal gland may manifest in a variety of ways. They may be painful or painless, palpable, and associated with swelling of the lid and ptosis. Enlargement of the lacrimal gland can be caused by tumor formation, such as the mixed tumor, adenoid cystic tumor or lymphoma, or by a granulomatous inflammation.

Tearing

Tearing may be the result of lacrimation, which is excessive tear formation of the lacrimal gland, or it may be caused by *epiphora*, which is defective drainage of tears. Lacrimation may result from psychologic stimuli (e.g., grief or depression), from irritation of the eye by wind or dust, or from irritative inflammatory disorders of the conjunctiva, cornea, or lids. These causes of lacrimation usually are self-evident and desist once the stimulus has stopped.

Persistent tearing, with overflow onto the cheek, is usually caused by obstruction somewhere in the lacrimal drainage system from the punctum situated on the medial aspect of the lower lid to the nasolacrimal duct. The patency of tear elimination can be tested in several ways. Fluorescein solution 2% instilled in the conjunctival sac normally disappears within 1 minute. A cotton swab placed in the nasal passages can usually prove the patency of the system, as it becomes stained with fluorescein. Irrigation of the lacrimal system with saline solution is less physiologic, but can at least demonstrate that tears will flow from the punctum to the nasolacrimal duct and empty into the nasal passages. If there is obstruction of the nasolacrimal canal, the tears forced through the lower canaliculus will reflux out through the upper punctum. This reflux of tears through the upper punctum is plainly visible. An additional point is that the person being tested will not taste the saline solution, which should be coming through the nose. Another test of tear function uses saccharin solutions placed in the conjunctival sac. If tears are being eliminated, 1 or 2 minutes later, the patency is proved by the patient indicating the taste of something in the throat.

It is also important to note the presence of apposition of the lower lid against the globe. Tearing can occur if the lower lid is not in contact with the globe, as can be seen with medial ectropions.

Regardless of the cause, the treatment of tearing caused by defective drainage is largely surgical. No one has ever died from a bit of tearing; thus the decision to operate depends on the distress of the patient created by the mechanical reflux of tears and the association of secondary infections (Box 23.1).

Dacryocystitis

Dacryocystitis, an inflammation of the lacrimal sac, is indicated by an inflammatory swelling at the site of the sac. This inflamed swelling is seen as a visible red lump just below the caruncle overriding the inframedial aspect of the orbital bone (Fig. 23.18).

Sometimes pressure over the sac causes pus or mucoid material to regurgitate through the punctum. This condition usually results from the effects of stricture of a nasolacrimal duct arising from chronic inflammation, usually of nasal origin. Obstruction of the lower end of this duct can be caused by the presence of a nasal polyp and extreme deviation of the septum, or by a marked congestion of the inferior turbinate. Surgery, called *dacryocystorhinostomy* (DCR), is required to establish a new canal for the tears, thus preventing stagnation.

Box 23.1 **Tear film function**

1. Hydrates and protects the ocular surface
2. Reduces friction on blinking
3. Enhances oxygen to the cornea
4. Removes waste and cell debris
5. Protects against infection

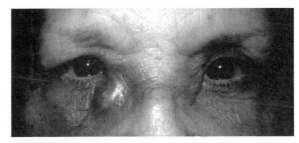

Fig. 23.18 Dacryocystitis. Note the marked swelling over the lacrimal sac.

Questions for review and thought

1. Describe the typical contact conjunctival allergic response to neomycin.
2. What is a nevus? What type should cause concern?
3. What is a xanthelasma plaque? Does it have any significance?
4. What influence do cortisone drops have on the herpes simplex virus?
5. Keratoconus affects the cornea and is revealed by a forward protrusion of the globe. Why does it impair vision?
6. What are the external signs and symptoms that distinguish herpes zoster ophthalmicus?
7. What would you see if you stained the eye of a patient who has two marginal corneal ulcers with fluorescein? What is the usual cause of such ulcers?
8. What glands lie in the eyelid and what are the conditions called when they become inflamed?
9. What causes repeated blinking in childhood?
10. Describe the typical picture of chronic blepharitis.
11. What is the treatment for a stye?
12. What causes persistent tearing?
13. What virus that produces cold sores on the lips can also cause a severe keratitis? What is the typical pattern of infection that it produces on the cornea?
14. Name three causes of purulent conjunctivitis of the newborn.
15. What is a basal cell carcinoma? Where is it usually located with respect to the lids? How is it treated? What is the prognosis after treatment?

Self-evaluation questions   Q

True–false statements

Directions: Indicate whether the statement is true **(T)** or false **(F)**.

1. Large cobblestones under the eyelid often are seen in vernal conjunctivitis. **T** or **F**
2. A pterygium is a vascular invasive area on the cornea. **T** or **F**
3. Keratoconus results in scarring and irregular curvature of the cornea. **T** or **F**

Missing words

Directions: Write in the missing word in the following sentences:

4. The virus that causes a dendritic pattern of the cornea is called _____.
5. When herpes zoster ophthalmicus involves the eye, the tip of the _____ is usually involved and blistered.
6. A fingernail injury to the cornea may result in recurrent _____ of the cornea a few months later.

Choice-completion questions

Directions: Select the one best answer in each case.

7. Ptosis or blepharoptosis is a drooping of the upper lid caused by a paralysis of:
   a. the levator palpebrae superioris muscle.
   b. Müller's muscle.
   c. the orbicularis oculi.
   d. a or b.
   e. none of the above.
8. A subconjunctival hemorrhage may occur in which of the following conditions?
   a. Trauma.
   b. Blood disorders.
   c. After sneezing.
   d. Perforating injury of the globe.
   e. All of the above.
9. Abrasion of the cornea is not caused by:
   a. entropion resulting from scarring of the conjunctiva.
   b. entropion resulting from spasm of the orbicularis.
   c. trichiasis.
   d. dacryocystitis.
   e. contact lenses.

Answers, notes, and explanations A

1. **True**. Although cobblestones or large papules on the undersurface of the eyelid are typically seen in vernal conjunctivitis, they may also occur in a number of allergic conditions. In addition, giant papillary conjunctivitis is seen with the use of both rigid and soft contact lenses, secondary to protruding corneal sutures and in poor-fitting ocular prostheses. It is believed in these cases to be caused by an allergic response to some protein constituent that builds up on the contact lens.

2. **True**. A pterygium is a locally invasive area that extends across the cornea and eventually may interfere significantly with vision. Once removed, there is a significant incidence of recurrence and each removal increases the risk of further recurrence. A number of surgical procedures have been advocated to try to overcome the recurrence rate of pterygia.

3. **True**. Keratoconus is marked by a cone-shaped protrusion of the cornea, resulting in irregularity of the spherical surface of the cornea. The cornea develops an irregularity that can no longer be corrected by spectacle lenses and requires correction by contact lenses. There are many microbreaks in the extremely thin cornea, resulting in scar formation and even hydrops of the cornea. Each small break in the cornea becomes devastating to the homogeneous regularity of the cornea and results in further scarring and reduction in vision.

4. **Herpes simplex**. The herpes simplex virus most commonly forms a dendritic pattern, usually in the central or paracentral area of the cornea. However, there is no set manner by which it manifests in the eye. It may appear as a conjunctivitis or may extend deeply into the stroma of the cornea and become a necrotic central ulcer that fails to heal. However, the dendritic pattern, which represents an involvement of the corneal epithelium, is the most typical manifestation of the herpes simplex virus.

5. **Nose**. When the tip of the nose is affected the ciliary ganglion is involved, through which the nasociliary branch of the fifth or ophthalmic nerve courses. Serious ocular damage can often be predicted if the tip of the nose is involved.

6. **Erosion**. Often, any abrasion of the cornea by objects, such as paper or a fingernail that involves the corneal epithelium also interferes with the basement membrane sufficiently to result in inadequate attachment of the epithelium to the basement membrane. During the night, the epithelium becomes relatively edematous. In the morning, on awakening, there is a tendency to dislodge the epithelium that is not firmly attached to the underlying basement membrane. This results in the typical symptoms of recurrent corneal erosion, with all the irritation and foreign body reaction that were present during the original injury.

7. **d. a or b**. The levator palpebrae superioris muscle may be affected in this condition, as occurs in most congenital ptoses and in many of the acquired paralytic ptoses. If Müller's muscle is paralyzed, such as occurs in Horner syndrome with paralysis of the sympathetic nerve, a slight ptosis is present.

8. **e. All of the above**. Whereas a subconjunctival hemorrhage is often harmless, it is important to be aware that it may be an ominous sign of a small perforating wound of the globe from a sharp flying missile. Thus radiologic studies and further detailed examination of the interior of the eye with a well-dilated pupil become important. In addition, the examiner should rule out medical conditions, such as blood disorders, hypertension, diabetes, and so on that may be responsible for a subconjunctival hemorrhage.

9. **d. Dacryocystitis**. Dacryocystitis does not cause abrasions of the cornea. Contact lenses result in the most serious type of abrasions of the cornea, either by incorrect insertion or by overwear syndrome. Trichiasis, or an abnormal row of eyelashes, may result in a constant irritation and abrasion of the corneal epithelium. Entropion also may result in irritation of the cornea by eyelashes.

Chapter | **24** |

Common retinal disorders

Parnian Arjmand, Hayley Monson, and Efrem D. Mandelcorn

As an ophthalmic medical assistant or technician, it is important to have a fundamental understanding of the common retinal disorders in clinical practice that are not readily visible on external examination. Detection of retinal disorders requires ophthalmoscopic examination and/or imaging. Although this assessment is not within the domain of the ophthalmic medical assistant or technician, patients with retinal disorders may ask questions to any member of the ophthalmic team to which they entrust the safety and health of their eyes. Therefore this chapter discusses some of the most common retinal disorders.

The clinical evaluation of the retina includes refraction, ophthalmoscopy (both direct and indirect), visual fields for peripheral and central vision, color vision assessment, dark adaptation studies, electroretinography, ultrasonography (to determine space-occupying lesions of the retina and the choroid), fluorescein angiography, optical coherence tomography (OCT), and OCT angiography (OCTA).

Retinal artery occlusion

Retinal artery occlusion is a true ocular catastrophe. If the central retinal artery is obstructed (i.e., central retinal arterial occlusion [CRAO]) by an embolus or thrombus, resulting in retinal nonperfusion, the nine layers of the retina undergo ischemic necrosis, resulting in a sudden and painless loss of vision to the affected eye.

Some studies suggest no detectable retinal damage if retinal blood flow is restored within 60 to 90 minutes; subsequent partial recovery may be possible if ischemia is reversed within 240 minutes.[1]

The diagnosis is based on the retinal finding of the classic cherry-red spot. The retina becomes gray from swelling or edema because the retina loses its normal transparency. The blood vessels become attenuated and segmented (Fig. 24.1). Ischemic changes make the entire nerve fiber layer of the retina gray except in the foveal region which is devoid of the nerve fiber layer. Consequently, the background in the fovea remains a normal red color from the underlying choroidal vascular supply, leading to the appearance of a cherry-red spot. The usual prognosis is total and permanent loss of light perception in the involved eye (Fig. 24.2).

If a branch of a retinal artery is involved, the prognosis is often better. Patient may have a permanent visual field deficit, or may not notice any changes in their vision.

In elderly patients, a retinal arterial occlusion (RAO) may be secondary to a life-threatening medical emergency, namely, giant cell arteritis (GCA). In patients over the age

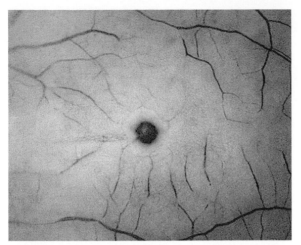

Fig. 24.1 Central retinal artery closure, acute. Note the graying in the macular area and the cherry-red spot.

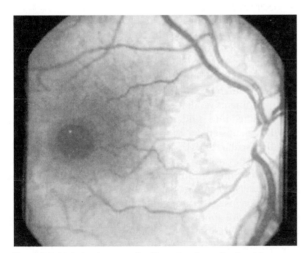

Fig. 24.2 Hole in the macula. Note the "punched-out" reddened area.

of 60 years with an RAO, GCA should be suspected and appropriate laboratory and medical workup should be done immediately. As well, patients presenting with an RAO should be urgently referred to a stroke center for appropriate systemic medical workup to diagnose and optimize their stroke risk factors.

Similar to retinal vein occlusions (see later), RAOs can lead to subsequent macular edema (swelling within the macula), development of abnormal neovascularization within the anterior and posterior segments, and lead to sequalae of glaucoma, vitreous hemorrhage, and retinal detachment. As such, patients with RAO should be examined every 3 to 6 months by the ophthalmologist or the retinal specialist to monitor for these findings.[2]

Retinal vein occlusion

Central retinal vein occlusion (CRVO) is generally caused by a thrombus in a central retinal vein. Conditions associated with an increased risk of retinal vein occlusion include diabetes, hypertension, polycythemia, glaucoma, and any other condition that causes stasis of blood flow.

Because there is no pain, the patient may not be immediately aware of the onset of the condition. The profound loss of vision may not be detected until the patient "discovers" it by rubbing or closing the good eye.

On ophthalmoscopic examination, the entire retina may be covered with superficial hemorrhages that appear flame shaped (Fig. 24.3). There may be scattered cotton-wool spots, which are microinfarcts of the retinal nerve fiber layer. The retinal veins appear dilated and tortuous distal to the site of occlusion. The macula is usually edematous and this leads to cystoid macular edema with loss of vision. If a branch of the vein is involved, only one sector of the retina will be affected so the vision may or may not be affected. The prognosis for visual recovery is significantly better with a branch vein occlusion than with a central vein occlusion.

The chances for significant visual recovery in an ischemic CRVO are generally poor. The most dreaded complication is neovascular glaucoma, which can result in a blind eye with severe pain that may eventually be managed by enucleation. With ischemia, there is proliferation of new blood vessels that can occur on the iris and extend over the trabecular meshwork, resulting in obstruction of aqueous outflow and elevated intraocular pressure, hence the term neovascular glaucoma.

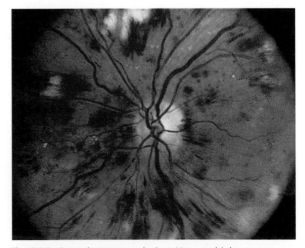

Fig. 24.3 Central venous occlusion. Note multiple hemorrhages and distended vessels. (Courtesy Mount Sinai Hospital, Toronto.)

Once the diagnosis of a CRVO is made, a fluorescein angiogram is usually performed to determine the degree of retinal ischemia. If there is significant ischemia, laser photocoagulation to all peripheral ischemic retina (i.e., panretinal) can be performed. This is thought to destroy areas of ischemic retina that are probably responsible for producing a chemical mediator that leads to neovascularization, the formation of new blood vessels. Although the initial studies looking at laser photocoagulation in the treatment for CRVO demonstrated no beneficial effect, more recent studies (CRUISE, COPERNICUS, and GALILEO) have demonstrated that the use of intravitreal antivascular endothelial growth factor (anti-VEGF) inhibitors results in rapid and sustained improvement in visual acuity and central foveal thickness for patients with macular edema secondary to CRVO.[3]

Similarly, if there is macular involvement in branch retinal vein occlusion (BRVO; see Fig. 24.3), then vision will be affected. Studies involving BRVO have demonstrated that if vision has been decreased for more than 3 months and fluorescein angiogram shows a leakage of fluid in the macula, laser photocoagulation in a sector distribution can improve the visual prognosis. The risk of neovascular glaucoma is generally less of a concern with BVO.

More recent studies (BRAVO, CRUISE, HORIZON, and VIBRANT) have shown that monthly injections of anti-VEGF (bevacizumab, ranibizumab, or aflibercept) improved both visual acuity and central foveal thickness in patients with macular edema secondary to branch vein occlusion.[4]

Patients with venous occlusive disease should have a general medical evaluation to rule out diabetes, hypertension, or blood dyscrasias. The ophthalmologist must evaluate the nonaffected eye to rule out glaucoma, which is commonly associated with vein occlusions.

Diabetic retinopathy

Diabetic retinopathy is currently a prominent cause of vision loss around the world. Diabetic retinopathy affects over 350 million individuals worldwide, particularly between the ages of 20 and 70 years old with an estimated 10,000 new cases of blindness per year in the United States. These numbers are projected to continuously increase with the increase prevalence of diabetes mellitus. Fortunately, numerous clinical trials (DCCT and UKPDS) have demonstrated a significant reduction in ocular complications with aggressive control of blood glucose, blood pressure, and hemoglobin A1C levels.

Diabetes may have a juvenile or adult onset. In general, the incidence of diabetic complications increases with the duration of the disease. Complications may include systemic and ocular problems. Systemic complications include microvascular and macrovascular complications.

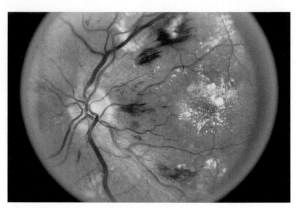

Fig. 24.4 Diabetic retinopathy. The retinal changes occur predominantly at the posterior pole with microaneurysms and "dot and blot" hemorrhages and hard exudates occur in the macular area.

Microvascular complications of diabetes include peripheral neuropathy and nephropathy, as well as diabetic retinopathy. Macrovascular complications include a heightened risk of stroke, myocardial infarcts, and other cardiovascular disease. Diabetic retinopathy is divided into nonproliferative and proliferative stages.

Nonproliferative diabetic retinopathy (NPDR) is further classified into mild, moderate, and severe retinopathy. NPDR is characterized by the presence of microaneurysms (small vascular buds), dot and blot hemorrhages, and lipid exudates from a serous leakage of the retinal vessels (Fig. 24.4). Other findings include the presence of cotton-wool spots (microinfarcts of the retina), irregular dilatation of retinal veins, and intraretinal microvascular abnormalities, which are abnormal capillaries within the retina as a result of ischemia.

Proliferative diabetic retinopathy is defined by the presence of abnormal blood vessel formation—that is, neovascularization on the optic disc, the surface of the retina, or the iris. These fragile aberrant blood vessels are easily ruptured, causing recurrent vitreous hemorrhage. These abnormal blood vessels can also contract to form fibrovascular scar tissue that can provide traction on the retina, resulting in tractional retinal detachment. Aberrant neovascularization within the anterior segment, including the iris with extension to the trabecular meshwork, can lead to neovascular glaucoma.

Ocular treatment modalities for diabetic retinopathy depend on the stage of the disease and the absence or the presence of a variety of complications. If neovascularization is present, then panretinal photocoagulation (PRP) is the treatment of choice. Approximately 2000 to 3000 photocoagulation spots are applied to the peripheral retina with the argon laser, essentially destroying the ischemic retina, which is thought to be the source of vasoproliferative factors. As well, laser photocoagulation to the peripheral retina reduces overall retinal oxygen demands and increases oxygen delivery to other portions of the retina, the macula, and the optic nerve. This treatment reduces and often resolves the neovascularization.

PRP can be done in the office, or intraoperatively if the patient requires vitrectomy surgery. In recent years, studies have indicated that anti-VEGF medications may be a good adjunct or alternative to PRP in patients with proliferative diabetic retinopathy who are reliable to follow up (see later).[5]

If vision is decreased by macular edema outside the fovea, photocoagulation of leaking microaneurysms in the macular area has been shown to improve vision. If the patient has a nonclearing vitreous hemorrhage, or if there are fibrovascular bands producing a tractional retinal detachment, a pars plana vitrectomy is the surgical procedure of choice. The vitrectomy infusion suction and cutting instruments are introduced over the pars plana and the vitreous hemorrhage is removed and replaced with saline. The tractional bands are also cut and released allowing the retina to reattach to its normal position.

Multiple studies have implicated VEGF as the main culprit in the pathogenesis of diabetic retinopathy and diabetic macular edema. The retina becomes ischemic because of capillary damage from diabetes. Ischemic areas of the retina produce VEGF and other chemical factors resulting in neovascularization, the proliferation of abnormally formed blood vessels. These abnormal blood vessels are fragile and may leak (causing macular edema), bleed (causing vitreous hemorrhage), and eventually form fibrovascular scar and traction, ultimately causing tractional retinal detachment and blindness. After decades of clinical trials, the use of recombinant antibodies specifically targeting VEGF has been shown to not only restore the integrity of blood-retinal barrier, minimizing serum leakage, but also to dramatically improve vision in the majority of patients with diabetic macular edema. The three most commonly used anti-VEGF medications are: bevacizumab (Avastin), ranibizumab (Lucentis), and aflibercept (Eyelea). Multiple pivotal studies (RESTORE, READ2, RISE/RIDE, DA VINCI, VIVID, and VISTA) and results released by Diabetic Retinopathy Clinical Research Network (DRCR.net) demonstrated that intravitreal anti-VEGF blocks the effects of VEGF and significantly improves vision loss from diabetic macular edema.[6-8]

The management of diabetes requires a coordinated effort between healthcare providers, including the ophthalmologist, general practitioner, endocrinologist, and dietician. Although technologic advances have been beneficial, diabetic retinopathy remains one of the leading causes of blindness in North America.

Educating diabetic patients regarding the sequelae of diabetic retinopathy and macular edema, and the importance of blood glucose and blood pressure control is of utmost importance for all eye care professionals.

Retinitis pigmentosa

Retinitis pigmentosa (RP) is a complex genetic disorder with a variable pattern of transmission. RP may be inherited as a sex-linked trait or as an autosomal dominant or recessive trait. RP can be classified into various subtypes, but symptoms common to many cases of RP include nyctalopia (difficulty seeing in dim illumination) and progressive loss of peripheral visual field. The subtype classification of a case of RP depends on the nature of the condition and its duration. RP may be mild or may progress to cause severe blindness. Disease severity is often worse in those who begin presenting symptoms in childhood or adolescence, as compared with those who initially present in adulthood.

It is not inevitable that each case will develop and cause constricting field loss. Some cases of RP remain stable for a lifetime.

The diagnosis can often be made with direct visualization of the fundus using ophthalmoscopy. The following findings are characteristic features:

1. Bone spicule-like pigment debris in the midperiphery of the retina (Fig. 24.5)
2. Retinal vessel attenuation

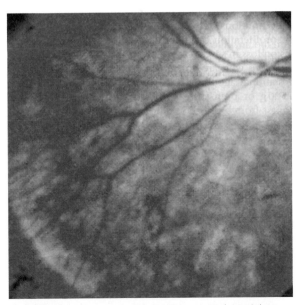

Fig. 24.5 Retinitis pigmentosa. Note attenuated arterioles, bone spicule pigment formation in the periphery, and waxy pallor of the optic disc.

Currently, there are trials investigating the role of post-delivery systems for anti-VEGF, retinal stem cell transplantation, and recombinant gene therapy. Several other studies are looking at the role of other proteins, such as angiopoietin, complement C3, C5, and the role of drugs with anti-inflammatory benefits, such as Doxycycline and metformin for the treatment of wet AMD. These modalities are currently investigational only.

New approaches to screening, early and noninvasive diagnosis, and treatment of AMD are rapidly evolving. Exciting new treatment modalities will help us meet the challenge of this devastating disease and improve the quality of life for patients with AMD.

Ocular manifestations of common systemic diseases

Retinal examination often reflects the status and severity of various systemic conditions. These will be reviewed later (Figs. 24.9–24.13).

Hypertension

Patients with high blood pressure, or malignant hypertension, may be diagnosed by the ophthalmologist. Elevated high blood pressure may be asymptomatic and can present with early microvascular damage and retinal vascular changes.

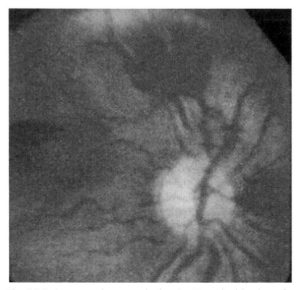

Fig. 24.9 Acute myelogenous leukemia. Note the blotches of hemorrhage.

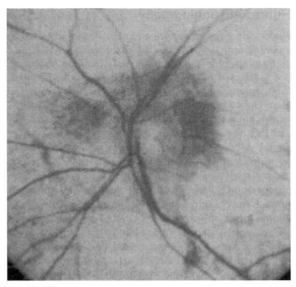

Fig. 24.10 Metastasis of breast cancer to the right eye. Note elevation of the peripheral retina.

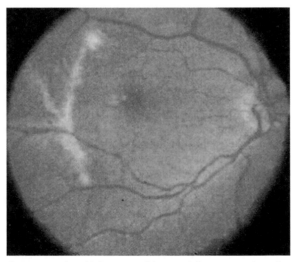

Fig. 24.11 Choroidal tear. A white scar follows contusion of the globe, resulting from rupture of the choroid.

In the early phase of hypertensive retinopathy, the only manifestation may be an attenuation of the retinal arterioles. This narrowing may be uniform, as found in older people, or focal, which may occur in a younger person.

In elderly persons, the changes may be mild as the retinal vessels become thicker, with a dulling of the light reflexes on the retinal arteriole surface. At the area of crossings, the retinal arterioles may appear to compress the underlying veins and cause *arteriovenous nicking* of the underlying blood column.

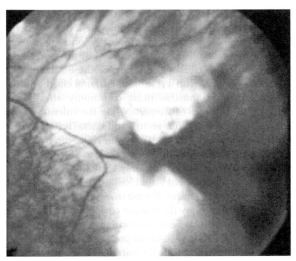

Fig. 24.12 Retinoblastoma. This is the most common retinal tumor in children, manifested by large, white lesions in the posterior pole of the eye.

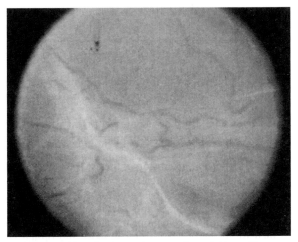

Fig. 24.14 Sickle cell retinopathy. Note the retinitis proliferans with underlying traction retinal detachment inferiorly. (Courtesy Mount Sinai Hospital, Toronto.)

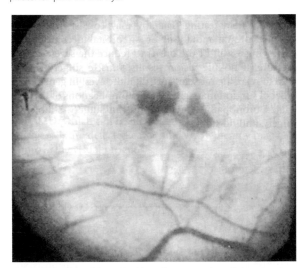

Fig. 24.13 Choroideremia. Hereditary atrophy of the vascular choroid reveals a white underlying sclera. The retina is also affected. It usually leads to blindness.

Younger patients with severe hypertension (malignant hypertension or eclampsia in pregnancy) may display a florid type of retinopathy with flame-shaped hemorrhages, exudates, cotton-wool spots, and marked narrowing of the retinal arterioles. The most ominous sign is edema, or swelling, of the optic disc.

Sickle cell disease

Sickle cell hemoglobinopathies are most common in patients of African and Mediterranean ancestry. The disorder is hereditary. The normal hemoglobin in the red cell is replaced by the sickle hemoglobin (hemoglobin S), which assumes an abnormally rigid sickle-like shape under various circumstances. The rigid sickle cells have difficulty passing through blood vessels, which often result in vascular occlusion (vasoocclusive crisis).

Retinal changes are common in this disease (Fig. 24.14). Early stages of sickle cell retinopathy include retinal hemorrhages and small retinal arteriole occlusions. As the retina becomes progressively more ischemic, neovascularization occurs on the surface of the retina—leading to retinal and vitreous hemorrhages—and preretinal membranes. Comma-shaped capillaries in the conjunctiva are part of the general vascular pattern. The final stages of sickle cell retinopathy, like proliferative diabetic retinopathy, include neovascularization and associated tractional retinal detachment.

Thyroid disorders

Ocular disease can be seen in patients with hyperthyroidism (excessive thyroid activity), hypothyroidism (depressed thyroid activity), and even euthyroidism (normal thyroid function after successful treatment for hyperthyroidism).

Persons with hyperthyroidism tend to have a rapid pulse, shortness of breath, and loss of weight. Those with hypothyroidism show a deceleration of activity and may be dull mentally, with a low voice, reduced pulse rate, dry skin, and weight gain.

Patients with a thyroid disorder and specific eye findings have a condition referred to as *Graves disease*. The etiologic factors of this condition are thought to be immunologic. A variety of tests can be used for diagnosis of the thyroid

then flows into the capillaries and from there into the veins. When there is partial venous filling (i.e., laminar flow), the arteriovenous phase is recognized. When the veins are filled with fluorescein, this is the venous phase. The dye is distributed throughout the blood (recirculation phase) 3 to 5 minutes after injection and early leakage and staining occur during this period. The elimination phase can be observed between 30 and 60 minutes after injection.

Damage to the endothelium of retinal capillaries or the RPE causes leakage into and beneath the retina. Diagnostic patterns include defects of the pigment epithelium (which act as windows to the underlying choroidal fluorescence), accumulation of dye between choroid and retina (e.g., serous detachment), staining within the retina (secondary to leakage from retinal capillaries), interference with visualization of choroidal fluorescence (by exudates, pigment, or hemorrhage), obstruction to filling (arteriole or venous occlusion), and abnormal vessels (e.g., neovascularization).

Fig. 24.21 shows the presence of dye leakage into the macula. This is associated with a decrease in vision and is consistent with the diagnosis of cystoid macular edema. This condition may be seen after any type of intraocular surgery, most commonly after cataract extraction, or it may be a consequence of an inflammatory condition of the posterior segment that causes leakage of the macular vessels.

Fig. 24.22A shows a diabetic fundus with microaneurysms, which appear as punctate areas of hyperfluorescence. A later stage of the angiogram (Fig. 24.22B) shows significant leakage of dye into the macula, which accounts for the decrease in vision.

Fig. 24.23 is an angiogram of a central retinal vein occlusion. One can appreciate the tortuous retinal veins, hypofluorescent areas that represent scattered hemorrhages, and

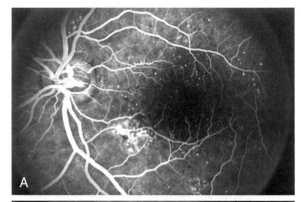

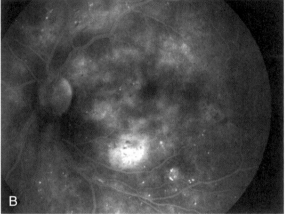

Fig. 24.22 (A) Fluorescein angiogram of a diabetic fundus. (B) Later angiogram phase of the same diabetic fundus as in (A). Areas of hyperfluorescence represent leakage of fluid into the macula.

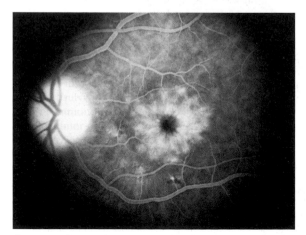

Fig. 24.21 Fluorescein angiogram that demonstrates cystoid macular edema.

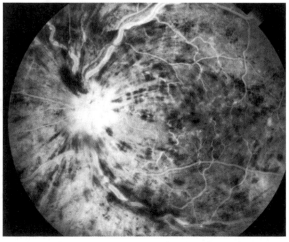

Fig. 24.23 Fluorescein angiogram of a central retinal vein occlusion.

hyperfluorescent areas that are a result of leakage from the vessels. This is in contrast to Fig. 24.24, which is an angiogram of a BRVO that shows blockage of the choroidal fluorescein by blood in a sector distribution. The patient has decreased vision as a result of macular edema from vessel leakage. Laser photocoagulation can be performed to improve the visual prognosis.

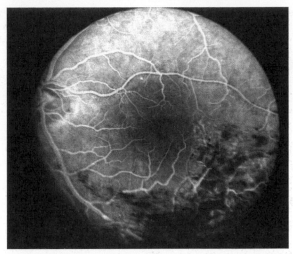

Fig. 24.24 Fluorescein angiogram of a branch retinal vein occlusion.

Questions for review and thought

1. Discuss the possible eye involvement of diabetes mellitus.
2. What is the use of the laser in ophthalmology?
3. What is the clinical picture of someone who has had a central retinal artery occlusion?
4. What symptoms suggest a retinal detachment?
5. What are the retinal findings that suggest retinitis pigmentosa?
6. What is retinopathy of prematurity? What is its cause?
7. An individual has a metallic foreign body that perforates the eye and enters the posterior chamber. What possible eye involvements may there be?
8. What are the clinical manifestations of hyperthyroidism?

Self-evaluation questions   Q

True–false statements

Directions: Indicate whether the statement is true (**T**) or false (**F**).

1. Retinopathy of prematurity occurs in one eye of premature infants exposed to high concentrations of oxygen. **T** or **F**
2. Every retinal hole should be sealed with either laser beam or cryosurgery. **T** or **F**
3. Drusen of the retina rarely cause any loss of vision. **T** or **F**

Missing words

Directions: Write in the missing word in the following sentences.

4. Central retinal vein occlusion can cause _____ 3 months after the event.
5. Diabetic retinopathy is more prevalent with diabetics whose disease is poorly controlled and who have had their disease at least _____ years.
6. Retinitis pigmentosa causes _____ field defect in the early stages.

Choice-completion questions

Directions: Select the one best answer in each case.

7. Retinal detachments are common:
   a. in high myopes.
   b. after contusion.
   c. with malignant melanomas.
   d. with retinal tears with an operculum.
   e. all of the above.
8. Central serous retinopathy is a disease of:
   a. elderly persons over 65 years.
   b. persons between 25 and 50 years.
   c. females.
   d. patients of African ancestry.
   e. absent symptoms.
9. Central retinal artery occlusion usually is caused by:
   a. a tumor of the optic nerve.
   b. a thrombus.
   c. an embolus.
   d. glaucoma.
   e. carotid artery stenosis.

Answers, notes, and explanations

A

1. **False**. Retinopathy of prematurity is a bilateral disease occurring in infants born before 36 weeks of gestation or weighing less than 4.2 pounds at birth and having a history of significant oxygen therapy. These infants develop three signs: peripheral neovascularization (especially on the temporal periphery), vitreous bleeding, and retinal detachment.

   Infants exposed to high doses of oxygen should be examined with the indirect ophthalmoscope before discharge from the hospital and every 2 months until the condition is considered stable.

   The treatment of this condition is still not satisfactory despite the use of lasers, cryotherapy, vitamins C and E (tocopherol), and encircling retinal buckles.

   The most serious complication of retinopathy of prematurity is retinal detachment, which may not be evident until the age of 10 to 20 years.

   The difficulty in evaluating treatment of this condition results from the fact that many infants have a spontaneous regression.

2. **False**. Every break or retinal hole should not be sealed with laser beam or cryosurgery. Many retinal holes are not through-and-through or do not have an operculum or lip developed through traction. It is true, however, that in many retinal detachments, a retinal break develops. A hole in the retina permits the accumulation of fluid between the pigment layer of the retina and the anterior nine sensory layers of the retina. The subretinal fluid that accumulates acts as a wedge between the retinal layers and further detachment results.

   Most retinal holes occur in the extreme periphery of the retina. They are quite common and most do not lead to detachment. If a retinal hole is found with a break in the retina, with evidence of traction or a serous wedge, these breaks are treated. Although most retinal holes do not cause a retinal detachment, most detachments (over 85%) reveal multiple holes.

3. **True**. Drusen of the choroid are basically excrescences of Bruch's membrane of the choroid. They appear as yellow deposits in the posterior pole of the retina, sometimes surrounded by a collarette of retinal pigment. Unless associated with macular degenerative phenomena, these drusen usually are harmless.

   Drusen of the optic nerve are quite another matter. They consist of hyalin or calcium and these deposits take up and compress tissue in the optic nerve. Field defects are common and may be quite varied depending on the size of the drusen, their location, and their development. In addition to causing visual field defects, drusen may simulate the appearance of papilledema or swelling of the optic nerve head.

Typically, drusen are glistening pearl-like bodies which, when visible, are seen in the surface of the optic disc. When they are buried, the disc is heaped up and its margins are quite blurred.

4. **Neovascular glaucoma**. Central retinal vein occlusion can cause a severe, intractable glaucoma within 3 months after the venous occlusion.

   The vascular ischemia of the venous occlusion causes neovascularization at the level of the retina and iris. In the retina, macroaneurysms and vascular buds appear. These can create retinal hemorrhage and lead to retinal detachment. In the iris, the vascular proliferation can sew up the angle structures with fibrovascular tissue. This leads to a permanent angle-closure type of glaucoma that cannot be satisfactorily treated medically or surgically. The term *hemorrhagic glaucoma* is a misnomer because it is not the presence of the blood in the anterior chamber that causes the glaucoma. It is caused by the growth of active fibrovascular bands that invade and occlude the angle structures.

5. **15**. Diabetic retinopathy is a major cause of blindness in North America. Initially, the retinopathy was thought to be a straight function of duration. Those with diabetes for 15 years or longer were the most susceptible to the disease. The duration factor is still valid inasmuch as it is uncommon to see diabetics of 25 years without some form of retinopathy. That is not to say that long-term diabetics invariably go blind but they show a few microaneurysms, perhaps some neovascularization of the retina, or turgid retinal veins. In addition to duration, most researchers believe that hyperglycemia by itself is toxic and proper control is important to minimize the disease. For years, this point was contentious but appears now to be settled. Another area of dispute is the relationship of age to retinopathy. It was believed that maturity-onset (40 years or over) diabetics were free of the complications of retinopathy. This is definitely not true. Approximately 20% of maturity-onset diabetics develop retinopathy. When this occurs, it usually is more severe than in the juvenile diabetics. Some physicians believe that the division of juvenile diabetes and maturity-onset diabetes should be abolished and replaced by insulin-dependent and noninsulin-dependent disease. Insulin-dependent diabetics are more prone to retinal complications of this disease.

6. **Tubular or signet ring**. Retinitis pigmentosa can cause tubular field defects. Such defects in the visual field also can be caused by syphilis, glaucoma, quinine poisoning, eclampsia and, on occasion, hysteria.

   The diagnosis of this disease can be made by observing the bone spicule pigment deposits in the retina at the

A   Answers, notes, and explanations—Continued

level of the midperiphery. Also an ERG can reveal the flat electrical response of the rods, which is abolished under dim light. There usually is a family history of the disease. This may not be obvious because the disease can be transmitted as a dominant, recessive, or sex-linked type of hereditary pattern.

Occasionally, vitamin A deficiency can be uncovered and this plus nutritional disorders, although rare in industrialized countries, may mimic retinitis pigmentosa. At present there is no cure for this disease. In many patients the evolution of this disease may be quite slow; thus blindness may not occur in all afflicted patients.

7. **a. In high myopes.** The typical high myope has a tilted disc with an oblique entry of the optic nerve through the sclera, an elongated eye sometimes with a large posterior staphyloma, and a stretched vascular system for both the retinal and the choroidal circulations. As a result, through vascular ischemia, retinal holes (some leading to retinal tears and subsequent detachment) are common. A retinal tear with an operculum is merely a large retinal tear with a lip or edge that is everting. Such tears cannot be sealed by laser therapy and represent a further stage in the development or evolution of a retinal detachment. A malignant melanoma can cause a detachment by virtue of this solid mass derived from the choroid pressing forward from behind and pushing the retina anteriorly. Diagnostically, the melanoma is one of the few instances in which a retinal detachment may be present without a retinal hole or tear. Injury also may cause retinal detachment as a result of the underlying presence of blood, edema fluid, and inflammatory debris. Injury is not the major cause, however, of most retinal detachments.

8. **b. Persons between 25 and 50 years.** Central serous retinopathy is a disease of young people. At times, it may be related to stress or a prolonged period of anxiety or to an allergic reaction to drugs, vapors, or chemicals but commonly it has no antecedent of any kind. The person invariably is made aware of the problem because of blurred and distorted vision. Lines appear curved, at times with missing pieces in the center, and color vision is depressed or darker in hue. The patient's symptoms are pathognomonic of this condition. However, support for the diagnosis can be made by the Amsler grid or by looking for the tell-tale macular blister, which usually is clinically evident. The treatment, depending on the severity of the condition, is systemic steroids, laser beam obliteration of the leaking vessel if possible, and tincture of time. Often, the condition improves without any drug or device. Angiography of the retinal and choroidal circulation should be done because simulating conditions include a small macular melanoma, histoplasmosis, hematoma, and an effusion of a hemangioma.

9. **c. An embolus.** Central retinal artery occlusion is invariably a result of an embolus from an atheromatous plaque of the carotid artery. It is commonly a mixture of fatty debris, platelets, and fibrin and appears as a glistening yellow plaque at the head of the optic nerve in the central retinal artery. At times, nothing is found at this location but fragments of the embolus may be visible in the retinal circulation. Such an event invariably causes blindness unless heroic measures, such as ocular paracentesis or heavy massage of the globe are undertaken within 5 minutes. Such patients should receive the benefit of a neurologic investigation to direct attention to the carotid artery on that side, which also may be stenosed or compromised by the presence of an atheromatous ulcer in the wall of the vessel.

Patients with this disease often worry about a similar event occurring in the other eye. Of course, it is possible, because atheroma in a person usually is not limited to a single vessel but is present more or less in all large blood vessels. Statistically, the chances of such a catastrophe being bilateral are extremely remote and highly improbable.

References

1. Rudkin AK, Lee AW, Chen CS. Ocular neovascularization following central retinal artery occlusion: prevalence and timing of onset. *Eur J Ophthalmol.* 2010;20(6):1042–1046.
2. American Academy of Ophthalmology. 2019-2020 BCSC (Basic and Clinical Science Course), Section 12: Retina and Vitreous. 2019. American Academy of Ophthalmology.
3. Brown DM, Campochiaro PA, Singh RP, et al. Ranibizumab for macular edema following central retinal vein occlusion: six-month primary end point results of a phase III study. *Ophthalmology.* 2010;117(6):1124–1133.
4. Campochiaro PA, Heier JS, Feiner L, et al. Ranibizumab for macular edema following branch retinal vein occlusion: six-month primary end point results of a phase III study. *Ophthalmology.* 2010;117(6):1102–1112.e1.
5. Sun JK, Glassman AR, Beaulieu WT, et al. Rationale and application of the protocol S anti-vascular endothelial growth factor algorithm for proliferative diabetic retinopathy. *Ophthalmology.* 2019;126(1):87–95.
6. Reddy RK, Pieramici DJ, Gune S, et al. Efficacy of ranibizumab in eyes with diabetic macular edema and

macular nonperfusion in ride and rise. *Ophthalmology.* 2018;125(10):1568–1574.

7. Gross JG, Glassman AR, Liu D, et al. Five-year outcomes of panretinal photocoagulation vs intravitreous ranibizumab for proliferative diabetic retinopathy: a randomized clinical trial. *JAMA Ophthalmol.* 2018;136(10):1138.

8. Furino C, Boscia F, Reibaldi M, Alessio G. Intravitreal therapy for diabetic macular edema: an update. Mencía-Gutiérrez E, ed. J. Ophthalmol. 2021;2021:1–23.

9. Lim JW, Kang SW, Kim YT, et al. Comparative study of patients with central serous chorioretinopathy undergoing focal laser photocoagulation or photodynamic therapy. *Br J Ophthalmol.* 2011;95(4):514–517.

10. Brown DM, Kaiser PK, Michels M, et al. Ranibizumab versus verteporfin for neovascular age-related macular degeneration. *N Engl J Med.* 2006;355(14):1432–1444.

11. Lalwani GA, Rosenfeld PJ, Fung AE, et al. A variabledosing regimen with intravitreal ranibizumab for neovascular age-related macular degeneration: year 2 of the PrONTO Study. *Am J Ophthalmol.* 2009;148(1):43–58.

12. Regillo CD, Brown DM, Abraham P, et al. Randomized, double-masked, sham-controlled trial of ranibizumab for neovascular age-related macular degeneration: PIER Study year 1. *Am J Ophthalmol.* 2008;145(2):239–248.

13. Rosenfeld PJ, Brown DM, Heier JS, et al. Ranibizumab for neovascular age-related macular degeneration. *N Engl J Med.* 2006;355(14):1419–1431.

Chapter | 25 |

Glaucoma

Michael S. Berlin, Jonathan Shakibkhou, Anne Nguyen, Omar Sirsy, and Harold A. Stein

Introduction

The ophthalmic technician is a critical member of the glaucoma patient management team. Responsibilities integral to the ophthalmic technician's role in the care of patients with glaucoma include:

- Identifying factors that may be indicative of glaucoma when taking a patient's history
- Performing key tests to define the glaucoma patient's status
- Aiding in glaucoma patients' treatment by teaching them about their condition, demonstrating treatment techniques (such as applying eyedrops), and monitoring their compliance and treatment efficacy in preventing progression
- Assisting in the preoperative preparation and especially in the postoperative care of glaucoma surgical patients

Each one of these aspects is essential to the complete care of the glaucoma patient.

An understanding of what glaucoma is, what glaucoma does to the eye, and what we can do about it enables the technician to become a key component of this glaucoma patient management team. It is the ophthalmic technician who has the potential to effect a positive outcome in the prognosis of glaucoma patients. More than 80 million people worldwide are afflicted by glaucoma. There are countless millions in whom glaucoma has not been diagnosed. For every person blinded by glaucoma, there are at least six individuals who have lost useful vision in one eye.[1]

Classification

Glaucoma is a localized ocular disease characterized by optic nerve cupping and visual field loss, and is usually associated with elevated intraocular pressure (IOP). The hallmark of glaucoma is a progressive optic neuropathy. Risk factors for glaucoma include:

- Elevated IOP
- Family history of glaucoma
- People of African or Hispanic ancestry
- Diabetes
- Myopia
- Trauma to the eye
- Advanced age

Glaucoma falls roughly into five classifications (Table 25.1):

1. *Primary open-angle* or *chronic glaucoma*. This condition is thought to arise from a progressive outflow obstruction

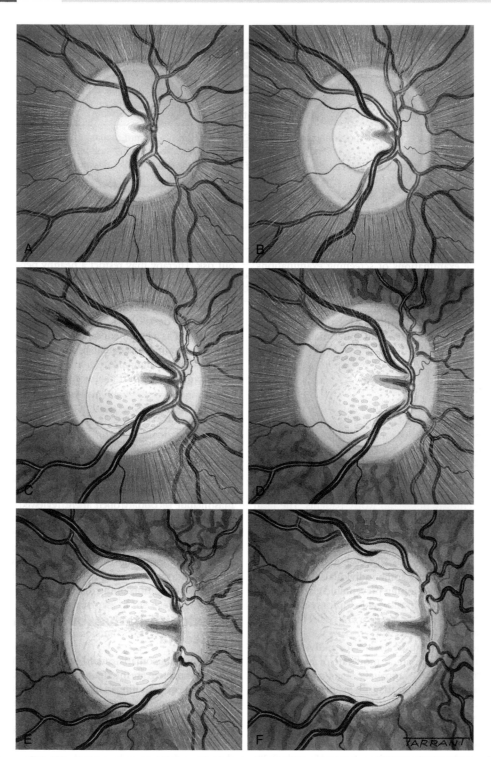

Fig. 25.3 Progression of optic nerve damage. (A) Normal, (B) Early, (C) Moderate (D) Advanced (E) Late (F) End stage with severe vascular impairment cupping.

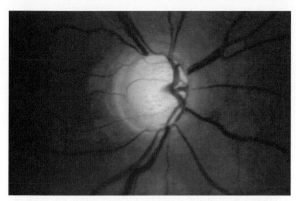

Fig. 25.4 End-stage glaucomatous cupping. (From Kanski J. *Clinical Ophthalmology: A Systematic Approach.* 5th ed. Oxford: Butterworth-Heinemann; 2003, with permission.)

Box 25.1 Diagnostic tests for glaucoma

Intraocular pressure: tonometry
Gonioscopy
Central corneal thickness
Structural: optic nerve
- Stereo disc photography
- Nerve fiber layer thickness (optical coherence tomography [OCT])
- Ultrasound biomicroscopy (UBM)
- Confocal scanning ophthalmoscopy (Heidelberg retina tomograph)
- Retinal nerve fiber layer assessment (GDx VCC)

Functional: visual fields (see Ch. 18)
- Standard automated perimetry (SAP; white on white)
- Short-wave automated perimetry (SWAP; blue on yellow)
- Frequency doubling technology (FDT)

Traditional IOP-lowering medications may be less effective in patients with exfoliative glaucoma, thus requiring additional therapy such as argon laser trabeculoplasty (ALT) or selective laser trabeculoplasty (SLT).

Pigmentary glaucoma

Pigmentary glaucoma occurs when iris pigment granules flake into the aqueous humor or other structures, such as the trabecular meshwork, and clog the drainage channels of the eye. This condition tends to occur at a younger age, usually in the 20s or 30s, and in near-sighted patients. It is more common in men than in women.

Patients are often treated with drops, such as a prostaglandin or a beta blocker, because these drops have a relatively low incidence of side effects and are well tolerated in younger patients. Miotics can be used to treat pigmentary glaucoma because it causes the pupil to constrict and prevents the iris from rubbing against the lens, thereby preventing release of pigment onto the surrounding structures. However, miotics often cause blurred vision and require more frequent dosing, thus limiting their use. Other options include laser iridotomy and ALT or SLT.

Neovascular glaucoma

Neovascular glaucoma is a severe form of secondary glaucoma. It is associated with the proliferation of vessels in the anterior chamber angle. The blood vessels generated through neovascular glaucoma are abnormal, and when new blood vessels form in the anterior chamber angle, the aqueous outflow can be compromised. Typically, the three most common conditions responsible for neovascular glaucoma are diabetic retinopathy, central retinal vein occlusion, and carotid artery obstructive disease.

Neovascular glaucoma is often treated with panretinal photocoagulation, which has been shown to reduce anterior segment neovascularization. Traditional IOP-lowering medications also can be used to lower the pressure, as well as trabeculectomy and aqueous drain implants.

Traumatic glaucoma

Traumatic glaucoma refers to any injuries to the eye that result in glaucoma. Blunt trauma, such as a direct injury to the eye or a blow to the head, usually as a result of sports, can cause an accumulation of blood and debris that clogs the drainage channels. In this case, glaucoma medications can be used to control eye pressure, and surgery may be necessary. In most cases, the elevated eye pressure is temporary.

When a penetrating eye injury occurs, such as by a sharp instrument, it can cause the eye to become swollen and bleed, leading to elevated eye pressure. In addition, drainage channels can be blocked by damaged tissue and scarring. Ocular trauma is often treated by topical corticosteroid therapy as an initial treatment to minimize permanent tissue damage and scarring.

Glaucomatocyclitic crisis

Glaucomatocyclitic crisis is a condition with self-limited recurrent episodes of markedly elevated IOP with mild idiopathic anterior chamber inflammation. It is most often classified as secondary inflammatory glaucoma.

In 1948 Posner and Schlossman first recognized glaucomatocyclitic crisis and described the features of this syndrome. For this reason, the entity is often termed Posner–Schlossman syndrome (PSS).

Most commonly, a "crisis" presents with slight discomfort. The patient may be pain-free even though the IOP is quite elevated. The patient may report blurred vision or halo vision if the IOP is high. A history of attacks of blurred vision lasting several days, which recur monthly or yearly, is usual. IOP is usually elevated in the range of 40 to 60 mm Hg.

The favored initial treatment for PSS is a combined regimen of a topical nonsteroidal antiinflammatory drug (NSAID; e.g., diclofenac) and an antiglaucoma drug, such as timolol or dorzolamide. Prostaglandins are often avoided initially. Surgery is never indicated.

Primary angle-closure glaucoma

Angle-closure glaucoma may be primary or secondary. Primary angle-closure glaucoma constitutes approximately 10% of all glaucoma cases and occurs in about 5% to 10% of the older adult population. In the general population, a higher incidence of angle-closure glaucoma occurs in association with shallower anterior chambers. Angle-closure glaucoma shows increased incidence among people of Asian and Inuit descent and is less common among people of African ancestry.

Patients with this disorder have essentially normal but often short (hyperopic) eyes with a shallow anterior chamber and a narrow entrance into the angle. Such crowding of the angle structure tends to occur more often in hyperopia and increases as the patient becomes older. The narrowing is mainly caused by the increased size of the crystalline lens as a cataract forms, which tends to push the entire iris diaphragm forward, narrowing the endocorneal angle of the anterior chamber to less than 20 degrees, thus enabling the term *narrow angle*.

A common trigger mechanism that brings about closure of a critically narrowed angle is dilation of the pupil. Pupil dilation relaxes the iris and causes its tissue to bunch up toward the base of the iris, thereby effectively blocking the angle outflow structures. Also dilation of the pupil may relax the periphery of the iris sufficiently so that the pressure in the posterior chamber exceeds that in the anterior chamber, resulting in further forward displacement of the iris and crowding of the angle structures. If the pupillary border of the iris is bound down (as a result of inflammation) to the anterior lens capsule, or if the pupil is blocked by a prolapsed vitreous body, a pupillary block mechanism exists. This may lead to bowing of the iris, or iris bombé (Fig. 25.5). In this situation, the pupil is blocked so that the aqueous pressure from the posterior chamber bows the iris forward, thus blocking the angle of the anterior chamber and preventing fluid outflow.

An attack of acute angle-closure glaucoma can become fully developed within 30 to 60 minutes. The abruptness of the onset is so characteristic that a presumptive diagnosis of acute angle-closure glaucoma can virtually be made over the telephone. The attack commonly begins under conditions that lead to pupillary dilation, for example, conditions of dark adaptation (movie theaters), fear, or emotional arousal. Such attacks are often precipitated by dilation during an eye examination.

The pain can vary from a feeling of discomfort and fullness around the eyes to a severe, referred pain that can radiate to the back of the head or down toward the teeth. With severe pain, the patient may be prostrate and nauseated and may even vomit. Vision is usually reduced and patients often report seeing halos as the result of a cloudy edematous cornea.

Certain drugs can also precipitate an attack, the most common being cyclopentolate and tropicamide. Other often used

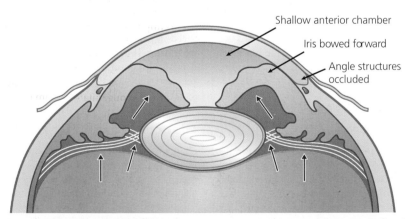

Fig. 25.5 Pupillary block glaucoma. The pressure in the posterior chamber exceeds that of the anterior chamber. The iris is bowed forward (iris bombé) and occludes the angle structures. Without treatment, the iris becomes permanently adherent to the angle structures and intractable secondary glaucoma ensues.

medications that can precipitate an attack are epinephrine derivatives. These drugs are frequently agents in common hay fever remedies, and the package insert indicates their contraindication in glaucoma; however, the phenylephrine derivative drugs are usually safe in open-angle glaucoma.

Examination reveals that the eyelids and conjunctiva are edematous and congested, especially around the limbus. The cornea appears steamy and hazy because of epithelial edema, which results from aggregations of tiny water droplets in the superficial layers of the cornea. The iris itself appears dull, gray, and patternless because of the edema. The pupil is typically middilated and may be oval. It does not respond normally to light. The IOP is often extremely high, in the range of 40 to 60 mm Hg or higher.

This type of ocular catastrophe is preceded in nearly half of cases by premonitory self-limiting episodes of aching blur, lasting a few hours each time and occurring with increasing frequency before an acute attack. Also the patient may report seeing halos or rainbows around lights, which are caused by the slight edema of the cornea in these premonitory periods. These halos, although not pathognomonic of glaucoma, are most significantly related to this disease and are caused by dispersion of light by the epithelial edema. They are typically composed of two colored rings: an inner blue-violet ring and an outer yellow-red ring (Fig. 25.6). Between attacks, little or no abnormality may be noted.

The halos caused by subacute attacks can be distinguished from the permanent halos caused by lens opacities by placing a stenopeic slit across the line of vision. A glaucoma halo remains intact but with diminished intensity behind the slit, whereas a lenticular halo is broken up into segments that revolve as the slit is moved. The halos that are sometimes caused by conjunctival debris can be swept away by movements of the lid.

Secondary angle-closure glaucoma occurs as a result of an underlying pathologic etiology.

The conditions that can lead to *secondary angle-closure glaucoma* are:

- Iritis or uveitis
- Lens dislocation
- Lens swelling
- Scar tissue or peripheral anterior synechiae between the iris and the trabecular meshwork
- Posterior synechiae to the lens
- Blockage of drainage channels by the accumulation of "flaky" protein or iris pigment

The most common cause of anterior synechiae is chronic angle-closure glaucoma and the most common cause of posterior synechiae is chronic, severe iritis.

Congenital glaucoma

Congenital glaucoma is an extremely uncommon disease. It is estimated that an average ophthalmologist is unlikely to see more than one new case of congenital glaucoma in 5 years of practice. Despite its rarity, the signs and symptoms of the disease are so characteristic that a diagnosis should not be missed.

Often the parents are aware that their baby has something wrong with the eye in the first few weeks or months of life. The child appears extremely sensitive to light and tears profusely. Many infants even keep their eyelids tightly closed most of the day to avoid the light. However, it is the corneal haziness caused by the corneal edema that makes most parents suspect that something is wrong with the child's eyes. Because the eyeball tissue is distensible in early infancy, the increased IOP causes progressive enlargement of the infant's eye and cornea. Most infant corneas measure less than 10.5 mm in horizontal diameter. A measurement greater than 12 mm is considered diagnostic of congenital glaucoma. These eyes, hazy and enlarged, appear so abnormal that the term *buphthalmos* has been commonly applied to designate this condition (see Fig. 25.1).

It is important that any child with a symptom of tearing is seen immediately because the earlier glaucoma is diagnosed and brought under control, the better is the prognosis. In most cases, tearing is caused by a blocked tear duct, but the ophthalmic assistant should always be aware of the possibility of congenital glaucoma.

Diagnosis

Screening and aids in diagnosis

Screening for glaucoma

A comprehensive screening program consisting of tonometry, optic disc examination, and screening perimetry, although costly, helps detect and initiate early treatment to prevent

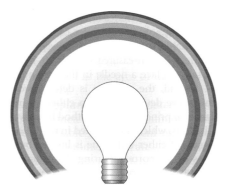

Fig. 25.6 Halos around lights. This is a prominent symptom in angle-closure glaucoma. These colors are related to the spectral colors of light through water droplets in the cornea.

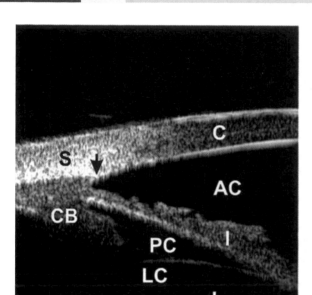

Fig. 25.36 Ultrasound biomicroscopic appearance of a normal eye. The cornea (*C*), sclera (*S*), anterior chamber (*AC*), posterior chamber (*PC*), iris (*I*), ciliary body (*CB*), lens capsule (*LC*), and lens (*L*) can be identified. The scleral spur *(black arrow)* is an important landmark to assess the morphologic relationships among the anterior segment structures.

horizontal line. The nerve fiber bundle defect is a prototype of glaucomatous field defects.

3. *Baring of the blind spot.* Baring of the blind spot is an arcuate or partial nerve fiber bundle defect emerging from the blind spot.

4. *Nerve fiber bundle defect or Bjerrum's arcuate scotoma.* This defect is a complete type of nerve fiber bundle defect emanating from the blind spot, arching over central fixation, and ending on the horizontal line. In its early stages, this defect may not be attached to the blind spot and may extend only partway around the macular region.

5. *Nasal depression of the field.* This type of defect may appear quite early in glaucoma and later merges with a nerve fiber bundle defect to create an area of considerable visual loss.

The presence of typical glaucomatous field defects is virtually diagnostic of glaucoma, irrespective of the IOP. The treatment of glaucoma is directed principally toward avoiding further field loss, not merely reducing IOP. If a patient is under treatment and the pressure has been maintained at a satisfactory level, visual fields should be examined approximately 2 or 3 times a year. It is important in field testing to use an adequate-sized test object; many glaucoma patients cannot see well because they have cataracts. The examiner should use the smallest detectable stimulus that can be seen temporal to the blind spot.

The last area of visual field loss in glaucoma is the central vision area. Thus the wave of darkness that comes from the blind spot first surrounds the central area, extends to the periphery, and leaves the individual at the end stage of the disease looking clearly straight ahead through a long tunnel of darkness, so-called *tunnel vision* (Fig. 25.37).

Changes of the optic nerve head often precede detectable visual field loss. It has been estimated that almost half of the near fibers of the disc have to be lost before reproducible early field defects can be found. The correlation between optic nerve changes as noted by alterations of the disc and changes in visual function as detected by visual field assessment is usually parallel. If the correlation is not there, then one has to look for other sources of visual field changes, such as other defects or disturbances of the optic nerve, retina, or even farther along the optic neural pathways in the brain.

Techniques of perimetry. Because perimetry is discussed in Chapter 18, the following points highlight only its importance in glaucoma.

Kinetic perimetry involves moving the test object from a nonseeing area to a seeing area, whereas *static perimetry* involves the use of stationary test objects presented at random. The points at which the patient fails to recognize the spot of light are noted.

Threshold static perimetry measures the intensity thresholds of visual acuity of the individual points within the field of vision. This is accomplished by gradually increasing the target light on the subthreshold intensity and recording the level at which the patient first recognizes the target. The process also can be approached from the other direction, that is, decreasing from the suprathreshold level and recording the lowest value found.

Static perimetry has been shown to be more sensitive than kinetic perimetry at detecting early glaucomatous field defects. Most commonly, white targets are presented on a white background (white-on-white [WOW]). In short-wavelength automated perimetry (SWAP), a blue target is presented on a yellow background. SWAP can often identify earlier field loss than WOW.

Cataracts can also cause visual field defects. In one study of 90 eyes with open-angle glaucoma and cataracts, 41% had a partial or complete scotoma reversed after the cataract was removed. Reduced ocular clarity from other causes, such as corneal scarring may also affect and reduce the visual field. A miotic pupil may depress central and peripheral threshold retinal sensitivity and exaggerate field defects.

The correction of myopia with glasses is not required with the use of a 300-mm perimeter unless the refractive error exceeds 3.00 diopters. With high myopia, refractive scotomas may appear that can be confused with glaucomatous field defects. Usually, they are eliminated with appropriate correction of the refractive error. Astigmatic errors should first be corrected before visual field tests unless they are less than 1.00 diopter. Increasing age also causes a reduction in retinal threshold sensitivity.

Psychologic factors may depress the visual field and create false pockets of visual field loss. The field test is definitely influenced by the state of the patient's alertness, anxiety, calm, and degree of cooperation. A lack of familiarity with the test and heightened tension about performing well often lead to a poor first-test result, which invariably improves on the second or third visual field test. This improvement is not a reflection of a change in optic nerve status; rather, it is a result of familiarity with the test and better response to the visual stimuli.

The frequency doubling technology (FDT) field technique works by flickering a coarse pattern of vertical dark and bright bars at a very high frequency. The advantages of the FDT are that it is a compact, transportable perimeter with tolerance to refractive errors and rapid test times.

The tangent screen is almost a historic relic of visual field testing (see Chapter 18). It suffers from the drawbacks of monitoring fixation and is limited by variations in background lighting. No visible record is automatically elicited, the area is strictly limited to the central 30 degrees, and the screen does not reveal the peripheral field where early glaucomatous defects may appear.

Approaches to glaucoma field testing. There are two approaches to glaucoma field testing. The first is a screening technique to detect the presence of a glaucoma field defect. The second is to measure accurately the breadth, depth, and density of the field defect so that it can be appropriately charted on subsequent dates to ascertain any progressive loss of field.

The goal in visual field testing for glaucoma is the earliest detection of visual field changes. Historical methods include the Goldmann perimeter, a technician-driven kinetic perimeter, which maps the size and shape of scotomas by means of both central threshold targets and peripheral targets and reveals glaucomatous defects with a high probability. However, the most commonly used perimeters today are the Humphrey field analyzer (Figs. 25.38 and 25.39), a static perimeter that is automated, monitors fixation, and is less technician-dependent than the Goldmann perimeter. However, by the time visual field loss is detected by standard automated perimetry, substantial structural damage may exist. For this reason, also in use is the Humphrey FDT visual field instrument, which provides suprathreshold screening tests that identify early visual field loss. SWAP may also detect functional loss earlier.

Pathophysiology and the longitudinal treatment plan for progressive primary-angle glaucoma

One of the first diagnostic indicators for a physician to consider a diagnosis of glaucoma is an elevated IOP, measured by the various tonometers mentioned earlier in this

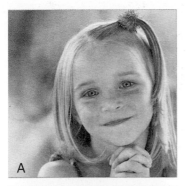
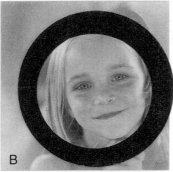
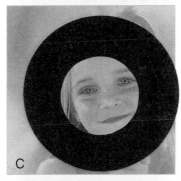
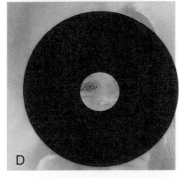

Fig. 25.37 Progressive constriction of visual field caused by advancing, irreversible glaucoma damage. Normal vision (A). Progressive constriction of visual field (B–D).

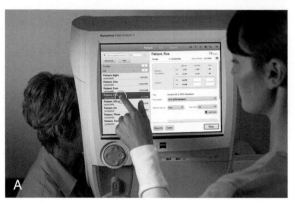
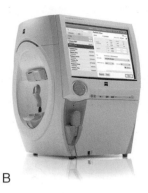

Fig. 25.38 Touchscreen programming of Humphrey Field Analyzer 3 (A). Humphrey Field Analyzer 3 (B). (Courtesy Carl Zeiss Meditec, Inc., Dublin, CA.)

chapter. A high IOP is often a cause of optic nerve degeneration and various interventions to reduce eye pressure are taken to lower the rate of progressive optic nerve degeneration. It is important to note that a patient's IOP is not a fixed pressure but rather fluctuates throughout the day. For this reason, ophthalmologists will often request that diurnal IOP information be obtained with the intention of finding the range of fluctuation in the patient's IOP over a 24 hour period. The range provides valuable data to the ophthalmologist which includes the time of day a patient has a peak in their IOP. This information may inform the physician on the most effective times for that specific patient to adequately control their IOP. A common finding in patients with open-angle glaucoma is greater fluctuation in IOP measured during the diurnal test when compared with nonglaucomatous patients.[6] In the field of ophthalmology, the progression and rate of change documented in data collected by the ophthalmic assistant is a critical factor for the patient's treatment plan and as such you play a vital role in the patient's health outcome.

In general, IOP ranges have been categorized into high, normal, and low IOP, however, this classification does not paint a full picture. The determination of a "high" IOP is dependent on the individual such that a normal IOP for one individual may be a high IOP for another; fundamentally a "normal" or target IOP is one where pressure induced optic neuropathy is negligible in the individual's lifetime. For instance, consider the pathology of normal tension glaucoma, where a "normal" IOP is too high for the individual and results in optic nerve degeneration. The example of normal tension glaucoma illustrates the significance of routine eye exams which include OCT. OCT allows for the measurement of the thickness of the RNFL; this nervous tissue layer is composed primarily of retinal ganglion cells and their projecting nerve fibers which collectively bundle in forming the optic nerve. OCT is effective in determining early-stage glaucoma, most notably in normal tension glaucoma, as decreases in the RNFL thickness are a result of neuronal degeneration, and signs of early neuronal degeneration may not manifest on a visual field test.[6] By definition, the diagnosis of mild stage glaucoma according to the American Academy of Ophthalmology, is described as "definite optic disc or RNFL abnormalities consistent with glaucoma as detailed earlier and a normal visual field as tested with standard automated perimetry (SAP)".[6] Glaucoma, in general, has been referred to as the "silent thief of sight" because it goes unnoticed as the brain nulls conscious awareness by making accommodation to the relatively slow progressive optic neuropathy.

To better understand the targets of treatment, it is important to understand the factors that determine IOP, most importantly inflow, outflow, and volume of aqueous humor. The volume of aqueous humor produced by the ciliary body per unit time will affect the total amount of aqueous humor present in the anterior and posterior chambers of the eye, as the volume of fluid increases, the IOP will also increase which may lead to optic nerve degeneration. The rate of aqueous humor production into the anterior and posterior chamber of the eye is often a target of antiglaucoma medications.

The next important factor is the volume of flow of aqueous humor from the angle found at the anterior chamber of the eye where the fluid passes through the trabecular meshwork into Schlemm's canal and subsequently into collector channels and aqueous veins. There are many pathologies that obstruct the flow through this path, and an obstruction in the outflow results in an accumulation of aqueous humor which will increase eye pressure. There are many antiglaucoma medications used to increase outflow from the anterior chamber. Further, many different surgical procedures have been designed to address the problem of flow by either creating channels that span the

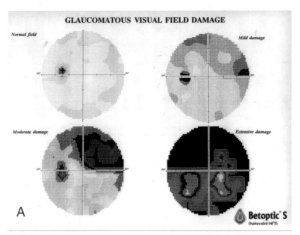

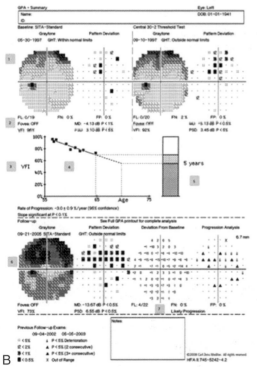

Fig. 25.39 Typical visual field progression because of glaucomatous optic neuropathy demonstrated per automated perimetry (A). Humphrey perimetry offers several printouts to assist in documenting and monitoring progression (B). (Courtesy Alcon; https://www.alcon.com.)

meshwork to allow drainage into Schlemm's canal or by creating an alternative path for fluid to drain by a fistula or tube shunt.

The first treatment plan for a patient that is diagnosed with glaucoma is the control of the factors discussed earlier

with antiglaucoma medications (Fig. 25.40). This can be challenging as the intervention is heavily dependent on the patient's compliance in using the medication(s) as prescribed and each medication has individual side effects. Further, even with compliance, there may not be adequate control of IOP. Although high IOP is often indicative of glaucoma, the damage and progression is assessed through diagnostic tools that allow the physician to visualize changes in the patient's optic nerve head, RNFL, and visual field over time. The progressive degeneration of the optic nerve as documented by progressive loss of visual field is often a result of nonadherence to the medication regimen which is an indication for a surgical intervention aimed to increase outflow and lower IOP.

As an ophthalmic technician, you play a vital role in gathering accurate data which will be evaluated to determine the patient's treatment plan. The ability to distinguish between representative or spurious data is important in patient management. The data gathered from the visual field is representative in many ways, but it is most useful for the ophthalmic technician to pay attention to the grayscale map. A basic understanding of the grayscale map is that an increased shading within the map translates into a patient's inability to detect light in that region of the retina (Fig. 25.41). Having a record of visual fields on a patient is useful for tracking progression and also may serve as a reference in understanding if the most recent visual field is reliable. A new change in any area of the visual field not seen in past recordings heightens suspension of patient error, new pathology or progressive disease (see Fig. 25.40). As an ophthalmic technician, it is important to closely monitor the patient during testing to ensure the patient is in the proper position with their testing eye(s) locked on the target. In general, a visual field should be performed at least every 12 months on a patient diagnosed with glaucoma, and a repeat visual field should be performed 3 months after noting any suspicious progressive change.[6]

Treatment

Open-angle glaucoma cannot be cured, but it can be adequately controlled so that further loss of visual function does not occur. Increased IOP is the primary modifiable risk factor for the progression to blindness in open-angle glaucoma; therefore reduction in IOP constitutes the principal goal of treatment. Every patient with cupping of the optic disc and visual field changes should be treated. Glaucoma therapy traditionally consists of topical medication, oral medication, laser procedure, and conventional surgery. In addition, recent advancements in microinvasive glaucoma surgeries have diversified treatment options for qualifying patients.

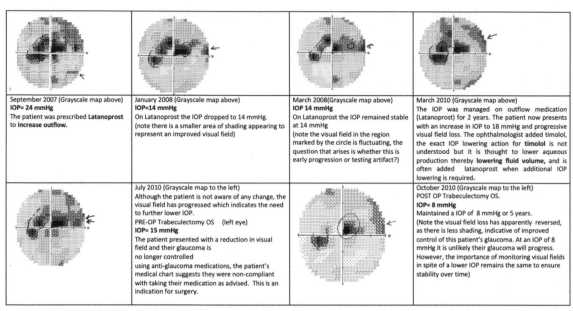

September 2007 (Grayscale map above)	January 2008 (Grayscale map above)	March 2008(Grayscale map above)	March 2010 (Grayscale map above)
IOP= 24 mmHg	**IOP=14 mmHg**	**IOP 14 mmHg**	The IOP was managed on outflow medication (Latanoprost) for 2 years. The patient now presents with an increase in IOP to 18 mmHg and progressive visual field loss. The ophthalmologist added timolol, the exact IOP lowering action for **timolol** is not understood but it is thought to lower aqueous production thereby **lowering fluid volume**, and is often added latanoprost when additional IOP lowering is required.
The patient was prescribed **Latanoprost** to **increase outflow**.	On Latanoprost the IOP dropped to 14 mmHg. (note there is a smaller area of shading appearing to represent an improved visual field)	On Latanoprost the IOP remained stable at 14 mmHg (note the visual field in the region marked by the circle is fluctuating, the question that arises is whether this is early progression or testing artifact?)	

July 2010 (Grayscale map to the left)
Although the patient is not aware of any change, the visual field has progressed which indicates the need to further lower IOP.
PRE-OP Trabeculectomy OS   (left eye)
IOP= 15 mmHg
The patient presented with a reduction in visual field and their glaucoma is
no longer controlled
using anti-glaucoma medications, the patient's medical chart suggests they were non-compliant with taking their medication as advised. This is an indication for surgery.

October 2010 (Grayscale map to the left)
POST OP Trabeculectomy OS.
IOP= 8 mmHg
Maintained a IOP of 8 mmHg or 5 years.
(Note the visual field loss has apparently reversed, as there is less shading, indicative of improved control of this patient's glaucoma. At an IOP of 8 mmHg it is unlikely their glaucoma will progress. However, the importance of monitoring visual fields in spite of a lower IOP remains the same to ensure stability over time)

Fig. 25.40 A clinical example in the longitudinal treatment of a patient who presented in the ophthalmology clinic with a high intraocular pressure (*IOP*) and visual field loss. (Courtesy Dr. Michael S. Berlin, Glaucoma Institute of Beverly Hills, Los Angeles, CA.)

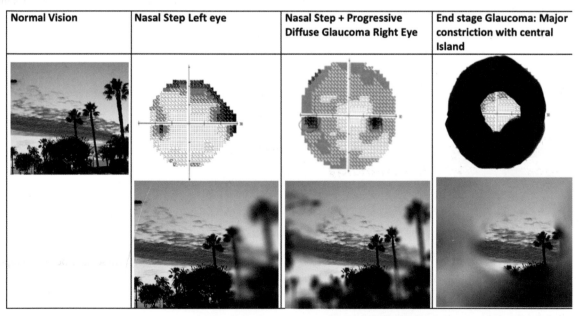

Fig. 25.41 Looking through the eyes of a patient with glaucoma. (Courtesy Jonathan Shakibkhou, Glaucoma Institute of Beverly Hills, Los Angeles, CA.)

The decision of when to treat and whom to treat is based on multiple factors that include medication effects, side effects, and costs; ability of the patient to comply with medication regimen; surgical risk–benefit issues; and quality of life issues. In glaucoma therapy, the goal is to buy time and delay the effects of a progressive, potentially blinding disease.

In every clinic or office, there is usually a large group of patients who have ocular hypertension. These are patients with ocular pressure values greater than 22 mm Hg, but who maintain normal discs with no detected visual field loss. The decision as to whether this type of patient should be actively treated requires individual consideration. These cases of suspected or borderline glaucoma can frequently be followed without treatment for many years. If follow-up examinations are difficult to obtain or if the ophthalmologist has poor rapport with the patient, the patient may be treated earlier.

Medical therapy

Glaucoma can usually be adequately controlled with topical medication. The past 3 decades have seen the development of numerous effective drops for glaucoma: prostaglandins, beta blockers, alpha agonists, topical carbonic anhydrase antagonists, and rho-kinase inhibitors. Prostaglandin analogs, used once daily, are generally the first agents to be used, followed by nonselective beta blockers to treat open-angle glaucoma. The nonselective beta blockers affect both beta-1 and beta-2 receptors and have the potential to cause serious cardiovascular and pulmonary side effects. They may be contraindicated in patients with actual or suspected compromised cardiovascular or pulmonary function because they can cause cardiac arrhythmias, bradycardia, or bronchospasm. Depression, dizziness, and impotence are well-recognized complications of beta blockers.

Certain older topical medications, such as pilocarpine contain benzalkonium chloride (BAK) as a preservative, which has a toxic effect on the cornea, particularly if used frequently during the day. Patients with some corneal toxicity may do better by switching to more costly preservative-free topical solutions. Combination therapies are also available. An advantage of combination drops is convenience and often improved adherence.

Pharmaceutical agents commonly used by class

Prostaglandins

Prostaglandins increase the outflow of the aqueous humor through the trabecular meshwork and the uveoscleral routes. Examples of these agents are bimatoprost (Lumigan RC®), latanoprost (Xalatan®), travoprost (Travatan Z®), tafluprost (Taflotan®), and latanoprostene bunod (Vyzulta®). Ocular side effects that have been observed include conjunctival hyperemia, ocular itching, and tearing. Prostaglandins have been reported to cause changes to pigmented tissue and adipose tissue. The most frequent reported changes have been increased pigmentation of the iris, eyelids, and increased pigmentation, growth of eyelashes, and sunken orbits. These changes may be permanent. BAK preserved, SofZia preserved, Polyquad preserved, and nonpreserved formulations are available.

Beta-adrenergic blocking agents

Beta-adrenergic blocking agents decrease aqueous secretion. Examples of these agents are betaxolol hydrochloride (Betoptic S and generic preparations), carteolol hydrochloride (Ocupress and generic preparations), levobunolol hydrochloride (Betagan and generic preparations), metipranolol (OptiPranolol and generic preparations), timolol (Betimol), and timolol maleate (Timoptic, Timoptic XE gel, and generic preparations). Beta-adrenergic blocking agents used in ocular therapy may affect beta-adrenergic sites throughout the body with systemic effects including slowing cardiac rates, lowering blood pressure, and exacerbating asthma and obstructive airway disease. Timolol maleate (Timoptic) solutions of 0.25% and 0.5% concentration are used once or twice daily, depending on the severity of the glaucoma. Timolol maleate and levobunolol hydrochloride (Betagan) have minimal side effects and can be used for most patients except those with asthma, cardiopulmonary disease, heart failure, or second- to third-degree heart block. Betaxolol hydrochloride (Betoptic S) is a more selective beta blocker with apparently fewer cardiovascular side effects and similar potency. This selectively affects only beta-1 receptors. Betaxolol hydrochloride, a cardioselective beta blocker, has a significantly lesser effect on the respiratory system and can therefore be used in some patients with respiratory diseases.

Alpha-2 selective agonists

Alpha-2 selective agonists reduce aqueous humor production and increase uveoscleral outflow. Examples of these agents are apraclonidine (Iopidine) and brimonidine (Alphagan P and generic preparations). Apraclonidine is mostly used in ALT to prevent early postlaser spikes in IOP. Brimonidine is used for patients with open-angle glaucoma.

Carbonic anhydrase inhibitors

Carbonic anhydrase inhibitors decrease the production of the aqueous humor. They are available as both oral and injectable systemic agents and as topical agents. Examples of topical agents are brinzolamide (Azopt) and dorzolamide hydrochloride (Trusopt). These have been developed to be used 2 or 3 times daily. They can be used in addition to other medications. Side effects include a bitter taste and headaches. Other side effects of the topical agents include superficial punctate keratitis and ocular allergic reactions.

Examples of systemic agents are acetazolamide (Diamox and generic preparations), methazolamide (Neptazane and generic preparations) and dichlorphenamide (diclofenamid [Daranide, Oratrol]). Although oral acetazolamide is effective in lowering IOP, it is used rarely and sparingly because of its side effects. Many patients develop tingling in their fingers and toes, diarrhea, nausea, loss of appetite, and general malaise.

Other side effects of systemic carbonic anhydrase inhibitors include paresthesias, gastrointestinal problems, and sodium and potassium depletion. Severe but rare side effects include renal stones, Stevens-Johnson syndrome, and blood dyscrasias. Patients sensitive to sulfa may be allergic to Diamox, a sulfa derivative. The systemic agents most commonly supplement other topical agents used to treat glaucoma.

Rho-kinase inhibitors

Rho-kinase inhibitors are another class of IOP lowering medications which lower IOP through relaxing the trabecular meshwork, contraction of the ciliary muscle, and decreasing the production of aqueous humor. Overall, this increases aqueous outflow. An example of these agents is Netarsudil (Rhopressa®). Combined with Latanaprost (prostaglandin), it is marketed as Rocklatan®. Side effects include redness and hemorrhage of the eye. Other less observed side effects include mild corneal staining, headaches, blurry vision, site pain, and redness of eyelid. There are no reported systemic side effects, which makes it an attractive option among practitioners.[7]

Combination drops

Combination drops are another option for patients who require more than one therapy to manage their pressure. These combinations include two different classes of agents, for example, timolol maleate and dorzolamide hydrochloride (Cosopt) is a combination of a beta blocker and carbonic anhydrase inhibitor. Other examples of combination medications include brimonidine tartrate and timolol maleate (Combiga), and brinzolamide and brimonidine (Simbrinza suspension).

Miotics

Miotics (parasympathomimetic agents) are rarely used as a topical therapy for glaucoma but have historical importance. They act by mimicking the action of acetylcholine on parasympathomimetic postganglionic nerve endings in the eye. Examples of these agents are carbachol and pilocarpine hydrochloride. Miotics are also used to control accommodative esotropia. However, pilocarpines and epinephrine derivatives have been used less commonly in recent years, because of their required frequency, as well as their well-known ocular surface complications.

Sympathomimetics

Sympathomimetics, also rarely used, improve the aqueous outflow within the eye and to a smaller extent uveoscleral output. Examples of these agents are dipivefrin hydrochloride (Propine and generic preparations) and epinephrine hydrochloride (Epifrin).

Hyperosmotic agents

Hyperosmotic agents produce an osmotic gradient between the intraocular fluid and the blood, decreasing IOP by causing ocular fluids to move from the globe into the bloodstream. These agents are used in the acute treatment of angle-closure glaucoma and rarely in intraocular surgery when IOP is very high. Examples of these agents are oral glycerin, oral isosorbide (Ismotic), intravenous mannitol (Osmitrol), and intravenous urea (Ureaphil). Side effects of hyperosmotic agents include cardiovascular overload, urinary retention and headaches, nausea, and mental confusion.

Adherence with medication

A medication regimen should be as simple as possible. It has been estimated that anywhere from 20% to 40% of patients prescribed medication for open-angle glaucoma miss some or all of their drop dosages. Those who were asked to instill 3 times a day were more likely not to use the drops than those told to use them twice a day. Other disturbing factors that lead to relative noncompliance or poor compliance are side effects of the medication, such as miosis and loss of focusing accuracy with pilocarpine, as well as failure to understand that the treatment preserves the visual field and the acuity already present. In many instances, these patients do not believe they are sick, especially if no other disease is present, and are reluctant to undertake a treatment of medication when they have only the physician's pronouncement that they need it.

Contraindications of medications and the risk of dry eyes in glaucoma

Dry eye disease is commonly seen in patients with glaucoma. Studies have suggested that 50% to 60% of glaucoma patients also have dry eye disease.[8] This could be a result of multiple factors. As people age, their risk for both dry eyes and glaucoma increases. In addition, pressure-lowering eye drops contain preservatives like BAK, which damages cells on the surface of the eye. Environmental conditions, such as looking at computer screens and air conditioning can exacerbate dry eye.

Dry eye disease is usually managed in multiple ways. Artificial tears can be in different forms, such as eye drops, gels, and ointments. They are long-lasting but can blur vision temporarily. Punctual plugs are devices that can be placed in the tear duct of the eye. They try to keep the tears on the eye from evaporating. Warm compresses and eyelid cleansing can keep glands from being clogged. LipiFlow is an in-office procedure that uses thermal pulsation to treat dry eye related to Meibomian gland dysfunction. For glaucoma patients, preservative-free glaucoma eye drops may be offered by the ophthalmologist.[9]

If a patient is using eye drops for dry eyes along with glaucoma medications, the patient must wait at least 10 minutes to administer eye drops after glaucoma medication to avoid dilution.

Office-based laser treatments

Argon laser trabeculoplasty

Laser treatment of the trabecular meshwork has been effective in controlling open-angle glaucoma and obviating the need for invasive surgery in many patients. The actual procedure involves treating the mid- to anterior portion of the trabecular meshwork with a thermal laser. A gonioprism is used to position the light into the trabecular meshwork. Approximately 80 to 100 spots of 50 μm size are equally spaced over 180 degrees of the angle. Often, the remainder of the angle will be treated at a later time.

The ALT reduces the IOP. Although the exact mechanisms are unknown, IOP most likely lowers secondary to both mechanical and biologic effects. Although the success rates vary for different types of open-angle glaucoma, there does appear to be a relationship between laser success and a patient's age and degree of trabecular meshwork pigmentation. In some patients, laser therapy is used as a first-line treatment. However, laser therapy is often an adjunct to medical therapy and does not ensure that medications may be stopped.

Selective laser trabeculoplasty (Fig. 25.42)

A less thermal laser treatment for managing patients with open-angle glaucoma, SLT is an improvement over ALT. SLT is a q-switched, 532-nm laser and has a 200 μm spot size. This procedure uses a very short laser pulse to irradiate and selectively target pigmented cells in the trabecular meshwork, thought to work by triggering a biologic response that stimulates an increase in the drainage of aqueous humor to ultimately reduce IOP within several weeks postprocedure. SLT has a distinct advantage in that it is less thermal; adverse scarring or damage to adjacent tissues is avoided with this treatment so the technique may potentially be repeated if necessary.

Although the use of prostaglandins has decreased the need for laser therapy, laser therapy may eliminate or at least reduce drop dependency, which can prove costly to patients. SLT often can eliminate the need for drops and the issue of compliance with drops in the management of glaucoma, especially when used as first-line therapy.

SLT has proven beneficial in early-stage treatment and has become a primary option for open-angle glaucoma patients who cannot tolerate or who are noncompliant with medical therapy. It is effective for those who have undergone prior argon laser treatments and may not interfere with the success of future surgical interventions. In fact,

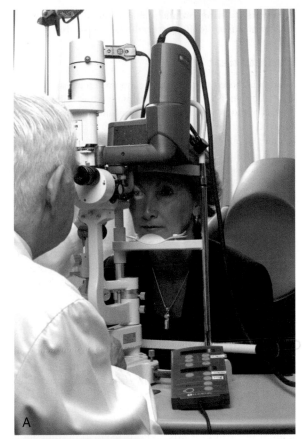

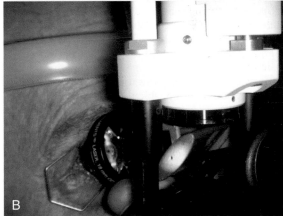

Fig. 25.42 Patient undergoing selective laser trabeculoplasty (SLT) (A). Gonio lens use for SLT may be performed with or without an additional eyelid speculum (B).

SLT may postpone or even preclude the need for additional medications or incisional surgery, thereby reducing the overall expense associated with treatment. An additional advantage of SLT to ALT is that significantly less trabecular meshwork scarring occurs such that later microinvasive glaucoma surgery (MIGS) procedures are possible.

When to treat

Newly diagnosed patients should be treated as early as possible to reach and consistently maintain a low IOP to reduce the risk of progression. Most clinicians initiate glaucoma therapy with medications before laser therapy is attempted. There has been a shift in thinking toward the use of laser therapy as an initial treatment, especially since the availability of the SLT laser. Laser therapy does not require compliance and is virtually free of significant complications from the procedure itself. It is performed on an outpatient basis during an office visit and requires no hospital stay. A rare problem with this treatment is a possible rise in IOP occurring in the first weeks after laser therapy. At this time, however, most ophthalmologists still use medical therapy first and reserve laser treatment for poor responders or those requiring long-term oral therapy.

Surgery for glaucoma

Common therapeutic regimens for the treatment of glaucoma are most often medications followed by office lasers (SLT and ALT) and then, reserved for patients in whom these attempts at controlling IOP to prevent permanent vision loss are not adequate, invasive surgical procedures, such as trabeculectomy and tube shunts. However, another option has become available; it is surgical but far less traumatic than trabeculectomy or tube shunts. This group of surgical procedures is MIGS and is likely to become more common, replacing some medication therapies and some of the more invasive surgical therapies.

Surgery has historically been used only if the patient continues to lose visual field despite attempts by the ophthalmologist to provide maximally tolerated medical- and office-based laser therapy. This usually means that the ophthalmologist has been unable to effectively lower the IOP with the most potent drugs available, either singly or in combination, or the patient is not compliant with medication use. Newer surgical procedures, such as MIGS, which are Schlemm's canal procedures, enable outflow restrictions to be bypassed within the eye. This is achieved by improving flow from the anterior chamber into Schlemm's canal instead of making a full-thickness hole in the sclera. Thus the surgical treatment of glaucoma, especially with MIGS, may come to be performed earlier in the course of the patient's glaucoma conditions as the risks of surgery and postsurgical eye conditions are significantly decreased with newer techniques and technologies.

Surgery may come to be performed earlier in the course of the patient's glaucoma condition as the risks of surgery and postsurgical eye conditions are significantly decreased with newer techniques and technologies.

Many types of invasive surgical procedures are performed for open-angle glaucoma. They are essentially fistulizing operations; that is, they attempt to create an opening between the anterior chamber and the subconjunctival space with and without implant devices (tube shunts, e.g., Ahmed, Molteno, and Baerveldt) or between surgically prepared layers of the sclera ("subscleral," "nonpenetrating," or suprachoroidal stent filtering procedures). In all glaucoma surgeries, the actual operation is a small part of the care that guarantees a successful outcome. Postoperative management is critical to successful glaucoma surgery. Recognizing and controlling postoperative complications is key. Hypotony, wound leaks, fluid shifts within the eye, infection, and inadequate pressure control are conditions often managed in the short-term postoperative period as the patient's wound healing is modulated to enable eventual controlled IOP lowering. Long-term risks include a more rapid progression of cataract and an ongoing risk for infection (e.g., endophthalmitis), the onset of which requires emergency attention and management.

Unlike cataract surgery, in which patients expect to see well within a short time postoperatively, glaucoma patients must understand that their surgery is not to improve current vision, but to preserve their vision over the long term. Immediately after glaucoma surgery, vision may be slightly worse than preoperatively, and patients will often need an eventual change in their glasses prescription. Because cataract and glaucoma often occur in the same older adult population, combined glaucoma and cataract surgery may be performed.

Glaucoma surgical procedures are being performed less often today because of the adequacy in most instances of medical management. However, if untreated or inadequately treated, *absolute glaucoma* with complete blindness and markedly elevated pressure in an eye is still a tragic entity.

Key to the success of all glaucoma surgery is the postoperative time period in which wound-healing modulation is necessary and stabilizing IOP is paramount. Teamwork among the surgeon, the technician, and the patient is essential to ensure successful outcomes of glaucoma surgical procedures.

Microinvasive glaucoma surgery (MIGS)

MIGS is a novel method for treating glaucoma that will likely replace and decrease the need for medications and will likely replace or delay the need for more invasive surgical procedures. MIGS includes various methods of increasing aqueous outflow via device implantation or physiologic tissue alteration, such as excimer laser trabeculostomy (ELT), canaloplasty, and iStent techniques. Clinical trials are being conducted with these and several other MIGS devices. MIGS have the ability to provide a safe alternative to traditional medications, especially in early or midstage glaucoma patients who are not able to comply with more traditional medication therapies.

Excimer laser trabeculostomy (Fig. 25.43)

ELT is an innovative glaucoma laser surgery based on LASIK technology. It is the first of what is now called MIGS, an outpatient procedure which results in long-lasting IOP reduction by improving outflow resulting in lowering IOP without creating healing, scarring, or requiring implantation of stents. This procedure, which is sometimes referred to as "LASIK of the trabecular meshwork," enables an essentially nonthermal laser to create channels within the trabecular meshwork, which significantly reduces outflow resistance. A 308-nm xenon chloride excimer laser is used because of its precise and effective nonthermal interaction with tissues. A small excimer laser probe is passed through a clear corneal incision to contact the trabecular meshwork to remove tissue thereby creating outflow channels from the anterior chamber to Schlemm's canal. The nonthermal energy of the laser results in far less tissue destruction, whereas alternative

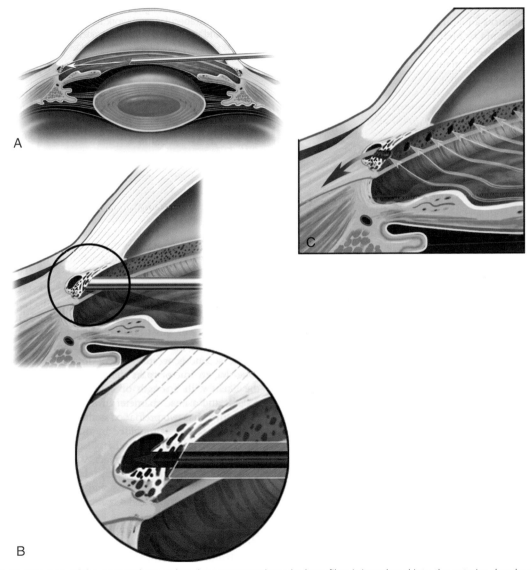

Fig. 25.43 Diagrams of the excimer laser trabeculostomy procedure: the laser fiber is introduced into the anterior chamber through a clear cornea paracentesis incision and advanced across the anterior chamber to the trabecular meshwork of the opposite quadrant (A). When the fiber tip is in contact with or slightly compressing the trabecular meshwork laser pulses are initiated (B). A series of laser channels enables flow from the anterior chamber into Schlemm's canal (C).

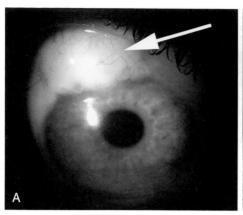
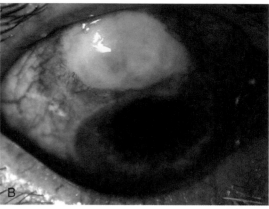

Fig. 25.48 The newly formed bleb (*arrow*) after trabeculectomy (A). An infected bleb (bleibitis) (B). (B, From Shah P, Chiang M, Lee G. Blebitis and Endophthalmitis. In: Glaucoma, 2nd ed. Shaarawy, T. M. et al. Elsevier; 2015.)

hypotony, cataract, and the need for subsequent surgery. At 2.5 years, the probability of bleb-related infections is 1.5%. The major risk factors for infectious complications of filtering blebs are leaks, thin/avascular blebs, the use of antimetabolites, and blepharitis/conjunctivitis.[9] All trabeculectomy patients must be taught to carefully monitor their postsurgical eye for any sign of redness or discharge and immediately inform their ophthalmologist. When detected and treated early, blebitis can be prevented from becoming endophthalmitis, with inherent risks of blindness prevented.

Tube shunts (Fig. 25.49). Tube-shunt surgery involves placing a flexible tube covered by eyebank sclera, cornea, or pericardial tissue to prevent erosion with an attached drainage plate in the eye to help drain fluid (aqueous humor) from the eye. Like trabeculectomy, its aim is to create a filtering bleb more posterior than a traditional limbal trabeculectomy, which often closes from scarring. Glaucoma tube-shunt surgery may be needed in patients with glaucoma that is not controlled by medications or laser treatment. It is useful either after failure of previous trabeculectomy surgery or in certain types of glaucoma in which traditional trabeculectomy surgery would almost certainly fail. Examples of such patients are those with neovascular glaucoma and patients who have corneal transplants.

During the first few weeks after surgery, a bleb of fibrous tissue and collagen forms around the plate of the implant. The thickness of the bleb determines the rate at which aqueous flows out of the anterior chamber of the eye. The excess aqueous fluid is shunted through the tubing of the implant, and passes through the space that develops between the bleb and the plate. By diffusion, the fluid flows into the capillaries, where it exits the eye and enters the general circulation. The IOP is lowered as a result of this increase in outflow. The device is partially visible behind the upper eyelid after the surgery.

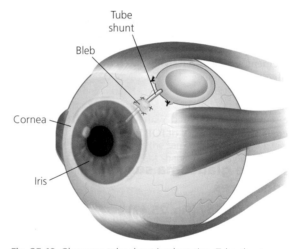

Fig. 25.49 Glaucoma tube shunt implantation. Tube-shunt surgery involves placing a flexible tube covered by eyebank sclera, cornea, or pericardial tissue to prevent erosion with an attached drainage plate in the eye to help drain fluid (aqueous humor) from the eye.

The types of implants used in glaucoma surgery fall into two categories: nonvalved (e.g., Molteno, Baerveldt) or valved implants (e.g., Ahmed). Restrictive implants have valves to limit fluid flow in one direction and prevent the IOP from being too low.

The major complications of tube-shunt surgery are bleeding, double vision, retinal detachment, IOP too high or too low, and corneal decompensation.

Cyclophotocoagulation and cyclocryopexy

Cyclophotocoagulation and cyclocryopexy are used to treat the ciliary processes with thermal laser radiation or freezing, respectively, to create scar tissue in the ciliary body to reduce the production of aqueous humor and thus lower the IOP. Cyclophotocoagulation can be performed either by transscleral cyclophotocoagulation or endoscopic cyclophotocoagulation (ECP). ECP allows the surgeon to view the area through an endoscopic camera, which aids in the very precise placement of the laser beam used for treatment of individual ciliary processes.

Treatment of angle-closure glaucoma

The procedure of choice is laser iridotomy (Fig. 25.50). A peripheral iridotomy is accomplished to relieve the pupillary block and allow the anterior chamber to deepen. A thermal or photodisruptive laser is used to create a small opening in the iris, which creates an additional pathway for fluid to flow. The procedure is curative if the attack has not caused adhesions between the iris and the angle structures. An iridotomy should be performed eventually in both eyes of patients with narrow angles because it has been shown that 50% to 70% of patients with angle-closure glaucoma in one eye will have an attack in the fellow eye within 5 to 10 years despite miotic treatment. For this reason, most surgeons prefer to do a prophylactic iridectomy on the healthy eye to avoid the hazards of acute-closure glaucoma. The risks of an iridectomy are far lower than the risks of a second angle-closure attack.

Medical therapy for angle-closure glaucoma is used only as a prelude to laser iridotomy. The purpose is to reduce the pressure and eliminate the corneal edema so that an effective laser procedure can be accomplished with greater safety and ease.

If the attack is not aborted early, permanent scar tissue can result in secondary glaucoma and vision can be permanently affected by damage to the optic nerve.

Acetazolamide (Diamox) or methazolamide (Neptazane), carbonic anhydrase inhibitors, are used to temporarily lower the IOP. Acetazolamide may be given orally, intramuscularly, or intravenously. Beta blockers, such as timolol, levobunolol, and betaxolol work in concert with carbonic anhydrase inhibitors to lower IOP. Miotic agents are used to mobilize the iris away from the peripheral angle.

In addition, various hypertonic solutions have been used to gain a more prompt and rapid reduction of IOP. The agents most commonly used today are mannitol, given in a dose of 1 to 2 g/kg of body weight (intravenously over 30–60 minutes), and glycerin, given in a dose of 1.5 g/kg of body weight (orally). Usually, 1.5 to 2 ounces (32–55 g) of glycerin is mixed with orange juice or lemon juice to avoid nausea caused by the sweet taste of the glycerin. Because the use of such agents can cause wide fluctuations in systemic blood pressure and in electrolyte balance, patients must be monitored closely during and after the use of these agents.

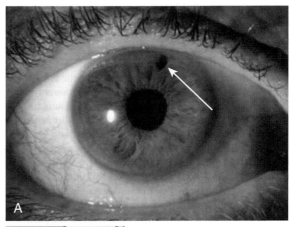

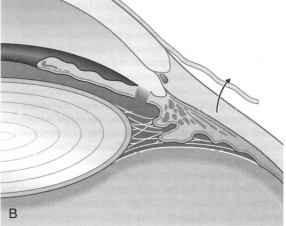

Fig. 25.50 Peripheral iridotomy (A) eliminates pupillary block (B). (B, From Shields MB, ed. *Textbook of Glaucoma*. 4th ed. Baltimore: Williams & Wilkins; 1998.)

The ophthalmic assistant should be familiar with angle-closure glaucoma because it constitutes a true ocular emergency. The abruptness of its onset is its most obvious clue. The patient may complain of intense eye pain, redness, or blurred vision. The pain can be so severe that the patient may experience headaches, nausea, or vomiting. There may have been earlier symptoms of pain and blurred vision lasting 15 to 30 minutes and then subsiding over a period of several months. This is because the acute rise in pressure subsided between pressure rises.

On examination, the dilation of the pupil fixed to light, combined with a steamy (clouded) cornea, is its most imposing sign. Such patients must be examined as soon as possible. Because treatment should begin as soon as the diagnosis is made, the ophthalmic assistant should keep all the medications for the treatment of this condition available for immediate use.

company. Disposable chin rest and forehead contact surface protectors should be replaced after each patient.

6. The virus's potential for aerosolized spread makes tonometry use difficult.[15,16] If available, a single-use, disposable tonometer tip for Goldman applanation tonometry (GAT) is recommended. A component that must be thoroughly cleaned is the reusable GAT prism. The GAT prism comes in contact with the tear layers and corneal surface, thereby requiring thorough cleaning with diluted bleach to prevent infection.[19] Noncontact tonometers should be used only with caution and preferably not at all as they create aerosolized microparticles. The Icare® tonometer has a disposable sleeve that should be replaced for every patient. The Perkins tonometer, mainly used for pediatric patients, may be used if Tono-pen and Icare® tonometers are unavailable. The Schiøtz tonometer has very specific instructions for cleaning which is referenced in this chapter.

7. During each patient examination, there are many considerations to be made. Ensure that breath shields have been installed for the slit lamp and that during slit lamp examinations when close proximity is necessary, instruct patients to minimize speaking. This will reduce the chance of contact with patients' respiratory droplets. After each patient, resterilize the slit lamps and other equipment. For gonioscopy, use is based on the ophthalmologist's discretion. Gonioscopes can often be cleaned with soap and water, dried and wiped with 70% isopropyl alcohol. Assure the gonioscope is dry of all alcohol residue before returning it to a case or holder and that the case/holder has been cleaned before use. Gonio lenses can be soaked in 0.5% hypochlorite/bleach and rinsed with distilled water and dried properly. Fundus evaluation with indirect ophthalmoscopes which are cleaned after each use as are the required lenses.

8. The use of single-drop eyedrops is preferred over multiuse drop bottles to avoid infected aerosolized exposures from cross-contaminating to other patients. If multiuse bottles are used, wash each after touching.

9. UBM should be performed only when mandatory (when the vision condition is threatening). Always use gloves and avoid using reusable cups. However, if not possible for disposable cups, the UBM cups may be sterilized with ethylene oxide (ETO) sterilization. The UBM probe may be cleaned with 70% isopropyl alcohol or covered with a disposable glove to be discarded after use.

10. During laser treatments, the use of gloves, three-layered masks that enclose the nasal region, slit lamp breath shield, disinfection of all lenses (like gonio lenses), and laser console with slit lamp should be performed.

11. Evaluate the necessity for surgery. Follow all recommended operating room guidelines.

The guidelines described in this section are recommendations for cleanliness during the pandemic, but also apply for any infectious agents with known similar transmission. These safety protocols have an impact on office economics and sustainability. Increased utilization of disposable equipment and changes in patient flow will affect the ophthalmic practice.[20] The pandemic has sparked encouragement for future research into eye care paradigms that will help eye care providers and researchers meet the challenges of future outbreaks. The current trends in glaucoma patient management encourages the use of less invasive surgeries like MIGS procedures which require less intensive postoperative care than do trabeculectomy and tube-shunt procedures, which require reduced on-site patient care times.

Summary

Glaucoma is one of the most common treatable ocular diseases, second only to cataract. Although early diagnosis and proper management remain the responsibility of the eye care professional, the ophthalmic assistant plays a key role in patient understanding, management, and especially adherence to the treatment regimen. The ophthalmic assistant must be aware of the signs and symptoms of acute angle-closure glaucoma, and should understand that glaucoma is treatable and blindness preventable when patients control their condition on a daily basis. Because vision lost to glaucoma is irreversible, the importance of early detection should be stressed. It is the ophthalmic assistant's duty to help glaucoma patients understand the nature of their disease, as well as the therapeutic regimens necessary for management. It is also the ophthalmic assistant's duty to encourage adherence, especially because glaucoma, in a similar manner to systemic hypertension, presents without symptoms and is therefore easily ignored by patients.

Recent and ongoing innovations have provided ophthalmologists and their patients improved techniques and technologies for diagnosing and monitoring glaucoma. New scanning devices can detect optic nerve abnormalities and narrowing angles earlier. Potential neuroprotective agents that may slow the progression of glaucoma independent of controlling the IOP, which is today's standard of treatment, are being evaluated. This research, as well as new classes of IOP-lowering medications, long-acting sustained-release medications, stem cell research, gene therapy, antioxidant therapy, and vasoactive medications further increase the likelihood of even more successful management of glaucoma. In addition, self-test devices for monitoring IOP and "home" visual field tests will soon become available, enabling patients to better monitor and manage their glaucoma with improved efficiency. The ophthalmic assistant's ultimate goal of providing early glaucoma detection, patient education, and a well-monitored treatment plan is becoming increasingly more viable with the advent of new medications, microsurgical techniques, automated diagnostic devices, home monitoring, and increased patient awareness.

Questions for review and thought

1. What causes angle-closure glaucoma?
2. List the classic symptoms that might suggest angle-closure glaucoma in a patient telephoning the office for an appointment.
3. What are the classic signs of angle-closure glaucoma?
4. Outline the medical treatment for an acute attack of angle-closure glaucoma.
5. What causes open-angle glaucoma?
6. What are the classic signs of damage from open-angle glaucoma?
7. What is the principle of applanation tonometry? How is applanation tonometry performed?
8. Discuss the usefulness of handheld applanation tonometers.
9. Outline visual field changes that may occur in open-angle glaucoma.
10. Outline a plan for the medical therapy of open-angle glaucoma.
11. Why does the eye enlarge in congenital glaucoma?
12. What causes pupillary block glaucoma and how does this mechanism come about?
13. Why does the eye enlarge in congenital glaucoma?
14. List ways to promote patient compliance with medications and proper drop instillation.

Self-evaluation questions   **Q**

True–false statements

Directions: Indicate whether the statement is true **(T)** or false **(F)**.

1. Patients with acute angle-closure glaucoma complain of halos or rainbows around lights. **T** or **F**
2. Primary angle-closure glaucoma occurs more commonly in males than in females. **T** or **F**
3. All patients with a high IOP (greater than 21 mm Hg) have glaucoma. **T** or **F**

Missing words

Directions: Write in the missing word in the following sentences:

4. In children with congenital or infantile glaucoma, distension of the eyeball is referred to as _____.
5. _____ is the most common cause of posterior synechiae.

Choice-completion questions

Directions: Select the one best answer in each case.

6. Chronic open-angle glaucoma is *not* characterized by:
   a. raised IOP.
   b. sudden loss of vision associated with excruciating pain.
   c. slow erosion of the visual field.
   d. slow progressive loss of visual acuity.
   e. cupping of the temporal aspect of the optic disc.
7. Which of the following are provocative tests available for the diagnosis of primary angle-closure glaucoma?
   a. Miotic test using pilocarpine.
   b. Mydriatic test using hydroxyamphetamine.
   c. Dark room provocative test.
   d. Pupillary dilation plus gonioscopy.
   e. All of the above.
8. Which of the following field defects is *not* commonly seen in patients with chronic open-angle glaucoma?
   a. Nerve fiber bundle defect.
   b. Loss of central vision (central scotoma).
   c. Paracentral scotoma.
   d. Nasal depression.
   e. Peripheral constriction.

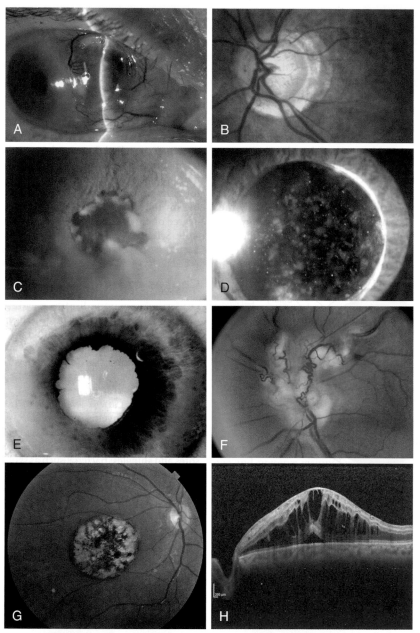

Fig. 26.3 Examples of uveitis complications that may result in vision loss. (A) Necrotizing scleritis in a patient with systemic autoimmune vasculitis. (B) Optic nerve damage in uveitic glaucoma. (C) Posterior synechiae, iris nodules. (D) Inflammatory deposits on the intraocular lens. (E) Uveitic cataract with corneal opacity, band keratopathy. (F) Optic disc edema. (G) Retinal scar. (H) An optical coherence tomography (OCT) image of cystoid macular edema. (A, From Tarabishy AB, et al. Survey of ophthalmology. 2010;55(5):429–444. B, From Bowling B. Glaucoma. In: *Kanski's Clinical Ophthalmology*. p. 305–394. ©2016. C, E, F, From Bowling B. Uveitis. In: *Kanski's Clinical Ophthalmology*. p. 395–465. ©2016. D, From Afredo A. Explantation of intraocular lenses in children with juvenile idiopathic arthritis–associated uveitis. *J Cataract Refract Surg*. 2009;35(3). Copyright © 2009 ASCRS and ESCRS. G, From Vasconcelos-Santos DV. Ocular Toxoplasmosis. In: Yanoff M, Duker J. *Ophthalmology*, 4th ed. © 2014 Elsevier Inc. H, From Witmer MT, Kiss S. Cystoid macular edema. In: Yanoff M, Duker J. *Ophthalmology*. 4th ed. © 2014 Elsevier Inc.)

Table 26.1 The SUN Working Group anatomic classification of uveitis

Type	Primary site of inflammation[a]	Includes
Anterior uveitis	Anterior chamber	Iritis
		Iridocyclitis
Intermediate uveitis	Vitreous	Pars planitis
		Posterior cyclitis
		Hyalitis
Posterior uveitis	Retina or choroid	Focal, multifocal, or diffuse choroiditis
		Chorioretinitis
		Retinochoroiditis
		Retinitis
		Neuroretinitis
Panuveitis	Anterior chamber, vitreous, and retina or choroid	

[a]As determined clinically. Adapted from the International Study Group anatomic classification.
SUN, Standardization of Uveitis Nomenclature.
From Albert DM, et al. *Albert & Jakobiec's Principles & Practice of Ophthalmology*. 3rd ed. Philadelphia: Saunders; 2008. Adapted from Jabs DA, Nussenblatt RB, Rosenbaum JT. Standardization of uveitis nomenclature for reporting clinical data. Results of the First International Workshop. *Am J Ophthalmol*. 2005;140(3):509–516.

Table 26.2 The SUN Working Group descriptors of uveitis

Category	Descriptor	Comment
Onset	Sudden	
	Insidious	
Duration	Limited	≤3 months' duration
	Persistent	>3 months' duration
Course	Acute	Episode characterized by sudden onset and limited duration
	Recurrent	Repeated episodes separated by periods of inactivity without treatment ≥3 months in duration
	Chronic	Persistent uveitis with relapse in <3 months after discontinuing treatment

SUN, Standardization of Uveitis Nomenclature.
From Albert DM, et al. *Albert & Jakobiec's Principles & Practice of Ophthalmology*. 3rd ed. Philadelphia: Saunders; 2008. Adapted from Jabs DA, Nussenblatt RB, Rosenbaum JT. Standardization of uveitis nomenclature for reporting clinical data. Results of the First International Workshop. *Am J Ophthalmol*. 2005;140(3):509–516.

hospitalized patients, or IV drug users); and parasites, such as the tiny intracellular toxoplasmosis organism transmitted from undercooked meat or exposure to cat feces.

Inflammatory causes can be linked to systemic autoimmune diseases, such as juvenile idiopathic arthritis, multiple sclerosis, ankylosing spondylitis, and sarcoidosis, or they can be isolated to the eye, as is the case with sympathetic ophthalmia and birdshot chorioretinitis. Blunt trauma, occult penetrating trauma, or a retained intraocular foreign body can cause chronic intraocular inflammation. In rare cases, uveitis can be caused by an inflammatory reaction to certain systemic medications. Finally, some cancers, such as lymphoma can mimic or "masquerade" as uveitis, with deposition of abnormal white blood cells in various structures of the eye. See Table 26.3 for a more complete list of uveitis causes.

Approach to the patient with uveitis

In clinical practice, distinguishing between infectious and noninfectious causes may not be possible initially, because both can present with intraocular inflammation that looks

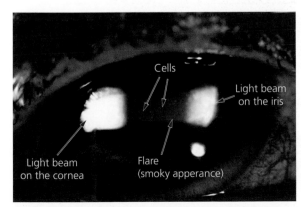

Fig. 26.4 Clinical appearance of anterior chamber cell and flare at the slit lamp. (From Witmer MT, Kiss S. Cystoid macular edema. In: Yanoff M, Duker J. *Ophthalmology*. 4th ed. © 2014 Elsevier Inc.)

Table 26.3 Selected causes of uveitis

Noninfectious	Infectious
With systemic disease	**Viral**
Systemic lupus erythematosus	Herpetic (HSV, VZV, CMV, EBV)
Sarcoidosis	Fuchs heterochromic iridocyclitis (rubella)
Systemic vasculitis	Measles virus
Juvenile or rheumatoid arthritis	West Nile virus
Behçet disease	**Bacterial**
Inflammatory bowel disease (Crohn/ulcerative colitis)	Syphilis
Ankylosing spondylitis, psoriatic arthritis, HLA-B27 diseases	Tuberculosis
Without systemic disease	Cat scratch disease (*Bartonella henselae*)
Vogt–Koyanagi–Harada (VKH) syndrome	Lyme disease (*Borrelia burgdorferi*)
Sympathetic ophthalmia	Brucellosis
Inflammatory chorioretinopathies (white dot syndromes)	Rickettsial diseases (e.g., Rocky Mountain spotted fever)
Drug induced	**Fungal**
Rifabutin	*Candida* species
Cidofovir	*Aspergillus* species
Osteoporosis drugs (bisphosphonates)	Histoplasmosis
Select antibiotics: sulfonamides, fluoroquinolones	**Parasitic**
Select topical drops: brimonidine, prostaglandin analogs	Toxoplasmosis
Trauma	Toxocariasis
Blunt trauma	Diffuse unilateral subacute neuroretinitis (DUSN)
Occult foreign body or ruptured globe	Onchocerciasis (river blindness)
Masquerade	
Primary intraocular lymphoma	
Metastasis to eye from extraocular cancer site	

CMV, Cytomegalovirus; *EBV*, Epstein-Barr virus; *HSV*, herpes simplex virus; *VZV*, varicella zoster virus.

highly similar (e.g., white spots on the choroid caused by a tuberculosis infection or by an autoimmune sarcoidosis infiltration). Instead, the type of uveitis is categorized as described in the previous section: how does it behave and where is it located? Much like providing a description of a criminal to a forensic sketch artist, a good description creates an image that can then be cross-referenced against known suspects. In this scenario, the suspects are the known causes of uveitis, each of which with its own typical set of clinical characteristics. Matching the forensic sketch with the correct suspect (making the correct diagnosis) is aided by obtaining a review of systems and performing diagnostic tests, such as labs or imaging.

For example, a recurring uveitis that suddenly affects the anterior chamber of one eye could fit the description of ocular herpes simplex or that of anterior uveitis associated with a genetically associated inflammatory arthritis (human leukocyte antigen [HLA]-B27 arthritis or ankylosing spondylitis). A review of systems that reveals morning low back stiffness and a blood test showing a positive marker for the gene HLA-B27 allows us to pick the right suspect from the line-up.

History

Listen to your patient. He is telling you the diagnosis.

William Osler, MD (1849–1919),
"Father of Modern Medicine"

Eye symptoms

Patients with anterior uveitis are likely to complain of redness, light sensitivity, decreased vision, or pain. They may notice a change in the size or shape of their pupil if there is scar tissue formation (posterior synechiae). Patients with intermediate or posterior uveitis are more likely to describe blind spots, floaters, or flashes instead of redness or pain. Ask the patient how long the symptoms have lasted, if they occurred suddenly or gradually, whether they have occurred previously, and whether they are in one or both eyes.

Medical history

Obtaining a complete medical, family, and social history is critical to the evaluation of the patient with uveitis. Emphasis on personal or family history of autoimmune, inflammatory, or infectious diseases is useful. In addition, understanding a patient's comorbid conditions is necessary when considering local ophthalmic or systemic medications. Smoking can make uveitis worse. IV drug use or unprotected sex can increase risk of certain bacterial and viral causes of uveitis. Occupations or hobbies involving the handling of animals increase the risk of certain zoonotic infections. Infectious uveitis has been linked to exposure to household pets or travel to countries with high levels of endemic infections. A complete list of medications, including recent changes or additions can reveal use of a prescription drug known to cause uveitis (including rifabutin, pamidronate, or certain newer chemotherapy drugs, such as ipilimumab). A history of ocular trauma or surgery can cause uveitis in some cases.

Review of systems

A variety of systemic symptoms can be manifestations of diseases also known to cause uveitis. Skin changes, such as peeling, redness, or loss of pigment can be seen in conditions, such as lupus, sarcoidosis, vasculitis, HLA-B27 arthropathies, syphilis, or Vogt–Koyanagi–Harada (VKH). Joint pain, swelling, or stiffness is another common feature of certain autoimmune diseases. Bloody diarrhea can be

Table 26.4 Example uveitis patient questions

Symptoms	Exposures
Oral or genital ulcers	Sexually transmitted diseases
Cold sores	Dogs, cats, or other pets at home
Ringing in ears	Farm animal exposures
Weight gain or loss	Raw meat consumption
Numbness, tingling, weakness	Unpasteurized milk, unwashed fruits and vegetables
Bowel or bladder incontinence, blood, frequency	Tick bites, mosquito bites
Skin rashes, spots, or depigmentations	Tuberculosis (TB) risk factors: travel to endemic areas, homelessness, incarceration
Joint pains or arthritis	Intravenous drug use
Shortness of breath	

seen in inflammatory bowel disease, neurologic changes in multiple sclerosis, oral and genital ulcers in Behçet disease, cold sores or shingles in herpetic uveitis, and fevers or lethargy in a variety or infectious and noninfectious uveitic diseases. Most uveitis specialists have a questionnaire specific to the investigation of social, behavioral, and symptomatic clues to the cause of uveitis (Table 26.4).

Physical examination

I have made a discovery…by means of which it is possible to see the dark background of the eye.…

Hermann von Helmholtz (1821–1894),
inventor of the ophthalmoscope

The ophthalmic technician is uniquely poised to acquire front-line physical examination data. The visual acuity, refractive state, intraocular pressure, pupils, confrontational fields, and extraocular motility are key components in evaluating the patient with uveitis. Identification of scleral redness (injection), corneal epitheliopathy, endothelial deposits (called *keratic precipitates*), and anterior chamber cell and depth are examination findings that may have a direct effect on what the doctor chooses as the next best step (gonioscopy, assessment of corneal sensation, endothelial cell counts, instillation of eyedrops, etc.). Table 26.5 lists uveitis physical examination signs that may be seen by the ophthalmic technician at the initial slit-lamp examination.

Case examples

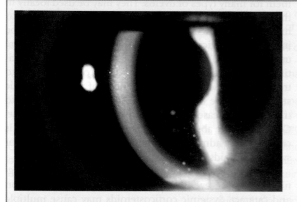

Case 1. Glaucomatocyclitic crisis Posner-Schlossman syndrome (anterior uveitis)

Unilateral, limited, recurrent unilateral anterior uveitis associated with small round keratic precipitates seen in the image. The patient has minimal discomfort, and intraocular pressure spikes to 40 to 50. A viral etiology, such as CMV, or other herpesviridae has been proposed. Treated with topical steroids and ocular antihypertensive drops. Consideration of antiviral medications. (Photo courtesy Thellea K. Leveque, MD, MPH.)

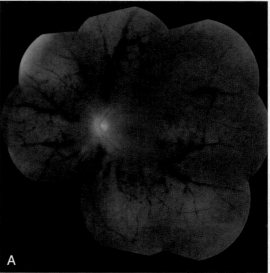

A

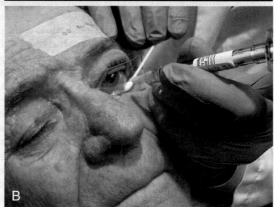

B

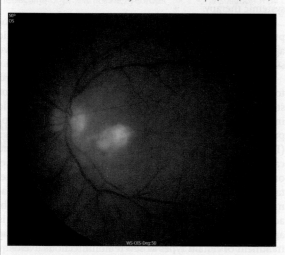

Case 2. Behçet disease (panuveitis)

Sudden onset of a central blind spot in the setting of mild redness and light sensitivity in a 41-year-old patient of Asian ancestry with oral and genital ulcers. Examination shows a relatively quiet eye with a small hypopyon, vitritis, and a branch retinal artery occlusion (white retinal infarct shown in the image). Clinicians perform a careful review for other systemic involvement. Treated with systemic steroids and long-term immunosuppression. (Photo courtesy Thellea K. Leveque, MD, MPH.)

Case 3. Acute retinal necrosis (panuveitis)

Sudden-onset unilateral redness, light sensitivity, decreased vision, and pain in the left eye of an otherwise healthy 67-year-old patient. Examination reveals elevated IOP, with anterior and intermediate uveitis and a rapidly progressive peripheral retinitis with occlusive retinal arteriolitis, shown in the image. Vitreous tap is positive at 10^6 copies/mL of varicella zoster virus (VZV). Treatment is with local and/or systemic antivirals with systemic corticosteroids. (A, Photo courtesy Thellea K. Leveque, MD, MPH. B, From Intravitreal injections. Bhavsar AR. *Surgical Techniques in Ophthalmology: Retina and Vitreous Surgery.* Philadelphia: Saunders; 2009:133–143.)

Case examples—Continued

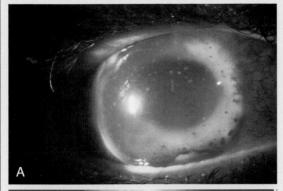

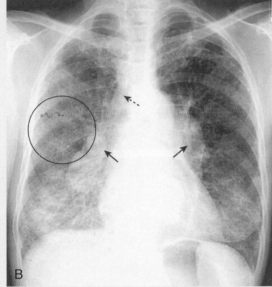

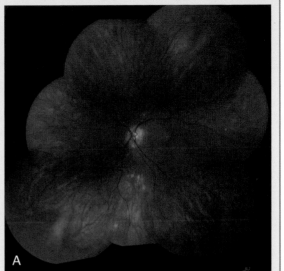

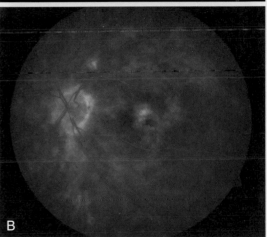

Case 4. Sarcoid uveitis (variable presentation)

Bilateral chronic iridocyclitis in a 55-year-old female with large greasy-appearing keratic precipitates shown in the slit-lamp image. Chest x-ray shows bilateral hilar lymphadenopathy, as shown by the *arrows*. Treatment varies with disease severity and other organ system involvement. Treatment is with steroids and immunomodulatory therapy.

(A, From Nussenblat R, Whitcup S. *Uveitis: Fundamentals and Clinical Practice*. 4th ed. Philadelphia: Mosby; 2010. B, from Herring, W. *Learning Radiology: Recognizing the Basics*. 3rd ed. Philadelphia: Saunders; 2009.)

Case 5. Birdshot chorioretinopathy (panuveitis)

A 60-year-old White female with Western European ancestry presents with insidious onset of bilateral floaters and photopsias. Dilated funduscopic examination reveals multiple yellow choroidal spots (noted in the image), panuveitis, and cystoid macular edema. Retinal vasculitis noted on fluorescein angiography. Blood test positive for HLA-A29. Treat with slow-release local steroids or systemic immunomodulation. (A, B, Photos courtesy Thellea K. Leveque, MD, MPH.)

Case examples—Continued

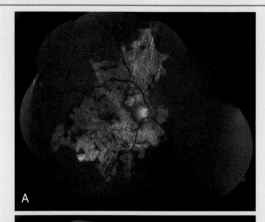

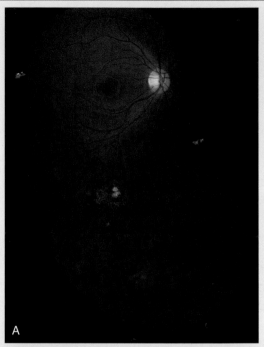

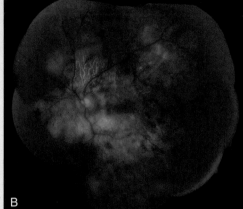

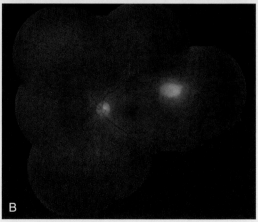

Case 6. Serpiginous chorioretinopathy (posterior uveitis)

A 40-year-old male with bilateral rapidly progressive field constriction, absent anterior, and vitreous inflammation with a negative uveitis workup. Dilated funduscopic examination reveals nearly confluent, atrophic chorioretinal lesions with serpent-like borders. Treated with systemic immunomodulation. (A, B, Photos courtesy Thellea K. Leveque, MD, MPH.)

Case 7. Toxoplasmosis reactivation (panuveitis)

Insidious onset of redness, pain, floaters, and decreased vision in the left eye of a 12-year-old girl born in Brazil. The right eye has an inactive scar. The images show that the right eye (A) has an inactive scar, and the left (B) has panuveitis with a fluffy white patch of retinochoroiditis. Toxoplasmosis serum IgG is positive. Treatment with short-term antibiotic therapy and adjunctive corticosteroids. (A, B, Photos courtesy Thellea K. Leveque, MD, MPH.)

Questions for review and thought

1. What is uveitis?
2. Can you identify some of the vision-threatening complications of untreated uveitis?
3. Why is it important to carefully classify and describe uveitis?
4. What are some of the broad categories that cause uveitis?
5. What are some of the symptoms that typify anterior uveitis? Intermediate and posterior uveitis?
6. What are some reasons to take a careful medical family and social history?
7. What role does the technician play in gathering physical examination data?
8. Why is there no single set of laboratory tests specific to the uveitis workup?
9. What is the role of corticosteroid therapy in uveitis? Why is it good, and why is it bad?
10. How do we decide when to treat systemically or locally?
11. When is surgery indicated in the treatment of uveitis?

Self-evaluation questions

Q

True–false statements

Directions: Indicate whether the statement is true (**T**) or false (**F**).

1. Uveitis is an eye disease best treated with topical steroids. **T** or **F**
2. All patients with uveitis complain of redness, light sensitivity and pain. **T** or **F**
3. Uveitis can affect males and females of all ages, and may have systemic manifestations or be isolated to the eye. **T** or **F**

Missing words

Directions: Write in the missing word in the following sentences:

4. Cellular deposits on the corneal endothelium are called _____.
5. _____, or iris adhesions to the anterior lens capsule, may cause pupillary irregularities.
6. Because sympathetic ophthalmia affects the anterior, intermediate, and posterior eye segments, it is best classified as _____.

Choice-completion questions

Directions: Select the one best answer in each case.

7. Which of the following is *not* typically included under the umbrella term "uveitis"?
   a. Retinitis.
   b. Intermediate uveitis.
   c. Scleritis.
   d. Conjunctivitis.
8. Which of the following is true regarding the workup, diagnosis, and treatment of uveitis?
   a. The patient history is typically not important in the diagnosis of uveitis.
   b. Most uveitis patients should get the same set of laboratory tests and in-office imaging studies to aid in diagnosis.
   c. Topical and systemic steroids are effective, safe, and have few side effects.
   d. None of the above.
9. Which of the following is *not* a known cause of uveitis?
   a. Parasite infection.
   b. Autoimmune disease.
   c. Primary open-angle glaucoma.
   d. Certain medications.
   e. Eye trauma.

Answers, notes, and explanations

A

1. **False.** Uveitis is an eye disease best treated with topical steroids. Uveitis refers to a diverse group of inflammatory eye diseases. Topical steroids are a common treatment but are inadequate to treat posterior segment disease, uveitic disease with systemic manifestations, or uveitic disease with an infectious etiology.

2. **False.** All patients with uveitis complain of redness, light sensitivity, and pain. Most patients with anterior uveitis describe some combination of redness, light sensitivity, decreased vision, and pain. However, patients with intermediate or posterior uveitis may have a painless, quiet eye with floaters and/or photopsias. Sometimes uveitis has no symptoms.

Answers, notes, and explanations—Continued

A

3. **True**. Uveitis can affect males and females of all ages, and may have systemic manifestations or be isolated to the eye. The wide diversity of patient features and of disease manifestations is part of what makes the diagnosis of uveitis challenging and exciting. The inflammatory chorioretinopathies ("white dot syndromes") are more likely to affect young myopic females. The panuveitis with occlusive vasculitis of Behçet disease is more likely to affect individuals with ancestry in southern Europe, the Middle East, and central Asia. Children suffer from the severe anterior uveitis of juvenile idiopathic arthritis. A detailed description of the characteristics of the patient and of the uveitis allows the diagnostician to choose the right uveitis suspect from the lineup.

4. **Keratic precipitates**. These are cellular deposits on the corneal endothelium.

5. **Posterior synechiae**, or iris adhesions to the anterior lens capsule, may cause pupillary irregularities.

6. **Posterior uveitis**. Because sympathetic ophthalmia affects the anterior, intermediate, and posterior eye segments, it is best classified as posterior uveitis.

7. **d. Conjunctivitis**. Uveitis is an umbrella term used to describe inflammatory diseases of the deep inner coat of the eye known as the uvea: the iris, ciliary body, and choroid. Because adjacent structures are often involved, uveitis has grown to include inflammatory diseases of the retina, cornea and sclera. It is categorized into anterior, intermediate, and posterior disease, with the posterior component being retinitis or choroiditis. Inflammation of

the conjunctiva is not deep enough to be considered part of the uveitis family.

8. **d. None of the above**. As discussed in question 3, the patient history is critical because it may reveal symptoms, exposures, or diagnoses that contribute to our understanding of the nature of the uveitis at hand. There is no single laboratory workup for uveitis. Most uveitis is diagnosed on clinical grounds, with laboratory tests used to detect infectious diseases that cannot be identified by the clinical presentation, to detect systemic diseases with an effect on the patient's health, or to ensure the absence of unrelated underlying infectious disease before initiating an immunosuppressive regimen. Topical and systemic steroids are effective, but they may have dangerous side effects. In the eye, they cause cataract and glaucoma. Systemically, there are many side effects including insomnia, blood glucose abnormalities, mood changes, and weight gain.

9. **c. Primary open-angle glaucoma**. Parasitic infections may cause diffuse unilateral subacute neuroretinitis (DUSN), toxoplasmosis retinochoroiditis, toxocariasis granulomas, and others. Autoimmune diseases, such as Behçet, or the HLA-B27-associated spondyloarthropathies and many others have well-described ophthalmic manifestations. Cidofovir, rifabutin, and others can cause uveitis. Blunt or penetrating ocular trauma can cause inflammation. Rarely a penetrating injury to one eye can cause a cascade of inflammation that results in uveitis in the fellow eye (sympathetic ophthalmia). Primary open-angle glaucoma does not cause uveitis.

References

1. de Smet MD, Taylor SR, Bodaghi B, et al. Understanding uveitis: the impact of research on visual outcomes. *Prog Retin Eye Res*. 2011;30(6):452–470.
2. Gritz DC, Wong IG. Incidence and prevalence of uveitis in Northern California; the Northern California Epidemiology of Uveitis Study. *Ophthalmology*. 2004;11(3):491–500. discussion.
3. Acharya NR, Tham VM, Esterberg E, et al. Incidence and prevalence of uveitis: results from the Pacific Ocular Inflammation Study. *JAMA Ophthalmol*. 2013;131(11):1405–1412.
4. Nussenblatt RB. The natural history of uveitis. *Int Ophthalmol*. 1990;14(5–6):303–308.
5. Suttorp-Schulten MS, Rothova A. The possible impact of uveitis in blindness: a literature survey. *Br J Ophthalmol*. 1996;80(9):844–848.
6. Rothova A. Suttorp-van Schulten MS, Frits Treffers W, Kijlstra A. Causes and frequency of blindness in patients with intraocular inflammatory disease. *Br J Ophthalmol*. 1996;80(4):332–336.
7. Jabs DA, Nussenblatt RB, Rosenbaum JT. Standardization of uveitis nomenclature for reporting clinical data. Results of the First International Workshop. *Am J Ophthalmol*. 2005;140(3):509–516.
8. Dunn JP. Uveitis. *Prim Care*. 2015;42(3):305–323.
9. Jabs DA, Busingye J. Approach to the diagnosis of the uveitides. *Am J Ophthalmol*. 2013;156(2):228–236.
10. Samy A, Lightman S, Ismetova F, et al. Role of autofluorescence in inflammatory/infective diseases of the retina and choroid. *J Ophthalmol*. 2014;2014:418193.

Chapter | 27 |

Dry eye disease

Neel D. Pasricha, Masako Chen, and Rahul Singh Tonk

Introduction

Dry eye disease (DED) is one of the most common causes of visits to eye care professionals, with one in five eye care patients presenting with DED. Worldwide, the prevalence of DED is as high as 50%, with both signs and symptoms of DED increasing with age and occurring more frequently in women than in men. Furthermore, DED prevalence based on signs alone is as high as 75% in some populations. This makes DED a major global health concern with significant economic consequences for individuals and society through its detrimental effect on work productivity, quality of life, and vision, as well as the psychosocial impact of pain. In the United States alone, the average cost of DED management is over $10,000 per patient and $55 billion overall. The Tear Film & Ocular Surface Society Dry Eye Workshop II (TFOS DEWS II) was formed in March 2015 to achieve a global consensus concerning multiple aspects of DED from 150 clinical and basic science research experts around the world. Using the TFOS DEWS II report, published in July 2017, along with current DED knowledge, this chapter provides a comprehensive approach to the DED patient.[1]

Classification

The definition of DED, as defined by TFOS DEWS II, is:

> *Dry eye is a multifactorial disease of the ocular surface characterized by a loss of homeostasis of the tear film, and accompanied by ocular symptoms, in which tear film instability and hyperosmolarity, ocular surface inflammation and damage, and neurosensory abnormalities play etiological roles.*

Classification of DED can be split into two large pathophysiologic categories: aqueous deficient and evaporative (Fig. 27.1). Aqueous deficient DED describes conditions affecting lacrimal gland function, whereas evaporative DED describes conditions affecting the eyelid and/or ocular surface. These two categories exist as a continuum, and thus must both be evaluated and managed for every DED patient.

Subjective evaluation

The first step in evaluating a DED patient involves careful and thorough collecting of subjective information, which

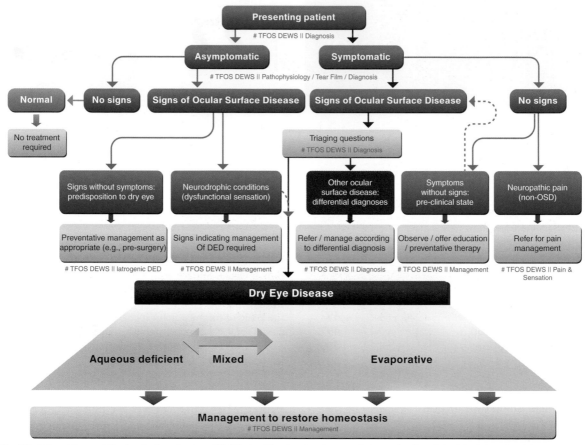

Fig. 27.1 Tear Film and Ocular Surface Society (*TFOS*) classification for dry eye. Schematic of a clinical decision algorithm to approach a patient with dry eye syndrome. (From Craig JP, Nelson JD, Azar DT, et al. TFOS DEWS II Report Executive Summary. *Ocul Surf.* 2017;15(4):802–812.)

can be separated into nonocular and ocular risk factors and stratified by consistent, probable, or inconclusive risk factors for DED. Basic demographic information of age, sex, and race is important, as DED risk increases with increasing age, female sex, and Asian race. Systemic conditions such as connective tissue disease, Sjögren syndrome, androgen deficiency, and history of hematopoietic stem cell transplantation have all been identified as consistent risk factors for DED, whereas diabetes, rosacea, viral infection, thyroid disease, and psychiatric conditions are probable risk factors for DED. Reviewing the medication list is important because antihistamines, antidepressants, anxiolytics, isotretinoin, and estrogen replacement therapy are all consistent risk factors for DED. Anticholinergics, diuretics, and beta-blockers are probable risk factors for DED. Social history is crucial in the evaluation of DED, with environment factors, such as pollution, low humidity, and sick building syndrome, as well as computer use, all as consistent risk

factors for DED and low fatty acid intake a probable risk factor for DED. Last but not least, a careful ocular history is necessary as contact lens wear is a consistent risk factor for DED, whereas pterygium and history of refractive surgery are probable risk factors for DED. Inconclusive risk factors for DED include Hispanic ethnicity, sarcoidosis, menopause, pregnancy, acne, history of botulinum toxin injection, multivitamins, oral contraceptives, smoking, and alcohol use (Fig. 27.2).

DED symptoms broadly include, but are not limited to, eye discomfort and visual disturbance. To help quantify DED symptoms, there are several validated questionnaires commonly used in clinical practice. One of the most comprehensive DED questionnaires is the National Eye Institute Visual Function Questionnaire 25 (NEI VFQ-25), which consists of 25 vision-targeted questions representing 11 vision-related constructs, plus an additional single-item general health rating question that takes approximately

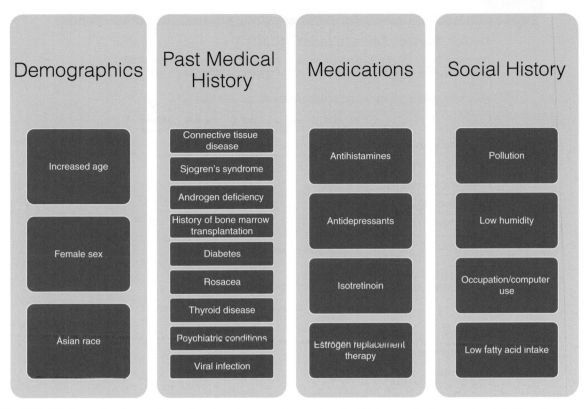

Fig. 27.2 Risk factors for dry eye disease based on demographics, past medical history, medications, and social history. These factors should be asked when eliciting a history from the patient.

10 minutes on average to administer in the interviewer format. Several shorter DED questionnaires exist, such as the Ocular Surface Disease Index (OSDI), which is a 12-item questionnaire designed to provide a rapid assessment of the symptoms of ocular irritation consistent with DED and their impact on vision-related functioning that provides a final score ranging from 0 to 100, which can stratify patients into normal (i.e., no DED), mild, moderate, or severe DED (Fig. 27.3). Another quick option is the Dry Eye Questionnaire 5 (DEQ-5), which queries eye discomfort, eye dryness, and watery eyes, with scores over 6 suggesting DED and scores over 12 warranting testing to rule out Sjögren syndrome. The Standard Patient Evaluation of Eye Dryness (SPEED), like its name suggests, is fast and evaluates both the frequency and severity of DED symptoms in eight questions, each scored zero (no symptoms) to four (intolerable symptoms) for a final score out of 28. For preoperative refractive surgery patients, the American Society of Cataract and Refractive Surgery (ASCRS) modified the SPEED questionnaire (SPEED II) to include extra questions relevant to identifying DED in preoperative patients.[2] The

importance of neuropathic-like ocular pain in DED has garnered more attention recently and can be quantified using the Neuropathic Pain Symptom Inventory (NPSI) modified for eye pain (NPSI-Eye) that is composed of 12 questions, with 10 of the questions scored, giving a total score range of 0 to 100.[3]

Objective evaluation

Given the multifactorial nature of DED, the objective evaluation likewise must be multifaceted. The TFOS DEWS II diagnostic approach to DED begins with triaging questions and risk factor analysis (see earlier), followed by diagnostic tests and subtype classification tests (Fig. 27.4). ASCRS recommends a focused clinical examination dubbed "Look, Lift, Pull, Push" to confirm the subtype, severity, and visual significance of DED.[2] Asia Dry Eye Society created a tear film-oriented dry eye classification which suggests three types of dry eye: aqueous-deficient, decreased wettability,

Ocular Surface Disease Index© (OSDI©)[2]

Ask your patient the following 12 questions, and circle the number in the box that best represents each answer. Then, fill in boxes A, B, C, D, and E according to the instructions beside each.

HAVE YOU EXPERIENCED ANY OF THE FOLLOWING *DURING THE LAST WEEK*:

	All of the time	Most of the time	Half of the time	Some of the time	None of the time
1. Eyes that are sensitive to light?	4	3	2	1	0
2. Eyes that feel gritty?	4	3	2	1	0
3. Painful or sore eyes?	4	3	2	1	0
4. Blurred vision?	4	3	2	1	0
5. Poor vision?	4	3	2	1	0

Subtotal score for answers 1 to 5 | (A)

HAVE PROBLEMS WITH YOUR EYES LIMITED YOU IN PERFORMING ANY OF THE FOLLOWING *DURING THE LAST WEEK*:

	All of the time	Most of the time	Half of the time	Some of the time	None of the time	
6. Reading?	4	3	2	1	0	N/A
7. Driving at night?	4	3	2	1	0	N/A
8. Working with a computer or bank machine (ATM)?	4	3	2	1	0	N/A
9. Watching TV?	4	3	2	1	0	N/A

Subtotal score for answers 6 to 9 | (B)

HAVE YOUR EYES FELT UNCOMFORTABLE IN ANY OF THE FOLLOWING SITUATIONS *DURING THE LAST WEEK*:

	All of the time	Most of the time	Half of the time	Some of the time	None of the time	
10. Windy conditions?	4	3	2	1	0	N/A
11. Places or areas with low humidity (very dry)?	4	3	2	1	0	N/A
12. Areas that are air conditioned?	4	3	2	1	0	N/A

Subtotal score for answers 10 to 12 | (C)

ADD SUBTOTALS A, B, AND C TO OBTAIN D (D = SUM OF SCORES FOR ALL QUESTIONS ANSWERED) | (D)

TOTAL NUMBER OF QUESTIONS ANSWERED (DO NOT INCLUDE QUESTIONS ANSWERED N/A) | (E)

Please turn over the questionnaire to calculate the patient's final OSDI© score.

Fig. 27.3 Ocular Surface Disease Index (*OSDI*). A 12-item questionnaire for rapid assessment of a patient's symptoms and functioning to stratify patients into normal, mild, moderate, or severe dry eye disease. OSDI was originally developed by the Outcomes Research Group at Allergan Inc. See https://jamanetwork.com/journals/jamaophthalmology/fullarticle/413145 for more information.

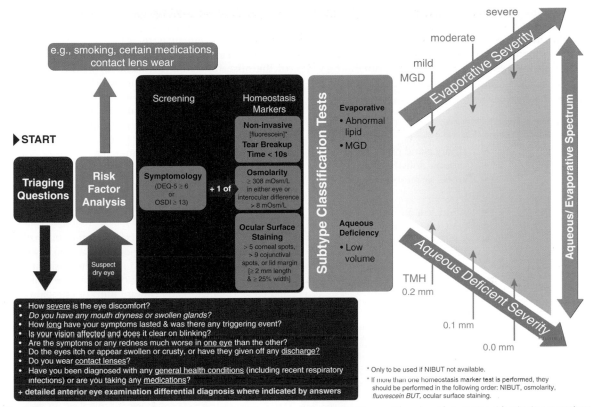

Fig. 27.4 Tear Film and Ocular Surface Society diagnostic approach to dry eye disease. The algorithm starts with triaging questions, followed by risk factor analysis. If the patient has dry eye disease based on screening questions, diagnostic testing will be indicated to allow classification into dry eye disease etiology and severity. (From Craig JP, Nelson JD, Azar DT, et al. TFOS DEWS II report executive summary. *Ocul Surf*. 2017;15(4):802–812.)

and increased evaporation, which can be practically diagnosed based solely on the patterns of fluorescein breakup.[4] Regardless of the diagnostic approach used, it is important to understand what to look for on examination and what diagnostic testing is available to assess DED.

Systemic

DED can be associated with Sjögren syndrome, which is an autoimmune disease affecting the minor salivary glands and causing the clinical triad of keratoconjunctivitis sicca (dry eye), xerostomia (dry mouth), and inflammatory arthritis. Thus it is important to ask DED patients about mouth dryness or swollen glands. Classic markers of Sjögren syndrome are anti-Ro/SS-A, anti-La/SS-B, antinuclear antibody, and rheumatoid factor. Early makers of Sjögren syndrome include antibodies against salivary protein 1, parotid secretory protein, and carbonic anhydrase 6,

and may be more accurate signals of early Sjögren syndrome.[5] A diagnostic test kit is commercially available (Sjö®) that incorporates both the classic and early markers of Sjögren syndrome (Table 27.1).

External

Several external signs exist that can help determine the etiology of DED. Periocular dermatitis, which can be associated with atopic dermatitis, is characterized by small red scaly papules and pustules around the eye. Allergic shiners, which can be associated with allergic conjunctivitis, appear as dark circles under the eyes from periorbital venous congestion because of swelling of tissues in the nasal cavity. Rosacea has a strong association with meibomian gland dysfunction (MGD) and can manifest as small, red, pus-filled bumps on the face or a large, red, bulbous nose (rhinophyma).

Autoimmune disorders that may cause DED can manifest as rashes, such as the malar rash in systemic lupus and the heliotrope rash in dermatomyositis. Herpes zoster ophthalmicus (shingles) is caused by reactivation of varicella-zoster virus in the ophthalmic (V1)

Table 27.1 Biomarkers for Sjögren syndrome

Biomarkers tested in Sjo® test	
Novel	• Salivary gland protein1 (SP-1) • Carbonic anhydrase VI (CA-6) • Parotid secretory protein (PSP)
Traditional	• Antinuclear antibody (ANA) • SS-A (Ro) antibody • SS-B (La) antibody • Rheumatoid factor (RF)

The Sjo test is a diagnostic test kit that assesses for both traditional and novel biomarkers of Sjögren syndrome. The novel biomarkers may help detect Sjögren syndrome earlier in the disease trajectory.

division of the trigeminal nerve, which can manifest as a dermatomal unilateral painful vesicular rash. Risk of ocular involvement is increased in the presence of Hutchinson's sign, which is vesicles present on the tip of the nose indicating involvement of the nasociliary nerve. Proptosis, which can be associated with a variety of diseases, such as thyroid eye disease, can cause exposure keratopathy and can be assessed rapidly by having the patient tip his/her chin up and viewing the eye position from a worm's-eye view, or can be assessed formally using an exophthalmometer.

Lids and lashes

Evaluation of the eyelid starts by examining the patient's blink for quantity (normal or hypometric) and quality (complete closure or lagophthalmos). Next, the positioning of the eyelid is assessed for lid retraction causing scleral show and presence of entropion (inward turn) or ectropion (outward turn) of either the eyelid or puncta. The puncta should

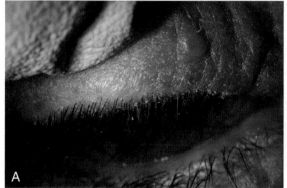
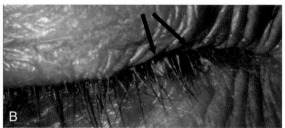
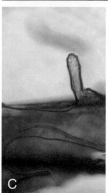

Fig. 27.5 Characteristic findings of patients with blepharitis. (A) Slit lamp photography of the right eyelid of a patient with scurf. Note the adherent debris and scale on the eyelashes. (B) Slit lamp photography of the eyelid in a patient with scurf, demodex, and makeup debris. The demodex can be seen adherent along the base of the eyelashes (*arrows*). (C) Demodex folliculorum under high power microscopy.

also be assessed for patency or stenosis. Checking the eyelid for masses, for example, benign lesions such as chalazia or hordeola, as well as malignant lesions, such as sebaceous cell carcinoma, is important and should include inspection, palpation, and lid eversion. Pulling on the eyelid can reveal floppy eyelid, which has been associated with obstructive sleep apnea and papillary conjunctivitis. The eyelashes should be assessed for loss of eyelashes (madarosis), inward turning of eyelashes (trichiasis), and various types of debris, including sleeves (Demodex), collarettes (Staphylococcal), and scurf (seborrheic blepharitis) (Fig. 27.5).

Meibomian gland dysfunction

MGD is the main cause of evaporative DED and thus warrants careful examination. One static approach is to score six different categories for a total score out of 15: abnormal lid margin findings of vascularity (0-3), plugging of gland orifices (0-3), lid margin irregularity (0-2), lid margin thickening (0-2), partial glands (0-3), and gland dropout (0-2) (Table 27.2).[6] A dynamic evaluation of MGD is also important and looks at meibomian gland expression in terms of both volume and quality of meibum expressed (Fig. 27.6). The structure of meibomian glands can be viewed with simple transillumination or using interferometry. There are multiple commercial devices available to help analyze meibomian gland dysfunction, including the Meibomian Gland Evaluator™, Meibox, LipiScan/LipiView®, OCULUS Keratograph® 5M, and HD Analyzer (Fig. 27.7).

Tear film

The tear film is composed of three layers: the inner mucous layer (secreted by conjunctival goblet cells), middle aqueous layer (secreted by the lacrimal gland and accessory lacrimal glands of Krause and Wolfring), and outer lipid layer (secreted by the meibomian glands, glands of Zeis, and glands of Moll) (Fig. 27.8). Assessment of the tear film starts by assessing tear volume. This can be objectively accomplished by measuring the tear meniscus height (<0.25 mm suggestive of DED). Schirmer's test can also be performed using a paper strip placed in the lateral third of the lower eyelid either without topical anesthesia (measures the combined basal and reflex tear secretion, abnormal <10 mm at 5 minutes) or with topical anesthesia (measures only basal tear secretion, abnormal <5 mm at 5 minutes) (Fig. 27.9). The phenol red threat test uses a cotton thread combined with phenol red, a pH sensitive dye that changes color from yellow to red when exposed to tears, which are slightly alkaline (<10 mm of red thread at 15 seconds suggestive of DED).

Table 27.2 Proposed grading scales for meibomian gland dysfunction

Abnormal lid margin findings of vascularity

0 = No or redness in lid margin conjunctive and no telangiectasia crossing meibomian gland orifices

2 = Redness in lid margin conjunctiva and telangiectasia crossing meibomian gland orifices with a distribution of less than half of the full length of the lid

3 = Redness in lid margin conjunctiva and telangiectasia crossing meibomian gland orifices with a distribution of half or more of the full length of the lid

Plugging of gland orifices

0 = No plugging of gland orifices

1 = Fewer than three pluggings of gland orifices

2 = Three or more pluggings of gland orifices with a distribution of less than half of the full length of the lid

3 = Three or more pluggings of gland orifices with a distribution of half or more of the full length of the lid

Lid margin irregularity

0 = No lid margin irregularity

1 = Fewer than three lid margin irregularities with shallow notching

2 = Three or more lid margin irregularities or deep notching

Lid margin thickening

0 = No lid margin thickening

1 = Lid margin thickening with or without localized rounding

2 = Lid margin thickening with diffuse rounding

Partial glands

0 = No partial glands

1 = Fewer than three partial glands

2 = Three or more partial glands and fewer than three glands with loss of half or more of the full length

3 = Three or more partial glands with loss of half or more of the full length

Gland dropout

0 = No gland dropout

1 = Fewer than three gland dropouts

2 = Three or more gland dropouts

From Arita R, Minoura I, Morishige N, et al. Development of definitive and reliable grading scales for meibomian gland dysfunction. *Am J Ophthalmol*. 2016;169:125–137.

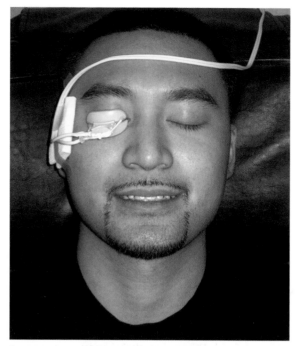

Fig. 27.16 External photograph of a patient undergoing Lipiflow treatment to his right eye. The device applies heat and pressure to the eyelids to relieve meibomian gland obstruction. The treatment is well tolerated and lasts 10 to 15 minutes per eye.

knowledge of DED continues to increase, allowing practitioners to detect this disease easier and earlier, leading to earlier intervention with improved patient outcomes. As of 2021, there are only four FDA-approved therapies for DED, each targeting only the inflammatory pathway and having

limited efficacy. Numerous innovative DED therapeutics are in the pipeline, however, with novel mechanisms of action and exciting clinical potential.

References

1. Craig JP, Nelson JD, Azar DT, et al. TFOS DEWS II report executive summary. *Ocul Surf.* 2017;15(4):802–812.
2. Starr CE, Gupta PK, Farid M, et al. ASCRS Cornea Clinical Committee. An algorithm for the preoperative diagnosis and treatment of ocular surface disorders. *J Cataract Refract Surg.* 2019;45(5):669–684.
3. Farhangi M, Feuer W, Galor A, et al. Modification of the Neuropathic Pain Symptom Inventory for use in eye pain (NPSI-Eye). *Pain.* 2019;160(7):1541–1550.
4. Tsubota K, Yokoi N, Watanabe H, Dogru M, Kojima T, Yamada M, et al. Members of The Asia Dry Eye Society. A new perspective on dry eye classification: proposal by the Asia Dry Eye Society. *Eye Contact Lens.* 2020;46(Suppl 1(1)):S2–S13.
5. Hubschman S, Rojas M, Kalavar M, Kloosterboer A, Sabater AL, Galor A. Association between early Sjögren markers and symptoms and signs of dry eye. *Cornea.* 2020;39(3):311–315.
6. Arita R, Minoura I, Morishige N, et al. Development of definitive and reliable grading scales for Meibomian gland dysfunction. *Am J Ophthalmol.* 2016;169:125–137.
7. Whitcher JP, Shiboski CH, Shiboski SC, et al. Sjögren's International Collaborative Clinical Alliance Research Groups. A simplified quantitative method for assessing keratoconjunctivitis sicca from the Sjögren's Syndrome International Registry. *Am J Ophthalmol.* 2010;149(3):405–415.
8. Takhar JS, Joye AS, Lopez SE, et al. Validation of a Novel confocal microscopy imaging protocol with assessment of reproducibility and comparison of nerve metrics in dry eye disease compared with controls. *Cornea.* 2021;40(5):603–612.

Chapter | 28 |

Examination of the newborn, infant, and small child

Alex V. Levin

Ocular examination of a newborn, infant, or small child presents unique challenges that require special techniques and particular knowledge of the normal variations in eyeball anatomy and function of this age group. Children may be unable or unwilling to participate voluntarily in the examination. The ophthalmic assistant must also remember that the child's caretaker is an integral part of the "patient team." Attention to the needs of both parent and child is essential for obtaining the desired information.

Approach to parent and child

Children are unique patients in that they are almost always accompanied by a caretaker who is their advocate, communicator, and guardian. The parent must be enlisted as a positive participant in the child's eye examination. In taking the ocular history, it is also important to distinguish between the parental concerns and the child's symptoms that led to examination. Sometimes the parent may have observed a visual behavior that is of concern. In other situations, the parent may not have observed a problem that

was noted by the referring pediatrician or family physician. One must never underestimate the value of parental observations, which should be noted on the patient's chart even if they contradict the physician's observation that initiated the referral. This is particularly important in assessing a baby who is thought to have poor vision or blindness. The question should be, "Do you think your baby sees?" Although some parents may deny that their baby's sight is poor, most will make an accurate assessment of the baby's ability to see objects and people, in particular the face of the parent during feeding. The parental assessment provides a most valuable piece of information.

Although it is important for ophthalmic assistants to introduce themselves to the parents, a self-introduction directly to the small child is also recommended. The child's individuality must be recognized and honored. Young children need to know that they have some control over the examination environment. They are often scared, unsure, or even tearful and combative. The initial introduction and conversation with the child may determine the success or failure of the remainder of the examination. Before conversing with the parents, the assistant can chat with the child about issues unrelated to the visit, inquiring about the youngster's age, siblings, pets, or a toy the child is clutching. Ask what game the child is playing on his or her tablet or smart phone and have the child demonstrate. Notice what is on the child's T-shirt, unusual jewelry, or a book he or she may be reading. If a teenager looks bored or unhappy, try to break the ice with some humor about the teen not wanting to be there. These comments often provide valuable reassurance to the child that the examiner has true interest and concern for the child's wellbeing. It is usually harmless to allow younger children to gain some feeling of control over this unfamiliar environment by asking if they want to sit alone or on the lap of a particular parent, allowing them to explore the room and touch equipment, and allowing them to play with toys or siblings in the room while the interview with the parent proceeds. It is essential for the ophthalmic assistant to have several toys available to distract the younger child both before and during the examination.

The assistant can make the examination a game by constantly carrying on a playful banter while presenting the child with tasks and toys. Banter about more mature matters, such as sports, dating, and extracurricular activities can even keep the teenager engaged. For younger and more fearful children, it is important to glean as much information as possible without touching the child. Often one can assess eye movements, pupillary reactions, external ocular anatomy, and even visual acuity with only the most minimal physical contact. When the child is asked to answer questions or perform visual tasks, such as visual acuity testing or binocular vision testing, one should always be positive when responding to the child's answer even if that answer is incorrect. If the child makes a mistake, one can simply say "good job" and move on to the next letter. Undermining a child's confidence by indicating a poor performance on a visual test may decrease compliance with the examination. It is also helpful if the examination is conducted without external interruptions, such as answering telephone calls or the movement of people walking in and out of the room. Because children in the younger age groups or older children with developmental challenges have very short attention spans, the examination must be conducted swiftly, in good humor, and with minimal extraneous distractions.

If the child becomes tearful or uncooperative, it often is best to back off and either undertake an unrelated conversation or ask the child how he or she would like to proceed. For example, some children prefer to hold the penlight or direct ophthalmoscope themselves. They can hold the instrument along with the assistant who is conducting the examination. It may be helpful to perform part of the examination on the parents or the child's toy (e.g., a teddy bear) in a mock fashion to demonstrate that it is painless before carrying out that step of the examination on the child.

Children have certain biologic needs that must be satisfied if an optimum examination is to be completed. If an infant appears cranky, one might inquire if the parent believes that the child needs to feed. Quite a bit of information can be obtained while the child is being examined during a feeding. A pacifier or favorite toy also should be allowed because it may increase the child's level of comfort and security. Interruptions for diaper changes and visits to the washroom must be permitted. If a sibling's behavior is distracting, the examiner can turn attention to that child and invite him or her to participate in the examination. For example, a sibling can be asked to flip the switch when the lights are being turned on and off or to hand the examiner toys and tools that are being used.

Vision assessment

Assessment of the visual acuity in neonates and infants is often limited to ascertaining whether vision is absent, present, or within normal limits for their age and equal in both eyes. Visual fixation is present at birth. The best visual target for the neonate is the human face. Normal infants should smile responsively and briefly follow a stimulus by 2 months of age. In the second and third months of life, infants develop the ability to follow a target beyond the midline, although it may not be until the fourth month that they can follow completely from one side over to the other (180 degrees). When the examiner presents an infant with a target, it is important to use a silent toy to ensure that any following or responsive behavior that is observed results from visual rather than auditory stimuli. High-contrast (black and white) targets are particularly helpful.

Children who are blind or have very poor sight often have wandering, purposeless, dysconjugate eye movements or nystagmus. The presence of nystagmus at birth, however, does not necessarily imply complete blindness. If a child has very poor sight, it is important to note if there is a response to light (light perception [LP]). One can look for the "eye-popping reflex" by abruptly turning off all illumination in the room. A sighted baby or infant will demonstrate a reflex opening of the eyes. When the lights are then turned on abruptly, both eyes should close. Even premature babies should respond to a bright light. If the child's eyes are closed, the bright light can be shone through the closed eyelid and a reflex contraction of the eyelid and surrounding muscles should be seen.

More formal technical tests are available to better quantify an infant's visual acuity, such as preferential-looking tests, and graded optokinetic nystagmus (OKN). The visual evoked potential (VEP) is a test designed to measure the ability of the occipital cortex in the brain to register a response to visual targets of increasingly difficult resolution by placing electrodes on the scalp that sense the passage of visual information from the eyeballs to the brain. The OKN drum (Fig. 28.1) will elicit nystagmus in anyone capable of seeing the stripes on the rotating drum. Preferential-looking techniques (Fig. 28.2) rely on the ability of an infant to distinguish between and favor a target that is variably different in terms of resolution (e.g., black-and-white stripes) compared with a bland gray target. The electroretinogram (ERG) is used to assess whether the retina is functioning in a child who is apparently blind or has poor sight. This test does not, however, measure visual acuity.

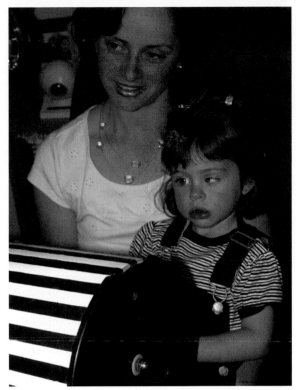

Fig. 28.1 The optokinetic nystagmus drum is rotated in front of the patient, inducing nystagmus in any patient who is neurologically normal and sighted. Note that this child has a crossed (esotropic) left eye. She is viewing with her preferred right eye. (Photograph by Leslie MacKeen.)

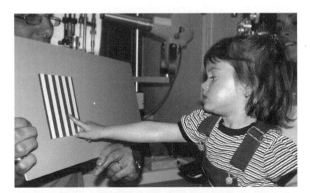

Fig. 28.2 Preferential-looking technique. Given the ability to distinguish between the stripes and the other side of the board, the child indicates the striped target. As the stripes get thinner and closer together, they become more difficult to distinguish from the homogeneous gray side, and the striped target becomes less preferred. (Photograph by Leslie MacKeen.)

If a significant difference exists in the visual acuity between the two eyes, the small child will object to the examiner covering the better eye. Although the eye can be covered by a piece of tape, the examiner's hand, or a commercially available occluder paddle, just using one thumb may be less frightening (Fig. 28.3). The child may become visibly uncomfortable or may attempt to remove the obstruction only when the better-seeing eye is covered. This test is best performed while presenting the child with a target of interest, such as a bright toy. A differential response on the covering of either eye is a critical sign of a difference in vision between the eyes.

The visual acuity in infants and preverbal children is usually recorded as central steady maintained (CSM) or good steady maintained (GSM). This indicates that the eyeball fixates with the fovea straight along the visual axis, nystagmus does not occur in the straight-ahead position, and there is no preference for either eye. If an eye is clearly unpreferred (i.e., not seeing as well as the other eye), but is otherwise straight and steady when it is fixating a target,

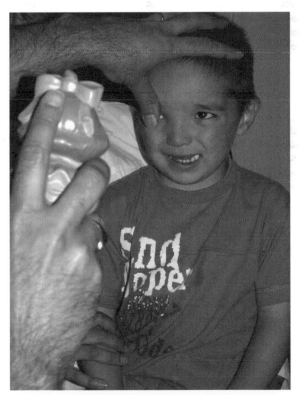

Fig. 28.3 The examiner covers the child's right eye while showing a toy for fixation. If the child has better vision in the right eye, he may become visibly upset or attempt to remove the examiner's thumb, indicating that the preferred eye is being covered. When the unpreferred eye is covered, the child may show no reaction at all. (Photograph by Leslie MacKeen.)

Box 28.1 Commonly used quantitative visual acuity tests for children

- Sheridan-Gardiner test
- HOTV matching test
- Allen picture test
- Snellen letter chart
- Tumbling E chart (not recommended, see text)
- Number chart

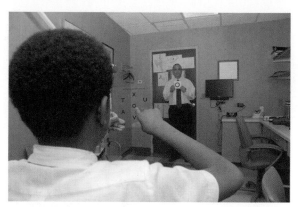

Fig. 28.5 Sheridan-Gardiner test. The child indicates the letter on the card that is being presented by the examiner. (Photograph by Jack Scully.)

the examiner may record the child's vision as CSNM: central, steady, but not maintained. Vision is not central when the patient appears to be fixating on a target although the eyeball is not pointing directly at what is being presented (eccentric fixation).

As children approach 3 to 5 years of age, they begin to be able to participate more voluntarily in the assessment of their visual acuity. Several types of charts that can be projected or posted for use in more formal visual acuity testing are listed in Box 28.1. The method chosen must be consistent with the child's developmental level and skills. For example, projected pictures (Allen pictures, Fig. 28.4) are a good test for a child who does not yet know letters. One might show the pictures to the child up close and ask that the figures be identified so that the examiner is aware of what interpretation the child gives to these somewhat abstract diagrams. For example, the birthday cake may be called a "bag of french fries" and the telephone a "butterfly." As long as the examiner knows what the child calls that picture, testing can proceed. At distance, even normally sighted children may have difficulty seeing pictures smaller than the 20/80 line.

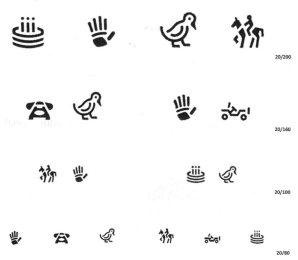

Fig. 28.4 Section of the near Allen picture card. (Courtesy the Franel Optical Supply, Apopka, FL.)

The use of recognition letter charts (Snellen letters) should be reserved for those children whose ability to identify letters is verified in advance by the parent. For children in the intermediate stage in which they recognize some of their letters, the Sheridan-Gardiner (Keeler, London, England) and HOTV tests may be helpful because they allow the child to match letter cards held by the examiner or projected letters with a cue card the child holds (Fig. 28.5). This approach also gives shy children more confidence and allows them to guess letters they might otherwise not feel secure enough to guess at orally. Children in these young age groups are often afraid of being wrong and, even with the greatest encouragement, will not read letters that they really are able to see. This underscores the constant need for building the child's confidence by indicating that the answer given is correct even when it is not. The tumbling E chart also can be used for children who do not recognize their letters. This test can, however, be difficult for small children to interpret because they may not know left from right and they may have trouble indicating with their hands in which direction the tumbling E is pointing, particularly when they are younger than 4 to 6 years old, the age range when handedness normally develops. At this age, they are almost always able to use other methods, rendering the tumbling E unnecessary.

When the visual acuity is tested, one eye must be covered at a time. Children will unconsciously make every effort to use their better eye if there is a difference between the visual acuity in their two eyes. Therefore the occlusion of one eye must be absolute. Children should never be allowed to hold their hand over their eye or to handhold a plastic occluder paddle. They may look around the occluder or look through tiny holes between their fingers, which can actually create a pinhole effect and improve the vision in the covered eye. It is recommended that 2-inch (5-cm)

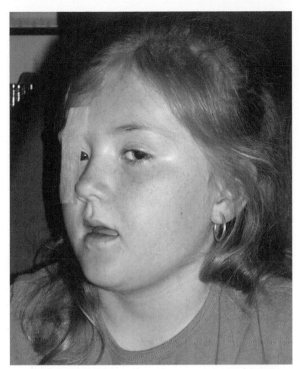

Fig. 28.6 Incorrectly applied paper tape occlusion allows the child to visualize the chart with the better right eye by peeking between the tape and the bridge of the nose. (Photograph by Leslie MacKeen.)

paper tape be applied over the eye that is not being tested to effect complete occlusion. Children must be observed constantly throughout the visual acuity examination to be sure that they are not peeking between the tape and their skin (Fig. 28.6). This can be accomplished either by the use of a "cheater's mirror" placed behind the child, which allows the examiner to view the projected target behind them while still facing the child, or by having the examiner stand next to the chart at the end of the examination lane while viewing the child and indicating which letters are to be read. If a child objects to the covering of one eye by tape, the examiner can hold a +5.00 or greater spherical lens in front of the eye not being tested. In most children, this sufficiently blurs that eye so that the child is actually viewing with the eye that does not have a lens in front of it even though both eyes are open. Having the parent use a hand to cover the child's eye invites the same problems as having the eye covered by the child's hand. If there is no other option, make sure the parent uses their palm rather than fingers to occlude the eye. If the child completely resists any form of intervention, ask him or her to read the chart with both eyes open and record the binocular vision.

To accommodate the child's short attention span, it is helpful to have the child identify only a few letters from each line. Most children have normal vision, so it may be advisable to start at the 6/9 or even 6/6 line rather than start at the top of a chart and work the child down through many lines of letters/pictures, which may lead to a loss of the child's attention and artificially poor results. It may be helpful to ask the parent to remain silent during this examination, because distracting comments, such as "you can do better," may serve to undermine a child's honest effort at good performance.

Remember, some children just are not ready to perform formal visual acuity testing. It is more important to forgo this part of the examination when one senses that the child's cooperation is being lost than to persist and develop a negative relationship with the child that would make the remainder of the examination difficult. Instead of a numerical acuity, one can revert to the CSM method described earlier.

Vision of 6/9 is considered acceptable up to grade 1, after which vision of 6/6 is expected on vision testing. If not, an explanation must be sought. That explanation may be poor compliance with testing if nothing else is found on examination. This conclusion, however, should be reached only after a complete ophthalmic examination has ruled out the presence of refractive error or anatomic problems. Ancillary testing may be requested by the ophthalmologist. A repeat visual acuity test performed later at a subsequent visit within a few months with a more confident and comfortable child also may be successful.

In most clinical situations, it is not necessary to test the near vision of children because it can be assumed that the remarkable accommodative abilities of young children allow for normal near vision in almost every child. Assessment of near vision is necessary only when there is subnormal (<6/18) distance vision in the better eye or a specific complaint about near vision. In the former situation, near vision should be tested with both eyes open simultaneously. If the vision is normal at near but abnormal at distance, one might suspect that the child is either nearsighted (myopic) or simply noncompliant with distance vision testing. In children who clearly have very poor vision at distance, the knowledge of the maximum near vision with both eyes open allows for proper educational intervention at school.

In children with nystagmus, the vision also should be tested with both eyes open, as well as with one eye fogged with a +5.00 sphere. Completely occluding one eye may make the nystagmus worse (latent nystagmus). Sometimes the visual acuity with both eyes open is better than with either eye individually. Some children with nystagmus may hold their head in an abnormal position while viewing straight ahead (Fig. 28.7). This abnormal position should be allowed because it is used unconsciously to help dampen the nystagmus (null point).

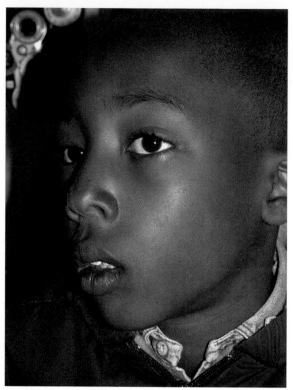

Fig. 28.7 This child has nystagmus. When his eyes are in left gaze the nystagmus is least (null point). Therefore he turns his face to the right when looking straight ahead so that his eyes are in left gaze. This keeps his nystagmus to a minimum and allows for better vision. (Photograph by Leslie MacKeen.)

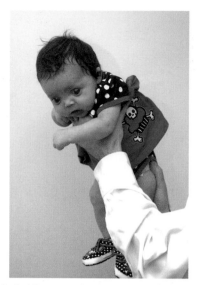

Fig. 28.8 By holding a newborn or young infant at a 45-degree angle with one hand on the baby's chest and the other on the buttocks, the baby's eyes will usually open when the buttocks are jiggled. Note that this child has very large eyes as a result of congenital glaucoma. (Photograph by Jack Scully.)

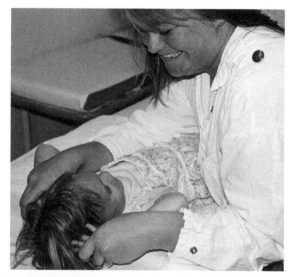

Fig. 28.9 Technique for restraining a small child. The parent or ophthalmic assistant leans over the child's abdomen while holding the child's hands next to the temples to immobilize the head. (Photograph by Leslie MacKeen.)

External examination

The anatomy of the eyelids, lashes, conjunctiva, cornea, and anterior segment should be no different from that of a normal young adult, except for size. Visualization of these structures, however, may be difficult because of the challenges with compliance or cooperation. In infants and newborns, eye opening can often be achieved by holding the child in the position demonstrated in Fig. 28.8. Sometimes it is necessary to restrain a child in a supine position (Figs. 28.9 and 28.10) and insert a lid speculum (Fig. 28.11). To obtain magnification, one can look through the direct ophthalmoscope, using it as a handheld magnifier by dialing in the black or green "plus" numbers and getting progressively closer to the child. With young children, this can be turned into a peek-a-boo game to allow the examiner to get close enough to visualize the front of the eye.

If more magnification is desired, the adult slit lamp can be used even for a small infant by holding the child in a horizontal position as the chin is placed on the chin rest. When doing this, it is important that the examiner be "in position," with all the necessary adjustments to the slit

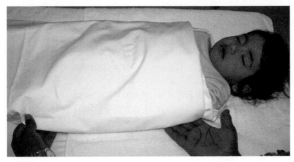

Fig. 28.10 Technique for restraining an infant. The child is wrapped in a towel with her arms at her sides. The parent or ophthalmic assistant can then lean over the child's abdomen while controlling the child's head at the temples. (Photograph by Leslie MacKeen.)

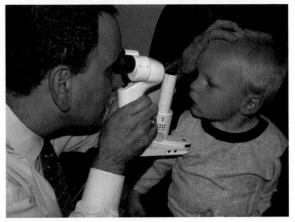

Fig. 28.12 Examiner using handheld slit lamp. (Photograph by Leslie MacKeen.)

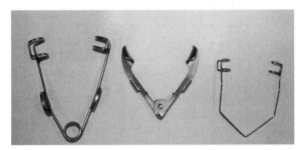

Fig. 28.11 Pediatric eyelid speculums. (Photograph by Leslie MacKeen.)

lamp already made for proper visualization, because the child may quickly become uncomfortable and tearful. A handheld slit lamp is invaluable for examining infants and small children (Fig. 28.12).

Pupils

The examination of a child's pupils is conducted in the same way as for adults. It is sometimes difficult, however, to obtain the distance fixation required to eliminate the normal miosis that occurs when a person focuses on a near target. To do this, many pediatric ophthalmologists have animated toys or movies on the far wall of their offices that can be controlled by a foot pedal. This distracts the child to the distant target while the pupils are being tested. One can even play a "magic game" by turning the child's nose while secretly stepping on the pedal that activates the toy or movie. Children then think that they can control the toy with their nose. This keeps them sufficiently amused while the examination continues. This trick is also useful for the examination of ocular motility and alignment.

The pupils should normally respond to light at birth, although the pupillary light reaction may be sluggish until the baby is 1 to 2 months old. The pupils of infants are relatively small compared with those of adults. In addition, because the eye examination of an infant may at times be conducted while the infant is asleep, it should be remembered that during sleep pupils are physiologically constricted. The consensual pupillary reaction is present at birth.

The red reflex is the yellow-orange-red reflection sometimes seen in the pupil in photographs. It can be elicited by looking through the direct ophthalmoscope while standing about 3 feet (1 m) away and keeping the face in focus while illuminating both eyes. The reflex should be equal in both eyes. This test plays an important role in the screening of newborns and infants for intraocular abnormalities, in particular a form of hereditary childhood eye cancer (retinoblastoma). A white reflex (leukocoria) may be the first sign of this potentially fatal tumor that is very curable if detected early. The presence of a black reflex (absent red reflex) may indicate an abnormality in the eye, such as cataract or vitreous hemorrhage that is blocking the light reflex. A falsely absent red reflex may be caused by the small pupils of newborns and infants that may not allow enough light in to create the reflex. In this situation, the testing should be repeated after pharmacologic dilation. The red reflex can also be used to assess pupil size, symmetry, position, and roundness.

Instillation of eyedrops

Eyedrops are feared by most children with the same vigor that they object to needles. In fact, some children will

515

immediately ask, "Am I getting drops?" when they walk into the room for their eye examination. Although one should never lie to a child, one might defer the answer to that question by saying, "Let's talk first and then decide."

Once the time comes for the instillation of eyedrops, the child must be informed, but it is preferable to wait to do so as the child is being positioned for this procedure. The child can be held securely in the parent's arms in a cradled position as if receiving a bottle or breast for feeding. The parent should be responsible for restraining the child's hands while the examiner controls the child's head and eyes. It is preferred that the child be told that the drops are going to sting. Well-meaning attempts by parents to alleviate a child's fears by indicating that "this won't hurt" should be corrected by saying that the drops might sting for approximately 15 to 20 seconds or one can tell the child to count to 10 as a means of distraction. Lying to the child can seriously undermine compliance and trust. It can be helpful to instill first a drop of topical anesthetic (proparacaine or tetracaine), immediately followed by the dilating drops. The onset of action of these topical anesthetics is quite rapid, which helps to lessen the pain of the mydriatic drops. Before eyedrops are instilled, the parents should be informed about the number of drops that are to be given and their purpose.

Relaxation of the pupillary sphincter and the ciliary muscles that govern accommodation can be much more difficult in children, particularly if they have heavily pigmented brown irides. Although different examiners may vary in their selection of mydriatic agents, it is usually safe to use some combination of phenylephrine 2.5% and tropicamide 1% or cyclopentolate 1% in all children except premature babies. Children who are corrected age before 36 weeks' gestation or those born small for gestational age at full term may require more dilute solutions of mydriatic agents, such as cyclopentolate 0.5%.

A repeat instillation of drops may be necessary if the pupils do not dilate well, particularly in darkly pigmented children. A full 20 to 30 minutes should be given for adequate paralysis of accommodation to occur. If there is any concern on the part of the ophthalmic assistant that a given child should not receive the standard eyedrop regimen, then instillation should be deferred until consultation with the ophthalmologist or pediatrician is sought. In particular, newborns and infants with hypertension, heart problems, seizures, or respiratory problems may require an alteration in the usual regimen.

Some children do not respond adequately to the eyedrops used in routine eye examination, or they may require stronger cycloplegic agents for assessing farsightedness (hyperopia) particularly as it relates to esotropia (accommodative esotropia). In these situations, a prescription may be given by the physician for atropine drops (0.5% for children <1 year, 1% for children >1 year) to be used twice daily for 3 days before a repeat examination. Parents should be cautioned to monitor their child for signs of atropine toxicity, such as feeling warm to the touch and redness (flushing). Although this protocol is generally safe, parents must be cautioned to keep this medication locked away because ingestion by a toddler or small child could be fatal.

When the child returns to the examination room for dilated eye examination, it is often helpful to begin that segment of the examination by announcing that no more drops will be necessary. If the discovery is made that the initial drops were insufficient, the examiner should adhere to the basic principle of being honest with pediatric patients, and perhaps prescribe the atropine drop regimen for home use before another visit rather than break the promise and instill drops again.

Refraction

Newborns, infants, and small children cannot participate in analysis and refinement of their refractions by sitting behind the phoropter and indicating which lenses give them better vision. Rather, the examiner uses the retinoscope and handheld lenses, as described elsewhere in this book, to determine the child's refractive error.

Most infants and small children are farsighted, although glasses usually are not required because the strong accommodative power of their eyeballs allows them to self-correct for their hyperopia. Higher degrees of farsightedness, however, can lead to esotropia (crossed eyes) and amblyopia (subnormal vision development). Likewise, myopia in the newborn and infant may be advantageous because their visual world is almost completely at near. Higher degrees of nearsightedness, however, may lead to ocular misalignment and amblyopia. Different ophthalmologists have different thresholds for the prescription of glasses. Contact lenses may be used in babies and small children with extremely high refractive errors or surgical aphakia after cataract extraction. Ophthalmic assistants can play an important role in teaching parents how to insert and remove contact lenses in their children.

Retina and optic nerve examination

Examination of the posterior segment of the eyeball through the dilated pupil in an infant or young child is essentially identical to that for an adult and requires the use of an indirect ophthalmoscope. In certain situations, such as the crying resistant toddler, it may be difficult to open the eyelids sufficiently to allow an adequate view. This may be best accomplished by the use of pediatric specula, which are commercially available (see Fig. 28.11). They are placed after the child has been restrained and a topical anesthetic applied. In some situations, examination under general anesthesia is necessary.

Although various commercially available papoose boards can be used, it is usually most reassuring and comfortable for the child to be restrained by having an adult, preferably the parent, leaning comfortably across the child's chest while holding the child's hands on either temple to keep the head still (see Fig. 28.9). The reassuring voice of a parent can often be quite helpful. Newborns and infants can be restrained by wrapping a towel or blanket around the child's arms and trunk (see Fig. 28.10). Some parents may feel quite uncomfortable about watching a speculum being placed into the eye. The examiner should explain the procedure first, giving the parents the option of staying, turning away, or stepping out of the room. The examination is virtually painless, but quite scary for a small child. Immediately after the examination is complete, the child should be allowed to seek solace in their parent's arms.

For older children who may sit cooperatively in their parent's lap, the introduction of the large and unusual indirect ophthalmoscope headpiece can be frightening. The ophthalmic assistant or examiner might reassure the child by giving this hat a silly name, such as a space hat or allow the parent to be mock examined first. Once the child knows that this imposing instrument is safe, cooperation may be enhanced.

Although the macula may not be completely developed in the first few months of life, the intraocular anatomy of a newborn and infant appears otherwise identical to that of an adult.

Common pediatric disorders

Amblyopia

Approximately 2% to 4% of all children have amblyopia. Because the visual system continues to develop through the first decade of life, any abnormality (e.g., unequal refractive error, ptosis, strabismus, cataract) that makes one eye less favored than its fellow eye may cause the brain to prefer the better eye. In doing so, the brain begins to neglect the visual development of the unfavored eye, causing its vision to become "lazy." Patching the good eye and correcting the underlying defect (e.g., glasses for anisometropia, surgery for ptosis) force the brain to use the unfavored eye and redevelop the vision properly. The ophthalmologist will decide the number of hours per day that the child should patch. Research has shown that patching may even be effective into the early teen years, but compliance may be difficult because of cosmetic concerns and teasing at school.

In some scenarios instilling atropine (atropine penalization) daily or weekly into the better eye can blur that eye sufficiently to allow the brain to redevelop vision in the amblyopic eye. Ongoing follow-up is essential to assess the progress of the amblyopic eye and to ensure that the patch or atropine is not causing impairment of vision in the better eye (occlusion amblyopia).

Strabismus

Any misalignment of the eyes is called strabismus. When one or both eyes are crossed, the condition is called esotropia (see Fig. 28.1). Some infants develop a form of severe crossing called infantile esotropia, whereas other children do not develop esotropia until later in childhood. Crossing of the eyes caused by uncorrected hyperopia is called accommodative esotropia. Prescribing glasses to "do the work" instead of the focusing muscles inside the eye (ciliary muscles) keeps the eyes straight, although they will still cross with the glasses off. If the crossing is particularly prominent when the child reads, bifocals may be prescribed.

Children with uncorrected nearsightedness may have an eye that drifts out (exotropia). If one eye is too high, it is called hypertropia. If an eye is too low, the term is hypotropia. Intermittent misalignment of the eyes, particularly intermittent exotropia, is common and within normal limits up to 3 to 4 months old and occasionally for longer. Most forms of strabismus that persist beyond infancy require eye muscle surgery, an outpatient procedure. This topic is covered in more detail elsewhere in this book.

Nasolacrimal duct obstruction

Many infants are born with an incompletely developed nasolacrimal drainage system such that the duct does not open completely into the nose. Sometimes referred to as blocked tear ducts, this unilateral or bilateral disorder is usually characterized by crusting on the eyelids, especially on waking, and by tearing and discharge in the absence of conjunctival injection. More than 95% of cases resolve spontaneously with the use of massage. One to four times daily, a finger is placed over the lacrimal sac, between the medial canthus and the nose, and pressure is applied posteriorly (towards the brain) to compress the sac and send pressure down the duct. Some ophthalmologists may also prescribe topical antibiotics if the discharge is copious or the conjunctiva inflamed. If symptoms persist after 3 to 6 months of proper massage and the child is more than 1 year old, surgical probing to open the duct may be considered. Some ophthalmologists practice in-office earlier probing, although others believe the usual spontaneous resolution of the condition should be allowed and probing conducted only if the symptoms and signs persist beyond 1 year, at which time general anesthesia is usually preferred for the procedure.

Cover test

A heterotropia, or tropia, is a constant manifest ocular deviation. Heterotropias must be differentiated from heterophorias, or phorias. A heterophoria is a latent ocular deviation kept in check by the power of fusion and made intermittent by disrupting fusion. Heterophorias are classified in a fashion similar to heterotropias. Esophoria is the tendency of the eyes to turn in, exophoria is the tendency of the eyes to turn out, hyperphoria is the tendency of one eye to turn up and hypophoria is the tendency of one eye to turn downwards. Any of these conditions may occur normally when fusion is disrupted.

The cover–uncover test is a reliable and easy method to detect and measure the angle of a heterotropia. This test is conventionally performed in the primary straight-ahead position, with and without glasses, with a viewing target situated at both distance and near. Subsequently, each of the eight other diagnostic positions of gaze are tested. To ensure fixation in young children, a flashing picture or a video displayed in the distance helps to capture their attention. A near fixation object should be an interesting and detailed article, such as a brightly-colored toy or a toy with a squeaker. Once the examiner is certain the child is looking at the fixation object, an occluder is used to cover one eye and the clinician looks for movement of the fellow uncovered eye. One of three situations may occur:

1. A manifest strabismus is revealed if the uncovered eye moves to take up fixation when the cover is placed over the fellow eye. If a child has manifest strabismus and the sound eye is occluded, the deviating eye may move horizontally or vertically. An outward movement of a nasally deviated eye is noted in patients with esotropia, whereas an inward movement of the laterally deviated eye is noted in those with exotropia. Likewise, a downward movement of the superiorly deviated eye can be observed in patients with hypertropia, whereas an upward movement of the inferiorly deviated eye is noted in those with hypotropia.
2. The uncovered fellow eye may wander, indicating that the fixation of the eye is defective or absent. This may occur in patients with significant amblyopia or blindness.
3. There may be no movement of the uncovered fellow eye, indicating that the eye is straight.

The alternating cover test, used to detect heterophorias, is performed by alternately covering each eye without allowing the patient to regain binocularity. The examiner looks for movement of the eye at the moment it is being uncovered. The occluder disrupts fusion and any latent tendency of the eye to drift is revealed if the eye deviates under the cover. The alternating cover test can also be used to measure the magnitude of strabismus. This is done by placing a prism over the strabismic eye with the apex of the prism oriented in the direction of the eye turn (Fig. 29.2).

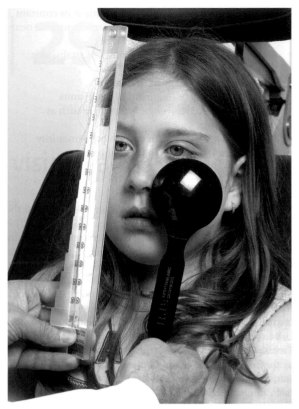

Fig. 29.2 Measurement of the angle of strabismus utilizing a prism bar.

The prism displaces the image of the fixation target onto the fovea of the deviated eye so that during the alternating cover test, there is no movement of either eye to take up fixation. Prisms of gradually increasing magnitude are introduced before one eye, as the other is occluded. The patient must maintain fixation on an accommodative target, such as a letter or number for an older child or an interesting toy or picture for a young child. For patients with limited cooperation, the examiner must exhibit ingenuity and patience to attract and maintain the patients' attention on a fixation target.

On occasion, a child is referred who appears to have an ocular deviation but has no detectable strabismus on further testing. This condition is called pseudostrabismus. Pseudostrabismus can be differentiated from true strabismus by means of the cover test. With pseudostrabismus, neither eye moves to pick up fixation with alternate occlusion because the eyes are straight. In most instances, the appearance of strabismus is caused by the presence of prominent epicanthal folds that extend from the upper lid to cover the inner canthal region. The child's eyes appear to be turned in because only a small amount of the sclera is visible medially when compared to the larger amount visible laterally. This false impression of an inward eye deviation (pseudoesotropia) is augmented when the child looks to either side, as the medial aspect of the adducting eye is further hidden by the epicanthal fold. Once pseudoesotropia has been detected, parents can be reassured that the appearance of the eye misalignment will improve over time as the child's face grows.

Sensory testing

Maddox rod

The Maddox rod is comprised of a series of red cylinders that distort a point of light into a fine red band, thereby changing the size, shape, and color of the point of light perceived by the eye. When a patient views the fixation light, one eye sees the light and the other eye, over which the Maddox rod is placed, sees a fine red line. The eyes assume a fusion-free position because these disparate images cannot be combined. The direction of the red line is perpendicular to the direction of the Maddox rod cylinders. If the Maddox rod is held so that the red cylinders are running horizontally before one eye, the vertical red line will appear either through the point of light (orthophoria) or to either side of the light (esophoria or exophoria). If the Maddox rod is held vertically, the red line will appear as a horizontal band either through the light (orthophoria), above it (hypophoria), or below it (hyperphoria). Measurement of a phoria's magnitude is determined by the amount of prism required to displace the red line so that the patient sees it running through the point of light. The Maddox rod can be used to measure the magnitude of vertical or horizontal phorias at either distance or near, although it is not as accurate as the alternating cover test.

Hess screen test, Lancaster red-green test, and Lees screen test

The Hess and Lees screen tests and Lancaster red-green test are similar in purpose but differ in the type of screen used and the method of charting. They are useful in the detection of paretic strabismus and are based on the fact that foveae of straight eyes project to the same point in space. In patients with strabismus, the foveae do not project to the same point in space and the measurement of this difference is a measure of the deviation.

The Hess screen is a three-foot square grid with small red lights at points in the grid such that the lights make up two squares, one inside the other. Each red light is individually controlled by the examiner and the patient, wearing red-and-green glasses, holds a flashlight that projects a green light. The patient fixates on the examiner's red light with the eye viewing through the red lens and projects the green flashlight in the direction towards which the eye under the green lens is pointing. The patient then tries to place the green light over each red light. If the eyes are not straight, the displacement of the green light in relation to the red light is a measure of the deviation (Fig. 29.3).[2] The Lancaster red-green test is similar to the Hess screen test, only the examiner uses a flashlight to project a linear red light at various points in the grid. The patient, wearing red-and-green glasses, tries to superimpose his or her linear green light overtop of the examiner's red light. The Lancaster red-green test can detect, but not measure, torsional differences between the eyes.[3]

The Lees screen test is plotted in the same way as the Hess screen test, although it is not as dissociating because the patient does not wear red-and-green glasses. The patient sits in front of two screens that are at right angles to one another. The eyes are dissociated via a two-sided mirror with an attached chin rest bisecting the junction of the two screens. The patient views the images from each fovea as though they are straight ahead. The patient is shown targets

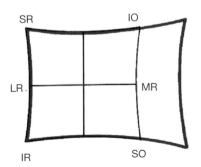
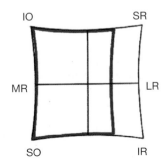

Fig. 29.3 Hess screen test results for a patient with a new right lateral rectus palsy. *IR*, Inferior rectus; *IO*, inferior oblique; *LR*, lateral rectus; *MR*, medial rectus; *SO*, superior oblique; *SR*, superior rectus. (Reproduced from Kanski J, Bowling B. *Clinical Ophthalmology.* 7th ed. Philadelphia: Saunders; 2011.)

a low-intensity light source for the illumination of the slides, and a high-intensity light source for creating after-images. Some synoptophores also contain a device called Haidinger's brushes, which is used to test macular function and projection.

Binocular vision is graded based on patient responses to disparate targets presented during testing. Parafoveal, foveal, or macular slides may be used in the synoptophore, depending on the patient's visual acuity. Grade 1 binocular vision requires simultaneous perception. Dissimilar targets, such as a lion and a cage, are presented to each eye. A patient with grade 1 binocular vision sees the lion in the cage (Fig. 29.8), but one image disappears intermittently if suppression is present. Grade 2 binocular vision requires fusional ability. Similar targets with missing elements are presented to each eye and must be fused before a complete picture is identified. For example, a picture of a rabbit with no tail holding a bouquet of flowers is presented to one eye. The other eye is presented with a picture of the same rabbit with a tail holding the base of some stems without flowers.

Grade 2 binocular vision is present if a patient fuses these images and reports seeing a tailed rabbit clutching a bouquet of flowers (Fig. 29.9). Suppression of one eye causes one of the controls, either the tail or the flowers, to disappear. With grade 2 targets, fusional reserves can be measured by moving the viewing tubes in or out to stimulate fusional convergence and divergence. The breaking point is reached when the patient complains of diplopia (two rabbits) or suppression (flowers or tail disappear). Grade 3 binocular vision requires the coordinated use of both eyes together to yield depth perception, or stereopsis. Grade 3 images are not quite superimposable and the fusion of these slightly disparate images by the brain creates the sensation of depth. In one example of Grade 3 targets, one seahorse appears distinctly in front of the others when the images are fused correctly (Fig. 29.10).

To measure strabismus, the patient rests his or her chin on the chin rest of the synoptophore, which has been adjusted so that each eye looks straight into each tube. All the readings on the synoptophore are set to zero. Consider

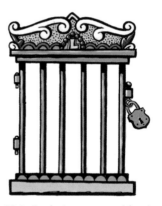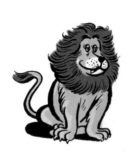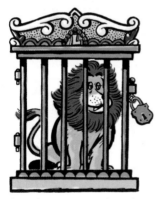

Fig. 29.8 Grade 1 targets used for determining the presence of simultaneous macular perception. The targets are dissimilar and cannot be fused, but the brain superimposes the images.

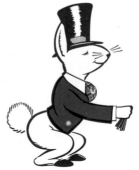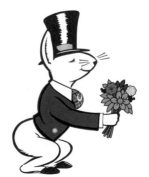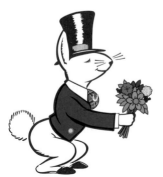

Fig. 29.9 Grade 2 targets used for determining the presence of simultaneous macular perception and fusion. The targets are similar and present a complete picture when fused.

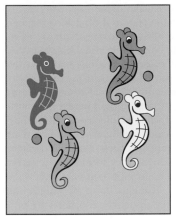 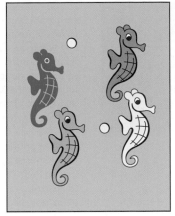 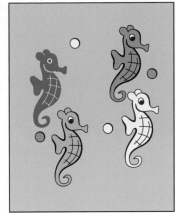

Fig. 29.10 Grade 3 targets used for determining stereopsis. The targets are similar but viewed at a slightly different angle, creating a sensation of depth. (Courtesy M. Blair, American Orthoptic Council.)

a patient with a left esotropia who fixates on a target placed in the right tube while the left eye is turned inwards. During the synoptophore assessment, Grade 1 targets are presented first to one eye and then to the other. To take up fixation, the deviated eye moves. The left tube is moved in the direction of the deviation until the left eye no longer moves when the target is presented. This measurement is called the objective measurement and corresponds to the amount of manifest deviation. Patients who fuse images when the full angle of strabismus is corrected have normal retinal correspondence. When anomalous retinal correspondence is present, the patient fuses even if the angle of strabismus is only partially corrected. The subjective angle is the angle where a patient reports that the targets presented to each eye are superimposed. The difference between the objective and subjective angles is referred to as the angle of anomaly. If the angle of anomaly is the same as the objective measurement of the deviation, harmonious anomalous retinal correspondence is present. If the angle of anomaly is less than the objective measurement of the deviation, the anomalous retinal correspondence is considered unharmonious.

Amblyopia

The estimated worldwide prevalence of amblyopia is 1.75%.[6] Amblyopia is a unilateral or bilateral decrease in visual acuity, typically equal or worse than 6/12 (20/40), caused by abnormal binocular interaction or visual deprivation. The three types of amblyopia are classified based on etiology: strabismic, refractive, or form deprivation. Strabismic amblyopia develops in esotropic patients more frequently than exotropic patients, because of the presence of persistent suppression scotomas. Asymmetric or bilateral high refractive error blurs the images cast on the retina and prevents normal visual processing of these images. Strabismic and refractive amblyopia usually respond well to treatment in children under 9 years of age, with higher success rates associated with younger age. This interval of reversibility, known as the critical period, is much shorter in stimulus deprivation amblyopia because it tends to be more severe and resistant to treatment. Stimulus deprivation amblyopia can occur because of ocular conditions that obstruct the visual axis, such as significant ptosis, cataracts, or corneal opacities. These underlying disorders must be treated aggressively within the first few months of life or the visual deficits may be permanent and irreversible. For this reason, early detection is fundamental in the management of amblyopia.

The treatment of amblyopia depends on the cause, with the goal of therapy being the restoration of equal and normal vision in each eye. In patients with strabismus, improvement or resolution of amblyopia allows for voluntary alternation between the two eyes. Any cause of stimulus deprivation must be corrected, often surgically, and appropriate refractive correction instituted. Significant refractive errors in one or both eyes are first corrected with glasses or contact lenses.[7] The most common method of amblyopia therapy for unilateral cases is the occlusion of the sound eye to force the use of the amblyopic eye. In the past, occlusion was maintained during the majority of a patient's waking hours. Although effective, this also increased the risk of occlusion amblyopia and the reduction in vision of the previously sound eye.[8] Part-time occlusion regimens, where the better-seeing eye is covered for 2 to 6 hours daily, have been shown to be as efficacious as full-time occlusion.[9] Occlusion is maintained until the vision in the affected eye is brought up to 20/25 or 20/20, or until vision no longer improves after months of

527

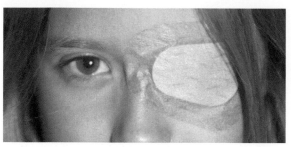

Fig. 29.11 An adhesive patch for the treatment of amblyopia. (Reproduced from Spalton D, Hitchings R, Hunter P. *Atlas of Clinical Ophthalmology*. 3rd ed. St Louis: Mosby; 2004, with permission.)

consistent or increased occlusion. It is important to reassess and modify the method of occlusion and increase the effort and daily duration of amblyopia therapy before concluding that therapy has failed. Once the decision has been made to stop amblyopia therapy, the daily hours of patching are tapered over several weeks and eventually discontinued as long as visual acuity is maintained.

Many types of patches are available for occlusion therapy. Adhesive patches seal off the eye and prevent children from peeking in any direction (Fig. 29.11). Although effective, this type of patch can be uncomfortable in hot weather as it can slip off moist skin and may cause contact dermatitis or skin sensitivity with prolonged repeated wear. Felt or fabric patches that extend underneath the lens and over the arm of a patient's glasses are available for those who do not tolerate adhesive patches. Similarly, rubber suction-cup occluders can be applied to the posterior lens surface and completely cover the eye because of a temporal extension that prevents peeking. Frosted lenses, clip-on occluders, or patches held in place with a strap around the head are not suitable because patients can peek around or shift them.

If a child is uncooperative and does not tolerate adhesive patches, atropine drops can be applied to the sound eye anywhere from 2 to 7 days a week. Atropine penalization is considered as efficacious as patching in the treatment of amblyopia.[10] Atropine can be extremely helpful in treating a hyperopic child as it blurs vision by paralyzing accommodation and impairs the child's innate ability to compensate for his or her refractive error. If a child is myopic, the benefit from atropine is negated because myopia provides the child with clear near vision in the penalized sound eye. The risks associated with atropine penalization include photosensitivity,[11] allergy, or rare systemic symptoms associated with atropine toxicity: fever, lethargy, hallucinations, and flushing. Atropine's long duration of action means that pupillary dilation and blurred vision persist for 2 weeks after instillation of the drops.

The success of occlusion therapy depends on the child's cooperation and adherence to the patching regimen. Older children are more likely to comply with amblyopia therapy when they are engaged in visual activities they enjoy. Activities, such as coloring, reading, watching television, or playing games can all be done using the amblyopic eye. Physical activities requiring spatial awareness are generally discouraged because of the lack of stereopsis resulting from monocular viewing while a child is patched. Some children may feel self-conscious or stigmatized when wearing the patch in public or amongst peers. On the other hand, some parents resist patching as they regard it as a sign of weakness in their child. To promote compliance, it is important to discuss concerns brought forth by families and help them understand the principles and necessity of amblyopia therapy. It should be emphasized to parents that poor compliance prolongs the duration of amblyopia therapy and that failure to treat amblyopia by age 9 years usually results in permanently reduced vision and stereopsis. Some children who have never been treated for amblyopia can respond slowly to therapy beyond the age of 9 years. For this reason, any child presenting with amblyopia should be given the opportunity for a patching trial, even those outside the window of neuroplasticity.

Eccentric fixation

Eccentric fixation is the culmination of damaging sensory habits in longstanding strabismus, primarily suppression and amblyopia. With this condition, the vision loss in the affected eye is usually profound because a retinal area other than the fovea is used for fixation. Visual acuity is typically less than 20/200 and the patient is unable to look directly at an object when the sound eye is covered. A decentered corneal reflex noted when the affected eye is viewing a target monocularly may be a clue to eccentric fixation, but retinal pathology, such as a dragged macula must be ruled out. Eccentric fixation can be detected by the use of a visuscope, which projects a target onto the retina and allows the examiner to visualize what part of the retina a patient uses for fixation.

Treatment of strabismus

The treatment of strabismus depends on the underlying etiology of the deviation and the age of the patient. Patients with well-controlled heterophorias or small heterotropias may need no treatment at all. Convergence insufficiency causing difficulty with near work often responds to orthoptic exercises. Other forms of strabismus can be temporary and may heal over time, but investigations as to the cause may be required in certain patient populations. For example, a sixth cranial nerve palsy in an older patient with diabetes can be observed for improvement over time. The same sixth nerve palsy in a healthy child with no preceding illness or trauma would require neuroimaging and close follow-up would be required because of the risk of amblyopia. In treating strabismus, it is imperative to eliminate any coexisting amblyopia. Augmented vision in the amblyopic eye promotes increased fixation stability and may reduce the angle of misalignment.[12] Spectacle correction of refractive error helps to improve both vision and alignment in strabismic patients with amblyopia. Older diplopic patients can be given permanent or temporary prism glasses to alleviate their double vision and regain fusion.

If conservative treatments are not indicated or are if they are only partly successful in treating strabismus, two further options are available. One option is the injection of botulinum toxin into an eye muscle, which paralyzes it and eventually allows the eye to straighten after a period of overcorrection.[13] The more common alternate option is eye muscle surgery, which can be performed on patients ranging in age from infancy to the elderly. Strabismus surgery involves strengthening weak eye muscles or weakening tight muscles to change the alignment of the eyes in relation to each other. In adults who undergo strabismus surgery with an adjustable suture technique, the alignment of the eyes can be further refined immediately after surgery while the patient is awake. Strabismus surgery can be repeated if a deviation returns or persists, or if an overcorrection is noted following surgery.

Summary

The main function of an orthoptist, working alongside an ophthalmologist, is to evaluate muscle balance and to promote binocular function through patient training and education. Orthoptics is an excellent adjunct in the preoperative and postoperative management of patients with strabismus. Orthoptic therapy improves a patient's quality of fusion and attempts to break down faulty sensory adaptations to strabismus, such as suppression and abnormal retinal correspondence. An ophthalmic assistant who is knowledgeable, adaptable, and enthusiastic is a great asset to an ophthalmologist or orthoptist working to diagnose and treat of strabismus.

Questions for review and thought

1. Many patients, particularly infants, have facial features that make them appear to have strabismus even though their eyes are orthophoric. What is this condition called?
2. What is the name of the condition where an eye deviates outward?
3. If the eye has a latent tendency to turn in, the condition is called esophoria. What is it called when there is a latent tendency for the eye to turn up?
4. Vision is depressed in one eye and the eye appears to turn in. However, when the fellow eye is covered, the eye does not take up fixation when a target is presented. What type of fixation is described in this scenario?
5. How does amblyopia develop? What are some of its causes?
6. The Hirschberg test is performed on a patient with strabismus. The light reflex is centered on one pupil but falls on the outer portion of the cornea of the fellow eye. What condition exists?
7. A patient complains of double vision. Describe a method for detecting which muscle or muscles are at fault and a method of measuring the amount of strabismus present.
8. The Worth 4-dot test is used to detect whether a patient fuses, experiences diplopia or suppresses of one eye. How is this test performed?
9. Discuss the treatment options and their limitations for a patient with amblyopia.
10. Describe three tests that can be used to test for sensory adaptations to strabismus.

Self-evaluation questions   Q

True–false statements

Directions: Indicate whether the statement is true (**T**) or false (**F**).

1. The primary difference between the alternating cover test and the cover–uncover test is the use of prisms. **T** or **F**
2. Anomalous retinal correspondence is a monocular adaptation to strabismus. **T** or **F**
3. To neutralize an exodeviation with prisms, the base of the prism is held toward the nose. **T** or **F**

Missing words

Directions: Fill in the missing word to complete the following sentences:

4. A term synonymous with binocular single vision is _____.
5. An alternating deviation is usually indicative of _____ visual acuity.
6. _____ are conjugate eye movements and _____ are disconjugate eye movements.

Choice-completion questions

Directions: Select the one best answer to complete the sentence.

7. When performing the alternating cover test:
   a. use a light for fixation.
   b. allow the patient to use both eyes at the same time.
   c. observe the occluded eye only.
   d. never have the patient wear his or her glasses.
   e. do not allow the patient to be binocular.
8. When a constant monocular deviation is present, the patient:
   a. may have anisometropia.
   b. may have fusion ability.
   c. has a deviation that cannot be neutralized.
   d. never demonstrates suppression.
   e. has an esodeviation.
9. Strabismus:
   a. is only monocular in nature.
   b. has motor and sensory adaptations.
   c. is always present when the corneal reflexes are not properly positioned.
   d. indicates that visual acuity is always lower in both eyes.
   e. requires surgical correction.
10. The Worth 4-dot test:
    a. is used to quantitate a deviation.
    b. is a test for color blindness.
    c. detects the presence and type of diplopia.
    d. detects the presence of amblyopia.
    e. is used to evaluate fusional amplitudes.

Answers, notes, and explanations   A

1. **False**. The primary difference between the alternating cover test and the cover–uncover test is binocularity. During the alternating cover test, the patient is never allowed to use both eyes at the same time to view the fixation target. When the cover–uncover test is performed, the patient must be allowed to regain binocularity between the occlusion of each eye.
2. **False**. Anomalous retinal correspondence is a binocular adaptation to strabismus. It is an abnormal relationship that develops between retinal elements in each eye.
3. **True**. To neutralize an exodeviation with prisms, the base of the prism is held toward the nose. In an exodeviation, the object of fixation stimulates the temporal retina and is therefore projected nasally. A prism displaces an image toward its apex. Therefore when a prism is held base-in in front of an eye, the object of fixation appears to the temporal side and the deviation can be neutralized.
4. **Fusion**. Fusion is the unification of visual input into a single image by the brain following the stimulation of corresponding retinal elements.
5. **Equal**. An alternating deviation is a condition in which one eye is used for fixation, followed by the other eye.

Because both eyes are used for fixation, the stimulation allows each eye to develop similar levels of visual acuity. Patients who develop amblyopia usually have a monocular fixation preference.
6. **Versions, vergences**. Versions are binocular eye movements in which both eyes move in the same direction, such as to the left (levoversion) or right (dextroversion). Vergence movements, such as convergence and divergence, are binocular movements in which both eyes move in opposite directions to attain and maintain fusion. Vergence movements are required when changing fixation distance.
7. **e. Do not allow the patient to be binocular**. By eliminating motor fusion, the mechanism that helps to keep the eyes aligned, the alternating cover test measures of the full amount of phoria and tropia present in a strabismic patient. To eliminate any attempts to fuse, the patient is constantly dissociated by alternate occlusion and is never allowed to become binocular.
8. **a. May have anisometropia**. Anisometropia, where the refractive error is unequal between the two eyes, can be an obstacle to fusion as one eye perceives an image that

Answers, notes, and explanations—Continued

A

is much clearer than the other eye. Anisometropia can be a precipitating factor in the development of amblyopia and strabismus.

9. **b. Has motor and sensory adaptations**. Strabismus is an abnormal condition in which there is a misalignment of the visual axes. Motor fusion is inadequate to maintain proper alignment of the eyes. Corresponding retinal elements are no longer simultaneously stimulated and the patient develops sensory adaptations that provide single vision, such as suppression or abnormal retinal correspondence.

10. **c. Detects the presence and type of diplopia**. An evaluation of the patient's macular and peripheral fusion status can be ascertained with the Worth 4-dot test. It is a subjective test used to determine the presence or absence of fusion, suppression, alternation, or diplopia. If diplopia is present, the type (homonymous or heteronymous) can be established by the position of the lights in relation to the position of the red-green filters in the glasses worn by the patient.

References

1. Lueder GT, Garibaldi D. Comparison of visual acuity measured with Allen figures and Snellen letters using the B-VAT II monitor. *Ophthalmology*. 1997;104(11):1758–1761.
2. Roper-Hall G. The Hess screen test. *Am Orthopt J*. 2006;56(1):166–174.
3. Christoff A, Guyton DL. The Lancaster red-green test. *Am Orthopt J*. 2006;56(1):157–165.
4. Timms C. The Lees screen test. *Am Orthopt J*. 2006;56(1):180–183. https://doi.org/10.3368/aoj.56.1.180.
5. Bagolini B. Sensorial anomalies in strabismus (suppression, anomalous correspondence, amblyopia). *Doc Ophthalmol*. 1976;41(1):1–22.
6. Hashemi H, Pakzad R, Yekta A, et al. Global and regional estimates of prevalence of amblyopia: a systematic review and meta-analysis. *Strabismus*. 2018;26(4):168–183.
7. The Pediatric Eye Disease Investigator Group. Randomized trial of treatment of amblyopia in children aged 7 to 17 years. *Arch Ophthalmol*. 2005;123(4):437–447.
8. Longmuir S, Pfeifer W, Scott W, Olson R. Effect of occlusion amblyopia after prescribed full-time occlusion on long-term visual acuity outcomes. *J Pediatr Ophthalmol Strabismus*. 2013;50:94–101.
9. The Pediatric Eye Disease Investigator Group. A randomized trial of patching regimens for treatment of moderate amblyopia in children. *Arch Ophthalmol*. 2003;121(5):603–611.
10. Li T, Qureshi R, Taylor K. Conventional occlusion versus pharmacologic penalization for amblyopia. *Cochrane Database Syst Rev*. 2019;8:CD006460.
11. Osborne DC, Greenhalgh KM, Evans MJE, Self JE. Atropine penalization versus occlusion therapies for unilateral amblyopia after the critical period of visual development: a systematic review. *Ophthalmol Ther*. 2018;7(2):323–332.
12. Repka Michael X, et al. The effect of amblyopia therapy on ocular alignment. *JAAPOS*. 2005;9(6):542–545.
13. Rowe FJ, Noonan CP. Botulinum toxin for the treatment of strabismus. *Cochrane Database Syst Rev*. 2017;3(3):CD006499.

Chapter | **30** |

Aseptic technique and minor office surgery

Aseptic technique

Aseptic technique in the office or hospital is an attempt to prevent infection by the elimination of microorganisms. Ophthalmic surgery demands maximum asepsis, particularly in operations involving the globe itself. Microorganisms that gain access to the interior of the eye can multiply and cause irreparable damage, often resulting in blindness. Aseptic technique demands:

- Proper sterilization of all instruments
- Sterilization of the skin adjacent to the operative site
- Sterilization of the hands of both the operator and the assistant
- Use of sterile solutions and ointments during and after the operation

For the most part, the following discussion of aseptic technique will be oriented toward ophthalmic surgery in the office.

Disinfection of eyelid skin

Office surgery for conditions involving eyelid skin requires carefully applied skin antiseptics (Table 30.1; spray packs of antiseptics are contraindicated.) Care must be taken that none of the antiseptic material enters the eye. This may be done with careful application by cotton applicators soaked in such solutions as tincture of iodine 2%, povidone-iodine (Betadine), Ioprep, alcohol, and cetrimonium bromide. It also may be done by scrupulous scrubbing of the area with hexachlorophene (Phisohex) or green soap. Betadine and alcohol are available in large, presoaked swabs.

Scrubbing (degerming of hands)

For many minor office procedures, scrubbing may be unnecessary if both the operator and the assistant adhere to a "no-touch" technique. In this technique, the tops of the sterile instruments are never touched by hands or laid down in a nonsterile area.

The skin of the hands contains normal bacterial inhabitants, as well as many transient microorganisms with which the individual may recently have come into contact. It is virtually impossible to scrub the hands sufficiently to get rid of all normal inhabitants, but the use of gloves overcomes this handicap. We tend to use powderless gloves, because particulate matter (e.g., starches) of powder can have a damaging effect in the eye.

Scrubbing with a brush degerms the hands by the removal of bacteria, and the dilution of the bacteria content is achieved by rinses and the use of antiseptic skin agents that are bactericidal. Before scrubbing, the fingernails should be cleansed with an orangewood stick. The various antiseptic agents available have their own scrubbing time, which should be followed rigidly. The fingers and nails should be carefully scrubbed and all hidden recesses of the hands scrupulously cleansed.

Instillation of eye medication

Eye medication can easily become contaminated by incorrect instillation. There is a right and a wrong way to instill eye medication both before and after minor office surgery (Fig. 30.1). With the patient's head tilted back, the dropper,

Table 30.1 Skin preparations and disinfecting solutions

Classification	Manufacturer	Type of bactericide
Tinctures		
Tincture of iodine 2%		Iodine-alcohol
Alcohol 70%		Alcohol
Zephiran chloride	Winthrop	Quaternary ammonium compound + alcohol
Merthiolate	Eli Lilly & Co	Sodium ethylmercurithiosalicylate + alcohol
Aqueous preparations		
Merthiolate	Eli Lilly & Co	Sodium ethylmercurithiosalicylate
Zephiran chloride	Winthrop	Quaternary ammonium compound
Hexachlorophene scrubs		
Gamophen	Arwood	Hexachlorophene
Septisol	Vestal	Hexachlorophene
Phisohex	Winthrop	Hexachlorophene
Iodophors		
Ioprep	Johnson & Johnson	Iodophor
Wescodyne	West	Iodophor
Betadine	British Drug Houses	Iodophor

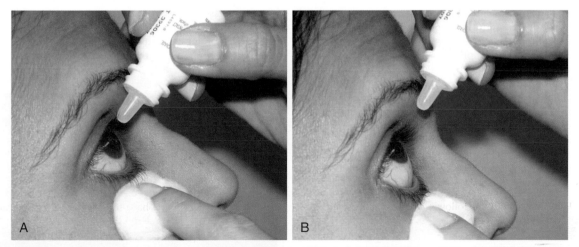

Fig. 30.1 Instillation of eyedrops. (A) Incorrect method; note contamination of dropper by lashes. (B) Correct method; note tip of dropper held free of globe and lashes.

dropper bottle, or ointment tube should be held about half an inch (1.25 cm) from the eye before the release of medication. When corneal anesthesia is required, the patient should be asked to look down so that the cornea will be completely covered by the medication. It is important that the tip of the dropper or dropper bottle never touches the eye or eyelid. Contamination will result, in which case the dropper and medication should be discarded. Alcohol and alcohol-type solutions must never enter the eye. They are damaging to the corneal epithelium.

Sterility of ophthalmic solutions

The sterility of eye solutions is desirable not only because of the obvious danger of ocular infection, but also because contaminated solutions may prove toxic and irritating to the eye. The sterilization of ophthalmic solutions may be performed effectively by pouring through bacterial filters. The addition of a preservative, such as chlorobutanol or benzalkonium chloride, aids in preventing contamination.

The ophthalmologist's office should have solutions that are well prepared and contain an added preservative. They should be kept in small bottles, never in large stock sizes. Individual-dose sizes are commercially available in disposable plastic containers. In addition, one must be careful about contamination of the eyedropper, particularly if it has touched an infected eye. If contamination is suspected, the solution should be discarded. One solution notorious for harboring microorganisms, particularly *Pseudomonas aeruginosa*, is fluorescein. However, fluorescein is available in dried sterile strips that are safe to use.

All solutions that enter the eye should be of the nonpreserved type (e.g., lidocaine 1% [Xylocaine], vancomycin). All solutions that are applied to an open wound should be made up fresh through micropore filters (e.g., mitomycin).

Disinfection of tonometer prism

Every tonometer prism should be cleaned and disinfected before use. The main purpose of this is to prevent the spread of infection from patient to patient, especially of the viruses that cause epidemic keratoconjunctivitis and acquired immunodeficiency syndrome (AIDS).

The Goldmann application tonometer prism is best cleaned and disinfected by soaking in 1:10 sodium hypochlorite solution (bleach) or 3% hydrogen peroxide. Some practices use 70% isopropyl alcohol soaks or wipe with an alcohol pad. After disinfecting, the prism should be rinsed in running water and dried. Detailed instructions are available on the manufacturer's website.

Several handheld applanation tonometers are available (e.g., TonoPen). These require a special sterile rubber cover for each individual.

Minor office surgery

Ophthalmologists vary in the amount and type of office surgery they perform. Such factors as the availability of outpatient facilities in a nearby hospital, the time spent at the hospital by the physician, the physical layout of the physician's office, and the presence of a trained and efficient ophthalmic assistant influence the decision whether to perform surgical procedures in the office or in the hospital outpatient department. When adequate physical facilities and a trained assistant are available, many minor procedures can be performed in the ophthalmic office in a special sterile operating room. Age may be a consideration for choice of patient.

Of fundamental importance is the general sterility of the area in which the surgical procedure is to be performed. Maintenance of adequate cleanliness and dusting of the surgical area should be performed regularly. The area should be segregated from the routine patient flow as much as possible. An office operating room will not achieve the same high standard of sterility that is found in a hospital operating room. Such factors as a separate scrub area, elimination of all street clothing, shoe covers, air filtration, and positive-pressure operating rooms are not generally found in an office minor-procedure operating room. In an office that one enters without a mask, airborne bacteria may remain active for hours. In all offices, emphasis must be placed on adequate sterilization of instruments, combined with personal measures to ensure that there is reasonable cleanliness and sterility in the surgical area.

Careful and complete cleanliness of instruments must precede all efforts at sterilization. It is useless to place a blood-stained curet into an antiseptic solution, heat oven, or autoclave because these dirty instruments can never be thoroughly sterilized. Scrupulous cleansing with a fine nailbrush or toothbrush and careful inspection of the instruments are essential. This inspection is done most efficiently with magnifying lenses or loupes. The cleansing may be done in soapy water or with one of the many detergents available. Protein enzyme solutions are available to remove blood and tissue debris from the instruments. Instruments with moving parts should be lubricated periodically or dipped into surgical instrument milk. After these instruments are carefully rinsed, they are sterilized (Fig. 30.2).

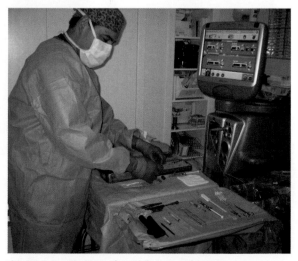

Fig. 30.2 Preparation of a sterile instrument tray.

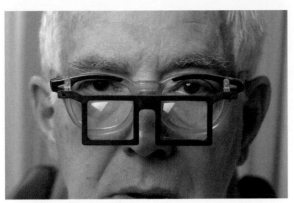

Fig. 30.3 Magnifiers for stereoscopic magnification when performing office surgery.

Sterilization of the instruments may be performed by one of the methods outlined previously. Small autoclaves are available for office use. They have their own timing device and will sterilize within 5 minutes. Disinfection of the patient's skin is performed for many lid procedures by applying an antiseptic solution, such as iodine, povidone-iodine (Betadine), or benzalkonium chloride.

The surgeon and the ophthalmic assistant should observe all rules of cleanliness, particularly for the more advanced procedures that may be performed in the office. Before handling sterilized instruments, the ophthalmic assistant should scrub, preferably with hexachlorophene soap. Gloves may be required for some of the minor operations. Powderless gloves are preferred. Assistants should not use nail polish or wear hand or wrist jewelry when assisting during minor office procedures. Masks and caps are often not necessary for most minor office procedures. More extensive operations, however, such as pterygium removal and plastic surgery on the eyelid, may require surgical care comparable to the standards used in a first-class hospital operating room. Minor surgery is often performed under magnification with loupes (Fig. 30.3).

Safety considerations

Defibrillator apparatus should be available in a conspicuous place (Fig. 30.4). All staff should be trained on this in association with regular cardiopulmonary resuscitation (CPR) courses.

Instruments and surgical materials for ophthalmic procedures

The following surgical instruments may be required in minor office surgery: forceps, scissors, needle holders, clamps, curets, scalpels and blades, and lacrimal instruments and

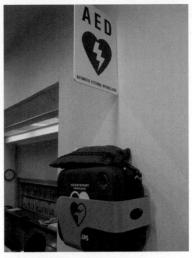

Fig. 30.4 An automatic external defibrillator should be visible in a conspicuous place.

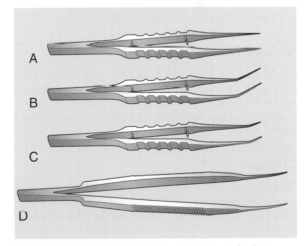

Fig. 30.5 Forceps. (A) Colibri 0.12 mm. (B) Capsulorrhexis. (C) Tying. (D) 0.5-mm teeth.

cannulas. The numerous individual variations of these instruments depend on the surgeon's choice.

Forceps

Forceps are used to grasp small tissues for either removal or suture insertion. The teeth of these instruments vary from 0.12 to 0.5 mm. The jaws may be rounded, flat, or serrated. Some forceps, called tying forceps, have no teeth. Others, called epilation forceps, also have no teeth and are used to remove eyelashes. Thus both tooth and nontooth forceps often are available in the office (Fig. 30.5).

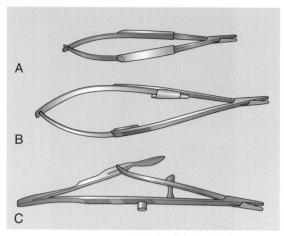

Fig. 30.6 Needle holders. (A) Small needle holder. (B) Medium-sized needle holder. (C) Large needle holder.

Scissors

Scissors may be blunt or sharp, curved or straight. They may have spring action or direct action.

Needle holders

Needle holders hold suture needles and provide good control for inserting needles. Some of these instruments are nonlocking, some locking; some handles are spring-loaded. Some needle holders for larger-size needles have a thumb release (Fig. 30.6).

Clamps

Clamps used in ophthalmic surgery may be round, with a guarded plate behind to provide hemostasis during removal of chalazia. Other clamps are used to hold eyelids during surgery, as well as to create hemostasis.

Curets

Curets are slim-handled and have a bowl-shaped end. The ends are either round or serrated and are used to remove chalazia and other small cystic material.

Scalpels, keratomes, and blades

Scalpels used by the physician depend on preference. Commonly used instruments are often disposable small blades, some angled blades, some keratomes for incising into the cornea, and the Bard-Parker scalpel used for skin cutting. Some tips are of gem quality (e.g., sapphire, diamond). Smaller and smaller keratomes are used to accommodate the newer foldable lenses.

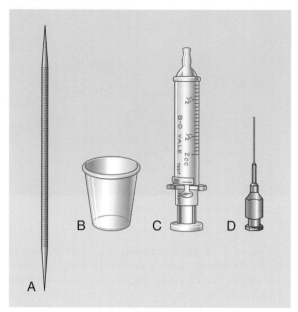

Fig. 30.7 Lacrimal set. (A) Punctum dilator. (B) Sterile medicine glass to contain either sterile normal saline solution or an antibiotic solution. (C) Syringe. (D) Lacrimal needle.

Lacrimal instruments

A lacrimal set consists of a punctum dilator, which enlarges the punctum; a sterile medicine glass to hold sterile saline solution or an antibiotic solution; and a disposable syringe with a blunt lacrimal cannula. The last introduces a solution into the canaliculus (Fig. 30.7).

Corrosion of stainless steel instruments

What is known as "'stainless steel" may contain a wide range of metals. These always include iron and chromium, but the alloy may also contain carbon, nickel, sulfur, tungsten, manganese, molybdenum, and other elements. Chromium imparts the stainless quality to the metal and the more chromium present, the more resistant it is to corrosion. Carbon provides hardness to the metal but reduces the corrosion-resistant effect of chromium. Special hardening processes are used by different manufacturers to try to produce a hardened instrument with low corrosion properties. Polishing also reduces the corrosive effect, but some areas, such as the knurled handles cannot be polished very well and consequently are the first to suffer corrosion.

The most common causes of corrosion are inadequate cleaning and drying after use, overlong exposure to sterilizing solutions, or too corrosive a sterilizing solution. The most important factor that causes corrosion is inadequate cleaning so that particles of material remain on the surface.

Fortunately, many sharp instruments today are available in disposable form. Where available, these usually are preferred because a sharp instrument is guaranteed every time.

Procedures

Chalazion surgery

A chalazion is caused by an obstruction of a meibomian gland of the eyelid. Because of this blockage, the gland becomes distended and ruptures, the oily contents being liberated into the substance of the lid. This results in a

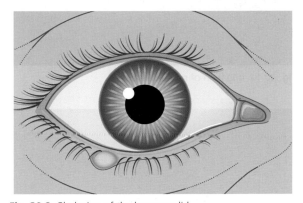

Fig. 30.8 Chalazion of the lower eyelid.

granulomatous inflammatory reaction that subsides spontaneously in some cases, but in other cases appears to remain as a chronic nodule on the eyelid (Fig. 30.8). The nodule may be removed under the eyelid through a vertical conjunctival incision or, occasionally, externally through the skin.

The ophthalmic assistant's help is essential in:
- Arranging the patient comfortably in the operating chair
- Anesthetizing the eye adequately with topical anesthetic drops
- Setting out the syringe and needle with the local anesthetic for infiltration into the eyelid
- Setting out a sterile towel with the instruments required
- Securing hemostasis by applying pressure directly at the operative site after chalazion removal
- Preparing the dressing, which usually consists of an antibiotic ointment and a firmly applied eye pad

The instruments required for the chalazion operation are shown in Fig. 30.9.

Eyepatch application

An eyepatch must be applied correctly if it is to perform the necessary function of preventing further bleeding and an accumulation of lid edema (Fig. 30.10). After the instillation of an antibiotic ointment, a recommended method is to immobilize the eyelid through pressure by applying an eye pad doubled in half over the site of the

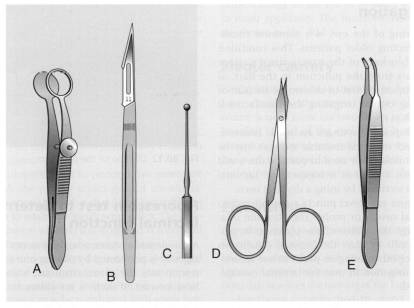

Fig. 30.9 Chalazion set. (A) Chalazion clamp. (B) Scalpel. (C) Curet. (D) Fine scissors. (E) Fine forceps.

fine needle is inserted along the pathway to the root of the lash. Magnification is essential in this procedure to see the tiny orifices through which the hairs emerge. Epilation is complete after the hyfrecator has been turned on for a few seconds and the lash can be removed without pulling. Cryotherapy is another useful method of permanently destroying hair follicles.

Electrosurgery

Electrosurgery is based on the principles of diathermy, which is the amplification of high-frequency alternating currents. This produces heat as a result of the resistance of the tissues. Frequencies used are between 2 and 4 MHz, which includes part of the radiofrequency spectrum. Because of this, as a precaution, these currents should not be used with individuals who have pacemakers or in the presence of any flammable or explosive gases or liquids.

A number of modes of electrosurgery are available for use in ophthalmology. The most familiar mode is wet field cautery. This is a bipolar cautery in which electrical current passes between two points in a wet field of saline and creates hemostasis. The two points are usually the two tips of a forceps. This is one of the methods of coagulating bleeding vessels during ocular surgery.

Fulguration or spark gap current is a form of electric current. Fulguration current produces a potent dehydrating effect on tissues that is destructive and self-limiting. The spark must jump across to the tissues, thereby producing a charring or carbon effect on the tissues. This procedure can coagulate heavy bleeders or destroy bases of tissue to prevent such things as recurrences of carcinoma.

A fully filtered current is a continuous flow of a high-frequency current that results in a nonpulsating flow of current. This produces a smooth cutting flow with a minimal amount of heat and tissue destruction. This type of current is ideal for cutting.

Fully rectified current produces a minute, but perceptible, pulsating effect that can, under certain conditions, reduce the efficiency of the cutting while producing some lateral heat. A benefit is that this heat can produce coagulation of the tissue surfaces and provide effective hemostasis.

Partially rectified current is an intermittent flow of high-frequency current. Because it is partially rectified, it produces more hemostasis and seals off bleeders. This type of current is commonly used in eyelid surgery.

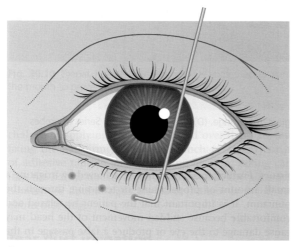

Fig. 30.14 Correction of entropion by Ziegler cautery.

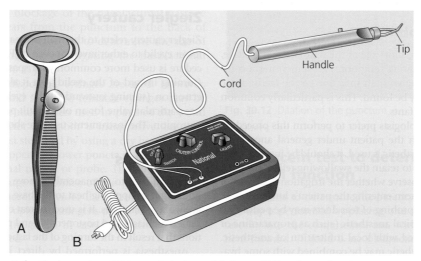

Fig. 30.15 Instruments for Ziegler cautery. (A) Large chalazion or lid clamp. (B) Fine thermal cautery.

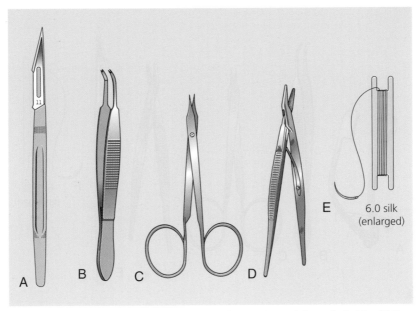

Fig. 30.16 Eyelid growth removal set. (A) Scalpel. (B) Fine forceps. (C) Fine scissors. (D) Needle holder. (E) Fine suture.

Eyelid growth removal

Patients with large growths of the eyelid may require hospital surgery for removal of the growth under adequate operating room conditions. However, many small papillomas, benign melanomas, verrucae, and other small lesions of the eyelids may be carefully and safely removed in the office. Specimen bottles that contain formaldehyde should be available from the local pathology laboratory so that the specimens may be stored and microscopically examined. Many of these lesions on the eyelid may be removed and the base cauterized. Others may require sutures. Fig. 30.16 shows the instruments that are required and that should be available when eyelid procedures are performed.

Pterygium removal

A pterygium is a fibrovascular membrane that extends from the medial aspect of the bulbar conjunctiva and invades the cornea (Fig. 30.17). It tends to be progressive and in time can make its way to the central portion of the cornea and interfere with vision. Pterygia are most common in southern climates where people have greater exposure to ultraviolet light, which appears to promote growth. In northern areas, people who have outdoor vocations, such as farmers, sailors, and postal workers, are most prone to develop this growth.

The purpose of pterygium removal is to excise the membrane before it can significantly interfere with vision. Because this operation requires incision into the cornea, as

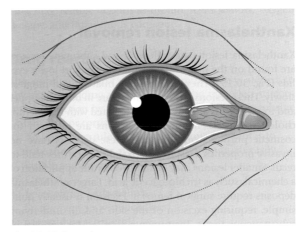

Fig. 30.17 Pterygium.

well as the conjunctiva, scrupulous cleanliness, disinfection of the patient's skin and the surgeon's hands, and sterilization of the instruments are required. The anesthesia is usually provided by topical drops, either alone or combined with subconjunctival injection. Placing the patient in a horizontal position is the preferred method for the surgical removal of the pterygium. Application of mitomycin solution is often helpful in preventing recurrence. Amniotic membrane graphs are used for recurrences. The instruments for a pterygium procedure are shown in Fig. 30.18.

541

procedure has been presented. The ophthalmic assistant who has been given this challenging responsibility must become familiar with the basic routine of the ophthalmologist. The assistant will then become a necessary and invaluable aid in the smooth performance of these minor surgical procedures and will derive a great deal of personal satisfaction from the work.

Questions for review and thought

1. What is meant by asepsis? When is aseptic technique of particular importance in eye surgery?
2. Outline ways in which the operative field may be contaminated at the time of surgery.
3. Outline ways in which wound contamination may be prevented.
4. Discuss the methods by which skin may be prepared for surgery.
5. How are tonometers sterilized?
6. How are eye medications rendered sterile and how is contamination of such medications avoided?
7. What are the main functions of the ophthalmic assistant with respect to minor office surgery?
8. List several minor ophthalmic procedures commonly performed in the office.
9. Discuss the procedure for nasolacrimal irrigation in an adult.
10. What instruments should be set out for the surgical removal of a chalazion?
11. What are general complications that may result from minor office surgery?
12. What emergency supplies should be on hand to deal with such complications?
13. How would you handle a patient who faints in the office?
14. What instruments are available for removing a corneal foreign body?
15. What is the purpose of an eyepatch after a corneal abrasion?
16. What is the advantage of fluorescein strips over solutions?
17. What reactions may occur after injection of a local anesthetic?

Self-evaluation questions   Q

True–false statements

Directions: Indicate whether the statement is true (T) or false (F).

1. In office practice, fluorescein in paper strip form is preferable to the large solution form of 2% fluorescein. **T or F**
2. Ophthalmic solutions are always sterile. **T or F**

Missing words

Directions: Write in the missing word(s) in the following sentences:

3. A technique that results in absence of microorganisms is called _____ technique.
4. Excitability, tremors, and convulsions are indications of _____ stimulation.
5. An agent that may be used to relieve immediate serious allergic reactions to drugs is _____.

Choice-completion questions

Directions: Select the one best answer in each case.

6. Which of the following is not necessary for a chalazion procedure?
   a. Scalpel blade
   b. Curet
   c. Forceps
   d. Speculum
   e. Clamp
7. Which of the following is incorrect? Tear duct irrigation for epiphora may be used to identify:
   a. blockage of the punctum.
   b. stenosis of the canaliculus.
   c. blockage of the nasolacrimal duct.
   d. ectropion.
   e. presence of a stone in the lacrimal sac.

Answers, notes, and explanations

A

1. **True**. Fluorescein in large bottle solutions can easily become contaminated, particularly with *Pseudomonas aeruginosa*, and consequently one may be introducing a new organism into the eye. Paper strips are far safer for office use. However, individual sterile dropper units are available and, although these are relatively expensive, they may also be used.

    The technique of applying fluorescein paper is to wet the fluorescein strip with saline solution or touch the wet conjunctiva so that a thin film of fluorescein will spread over the corneal surface. Any defect in the epithelial cells will be stained by fluorescein and become more easily visualized. It is advisable in record keeping to make a sketch of the staining area on the patient's record for later comparison and to follow the progress of healing. This may become important in recurrent corneal abrasion to identify the site of initial injury.

2. **False**. Although manufacturers provide preservatives, such as chlorobutanol, thimerosal, ethylenediaminetetraacetic (EDTA), and benzalkonium chloride to prevent the solutions becoming contaminated, there is no fail-safe method. Once a bottle has been opened and used on any patient, organisms can enter the solution and not be destroyed by the preservative. The longer the bottle remains on the shelf of the ophthalmic office, the more likely this is to occur.

    As a consequence, safeguards for ophthalmic drugs should be put into action once the bottle has been opened. These bottles should not remain on the shelf for any length of time. Second, when introducing drops into the eye, one should avoid contaminating the tip of the bottle or the tip of the eyedropper by touching the lashes or eyelid of the individual receiving the drops. If contamination is suspected, the solution should be discarded.

3. **Aseptic**. Aseptic technique refers to a method of surgery in which there is an absence of all living microorganisms. This technique involves sterilization of instruments, disinfecting the skin of the patient and the hands of the operator, and the use of sterile solutions, drapes, and medications so that nothing reaching the operative site has any microorganisms that will cause contamination.

4. **Central nervous system**. Some drugs reach the central nervous system and induce this type of excitability, tremors, or convulsions. Cocaine may be such an offending agent.

5. **Epinephrine (Adrenalin), cortisone**. Both agents may be used in certain situations to relieve an acute anaphylactic reaction in which the body responds adversely to some drug. Both of these agents should be kept on hand and be readily available for such emergencies.

6. **d. Speculum**. A chalazion clamp is usually satisfactory for holding the lid and creating hemostasis during the procedure. Chalazion clamps can be small or large and can be selected to suit the size of the chalazion.

7. **d. Ectropion**. The diagnosis of ectropion is usually made from external examination and does not require probing or tear duct irrigation to identify the problem. However, these procedures might identify any stenosis of the canaliculus that might have occurred as a result of the ectropion.

    In other situations, such as occlusion, stenosis, or presence of a stone of the lacrimal sac, there will be a resistance on irrigation of the nasolacrimal system.

Box 31.1 What to do before and after cataract surgery (handout to patient)

Be sure to bring your insurance details with you.

If you are currently taking medication, please bring these to the hospital with you. A nurse will inquire about all the medication you are taking.

Obtain a good night's sleep before admission to hospital.

Shampoo your hair the night before entering hospital.

Women: Please do not wear makeup, particularly mascara and facial preparations.

Do not wear or bring valuable jewelry.

Special relaxing medication may be given to you on the morning of surgery.

For local anesthesia

Eyedrops and occasionally a small local freezing injection may be given to you just before surgery.

In the operating room, you may see the usual lights and sterile equipment and a special microscope. You will not see anything of the surgery during the operation.

Surgery lasts about 15 minutes. Soon after, you will be able to sit up in bed.

After cataract surgery, you may have a bandage over only the operative eye. This will be removed soon after surgery and no eye bandage need be worn.

A small plastic shield may be placed over the eye at bedtime to prevent unconscious rubbing of the eye when asleep.

You will be out of bed soon after surgery.

Although you need not restrict your movements after surgery, please be careful of heavy lifting and excess bending.

Avoid bright window sunshine. If bright, wear sunglasses.

On the first night, there may be some discomfort. If so, take a mild pain-killing pill.

On discharge you will be given a two-page list of do's and don'ts.

24 hours to 2 weeks after surgery

- Go back to normal activities using caution. If you have pain, call the office. You may bend over gently to put on shoes. You may read and watch TV as you wish. You can do anything you were doing before surgery with the following exceptions:
  - No contact sports.
  - Avoid getting water in eye while swimming.
  - No swinging of golf clubs; however, chipping and putting should be safe.
  - No strenuous exercise.
  - You may wash your hair gently, or go to the beauty parlor, but avoid getting water in the eye.
    Just remember to use common sense!

After 2 weeks

You can function as you had before surgery and it is hoped, with much better vision. Medication may be stopped soon after this point.

Common symptoms after surgery

The following common symptoms may occur after surgery and should not cause alarm:

- Light sensitivity, especially to sunlight; be sure to use dark glasses.
- Do not be surprised if color perception is improved with your operated eye.
- Mild irritation, redness, itchiness, or watery eye may occur for the first several days following surgery.
- Your vision may be fuzzy for several weeks. Patients vary as to the time required before their vision returns.
- There may be some bruising around the eyelids or the side of your head, which will soon fade.
- A small amount of residue may collect in your eyelids or the corner of your eye on awakening in the morning. (This is most likely caused by eyedrop residue.)
  You should report any sudden onset of severe pain, loss of vision, or marked redness in the operated eye.

As soon as arrangements for the operative time and date have been completed, the patient should be notified by telephone to be sure that the time is suitable. Occasional adjustments may have to be made for illness, holidays, work, and special requests of the patient. A well-run ophthalmic practice, emphasizing goodwill, permits some latitude in this direction, depending on the urgency of the problem.

For previous retinal surgery

Often more conservative instructions may apply for cataract surgery:

1. Preoperative assessment is often scheduled directly or emailed.

2. Aspirin and other blood thinners do not need to be stopped if surgery is under topical and intracameral anesthesia.

3. Patching of one eye is only required at bedtime.

Our practice has been to follow the telephone call with a confirming letter outlining the date and time of admission to the hospital and requesting confirmation by return call or letter. The purpose of having the patient provide a return call or letter is to ensure that the date of surgery is suitable and that the patient's schedule has been altered accordingly.

The confirmation should always be double-checked and those patients who have not confirmed should be contacted.

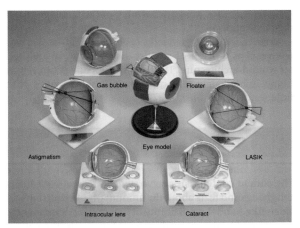

Fig 31.2 Visual aids, such as eye models, are available for demonstration purposes. (Courtesy Gulden Ophthalmics, Elkins Park, PA, USA.)

assistant or surgeon. The ophthalmic assistant double-checks that the signed form is available before patients come for surgery. In some cases and in some centers, a more detailed consent and acceptance is indicated, supported by video explanation.

A simplification of this routine may be followed when the patient has outpatient surgery. With outpatient surgery today, a physical examination may be arranged ahead of time. The patient may be asked to return to the office to pick up blood test forms. In addition, intraocular lens (IOL) implant power will be required for all cataract procedures. The power of the IOL is determined by the IOL Master or Lenstar and this typically performed before surgery. These measurements are usually performed on both eyes at the same time. In some cases, a B-scan may be required if the cataract is dense and the practitioner wishes to view the vitreous cavity and the status of the retina. Other investigational tests may be performed. Visual aids are available for demonstration purposes (Fig. 31.2).

Patients may be asked to have a physical check-up and a report from their doctor.

Consent form

Today consent forms are mandatory for all surgical procedures, whether minor procedures, such as yttrium aluminum garnet (YAG) laser iridotomy or capsulotomy, or major procedures, such as cataract removal, laser-assisted in situ keratomileusis (LASIK), photorefractive keratotomy (PRK), or other refractive procedures.

The contents of a proper consent form are outlined in Box 31.2. The patient should carefully review and understand this material. The surgeon should personally review significant risks, note these in the medical record, and permit the patient to ask questions. Duly signed consents onsite have been challenged in the courts!

We provide a simplified form that is mailed to patients. This permits them to discuss it at home. They bring this form back in and can ask questions of the ophthalmic

Preparing the child and parent for surgery

The child who is about to enter the hospital will have a great deal of apprehension. If this is the second or third hospital visit, the child's apprehension may have been increased by previous experiences. For many children, this will be the first experience away from their parents in strange surroundings.

Some hospitals have facilities for admission of the mother to the same room so that she may stay with the child the night before surgery and the night after. This is good practice because it diminishes the child's sense of insecurity and abandonment. If dual admissions are not possible, the child should be admitted to a room with other children where the child would feel more comfortable. The child may be terrified if placed with a sick adult given to groaning or erratic behavior.

It is important that the child be given some explanation about the purpose of the visit to the hospital and the routines to be expected. Virtually, every hospital requires some preliminary investigations, including a chest x-ray, urinalysis, hemoglobin determination, and temperature reading. The child should be told that a few simple painless tests will be performed the day before surgery. The child should be informed by the parent that he or she will go to sleep and, on awakening, will find a bandage over one eye.

The parent should be instructed as to the time of discharge and the necessary office visits that may be required afterward. A fully informed parent will be a cooperative parent after surgery.

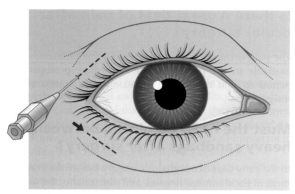

Fig 31.3 Subcutaneous infiltration anesthesia. The needle is pointed under the skin along the lower eyelid and the upper eyelid to anesthetize the skin and inactivate the orbicularis oculi muscle. (Modified from Berens C, King JH. *An Atlas of Ophthalmic Surgery*. Philadelphia: JB Lippincott; 1961.)

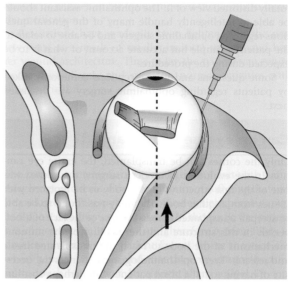

Fig 31.5 Advancement of needle in retrobulbar block. (From Allman KG. In: Yanoff M, Duker J, ed. *Ophthalmology*. 4th ed. Philadelphia: Elsevier Inc; 2014. All rights reserved.)

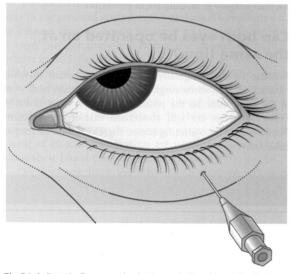

Fig 31.4 Retrobulbar anesthesia through the skin of the lower eyelid. The patient is asked to look up and away from the site of penetration of the needle. The needle penetrates the muscle cone behind the eye to paralyze the intraocular and extraocular muscles. (Modified from Berens C, King JH. *An Atlas of Ophthalmic Surgery*. Philadelphia: JB Lippincott; 1961.)

Retrobulbar anesthesia provides complete anesthesia of the globe and temporary paralysis to the muscles attached to the globe so that unwanted eye movements cannot occur during the procedure. The site of the penetration can be either through the skin (Fig. 31.4) or the conjunctiva (Fig. 31.5), the

needle coursing under the globe itself and the point of the needle emerging in the muscle cone of the eye (Fig. 31.6).

Peribulbar anesthesia has become increasingly popular as a result of occasional compression damage to the optic nerve caused by retrobulbar injections. In peribulbar anesthesia, a needle is directed down to the floor of the socket (or to the roof of the orbit) so that the anesthetic surrounds the soft tissue of the globe rather than being placed in the muscle cone itself.

Infiltration anesthesia may not be necessary with the new small incision and corneal incision surgery for cataracts. In intraocular (intracameral) anesthesia, developed by Dr. James Gills, an injection may be given into the anterior chamber at the start of cataract surgery to enhance patient comfort under topical anesthesia. The injection of 0.5 mL of preservative-free 1% lidocaine (Xylocaine) has resulted in a dramatic improvement in patient comfort, with a decrease in light sensitivity. This advance has led to essentially painless cataract surgery without the use of retrobulbar or peribulbar injections. Moxifloxacin and other unpreserved antibiotics may be used at the end of case by injection in the anterior chamber or behind the previously placed implant. In the rare case of endophthalmitis following cataract surgery, then antibiotics can be injected in the vitreous.

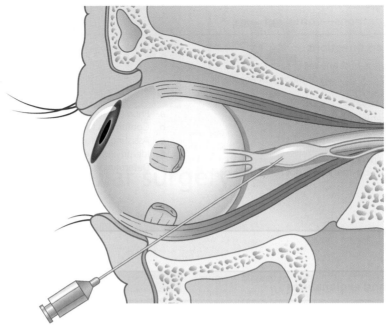

Fig 31.6 Point of destination of the retrobulbar injection. Note the needle point is in the muscle cone and amid the delicate nerves extending toward the eye. Injection of the anesthetic at this point paralyzes the muscles of the eye. (Modified from Berens C, King JH. *An Atlas of Ophthalmic Surgery*. Philadelphia: JB Lippincott; 1961.)

Questions for review and thought

1. Outline a routine to be followed in booking a patient for surgery.
2. Discuss the psychologic handling of a child who has to enter the hospital for strabismus surgery.
3. What forewarnings should be given to the adult patient before admission for major ocular surgery?
4. Discuss various types of anesthesia for cataract surgery.
5. What are the advantages of a local anesthetic over general anesthesia for cataract surgery?
6. What is the cataract-suturing technique in your center?

Self-evaluation questions   Q

True–false statements

Directions: Indicate whether the statement is true **(T)** or false **(F)**.

1. An important factor in scheduling patients for surgery is the length of the surgical procedure. **T** or **F**
2. An individual requests a certain date for surgery because of a forthcoming wedding in the family. This is considered an urgent booking. **T** or **F**
3. In advanced glaucoma, corneal transplantation may offer some hope in restoring vision. **T** or **F**

Missing words

Directions: Write in the missing word in the following sentences:

4. A lacerated globe is considered an _____ operation.
5. Children's surgery most often is performed under _____ anesthesia.
6. Anesthetic drops instilled in the eye are called _____ anesthesia.

Preparation

Patients are often seen by the family physician or internist at least 1 week before cataract surgery to ensure that medical conditions, such as diabetes and hypertension are under control. Also the ophthalmic surgeon should be provided with the names and dosages of the medications the patient may be taking.

Patients should be instructed to wash their hair before entering the hospital because hair washing is avoided during the first few postoperative days to prevent contamination of the wound by dirty rinse water. Smoking, of course, should be discouraged because a heavy cough can easily disrupt a fresh wound or initiate bleeding. With clear corneal microincisions performed under topical anesthesia, it is not necessary to discontinue aspirin or warfarin (Coumadin). If a peribulbar or retrobulbar block is given or a scleral incision is made, it is usually best to discontinue medication as this could result in bleeding.

Surgery

The object of cataract surgery is to remove the crystalline lens of the eye that has become cloudy. This is performed under an operating microscope that permits magnification. The technique of phacoemulsification is the most common method of removing cataracts today. An ultrasonic probe that vibrates rapidly can liquefy a lens through a microincision. This small-incision surgery has resulted in an incision size that has been reduced from 10 mm for extracapsular surgery to 1.8 to 2.2 mm for phacoemulsification. Special incision construction generally eliminates the need for sutures. This leads to minimal induced astigmatism and a rapid recovery. Most surgeons today perform cataract surgery in freestanding surgical centers on an outpatient basis (see Ch. 34).

Phacoemulsification

In 1963 Dr. Charles Kelman commenced research to ascertain the possibility of removing a cataract through a small incision. After attempting many preliminary techniques, including crushing, cutting, and drilling the lens, he finally perfected an apparatus and tip that he used to apply an oscillating and ultrasonic frequency to emulsify the cataract. He was attempting to improve on the system of cataract surgery that, in that era, consisted of freezing with a cryoprobe or by using a capsule forceps. With the phacoemulsifier, a microincision of less than 3 mm is required. This means less tissue destruction, less wound reaction, a quicker operation, less chance of wound disruption and its attendant complications, less astigmatism, and earlier ambulation and visual recovery (Box 32.1). In most cases, the patient is able to resume normal activities immediately after the operation.

Box 32.1 **Phacoemulsification**

Advantages

Small incision
Fewer wound problems
Less astigmatism
More rapid physical rehabilitation
Less risk of expulsive hemorrhage
Faster surgery
Quicker visual recovery

Disadvantages

Machine dependent
Longer learning period
Complications while learning
Expensive equipment
Difficult with hard nucleus
Need good pupil dilation
Difficult with small pupils

Skin and eye preparation

Before surgery, the skin around the eyelids is prepared with an antiseptic, most commonly povidone-iodine (Betadine) preparation. The eye is irrigated with a dilute solution of Betadine and balanced saline.

Anesthesia

Advances in anesthetic techniques have resulted in a dramatic change for both patients and surgeons. Retrobulbar injections into the orbit work well at providing anesthesia and akinesia. Unfortunately, the injections may be associated with complications that can include retrobulbar hemorrhage, intraocular penetration, and optic nerve penetration. The development of peribulbar injections decreases the chance of intraocular or optic nerve problems, but still can result in an orbital hemorrhage and discomfort. The use of topical anesthesia combined with intraocular lidocaine has revolutionized the way that surgery can be successfully performed.

After the superficial ocular structure is anesthetized with a topical anesthetic (e.g., tetracaine), a paracentesis is performed into the anterior chamber and 0.25 to 0.50 mL of 1% preservative-free lidocaine is injected into the anterior chamber. This results in dramatic anesthesia and usually eliminates all discomfort for the patient. The advantages of topical anesthesia are that it avoids all complications from orbital injections, provides increased safety for patients on anticoagulants, and results in an immediate recovery of vision because the optic nerve is not affected by this form of anesthesia.

Incision construction

Incision size has reduced with changes in techniques. The incision size for intracapsular cataract extraction was approximately 12 mm, with extracapsular cataract extraction 10 mm, and with phacoemulsification of around 2.5 mm. The advantages of a smaller incision are primarily less trauma to the eye, less astigmatic effect, and a quicker return to the former lifestyle. A self-sealing incision can be created in which there is an internal corneal lip of tissue that is closed off by the normal intraocular pressure. Sutures are not usually required. The induced astigmatism is minimal.

Continuous curvilinear capsulorrhexis

The technique involves making a small opening in the limbus or in the clear cornea and introducing a cystotome to cut an opening in the anterior capsule of the lens (Fig. 32.6). Previously, the opening into the anterior capsule was made with a capsulotomy needle by a series of jagged punctures that converted the central capsule into a series of postage-stamp cuttings. Currently, a continuous tear opening, often called *continuous curvilinear capsulorrhexis (CCC)*, is made by tearing the capsule so that the edges remain sharp, well demarcated, and very strong. This prevents extension into the periphery of tears of the capsule and permits the capsule

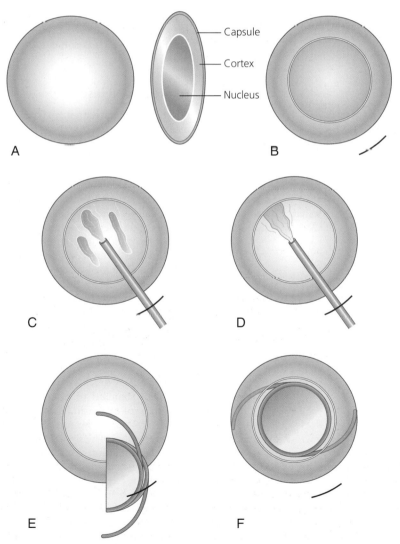

Fig. 32.6 Phacoemulsification. (A) Cataract. (B) Continuous curve capsulotomy. (C) Removal of nucleus. (D) Cortex aspiration and enlargement of incision. (E) Insertion of intraocular lens. (F) Wound closure.

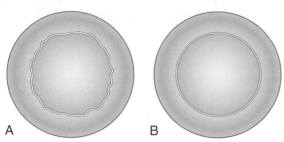

Fig. 32.7 (A) Can-opener capsulotomy. (B) Continuous curve capsulorrhexis.

to hold the lens implant securely (Fig. 32.7). This can be performed with better centration and circularity with the FS laser. The capsulotomy with a laser can be done on the line of sight, which allows the implant to be centered in the capsular bag.

Hydrodissection and hydrodelineation

Balanced saline can be injected into the lens to separate either the cortical material from the capsule *(hydrodissection)* or the nucleus from the epinucleus *(hydrodelineation)*. This allows the nucleus to be rotated freely within the capsular bag during the phaco technique. Separation of the nucleus from the epinucleus allows removal of the nucleus with phacoemulsification, leaving an underlying cushion of epinuclear tissue to protect against inadvertent rupture of the posterior capsule.

Machine design

Phaco equipment consists of a phaco tip that is inserted into the eye, a phaco handpiece that allows rapid vibration of the tip to liquefy the nucleus, and the machine that allows adjustments of a variety of parameters. The parameters that can be varied during each case include the amount of fluid infused into the eye, a vacuum level that allows suction of lens material, and the phaco energy that controls vibration frequency of the tip.

Phaco technique

There are a variety of techniques to emulsify and remove the nucleus, which may vary depending on the density of the cataract. A chopping technique uses a "chopper" to divide a nucleus into small segments before being emulsified. The phaco tip with high vacuum impales the nucleus and the chopper is used to divide the lens into fragments. A "divide and conquer" approach may be used in which a deep trench is created in the nucleus, and instruments are used to crack the nucleus into multiple pieces that can be

safely removed from the eye. A "flip" technique involves lifting or floating the nucleus above the capsule before emulsification is performed.

Sutures

The sutureless closure has resulted in more rapid rehabilitation after cataract surgery. The basic principle of sutureless incision is the creation of a valve-like self-sealing wound that is relatively small. The valve permits the incision to withstand unusual stress or intermittent raised intraocular pressure, which may follow in the postoperative period. The most common incision is made into clear cornea. If a scleral incision is made, various shapes of design have been advocated that lessen the degree of induced astigmatism. These include variations of straight incisions or a curvilinear incision, which is sometimes labeled the "frown and smile" incision.

Femtosecond laser

Advancements in technology have resulted in the development of laser cataract surgery (Fig. 32.8). Combining an FS laser (see following text) with a sophisticated imaging technique of optical coherence tomography (OCT) allows the laser to perform corneal wound construction (main incision and side-port incision); corneal relaxing incisions to reduce astigmatism; capsulorrhexis of an exact size, shape, and centration (Fig. 32.9); and fragmentation of the nucleus. The laser procedure is typically performed outside of the surgical operating room. After this procedure, the patient is taken to the surgical suite, where the eye is prepped and draped in the usual manner. A dull instrument is used to open the corneal wound incisions, and a viscoelastic substance is placed in the anterior chamber. A forceps is then used to grab the central capsule and pull this out from the eye. Hydrodissection and occasionally, hydrodelineation are performed. A phaco tip is then placed into the eye, and the nucleus, which was previously dismantled by the laser, is removed from the eye. The amount of phaco energy to remove the nucleus is significantly lower than with standard phacoemulsification. In fact, a high percentage of cases can be performed without any phaco energy. The remaining cortical material is aspirated from the capsular bag. The implant is then inserted through the small phaco incision, typically around 2.2 mm.

The main advantages of laser cataract surgery include less dexterity required on the part of the surgeon, an easier learning curve for beginner surgeons, more accurate and consistent corneal incisions, corneal relaxing incisions, and a perfectly round capsulorrhexis. In addition, because there is less energy used to liquefy the cataract, there is less intraocular turbulence, which can result in clearer postoperative corneas and a quicker visual recovery.

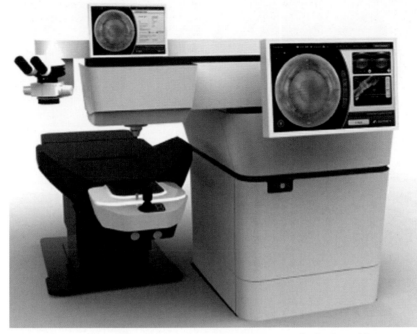

Fig. 32.8 Laser cataract unit for wound construction, limbal relaxing incisions, capsulorrhexis, and fragmentation of the nucleus. (Courtesy Optimedica, Santa Clara, CA.)

Intraocular lenses

Historically, one of the major problems after cataract surgery was the use of aphakic spectacles. Older adult patients had to bear the attendant magnifications and distortions by spectacles following cataract surgery. Contact lenses were developed, especially those that can be worn overnight or for extended wear, to avoid the handling difficulties of insertion and removal that are a constant hazard to the insecure older adult aphakic patient. The solution today has been in the direction of intraocular lens implants, which Ridley introduced in 1949. Through the pioneering efforts of Cornelius Binkhorst of Holland, Peter Choyce of England, Edward Epstein of South Africa, and Fyderov of Russia, the intraocular lens has become the major form of visual rehabilitation after cataract surgery. With the use of sodium hyaluronate (Healon) and other viscoelastic substances, endothelial damage is minimized during implant surgery. Magnification induced by spectacles and contact lenses has been reduced to zero with intraocular lenses through the positioning of the implant within the eye (Fig. 32.10).

The present-day success of intraocular lenses is a result of more skillful microsurgery, as well as better design, finish, and fixation of the lenses. In addition, a better understanding of positioning of the lenses within the capsular bag,

the use of the YAG laser for capsular opacification, and the better management and minimization of complications have led to significant success with intraocular lenses. Their use is indicated in virtually all patients undergoing cataract surgery.

Lens materials and design

Intraocular lenses are composed of an optical portion, called the "optics" of the lens, and the "haptics" (Fig. 32.11). The optics portion has a dioptric power that permits focusing light from afar onto the retina. The "size" of the optics varies from 5 to 7 mm in diameter. The term *haptics* is from the Greek word *haptesthai* meaning "to lay hold of." The haptics refer to the method of holding the optical portion in place in the human eye, which consists of loops that are made of either polymethyl methacrylate or Prolene. Polymethyl methacrylate is noteworthy as a hard, firm, inert material that has been singled out for the manufacture of quality intraocular lens optics and is inert in the human body. Loops made of this material are commonly used instead of Prolene. Prolene is a suture material that is also relatively inert in the human body and provides a softness and pliability that permit its support of the optical portion of the lens. Acrylic and silicone lenses have been developed, which are also inert inside the eye and

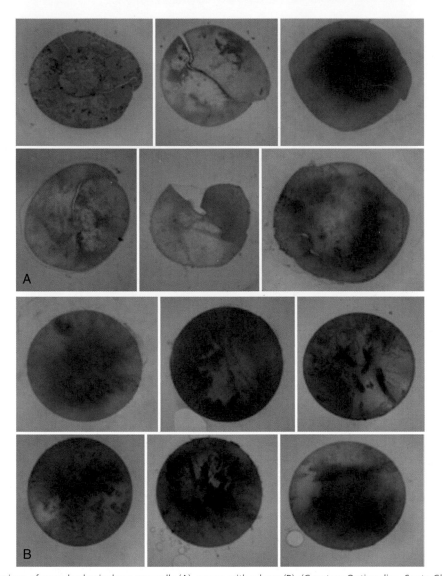

Fig. 32.9 Comparison of capsulorrhexis done manually (A), versus with a laser (B). (Courtesy Optimedica, Santa Clara, CA.)

can be folded so as to be inserted through a microincision. Titanium and metal loops have disappeared in the manufacture of intraocular lenses because of the adverse reaction they produce on the human retina. Loop designs are more flexible so as to permit greater adjustments within the structure of the eye itself to variations of the ocular changes that occur with each blink and contraction of the rectus muscles. This in itself has been a major step forward in the design of intraocular lenses.

The shape of the optical portion may be *planoconvex*, in which case the anterior portion of the lens is *convex*, whereas the back surface is flat. It may have reverse optics, in which the back surface of the lens is convex and the front surface is flat. It may alternatively be *biconvex*, in which both sides of the optical portion are convex. Some lenses are made *aspheric*, in which there is an alteration in power from the center of the lens to the periphery. Because of microincision surgery, foldable lenses are preferred.

Designs have incorporated an ultraviolet filter into the optical portion of the lens. This eliminates wavelengths in the ultraviolet spectrum less than 400 nm. The health of the cornea can be determined by specular microscopy on

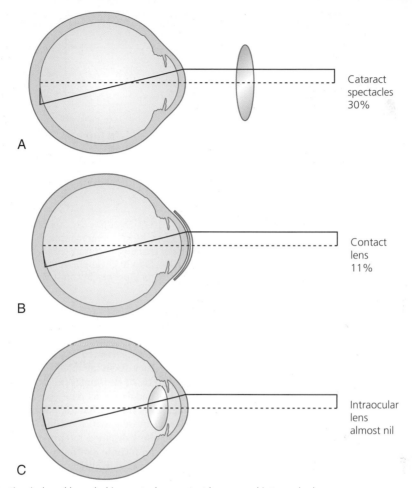

A

Cataract
spectacles
30%

B

Contact
lens
11%

C

Intraocular
lens
almost nil

Fig. 32.10 Magnification induced by aphakic spectacles, contact lenses, and intraocular lenses.

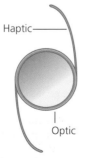

Haptic

Optic

Fig. 32.11 Intraocular lenses. (From Stein HA, Slatt BJ, Stein RM. *A Primer in Ophthalmology: A Textbook for Students*. St Louis: Mosby; 1992.)

corneal cell density (see Ch. 43) or by a guestimate using a × 1.6 objective lens with a slit lamp (see Fig. 32.5).

The power of the intraocular lenses varies from eye to eye. The use of optical coherence allows for the most accurate measurement of the axial length of the eye to determine the required power of the implant. The more common powers are about + 18.00 to + 22.00 diopters, but lenses are available for any power, including minus power and very high plus power.

Intraocular lenses also may be classified according to their position and their method of fixation. Anterior chamber lenses (Fig. 32.12) include lenses that lie in the anterior chamber of the eye. These may be angle-supported, in which case they are supported in the angle of the anterior chamber, or they may be iris-supported, in which case they may be attached with or without sutures to the iris. These lenses have almost become obsolete and are used only for

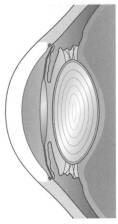

Fig. 32.12 Anterior chamber, angle-fixated intraocular lens.

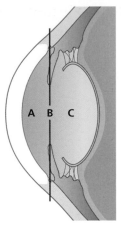

Fig. 32.14 Most common positions of intraocular lenses. (A) Anterior chamber. (B) Ciliary sulcus. (C) Capsular bag. (From Stein HA, Slatt BJ, Stein RM. *A Primer in Ophthalmology: A Textbook for Students*. St Louis: Mosby; 1992.)

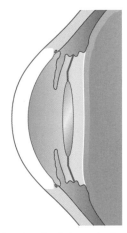

Fig. 32.13 Posterior chamber intraocular lens placed in the ciliary sulcus.

special purposes. Lenses are usually positioned in the posterior chamber and they may be supported by capsular support, in which case they may be called *in-the-bag lenses* (see Fig. 32.14C) because they are fitted directly into the capsular bag that contained the former crystalline lens, or they may be sulcus-supported (Fig. 32.13), in which case they lie in front of the remainder of the anterior capsule and are supported in the sulcus of the eye (Fig. 32.14B).

New developments in soft implants composed of silicone, hydrogels, and acrylic have heralded a new generation of implants, which may be folded and inserted through a much smaller incision. The development of *endocapsular* surgery with lens placement into the capsular bag has become state of the art.

Multifocal lenses *(bifocal intraocular lenses)* are another attempt to replace the human crystalline lens to provide a fuller range of vision. Bifocal intraocular lenses, which are sometimes referred to as *multifocal intraocular* lenses because they focus at many distances, have been introduced to try to eliminate spectacles entirely for the patient who has had a cataract removed. The advantage of multifocal lenses is simply that the patient does not require spectacles for most activities. Multifocal lenses separate rays of light to allow distance, intermediate, and near vision. Lens designs can include a diffractive optic, in which there are a series of rings with different step heights. Another design is a lens with different refractive zones. Because there is a separation of light rays with multifocal implants, there is an increased risk of glare and halos, as well as reduced contrast sensitivity. In many patients, the symptoms improve over 6 to 12 months. However, some patients can find night driving difficult.

Patient selection and expectations are critical to the acceptance of multifocal lenses. In general, the individual with type A personality is not a good candidate, nor are those who do a significant amount of night driving. In addition, patients with a limited visual potential are not good candidates, such as those with a diseased cornea (e.g., keratoconus or epithelial basement membrane dystrophy) or macular problems (e.g., age-related macular degeneration, macular hole, or epiretinal membrane). To achieve the best outcome, it is important to obtain the most precise biometric readings and to have the lens positioned in the capsular bag. Low postoperative astigmatism is also critical; this means correction of astigmatism at the time of surgery by limbal relaxing incisions or the insertion of a multifocal-toric implant.

Accommodating intraocular implants

An ideal implant would provide excellent vision at all focal distances. There is a great deal of research into the development of such a lens. The first lens approved in the United States was the crystal lens. This is a plate design with hinges that makes it capable of flexing. The proposed mechanism of action is that ciliary muscle contraction results in increased vitreous pressure that pushes the lens forward, with a resultant improvement in near vision. A YAG capsulotomy does not diminish the effectiveness of the lens.

The Restor implant and TECNIS multifocal implant use diffractive optics to provide distance, intermediate, and near vision. It is not uncommon for patients to experience some glare and halos, especially at night. These symptoms tend to decrease over time because of the mechanism of neuroadaptation. The TECNIS Symfony is an extended depth of focus implant that is designed with an elongated focal point to increase the depth of focus. This allows patients to have a broad range of vision and has been shown to have a lower risk of glare and halos.

The Panoptix (Alcon) is the latest diffractive multifocal that has shown improved results with a high patient satisfaction rate. It is considered a trifocal intraocular lens that is designed for distance, intermediate, and near vision. The Vivity lens (Alcon) is a nondiffractive implant that has a change in elevation to the central 2.5 mm of the lens to improve distance, intermediate, and some functional near. The incidence of halos and or glare with this lens is similar to a monofocal lens, and as a consequence, it can be used in those that drive frequently at night, type A individuals, or those with associated eye diseases like early macular degeneration or an epiretinal membrane.

A few new accommodative implants are under development. The FluidVision lens relies on liquid to make accommodative changes. By virtue of the natural human physiologic contraction and relaxation of the ciliary muscle, the fluid internal to the implant allows changes in shape like a pliable crystalline lens before the onset of presbyopia. The implant is acrylic and is filled with silicone oil. As the ciliary body muscle contracts and relaxes, forces are conveyed through the zonules and the capsule to the implant and the fluid in the haptics is pushed into the optic, causing the anterior curvature of the optic to increase. The lens is currently under clinical investigation.

Another prototype implant, the electroactive Sapphire AutoFocal, is an electromechanical lens equipped with a microscopic battery that stimulates shape change in the optic when sensing accommodation. As the pupil changes size and becomes smaller, the liquid crystals inside the lens are stimulated by electromechanical impulses, resulting in a change in the refractive lens to provide 3.00 diopters of reading. This implant does not rely on the muscles in the eye functioning and capsular bag contraction or hardening to be effective.

Corneal inlays for reading vision

An exciting new procedure for vision correction surgery is corneal inlays. These are small inserts placed under a LASIK flap or in a corneal pocket to enhance reading vision. The procedure is typically performed for presbyopic patients who have clear crystalline lenses and are interested in LASIK. However, pseudophakic patients, such as those following cataract surgery with a monofocal intraocular lens implant, may benefit from a corneal inlay to improve reading vision.

The Kamra corneal inlay was designed to increase the depth of field in the implanted eye. The inlay can enhance near and intermediate vision without a significant effect on distance acuity. Implantation can be combined with an excimer ablation to simultaneously address a refractive error and presbyopia. The inlay is implanted over the line of sight under a corneal flap or in a pocket. Unfortunately, the results have been disappointing over time because of an increased chance of corneal haze that may require explantation.

The Raindrop corneal inlay is intended to improve near and intermediate vision by changing the curvature of the cornea. The inlay steepens the central cornea for near vision and leaves the curvature of the more peripheral cornea unchanged for intermediate and distance vision. The material has a refractive index and water content similar to that of the human cornea. Distance acuity is minimally affected as light rays paracentral to the 2-mm inlay remain primarily focused on the retina, particularly with a middilated or dilated pupil. Pupil constriction creates a pseudoaccommodative effect using the steep and central cornea to focus light rays for near. Unfortunately, similar to the Kamra inlay a late inflammatory reaction has resulted in corneal haze in a high percentage of patients, and as a consequence the manufacturer is no longer in business.

A corneal inlay made from corneal tissue (allograft) offers the best potential to this method of presbyopia correction without an inflammatory reaction. Clinical trials look promising to date and should be available in the near future. One human cornea can provide around hundred corneal inlays.

Historical methods

Intracapsular cataract surgery

The intracapsular operation is rarely used today. If a lens is dislocated or has extremely poor zonular support, it is generally best to remove the entire lens through a large limbal incision. Because the capsule is completely removed with this technique, an anterior chamber lens or a sutured posterior chamber lens must be inserted. A cataract with weak zonules can undergo phacoemulsification with caution and with the insertion of a capsular tension ring that is placed into the capsular bag to expand its diameter before the insertion of an implant.

Extracapsular cataract surgery

This is becoming a historic procedure in North America, but in underdeveloped countries without the advantage of new technology, it continues to be a common procedure. A retrobulbar anesthetic or peribulbar injection is used to anesthetize the globe. Facial nerve paralysis may be produced by an O'Brien, Van Lint, or Nadblath anesthetic, but such anesthesia may not be necessary. The Honan intraocular pressure reducer or the superpinky ball, championed by Dr. James Gills, significantly lowers the intraocular pressure before surgery. Hand massage also may be used, but one should guard against excessive massage because of the possibility of central retinal artery or vein obstruction.

An incision is made at the superior limbus and a small opening is made into the anterior chamber. A viscoelastic substance is introduced. A small bent needle or cystotome is introduced and a cut is made into the anterior capsule in a circular can-opener, triangular, or D-shaped fashion (anterior capsulotomy) (Fig. 32.15). The wound is enlarged in extracapsular surgery to a chord diameter of 10 to 11 mm (approximately a 150-degree arc or smaller) to allow removal of the cataractous nucleus.

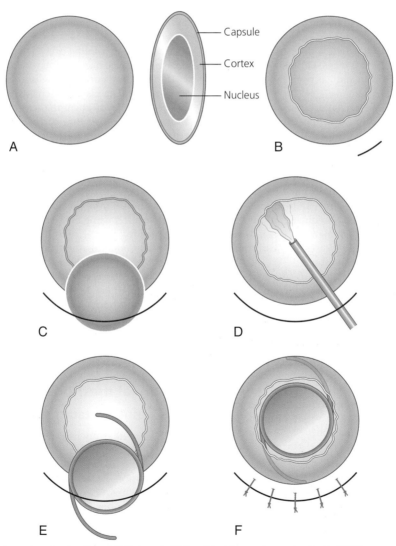

Fig. 32.15 Extracapsular cataract extraction. (A) Cataract. (B) Small incision and capsulorrhexis. (C) Phacoemulsification of lens. (D) Cortex aspiration. (E) Insertion of folded lens. (F) Rotation of lens in capsule.

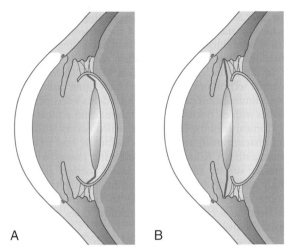

Fig. 32.16 Posterior chamber intraocular lens. (A) Capsular bag insertion. (B) Sulcus insertion.

The nucleus is then expressed from the eye. Sutures are inserted to maintain the anterior chamber so that the remaining cortex can be removed. The cortex may be removed by a manual method (e.g., Simcoe or McIntyre needle) or by an automated system. These are sometimes referred to as I/A units (irrigating/aspirating units). These instruments irrigate balanced salt into the eye in proportion to the amount of aspiration occurring. The automated systems are foot-controlled.

Once all of the cortex is removed from the capsular bag, the posterior capsule may be "polished" to remove any residual plaques. An intraocular lens is then inserted into the posterior chamber. This lens may be positioned either into the capsular bag (Fig. 32.16A) or into the sulcus (Fig. 32.16B). The capsular bag is preferred.

Sutures are then placed in the cornea or the corneoscleral wound. These may be radial interrupted sutures, a continuous suture, or a combination of the two. At the end of the procedure, an antibiotic (e.g., vancomycin) may be given intraocularly in the anterior chamber, or an antibiotic-steroid combination injection may be given subconjunctivally (Box 32.2).

The essential difference between intracapsular surgery and extracapsular surgery is that in the former the entire lens and capsule are removed from the eye, whereas in the latter the posterior capsule remains intact, permitting a pocket for an intraocular lens.

The large incision and sutures with extracapsular surgery usually result in induced astigmatism of a significantly greater degree than with phacoemulsification. Sutures may be removed at 4 to 6 weeks to reduce astigmatism. In general, the visual recovery may be more prolonged than with phacoemulsification.

Femtosecond laser cataract surgery

FS cataract surgery is considered to be one of the most significant advances in cataract surgery in 50 years. Laser cataract surgery has shown excellent results for accurate self-sealing corneal incisions; arcuate incisions to reduce astigmatism; highly circular, strong, and well-positioned capsulorrhexis; and potentially a safer and less technically difficult cataract removal with almost complete elimination of phacoemulsification. Laser technology may allow ophthalmologists to meet the demands of cataract patients to the same level that has been accomplished with laser vision correction.

The technology today recognizes clear corneal incisions. The benefits of clear corneal incisions are that they are well tolerated by patients, provide a rapid recovery of vision, preserve the subconjunctival space for future filtering procedures, and allow improved visibility during phacoemulsification as a result of the shorter tunnel. There are reports of an increased incidence of endophthalmitis that may be related to the use of clear corneal incisions. Although the incidence of endophthalmitis is only 0.13%, this remains the most feared complication of cataract surgery with a potential devastating effect. Endophthalmitis after cataract surgery with a permanent decrease in vision can affect an individual's quality of life, including productivity.

A clear corneal incision that is poorly constructed may result in leakage, hypotony, iris prolapse, or endophthalmitis. Cataract incisions created with a blade typically have a simple uniplanar configuration, with a suboptimal construction, and fluids may leak in and out of the eye. This increases the risk of endophthalmitis because bacteria from the tear film may enter the anterior chamber of the eye. Future studies will address the ideal architecture of the corneal incision to prevent leakage and minimize astigmatism induction. The FS laser has the potential to create a more

The postoperative loss of the anterior chamber may result from any of the following events:

1. Leaking wound diagnosed by Seidel test, that is, observing the escaping aqueous wash away fluorescein from the leak in the wound; the wound requires suturing
2. Inhibition of aqueous secretion in the treatment of glaucoma by acetazolamide and beta-blocker drops
3. Postoperative ocular trauma; patients should wear protective shields while asleep
4. Pupillary block (raised intraocular pressure); treat by immediate dilation or peripheral iridectomy

Iritis

In its mildest form, iritis may manifest as broad, thin, gray, or brown deposits on the intraocular lens precipitates, sometimes with cells in the anterior chamber or aqueous flare. The goal of treatment of iritis is to prevent synechiae (adhesions of the iris) implanting because they may be the precursors of retrolenticular membrane formation and glaucoma.

It is advisable to use mydriatic agents to promote gentle dilation and pupillary motion. Therapy depends on topical steroids to control the inflammation.

Retinal detachment

This occurs more frequently after cataract surgery and YAG laser treatment, especially in patients with a history of a high degree of myopia. This risk is increased if surgery is complicated by rupture of the posterior capsule with vitreous loss. A sudden loss of full or half vision is an important symptom.

Cystoid macular edema

This condition can be defined as an extracellular, intraretinal edema at the macula, which may be demonstrated by fluorescein angiography or with an OCT. Clinically, the patient manifests a reduction in visual acuity or distortion that may disappear over a period of time. A transient hyperopic shift in the refractive error usually occurs. The etiology of cystoid macular edema is unknown, but it may be precipitated by rupture of the posterior capsule and vitreous loss. In the majority of cases, the macular edema occurs in an otherwise uncomplicated procedure. The edema can occur in the early postoperative period, within 6 weeks, or later. The use of topical steroid and nonsteroidal drops promotes resolution of the edema. Rarely the cystoid macular edema may be chronic, resulting in a permanent loss of vision (Fig. 32.18).

Intraocular lens decentration

The implant occasionally can be noted to be decentered in a downward direction (*sunset syndrome*) or resting superiorly

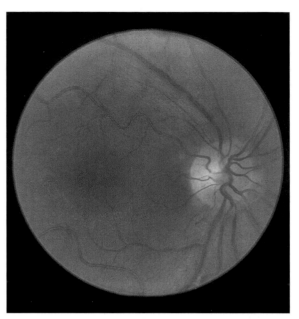

Fig. 32.18 Cystoid macular edema. (Reproduced from Spalton D, Hitchings R, Hunter P. *Atlas of Clinical Ophthalmology*, 3rd ed. St Louis: Mosby; 2004, with permission.)

(*sunrise syndrome*). If the decentration is associated with symptoms (e.g., glare, halos, or decreased vision), then surgical reposition or exchange of the implant is required.

Incorrect intraocular lens power

If the refractive error is significantly off from that intended and produces anisometropia, the implant can be exchanged. Other options include a secondary implant in the sulcus to correct the residual refractive error, or refractive surgery, such as LASIK or PRK.

Retained lens material (Fig. 32.19)

Occasionally, cortical material, recognized as fluffy white in appearance, can be noted in the anterior chamber. This usually resolves through absorption with time. Nuclear material, characterized as yellow or brown in appearance, also may be noted. If this is minimal in size, it will usually absorb with time. However, if there is more significant nuclear material, especially if a secondary uveitis occurs, surgical removal of the fragments is necessary.

Endophthalmitis (Fig. 32.20)

This is a true ocular emergency. Symptoms may consist of any or all of pain, redness, and decreased vision occurring in the first week postoperatively. The overall incidence is

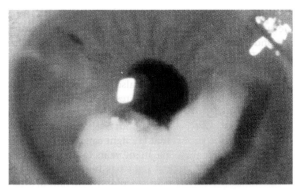

Fig. 32.19 Retained lens material.

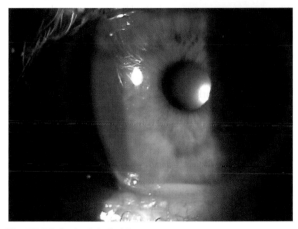

Fig. 32.20 Endophthalmitis.

0.01%, often associated with pain. Patients are often admitted to the hospital and treated with topical, intravitreal, and even intravenous antibiotics after specimens are taken from the anterior chamber and vitreous. If there is significant inflammation on initial presentation, a vitrectomy is often performed to improve the prognosis.

Final visual acuity is guarded unless the infection is recognized early and treated aggressively. The use of preoperative prophylactic broad-spectrum antibiotics, attention to surgical sterility, and the use of intraocular antibiotics into the anterior chamber at the conclusion of the procedure have further decreased the incidence of this complication in recent years.

Astigmatism

Significantly induced astigmatism with small incision and no-stitch phacoemulsification is uncommon. There is usually no induced astigmatism with an incision around 2.2 mm. There is typically a 0.50 diopter change in the astigmatism with a 3-mm incision. The larger the incision, the greater is the induced astigmatism. Temporal incisions also tend to induce less astigmatism than superior incisions. If significant preoperative astigmatism exists, limbal relaxing incisions or an astigmatic keratotomy can be performed at the time of surgery. Toric implants can be inserted and aligned in the eye to decrease astigmatism. If there is induced astigmatism and the patient is unable to tolerate this in a glass or contact lens, then incisional corneal surgery or laser vision correction can be performed.

Capsular opacification

If this is associated with diminished vision or symptoms of glare, then a YAG capsulotomy can be performed. Advances in intraocular lens designs with a square-edged optic have dramatically decreased the incidence of capsular haze. If a foldable silicone plate lens has been inserted, it is best to wait until at least 4 months after surgery to decrease the chance of dislocation of the implant into the vitreous following a YAG capsulotomy. Patients should be aware that there is an increased risk of a retinal detachment or cystoid macular edema following a YAG capsulotomy (Fig. 32.21).

Pseudophakic bullous keratopathy

Corneal decompensation may occur following cataract surgery, and this may be noted in the early postoperative period or typically months to years after the procedure. Preoperative risk factors include the presence of corneal guttata, Fuch's corneal dystrophy (guttata with edema), or a low endothelial cell count. Surgical risk factors include the insertion of an anterior chamber lens, prolonged phaco procedure time, or rupture of the posterior capsule. An endothelial graft or penetrating keratoplasty can be offered to improve both comfort and vision. An extended-wear bandage soft contact lens can improve the comfort if a patient is not interested in surgical repair or while waiting for keratoplasty. Hypertonic drops and ointment (Muro 128 5%) will decrease epithelial edema and enhance comfort (Fig. 32.22).

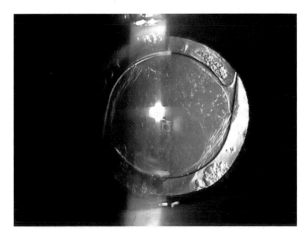

Fig. 32.21 Capsular opacification.

In ophthalmology, the *argon laser* can alter the trabecular meshwork and increase outflow of aqueous (see Glaucoma section earlier). It can be used for gonioplasty and for iridotomy because it can coagulate, retard, or destroy new vessel growth in the anterior and posterior segments of the eye. The nd:YAG laser also has a wide variety of uses in ophthalmology, but its most popular use has been that of opening the posterior capsule when it has become opacified.

The YAG laser is widely used today. Contrary to popular belief, this laser does not remove cataracts. Within months or years after a cataract has been removed, eye surgeons frequently use the YAG laser to clear cloudy secondary membranes. This results in restoration of vision by a noninvasive method of opening these membranes. The procedure is not painful and requires no hospitalization. The YAG laser is a "cold" type of laser and uses quick pulses of laser energy on clear tissues within the eye. It also is used for performing an iris iridotomy in cases of narrow-angle glaucoma.

Corneal transplantation

The cornea is the clear portion in the front part of the eye that is similar to the transparent covering on a watch. When injury, degeneration, or infection occurs that causes the cornea to become cloudy, vision is disrupted. Only by replacing a portion of the cornea with a clear window taken from a donor eye can vision be restored.

Not everyone with a corneal disease can be helped by corneal transplantation.

The cornea, because it is devoid of blood vessels, is one of the few tissues in the human body that may be transplanted from one human being to another with a large degree of success. The absence of blood vessels in both the donor and the host cornea reduces the allergic reaction, in which reactive immunoglobulins are carried through blood flow, and permits the body to retain and not reject the foreign cornea. Thus only those conditions in which the cornea is free of blood vessels are suitable for transplantation.

Two basic types of corneal transplantation are performed. One is the *lamellar* or *partial penetrating procedure*, in which a half thickness of cornea is transferred from the eye of a donor to that of the host (Fig. 32.27A). In this procedure, the anterior chamber of the eye is not entered and only the outer half or two-thirds of the cornea is transplanted. Union is made of the donor cornea with the host cornea by means of several interrupted fine sutures or a continuous suture around the periphery of the donor button. The donor button varies anywhere from 6 to 10 mm in diameter, depending on the extent of the disease involved. The second type of transplant operation is the *penetrating* or

full-thickness corneal transplant (Fig. 32.27B). In this operation, the full thickness of the cornea is removed from the donor eye and replaces the full thickness of the central portion of the host cornea. The surgery involves entering the anterior chamber, inserting the donor cornea, and establishing a tight fit by direct suture closure or a continuous suture (Fig. 32.28). A viscoelastic is often used to minimize endothelial damage.

In the postoperative period, the most common complications include a wound leak, suture breakage and wound dehiscence, infection, and graft rejection. If detected early and managed appropriately, these complications can be controlled or eliminated, enabling a high level of success for the operation. Thus careful monitoring by the doctor, nurse, or ophthalmic assistant is required.

In both the lamellar and full-thickness corneal transplant, the donor and the host buttons are trephined with a round cutting trephine, which cleanly and sharply removes the affected part. The cornea taken from a recently deceased person is then carefully sutured in place (Fig. 32.29).

New advanced corneal procedures to replace a diseased cornea caused by poor endothelial cell function include Descemet's stripping (automated) endothelial keratoplasty (DSEK/DSAEK) and Descemet's membrane endothelial keratoplasty (DMEK).

DSEK/DSAEK is a partial-thickness corneal transplant. The procedure involves replacing a patient's own Descemet's membrane and diseased endothelial cells with a thin graft of posterior corneal stroma, Descemet's membrane, and healthy endothelium from a donor. This means that the rest of the patient's cornea is left intact as opposed to the entire tissue being replaced as with a traditional penetrating keratoplasty or full-thickness corneal transplant. The DSEK procedure is indicated in patients with diseased or damaged endothelial cells, such as in Fuchs dystrophy or pseudophakic corneal edema. In cases where only the back-most part of the cornea is diseased or damage, it is not always necessary to perform a full-thickness transplant. Partial-thickness transplants by and large have a quicker visual recovery time and are more comfortable for the patient. Because less of the tissue is transplanted, there is also a greatly reduced risk of rejection.

A DMEK is performed in much the same way as the DSEK/DSAEK, with the main difference being that the graft used is only 5 to 10 microns thick. This makes the tissue much more delicate and even more difficult to handle. Surgeons have to take extra precautions and find unique ways to manipulate it to move it into position. Because the DMEK tissue does not contain stromal tissue, the grafts are typically able to mold to the host tissue with less unevenness at the juncture where the edge of the graft tissue and the host tissue meet. This leads to quicker visual recovery and less induced refractive error post operatively.

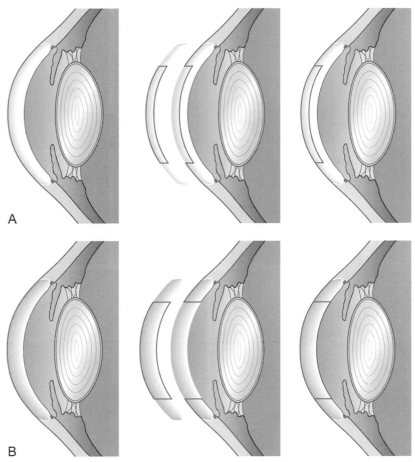

Fig. 32.27 Corneal transplant. (A) Lamellar, or partial penetrating, corneal transplant. The clouded outer portion of the cornea is removed and replaced with clear donor cornea. (B) Penetrating, or full-thickness, corneal transplant. The entire central portion of clouded cornea is removed and replaced with clear donor cornea.

Eyelid surgery

Entropion is a condition in which the eyelashes roll in and rub against the cornea. Numerous types of eyelid operations are performed for the correction of this condition. One of the simplest is Ziegler cautery, in which the cautery is applied to the area just below the eyelashes. Other procedures include tightening the underlying muscles of the eyelid or removing a wedge of tarsus from the inner aspect of the eyelid.

Ectropion occurs when the eyelid rolls outward. This may be the result of scarring from burns, and insertion of skin grafts taken elsewhere is required to reduce the pull from the scar tissue. Grafts of skin for the eyelids may be taken from upper eyelids or from behind the ears. In some cases, ectropion results from a laxity of the skin and underlying structures. This requires surgical removal of these tissues to properly evert the lid so that the lid margin lies in its correct position against the globe.

Ptosis occurs when the eyelid droops to cover the upper portion of the pupil (Fig. 32.30). Investigation in the adult should rule out medical causes before surgery is undertaken. If the levator muscle still functions, a resection of this muscle will be performed, either from the undersurface of the eyelid or through the eyelid skin. In this procedure, the muscle is identified and shortened by a measured amount of millimeters. When the levator muscle is completely paralyzed, the eyelid may be suspended from the brow muscles to the tarsal plate by use of fascia lata taken from the thigh or from cadavers, by collagen tapes, or by white silk sutures.

Answers, notes, and explanations   **A**

1. **False**. In recession of a muscle, the reattachment is made at a point toward the posterior portion of the eye and away from the cornea. This in effect weakens the pull of the muscle so that it has a less effective contraction. In convergent strabismus, the medial rectus may be recessed, whereas in divergent strabismus, the lateral rectus is recessed.

2. **True**. Cryosurgery involves the use of a probe cooled by liquid nitrogen, carbon dioxide, or Freon, so that the temperature ranges anywhere from − 20°C to − 70°C. By so lowering the temperature, a small probe can be applied to the lens of the eye to create an iceball formation and adhesion of the lens to the probe. This forms a bond that is useful in extracting the cataract. Cryotherapy is also used to destroy lashes and hair follicles. It is used in retinal detachment repair to create adhesions of the tissues themselves. It may be used in glaucoma to shrink the vascular coat of the eye.

3. **True**. In this procedure, which has gained widespread acceptance throughout the world, ultrasound is used in a small probe that enters the eye. By means of high-frequency sound waves, the cutting edge impinges on the cataractous lens and emulsifies it so it can be easily removed by aspiration.

4. **Enucleation**. Enucleation is performed whenever an eye is diseased and painful, or a malignant tumor is present. During enucleation, all muscles are severed from the globe and then the optic nerve is severed and the globe removed. An implant of plastic, glass, or silicone is placed in the socket to fill the defect left by removal of the eye. An artificial eye is then fashioned that moves with the implant and simulates the appearance of a normal eyeball.

5. **Trabeculectomy**. Trabeculectomy is the removal of a portion of the trabeculum to improve the outflow of fluid from the eye. It thereby reduces the devastating destructive effect that the elevated intraocular pressure of glaucoma creates.

6. **Ectropion**. An eyelid that turns out is called an *ectropion*, from *ec-* meaning "out." This may occur as the result of scarring of the overlying eyelid tissue (cicatricial ectropion) or from the laxity of the muscles (senile ectropion) as occurs in older adults. Surgical correction is the only means to repair an ectropion.

7. **c. Giving systemic antibiotics**. An operation, such as strabismus surgery, performed in a sterile environment requires no systemic antibiotics. Topical antibiotics may be given at the time of surgery and may even be given by some ophthalmologists in the postoperative period. This is usually satisfactory to overcome any invading organism. The rich blood supply of both the vascular coat and the muscles of the eye is usually sufficient to take care of any inflammation that may arise. This situation, however, may not be true for intraocular surgery when there is an absence of blood vessels and thus an absence of the vascular response to an invading microbacterial organism. In these intraocular cases, antibiotics may be preferred to raise the intraocular level of the antibiotics to prevent infection.

8. **e. Ziegler cautery**. All the procedures except Ziegler cautery are used for either narrow-angle or wide-angle glaucoma. Ziegler cautery is used to correct a spastic entropion of the eyelid.

9. **d. Keratoconus**. Keratoconus is a progressive out-pouching and thinning of the cornea with rupturing and scar formation. A corneal transplant is required when the cone has reached the point at which contact lenses or spectacles can no longer satisfactorily correct vision. The cornea eventually may become extremely thin, in which case a penetrating corneal transplant is required.

Assisting the surgeon

Most surgical procedures for the eye are performed on an outpatient basis. However, some procedures (e.g., retinal surgery, high-risk patients, cardiac surgery) are still performed in the hospital. This chapter highlights those patients who are admitted. Chapter 34 covers ambulatory or outpatient surgery.

Bedside ophthalmic assistant

One of our most important senses is that of sight. A blind or partially sighted individual is considerably impaired in the ability to move about freely, perform work, and function effectively. Daily living is seriously jeopardized. Consequently, any threat of loss or impairment of these abilities is a threat to an individual's independence.

Without sight, no longer can drivers drive their cars, pilots fly their planes, or surgeons perform their work. Because of the consequences of blindness and the fear associated with this threat, the nursing care of patients with eye disorders demands extraordinary skill.

The background for ophthalmic nursing requires a good understanding of people and their management. Psychologic problems induced by the emotional havoc created by the threat of losing one's vision must be dealt with effectively. Ophthalmic assistants interested in eye nursing will become involved in these emotional reactions.

General nurses are expected to increase their knowledge of the eye and eye disorders. They must become familiar with the terminology and acquainted with various diagnostic tests and surgical procedures. They also must become aware of the relationship between disease of the eye and disease of the body. A gentle touch and fine dexterity are prerequisites in caring for patients, particularly when administering eye medications and treating eyes that have undergone recent surgery. Nurses must move about quietly in the rooms of such patients, not dash into the room, bump into beds or chairs, or in any way startle patients who could become alarmed because they cannot see anyone's movements. Ophthalmic nursing is essentially "quiet" nursing. The successful restoration or, indeed, improvement in eyesight often provides a stimulating and rewarding experience for ophthalmic nurses.

Visually impaired patient

Blindness is considered to be a total lack of vision or vision insufficient to conduct the ordinary activities of life. It is defined as a central visual acuity of 20/200 or less in the better eye with corrective glasses or a field defect in which the peripheral field is contracted to such an extent that the widest diameter of the visual field subtends an angle not greater than 20 degrees.

With both these limitations, a person is *economically* blind. A vast majority of the blind are in the group just below this threshold. Some are able to read newspaper headlines and some can identify distant objects. They may see light in various directions—in the corridors and the windows and in the streets. Only in the most severe form is the blind person completely devoid of any light sensation.

Some blind patients live in false hope of a possible cure and refuse to adjust to their decrease in vision. Others withdraw from society and lean heavily on their visual defect.

Table 33.1 Hospital chart abbreviations

Abbreviation	Meaning	Abbreviation	Meaning
Aa	of each	mg	milligram
Ac	before meals	non rep	do not repeat
ad lib	as desired	ocul	eye
Amp	ampule	od	right eye
Bid	twice a day	os	left eye
c or cum	with	ou	each eye
Caps	capsule	pc	after meals
Cc	cubic centimeter	po	by mouth
Collyr	eyewash	prn	as needed
Dr	dram	qh	every hour
G	gram	qid	four times a day
Gr	grain	qs	sufficient quantity
Gt	drop	s	without
Hs	at bedtime	ss	half
Ic	between meals	stat	immediately
IM	intramuscular	tab	tablet
IV	intravenous	tid	three times a day
Lot	lotion	ung	ointment

Any evidence of small amounts of whitish material in the lower portion of the anterior chamber is an ominous sign and should be brought to the attention of the ophthalmologist immediately. It indicates a developing hypopyon, which may arise from an intraocular infection. If accompanied by severe pain, it is even more ominous and should be brought to the immediate attention of the surgeon or doctor on call.

Marked swelling of the eyelids combined with excoriation of the skin should be noted. This is a common sign of allergy to the medication that is being introduced or of an infection that may be starting. Unusual complaints of pain in the immediate postoperative period should be quickly brought to the attention of the ophthalmologist because occasionally, wound rupture or infection does occur, which is marked by severe pain. Evidence of a purulent discharge postoperatively is a warning sign.

Instructions to patient on discharge

When the patient is discharged from the hospital, or even if an outpatient, he or she should be given instructions that will ensure the continuing success of the eye surgery. Eyes that have had surgery require cautious care for the first few weeks after operation (Box 33.1).

Each ophthalmologist has specific individual methods of dealing with patients. The physician's input is most important in giving directions to patients. Typed discharge instructions similar to those in Box 33.1 are helpful.

Operating room assistant

Many ophthalmic assistants working in offices and clinics have the privilege of accompanying the ophthalmologist to the operating room. Here a new challenge awaits.

The drama of the operating room, the exactness, care, and detail required in eye surgery and the satisfaction resulting from a successful procedure instill a sense of accomplishment in the assistant at the end of each operating period. Here, the operating room assistant is expected to fulfill his or her role with the utmost gentleness, care, and attention.

Box 33.1 **Directions for patients leaving the hospital after cataract surgery**

1. Your wound is healing, but it will not be firm enough to stand much pressure. You may feel that something is in your eye. This is because of the stitches or the incision. This feeling will go away. Continue to be careful.
2. Avoid closing the eyes tightly. One often closes the eyes tightly when laughing, talking, sneezing, coughing or yawning, or if irritated. At these times, you should be particularly careful not to close your eyes tightly. Never rub or touch the eye.
3. Avoid stooping, straining, lifting, and bending over.
4. If there is much secretion then wipe off the lids with cotton, but avoid exerting pressure on the eye, particularly the upper lid.
5. You will be given drops to use in your eye. Please follow these directions carefully. When the drops are gone, fill your prescription and use those drops.

How to instill drops

a. Wash your hands thoroughly before and after putting in eyedrops and ointments.
b. Clean the edges of your eyelids, using a clean cotton ball or washcloth that has been moistened with tap water. Do not press on the upper lid.

c. Pull your lower lid down with one hand, forming a pouch. Look up.
d. Put one drop of medicine in the pouch. Do not touch the tip of the bottle to your lid, eyelashes, or any other place.
e. Close your eye for 1 full minute after each drop.
f. If you find the preceding difficult, lie on the bed and repeat the instructions while looking up at the dropper.
g. Never use eyedrops that are more than 2 months old. Discard them.

6. You may watch television and read.
7. You may go outdoors for a walk or drive. It is not necessary to cover the eye, but it is preferable to shield it from bright sunlight by wearing sunglasses with ultraviolet protection.
8. You may wash your hair 1 week after surgery, but do not get soapy water in your eye.
9. Mild pain and discomfort may be relieved by aspirin. If there is more severe pain, please contact us.
10. You may have the feeling of something in the eye because of the incision, but do not close it tightly. This feeling may persist for a few weeks.
11. Glasses or contact lens may be prescribed when the eye is fully healed and the prescription is stable.

The ophthalmic nurse probably will be responsible for the selection, care, handling, and sterilization of the many ophthalmic instruments required. A meticulous scrub and gown routine must be followed. One should be exceptionally careful that the exact sterile technique in scrubbing, gowning, and draping in the operating room is not broken by any member of the team, lest an infection develop that not only may cause irreparable damage but also result in blindness and even removal of the eye itself (Fig. 33.1).

The use of powderless gloves has been a major help in reducing airborne particles.

The operating room must be quiet except for background music; CD players or tapes are helpful. Sudden loud noises might make the patient move unexpectedly and endanger the eye. All those who assist the ophthalmologist must ensure that the environment is pleasant and quiet from the time the patient is brought into the room until he or she leaves. Personal talk, such as politics, vacation, sports, and other patients should be avoided.

Aseptic technique in the operating room

Although surgery has been practiced since ancient times, the practice of asepsis is recent. As long ago as 3000 BCE, Egyptians bored holes in skulls to let evil spirits out. Even in 700 BCE, the Hindus performed cataract and eyelid surgery. Those who performed the surgery learned to keep their fingernails short, take daily baths, and wear white clothing. It was only in the 19th century that Joseph Lister introduced modern surgical aseptic techniques. Lister recognized that results of surgery improved 10-fold if microorganisms could be kept out of the wound. Thus many methods of sterilization of instruments and preparations for cleansing and disinfecting the skin came into being, until today's modern methods were attained. Aseptic technique is discussed in Chapter 30. Strict adherence to the principles of instrument sterilization, skin disinfection, and eye preparation is essential to eliminate ocular infections, which can be visually devastating (Box 33.2).

Routine procedure for the operating room assistant

Before scrubbing

Assistants must know the operative procedure well, even if it requires additional reading for them to become familiar with the technique. There should be a regularly updated card or page listing the surgeon's preferences

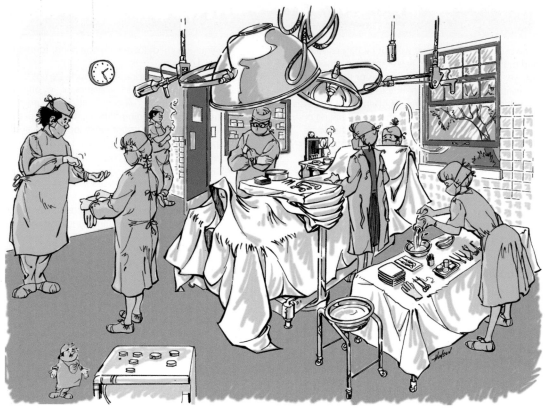

Fig. 33.1 Errors in aseptic techniques. Identify all errors of aseptic technique.

in instruments, sutures, and preparation of the patient. Assistants should question other operating room personnel who have worked with the surgeon to understand his or her special variations. If all are unfamiliar with the procedure, assistants should not hesitate to contact the surgeon a day or two before surgery to ensure that all necessary equipment is available.

Bringing the patient to surgery

The patient should be as relaxed as possible. A cheerful but quiet manner will provide an atmosphere of relaxation. Assistants should try to instill optimism and confidence in patients and should be particular to point out that everything will go well. They should always express confidence in the skill of the surgeon. It has been our habit to play soft music in the operating room throughout the procedure to ensure relaxation. Coming to the operating room for surgery is a unique and often terrifying experience for the patient. Each patient should be treated as if he or she were the only one and not one of many who pass through each day.

Cutting the eyelashes is not routinely performed for all procedures and may be abandoned by many surgeons since the advent of newer draping techniques. However, when it is necessary, the eyelashes should be cut before skin preparation. A thin film of ointment is placed on the cutting edge of an eyelash scissors so that the free lashes will adhere to the blades and be prevented from falling into the eye. The patient should be reassured that the lashes will rapidly regrow.

Scrubbing

Assistants should carefully clean the area under their nails with a nail file or orangewood stick before scrubbing. The water should be at a comfortable temperature. Many sinks have elbow, knee, or foot controls so that adjustments can be made during the scrub technique. Assistants should adhere to the required time and the antiseptics used in any given hospital. They must be sure to follow a definite scrub routine so that no bare areas or blind spots occur on the sides of fingers, back of hands, or back of arms (Fig. 33.2). There should be at least 20 to 30 brush strokes for every portion of skin. The water and the debris should always be allowed

Box 33.2 Some common errors in aseptic surgical techniques (see Fig. 33.1)

Masks and caps

1. Mask covering only the mouth and not the nose
2. Mask tied too loosely
3. Hair permitted to protrude from the cap

Scrub

1. Fingernails too long (should not exceed 1 mm)
2. Allowing the runoff to drip from the hands, thus contaminating them (runoff should be from the elbow)
3. Too short a scrub time
4. Failing to develop a systematic scrub routine and thus leaving bare spots
5. Splashing the clothes, thus contaminating sterile gown later

Drying

1. Using wet section of towel to dry upper arms, thus contaminating dry fingers
2. Allowing towel to touch unsterile clothing

Gowning

1. Allowing gown to become contaminated by the hands or other unsterile objects

2. Allowing gown to touch unsterile objects by walking about the room

Powdering hands

1. Dispensing powder from the hands into the air
2. Not carefully cleansing powder from outside of gloves

Gloves

1. Touching outer portion of glove
2. Failing to detect perforations or breaks in the glove
3. Holding hands against the body while waiting

Skin preparation

1. Believing the manufacturer's claim for the product; check it out
2. Relying on aqueous antiseptics
3. Failing to realize that quaternary ammonium compounds (Zephiran) may be neutralized by even small traces of soap
4. In applying antiseptics, going back and forth from clean to contaminated areas and back to the clean area again (instead, ever-widening circles should be made, starting from the eyelid margin)
5. Forgetting to prepare the eyelashes, the eyelid margin, or the eyebrows

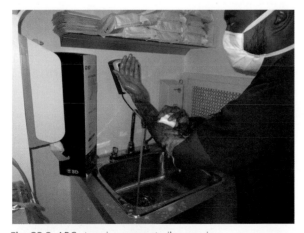

Fig. 33.2 ABC steps in proper sterile gowning.

to run down from the elbows into the sink and never to run back down over the hands, which have been scrubbed first.

Gowning

The gown must be folded so that the scrub assistant can unfold and put the gown on without touching the outer side with the bare hands. A towel placed on top of the gown should be used for careful drying of the hands before taking up the gown.

Gowns should be of sufficient thickness to provide protection from contamination by underclothing. Each sleeve should have a fitting wristlet. Many gowns now have wraparound backs to prevent the back area from contaminating instrument tables. Many doctors use disposable paper gowns that require no laundering and have no lint particles.

Gloving

Several techniques are available for putting on gloves under sterile operating room conditions. The *closed gloving technique* represents perhaps the best method available for the scrub assistant. Some advantages of the closed gloving technique are reduction of possible contamination of the gloves from the hands and free glove powder, which scatters in an operating room.

In the closed gloving technique (Fig. 33.3), the scrub assistant puts on the gown but slides his or her hands into the sleeves only until the sleeve cuff seams can be grasped between the fingers and thumbs. The hands do not protrude beyond the seam of the gown. The gloves are then laid out with the gown-covered hand. The glove is placed in the sleeve thumb down, with the fingers pointing toward

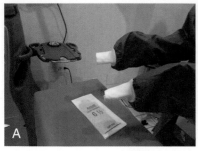
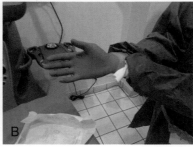
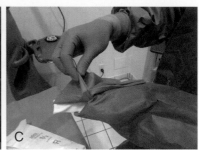

Fig. 33.3 Closed gloving technique.

the shoulder, and the wrist edge of the glove is level with the sleeve cuff seam. The cuff of the glove is then grasped against the sleeve with the thumb and forefinger, which are inside the sleeve. The upper edge of the glove cuff is grasped with the sleeve-covered fingers of the opposite hand and the glove opening is pulled down completely over the gown cuff of the hand being gloved. If the glove is being placed on the left hand, the glove cuff and the stockinette cuff are grasped with the right hand and both the cuff and the glove are pulled on at the same time. With the gloved hand, the other glove is now picked up and the same procedure is followed for gloving the other hand. Using this technique, the gloves are never touched with the bare hands.

Arranging the preparation table

A small table should be arranged to provide all the necessary solutions and supplies for preparing the skin and giving local anesthetic. These include antiseptic solutions, irrigation solutions, applicators, gauze, and local anesthetic solutions, as well as suitable syringes and needles. It is desirable that the sterile table be kept separate from the main instrument table and be removed once the eye and eyelid have been prepared.

Arranging the back table

The back table should be laid out in a definite order of use to provide necessary towels, gowns, and gloves for the surgeons, as well as drapes for the patient. Supplies, such as gauze and applicators should be placed here. The back table should include basins for solutions and basins for waste, in addition to required syringes for mixing and drawing up special solutions. Care must always be taken that solutions are never mixed or confused. Instruments are placed on the back of the table, leaving work space in front. Additional instruments that are seldom used but occasionally required may remain on the back table and not be transferred to the instrument, or Mayo, stand.

Arranging the instrument stand

The instrument, or Mayo, stand should be arranged according to a consistent pattern. Forceps are placed in one area, scissors in another, and needle drivers in another. Irrigating solutions, applicators, gauze, and so on have their own place on the instrument stand (Fig. 33.4).

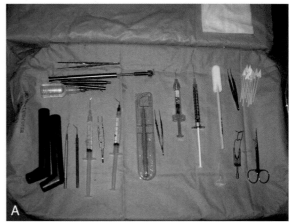
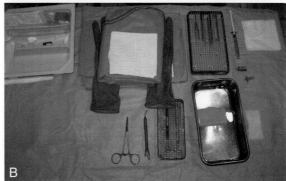

Fig. 33.4 (A) Typical instrument table for intraocular surgery. (B) Backup table for additional instruments.

Most ophthalmic surgical procedures can be classified in two main sections:

- Intraocular, which includes cataract extractions, corneal transplants, and corneal or scleral laceration repair
- Extraocular, which includes correction of strabismus and eyelid surgery

Each surgeon uses different instruments that he or she is comfortable with.

Example of a set of instruments for basic intraocular procedures.

One right and one left corneal section scissors
One pair Stevens scissors, curved
One pair spring scissors
One superblade or diamond blade
One pair iris scissors
One pair Vannas scissors
One straight and one angled fixation forceps (0.12 teeth)
Two fine-tying forceps
One anterior chamber irrigating cannula
One Sinskey hook
One eye speculum
Two straight and two curved fine hemostats
One muscle hook
One iris spatula
One synechia spatula or cyclodialysis spatula
One lens loupe
Two needle drivers, finely curved
Three anterior chamber irrigating tips (19, 27, and 30 gauge)
One irrigating cannula
Series of irrigating aspiration probes
Series of phacoemulsification tips and handpieces
Series of special keratomes, scleral blades for phaco incisions
Cautery cord and tip
One Hershman spatula
One intraocular lens-holding forceps

Instruments for extraocular procedures.

One no. 3 Bard-Parker knife handle (e.g., strabismus)
One pair Stevens scissors
One pair spring scissors
One straight and one angled fixation forceps
One double-pronged scleral forceps
Two muscle hooks
One caliper
One right and one left muscle clamp
Two straight and two curved fine hemostats
Two towel clips
Two skin hooks, fine
One anterior chamber irrigating tip, 19 gauge
One speculum

Special instruments for procedures, such as intraocular lens implants, corneal transplants, and enucleation may be sterilized in separate packages and dispensed as necessary in addition to the basic instrument tray. This method avoids unnecessary handling and sterilization of instruments not needed for routine surgery. It applies specifically to the delicate and expensive microsurgical instruments.

Demagnetization

Poor and frustrating surgical technique may be brought about by magnetization of microsurgical instruments, which in turn magnetizes the fine needles commonly used today. This may occur in the operating room or by exposure to larger surgical instruments while being sterilized with ethylene oxide. It is most frustrating to have to dislodge a fine needle from a needle driver during a critical point in a delicate eye operation.

A number of inexpensive methods are available for demagnetization of instruments and needles (Fig. 33.5). A tape head demagnetizer also can be used.

Diamond knives

The diamond blade is made from a gem-quality diamond, which is the hardest element known. Diamond knives are used in ocular surgery because of their extreme sharpness and ability to make a corneal or corneoscleral incision with ease and without tissue destruction. They are far superior to steel blades (Fig. 33.6A). This extension of the knife may be measured by the caliper on the handle, but should also be checked against a coin gauge (Fig. 33.6B), a ruler, or a microscope. Diamond knives used for cataract surgery are usually unguarded.

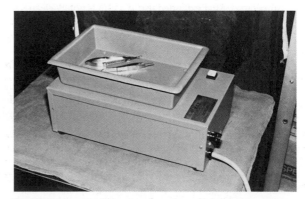

Fig. 33.5 Demagnetizing tray for microsurgical instruments and needles.

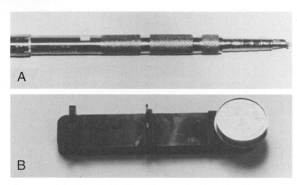

Fig. 33.6 (A) Diamond knife with guarded handle. (B) Coin gauge used to check calibration of the diamond knife.

To care for the diamond knife, one should use the following procedure:
1. Immediately after surgery, advance the knife blade sufficiently to be exposed, but not beyond the feet, and rinse thoroughly with sterile distilled water squirted with force through a syringe.
2. Visually examine the blade under a microscope for possible dirt or residue, which can be removed by extending the diamond beyond the feet and lightly plunging the blade into Styrofoam. Caution: cleaning should always be done by making fresh insertions into Styrofoam. Never apply excessive side motion to the diamond. Rinse thoroughly.
3. Visually examine the blade under a microscope for any remaining dirt or residue. If there is residue, repeat steps 1 and 2.
4. Retract the diamond blade.
5. Proceed with any method of sterilization normally used; 275° F (135° C) as maximum temperature for 3 to 5 minutes is an acceptable sterilization method for diamond knives and coin gauges. Try not to let blood, tissue, or saline solution dry on the blade, which causes susceptibility to cracking and edge chipping when the blade is autoclaved. After extended use, if a film is noted, clean the diamond blade by immersing it in a pan of distilled water with one tablet of an enzyme cleaner used for contact lenses. This proteolytic enzyme cleaner removes the protein that adheres to the surface of the diamond. Then rinse with distilled water and repeat the cleaning procedure.

Sapphire blade

The sapphire blade is made of crystal sapphire and is extremely sharp and delicate. Like the diamond blade, it is subject to chipping. The same requirements apply for cleaning with distilled water and use of an enzyme film. Before the film develops, it may be appropriate to insert both the diamond blade and the sapphire blade into a wet sponge or fiberglass packing material. One should not expose the sapphire blade to ultrasound cleaning. It may be sterilized by means of steam autoclave, ethylene oxide gas, or dry heat (see following text).

Ruby blade

The ruby blade should be stored in a retracted position until it is used. Any wiping motion against the blade will dull the cutting edge. The blade should be flushed with distilled water squirted with force through a syringe. Blood, saline, or tissue should not be allowed to dry on the blade. The blade may be cleaned with contact lens enzyme cleaner. It also may be cleaned in an ultrasonic cleaner.

Special care of gem blades

The following procedure should be used to care for gem blades:
1. Always protect the tip of the blade and store it in a retracted position.
2. Use a rest when laying an extended blade on a Mayo stand.
3. Observe the blade for cleanliness and chips under high magnification with retroillumination.
4. Immediately after use, flush the blade with a steady stream of distilled water with a syringe and needle.
5. The surgeon may gently wipe the side of the blade with a wet Merocel sponge.
6. Diamond and ruby blades can be cleaned after each use by ultrasound with hydrogen peroxide. Rinse thoroughly.
7. Clean baked-on protein as follows:
   a. Expose blades as far as possible
   b. Use a soft wet Styrofoam packing peanut; stab the blade and work it through incisions for 20 to 30 seconds in the direction it is designed to cut
   c. Rinse thoroughly with distilled water
8. Inspect with a calibration scope.
9. Dry the instrument immediately with a hot air blower. Blow drying removes excess moisture from hard-to-dry areas that are most susceptible to rust. It is a method preferred over towel drying because it prevents lint, keeps edges and tips sharp, and prevents accidental breakage or bending of delicate tips. Drying is not necessary if it is immediately followed by steam sterilization.
10. Avoid sudden hot or cold changes. Always allow the knife from the autoclave to cool in the air. Do not put it in a basin of water if in a hurry because blade damage can result.

Sutures

Sutures are available from the manufacturer in packets consisting of two parts: a primary packet enclosing the suture and a peel-apart overwrap enclosing the inner sterile packet.

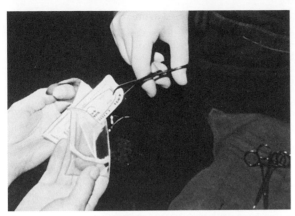

Fig. 33.7 Removing suture from sterile packet.

Table 33.2 Origin of suture materials used in ophthalmology	
Suture	**Raw materials**
Surgical silk	Raw silk spun by silkworm
Catgut (plain or chromic)	Submucosa of sheep intestine or serosa of cow intestine
Collagen (plain or chromic)	Flexor tendon of beef
Nylon	Polymeric amide derived from chemical synthesis
Mersilene (polyester fiber)	Polymer of terephthalic acid and polyethylene

The inside packet is sterile as long as the overwrap remains intact and undamaged. The circulating nurse must deliver the sterile inner packet to the sterile field without touching it or permitting the inner packet to touch unsterile surfaces. The nurse may use one of three methods to accomplish this:

1. The two flaps of the overwrap may be grasped between the thumbs and forefingers and peeled back to offer the packet to the scrub assistant, who may remove it with a sterile instrument (Fig. 33.7).
2. The inner packet may be flipped out onto the sterile table.
3. After the outer packet is opened, a transfer forceps may be used to place the inner packet on the instrument table.

The scrub assistant will then take the suture packet and open it. Many absorbable sutures contain a preservative, which must be carefully rinsed before the suture can be used. The suture should then be laid out on the tray in preparation for use.

Types of ophthalmic sutures. Ophthalmic sutures are made of a variety of materials, each material having specific advantages that can be tailored to the individual surgeon's likes (Table 33.2). The broad categories include the following:

1. *Plain surgical gut.* This is commonly referred to as *plain catgut*, a term believed to have originated from the Arabic word *kitgut* or *kitstring* signifying a fiddle string. The Arabian dancing masters used a three-string violin called a *kit* and ancient instrument makers created these strings from the intestines of a variety of animals. This material is absorbable. It eliminates the need for suture removal, which is of prime importance in children and uncooperative individuals. The disadvantages are, in time, variability or loss of tensile strength and absorption, an increased tendency to neovascularization, and some reaction to the material with granuloma formation.

2. *Chromic surgical gut.* This is gut that is chromicized to retard the tensile strength loss and lengthen the time of absorption permitting the suture to last longer. The disadvantage is that, like any natural suture, it causes some moderate tissue reaction.

3. *Vicryl or Dexon.* This is a synthetic absorbable suture that has strong tensile strength, elicits less tissue reaction than gut, and provides excellent knot security. Because of the hydrolytic absorption process, it is more predictable in terms of tensile strength retention and absorption than are the natural absorbable sutures. There is significant absorption in 30 days and maximum absorption in 60 to 90 days. These synthetic absorbable sutures, in sizes 4-0 through 8-0, are of a braided construction to maximize the handling properties. To further improve the passage through tissue and the knot-tying characteristics, an absorbable coating has been added to Vicryl sutures. The coating affects neither the absorption nor the degree of tissue reactivity elicited by the suture.

4. *Nylon.* This is a synthetic monofilament suture commonly used in anterior segment ophthalmic surgery. It maintains its tensile strength and does not irritate the tissues or support bacterial growth. The suture degrades, however, losing approximately 10% to 15% of its strength yearly and it is more difficult to tie than silk. It is available in a variety of sizes for ophthalmic use.

5. *Silk.* This is a natural protein material derived from the silkworm but treated with resins and waxes. This handles the best of all sutures and has excellent knot-tying security. It evokes a slight tissue reaction.

6. *Polypropylene* (Prolene). This is a strong, inert suture that ties well and does not degrade with time. This suture causes minimal inflammatory reaction, is not absorbed, and is not subject to biodegradation or weakening by the actions of tissue enzyme. Because of its relative

biologic inertness, there are no known contraindications. This suture is pigmented with copper phthalocyanine blue. It has more elongation than nylon and because of its hydrophobic nature and inertness in the eye, it has become increasingly useful in suturing intraocular lenses, in iris repair surgery, and in anterior segment wound closure.

7. *PDS* (polydioxanone) suture. This is a monofilament absorbable suture for corneoscleral closure. Wound-holding tensile strength is 56 days. The monofilament nature of this suture allows for easy passage through ocular tissue. Available in size 9-0, it is attached to a wide range of fine ophthalmic needles.

8. *Mersilene* polyester fiber suture. This is a monofilament polyester suture for corneoscleral closure. This suture is nonbiodegradable and has 50% more tensile strength than nylon. Mersilene is 20% less elastic than nylon; therefore it is said to create less suture-induced astigmatism. Available in size 10-0, it is attached to a wide range of fine ophthalmic needles.

Suture evaluation. Uniform standards are required in sutures for microsurgery. The *needles* should be sharp and should not dull easily with repeated passage. They must be securely swaged onto the suture. The *appearance* is important because colored sutures are more easily seen. The suture should be reasonably *pliable* to permit ease of handling. The tensile strength should be adequate for the area and should not crack or break with normal handling. The *pull-through* effect should be smooth and should not drag tissue. *Tying* should be performed simply. The knots should remain secure and the suture should not *fray*.

The knots should remain secure postoperatively. There should be no marked reaction to the suture, although a minimal reaction may accelerate wound healing. With absorbable sutures, the absorption time should be sufficient to maintain closure until wound healing is secure.

Ophthalmic needles

Needles have a variety of shapes, points, and curvature, each designed to perform a special task and each related to the type of material that the suture will be required to track through. The needles are attached directly to the suture.

Preparing the patient's eyelids

In ophthalmic surgery, skin antiseptic agents should be carefully applied, beginning at the lash margin and carefully including the lashes. Ophthalmic personnel should avoid having any of the solution enter the eye. A dry applicator is preferred for skin preparation. Beginning in increasing circles from the eyelid margin, the assistant prepares a large area above the eye. Special care must be taken that the eyebrow and underlying skin are adequately prepared with the antiseptic solution. The eye should then be flushed with saline, diluted povidone-iodine (Betadine) solution, or self-sterilizing aqueous antiseptic solution by use of an irrigating bulb or an asepto syringe.

Draping the patient

A large folded sheet is used to cover the patient's body. The head is commonly draped with a double-thickness sheet or double towels. An eye sheet, preferably with a small opening, or a disposable eye sheet is then placed over the operative site.

Amoric environment

The room for operating must be amoric (Greek *a* means "no"; *morion* means "particle"). This term was coined by Dr. José Barraquer to indicate that particulate matter can be as devastating to the visual performance of an eye as infected material. To obtain this amoric environment, it is ideal if the operating room is limited to eye surgery only and has positive pressure. The number of personnel in the operating room should be minimized, as well as movements in and out. All talcum powder should be eliminated by using powderless gloves. All cotton balls should be eliminated. All syringes, cannulas, needles, and Petri dishes should be washed at least 5 times. Ideally, Millipore filters should be used for any solution irrigated into the anterior chamber. A lint-free type of drape, such as plastic or paper, should be used. Instrument tips must be examined under the microscope and, if particulate matter is present, cleaned with a lint-free wipe. After any instrument has been used, it should be rinsed in saline and wiped well.

Care and handling of surgical instruments

Manufacturers of quality stainless steel instruments (both in the United States and in Germany) have always done their best to produce surgical instruments that are extremely resistant to rust or corrosion. The stainless alloys used in the manufacturing are subject to strict industry and government standards. Their composition may vary to enhance certain desired qualities in the final product. For instance, to guarantee an extra hard cutting edge in scissors, the manufacturer will select a type of stainless steel that contains a higher percentage of carbon molecules, thus making the steel extra hard after hardening and tempering. For some eye instruments that need to be nonmagnetic and in which hardness is not of prime importance, the stainless steel selected will contain little carbon and more chromium and nickel. As a general rule, the greater the carbon content, the harder the steel can be made by the instrument maker. However, it is exactly the carbon content of the stainless steel that can later present a corrosion or rusting problem if the instrument was not properly manufactured or is incorrectly used by the consumer.

To increase its corrosion resistance, a properly manufactured surgical instrument will have passed through two special processing steps. The first is called *passivation*. In this process, the instrument is treated with an electrochemical process to thoroughly clean its surfaces, thereby reducing its tendency to corrode. The same process can be achieved through immersing it in a bath containing a heated aqueous solution of 30% nitric acid.

The second special processing step is *polishing*. This creates an extremely smooth surface that removes areas of possible corrosive action. It actually builds a fine layer of chromium oxide on the instrument. This layer is highly resistant to corrosion and will actually continue to build up with regular handling and sterilizing of the item. Naturally, incorrect cleaning and handling may cause this layer to become damaged or disappear, thus increasing the possibility of corrosion problems.

Surfaces that cannot be effectively polished, such as knurled or serrated handles and glare-reducing satin finishes, are more prone to corrosive attack. Because this corrosion does not penetrate deeply, it may be removed by scrubbing with a brush or detergent. As an alternative, the instrument can be returned to as-new condition by passivation and repolishing by the manufacturer or a professional instrument repair service.

Use of shortcuts in instrument care can lead to rust, corrosion, stains, and spotting. Corrosion, the gradual wearing away of material, eventually impairs an instrument's function. The most common causes are:

- Inadequate cleaning and drying after use
- Corrosive chemicals or sterilizing solutions
- Use of ordinary tap water rather than distilled or softened water in the cleaning process
- Laundry detergent residue remaining in operating room linens
- Harsh detergents
- A malfunctioning autoclave

Cleanliness, lubrication, and correct handling and storage procedures ensure an instrument's proper performance. In addition, inspection, troubleshooting, and a professional instrument maintenance program can actually lengthen the serviceable life of surgical instruments. To that end, the following instrument care habits are recommended:

Rust

If the problem is one of real rust (which is rare), it is necessary to determine whether the rust originated from the instrument itself or whether it was transferred from another source. To check whether the item itself is rusting, a pencil eraser is used to remove the rust, then the surface beneath the rust is checked to see if it is pitted. A pitted and rusting instrument must be taken out of a set of instruments immediately because it can cause a rust problem for the entire set. The item is returned to the manufacturer (provided it is not too old), who, in many cases, will replace it at no charge.

If the instrument is not actually rusting but shows some rust deposits, it must be refinished by the manufacturer or a competent repair facility. An attempt should then be made to find the source of the rust. There are several possibilities, the most common one being that one or more instruments in the set are rusting because they are old and of the chrome or nickel-plated type. When this plating wears off through use or sharpening, the carbon steel below it becomes exposed and is subject to immediate corrosion during autoclaving or immersing in cold sterilization solutions.

Inexpensive instruments sometimes rust because they have not undergone the passivation process; thus the surfaces contain carbon molecules. High-quality stainless steel instruments will pass certain tests (boiling, copper sulfate), whereas some of the lesser-grade instruments will not. It is the latter that can cause a problem. The fact that these instruments were stamped "stainless" does not always guarantee that they were made corrosion-resistant by the manufacturer. The buyer must be aware of this.

Another source of rust can be the water used in the autoclave. It is recommended that distilled deionized water be used because this has been stripped of all minerals and metals. Distilled water alone may not be pure enough, because many marketed distilled waters still contain many essential minerals for plant growth or human consumption. These minerals sometimes tend to stain the instrument. Thus deionized distilled water is best.

How to avoid a stained appearance

Stains are deposited onto the instrument's surface, plated on, or, in the case of rusting, develop from the instrument itself. The most common discoloration is a result of deposit stains that commonly occur during autoclaving. Instrument stains appear in a variety of colors, and in most cases the colors suggest the origin of the stain.

Brown or orange stain

The most common stain is also the one most often mistaken for rust. After removing the stain with an eraser, which usually is not difficult, the ophthalmic assistant should check the surface of the instrument for porous signs (pits). If none is found under the stained area (usually the instrument surface is smooth), proceed to locate the cause of the staining.

With the brown or orange stain, the problem is most often a phosphate layer (brown to light orange) on the instrument, which develops as a result of the following causes:

1. *Detergents used to wash and clean instruments.* Many of the detergents sold are highly alkaline and contain polyphosphates that aid in breaking down fats and blood. Hands are also left softer after prolonged use of these detergents. However, this high alkaline content produces the brown or orange stain during the autoclave cycle. The best detergents for instrument washing are those that are neutral pH 7 (on a pH scale of 0–14). These are available from hospitals and surgical suppliers and do not cost much more than regular detergents. Also, often the instruments are not rinsed long enough to neutralize the detergents. A thorough rinsing ensures that the detergent is no longer on the instrument.

2. *Water source.* Traces of minerals or metals (or both) may be contained in the tap water in a particular geographic area. The best way to check whether the water is the cause of the staining is to take a clean (or new) instrument that has no staining on it, wash it thoroughly in distilled deionized water with neutral pH detergent, rinse it thoroughly in distilled deionized water, and put it through a sterilization cycle. Follow the same procedure with another clean instrument, but this time wash and rinse with tap water. If the second instrument shows staining, it could reasonably be assumed that the tap water contains elements that stain the instrument. If both instruments still show stains, then a check of the autoclave is necessary. In this case, clean the autoclave according to the manufacturer's instructions and run one or two cleaning cycles with a recommended cleaner.

3. *Dried blood.* This usually results in a dark brown stain that can be rubbed off. Blood should be removed from the instrument surface as soon as possible because it will break down the surface by chemical reaction.

4. *Surgical wrappings.* If the laundry uses too much detergent, or detergents that contain a lot of phosphates (which are the less expensive ones available), surgical wrappings may contain enough remaining detergents to cause a reaction during autoclaving. A telltale sign is the brown stain on the towel (the outline of the instrument in an orange stain on the towel may even be visible). This type of stain is difficult to remove and on many occasions, the instrument will have to be refinished by the manufacturer.

5. *Cold sterilization solutions.* Many times, these are high in pH (like detergents) and need to be rinsed off thoroughly before storing instruments or before autoclaving.

6. *Foreign matter inside steam pipes.* Rust-colored film is particularly prevalent in new hospitals as a result of foreign matter inside steam pipes during installation. Unfortunately, nothing can be done, but the situation is only temporary.

Light and dark spots

Light and dark spots are caused by the slow evaporation of condensation on instruments. Traced to mineral residue, such spots can be prevented by following the autoclave manufacturer's directions carefully and using distilled or demineralized water for all cleaning procedures and solution preparation.

Purplish black stains

Purplish black stains indicate exposure to ammonia. Thorough rinsing after use and cleaning in the usual manner should eliminate this stain.

Bluish black stains

These are usually a result of plating and are extremely hard to remove from the instrument's surface. The surface beneath the stain is always smooth, but the instrument may have to be refinished by the manufacturer to obtain good results. The cause of this staining is mixing of dissimilar metals in ultrasonic cleaners and during autoclaving.

Multicolor stains

These are caused mostly by excessive heat (chromium oxide stains) and actually show rainbow colors with a blue or brown overtone. When the instrument shows these heat stains, it may have lost part of the original hardness and may not perform as well (especially scissors, which need the extra hardness on their edges for cutting performance). Such instruments can usually be refinished by the manufacturer and the hardness can be tested. The stain can be polished off.

Black stains

The most common black stains are caused by an acid reaction. The eraser minimizes the stain, but the surface beneath remains slightly rougher than that of a normal instrument. Black stains may result from the detergents used. Similar to the brown stain caused by high pH in detergents, the black acid-type stain can be caused by low pH (<6) during autoclaving. The autoclaving temperature and pressure magnify the chemical effects of acid on steel many times, so the neutrality of the pH in the autoclave environment is of great importance.

Bluish gray stains

Bluish gray stains are indicative of cold sterilizing solutions. Following a manufacturer's directions explicitly will remedy the solution.

As described, stains are deposited onto the instrument surface, plated onto it or, in the case of rusting, develop from the instrument itself.

The most common discoloration results from deposit stains that commonly occur during autoclaving. To minimize such staining, it is important that the autoclave run perfectly and that it has a well-functioning drying cycle. The instruments should come out bone dry, whether in wrappers or loose on a tray. If any moisture is left in the pack or on the instruments, it will result in tiny water droplets that leave a circular stain on the instrument surface after drying.

An interesting fact in regard to plating stains or the stains that are a result of metal deposits is that the area of staining is always near the most magnetic parts of the instrument. New instruments are often highly magnetic in the locks, serrations, and ratchets because the carbon steel tools used to work on the instruments during production are highly magnetic themselves. This magnetism wears off gradually during handling and sterilization. This is why newer instruments tend to stain more visibly, causing the complaint that new instruments are showing stains but the old ones are not.

If there is any suspicion as to what might cause a staining problem, one clean instrument should be processed in the manner suspected of causing the problem and then autoclaved. A clean control instrument should then be processed by washing and rinsing it in distilled and deionized water only. This instrument should process without problems, whereas the first instrument will show the stain. All types of stains can be tested for in this manner, including water, detergent, wrapping, and cold sterilization solution left on the instrument.

Meticulous care during surgery will prolong the life of surgical instruments. Although blood and saline are the most common causes of corrosion and pitting, instrument contact with the following solutions should also be avoided if possible:

Aluminum chloride
Barium chloride
Carbolic acid
Chlorinated lime
Dakin's solution
Ferrous chloride
Lysol
Mercury bichloride
Mercury salts
Phenol
Potassium permanganate
Potassium thiocyanate
Sodium hypochlorite
Stannous chloride
Tartaric acid

Exposure to the following solutions is extremely detrimental:

Aqua regia (a mixture of nitric and hydrochloric acids)
Ferric chloride
Diluted sulfuric acid
Hydrochloric acid
Iodine (not to exceed 1 hour)

Steps in cleaning and sterilization

Cleaning

All instruments should be thoroughly cleaned immediately after use. Using a toothbrush is helpful. Blood or debris should never be allowed to dry on the instruments. Baked-on blood in a box lock or crevice can result in corrosion and subsequent cracking under stress. Therefore box locks should be opened and instruments with removable parts should be disassembled.

Cleaning solutions with a neutral pH level (7–8.5) are recommended. An extremely alkaline detergent (>9) may stain and might cause breaks and an extremely acid detergent (<6) may cause an instrument to pit.

After cleaning, the instruments should be dried quickly to avoid water stains. Of course, if they are to be autoclaved immediately, it is not necessary to dry them first.

Washer-sterilizers are ideally suited for washing and terminally sterilizing soiled instruments. However, it is imperative that the sterilizer itself be clean and functioning properly. Hospitals in hard-water areas should implement a water-softening or demineralizing system. Surgical wrappings must be free of any laundry detergent residue.

A helpful machine is the ultrasonic cleaner. For most offices, the medium-sized unit, 10 inches (25 cm) by 4 inches (10 cm) (6–8 inches [15–20 cm] deep) is usually adequate. Ultrasound is a form of acoustic vibration occurring at frequencies too high to be perceived by the human ear, usually greater than 20,000 Hz (i.e., 20,000 cycles per second). Ultrasonic cleaning uses acoustic vibration at high frequencies through a liquid medium. The vibration of the fluid is so rapid that it forms bubbles. This process is known as *cavitation*. The bubbles adhere to and collapse on the surfaces of instruments, causing the foreign matter on the surface to be dislodged gently but totally. Millions of microscopic bubbles or "vacuum cleaners" dislodge the foreign matter from the surfaces, blind holes, pores, tight joints, and places that cannot be reached by lengthy soaking and scrubbing. Ultrasonic cleaning accomplishes this in minutes and is so gentle it will not etch glass. The instruments are thoroughly cleaned and ready for sterilization, eliminating the possibility of "disinfected dirt." The minivacuum created by the exploding bubbles removes up to 90% of all foreign matter from the instrument, particularly in the hard-to-reach areas, such as the box locks, scissor locks, and other crevice-like areas.

Although an ultrasonic cleaner removes up to 90% of the soil, it does not preempt the need for sterilization. *Caution: microsurgical instruments must not come into contact with one another during ultrasonic cleaning.* The unit's vibrations may cause premature wear on their precision tips.

Lubrication

Ultrasonic cleaners remove all lubrication from instruments; therefore all clean instruments should be bathed in instrument milk or a similar product after ultrasonic cleaning. Instruments should be lubricated after every five procedures. It is also recommended that they be lubricated after every cleaning process to guard against mineral deposits and other water-system impurities that can lead to stains, rust, and corrosion. Previous vigorous cleaning removes all lubrication and may result in "frozen" lock boxes. To impede the growth of bacteria in the lubricant wash, only antimicrobial water-soluble lubricants are recommended. The manufacturer's instructions should be followed carefully.

Inspection

In addition to being completely clean and free-moving to ensure proper function and sterilization, instruments must be inspected before packaging for reuse.

Hinged instruments should be inspected for alignment of jaws, meshing of teeth, and stiff or cracked joints. Ratchets should close easily and firmly. To test ratchets, clamp the instrument on the first tooth. Holding the instrument at the box, tap the ratchet end against a solid object. Repair is required if the instrument springs open. Close the instrument to test its tension; when jaws touch, a space of $1/18$ to $1/16$ inch (1.6–1.4 mm) should exist between the Noratchet teeth of each shank.

Ring-handled instruments can be tested by holding one handle in each hand. Open the instrument and try to wiggle it. If the box lock is loose, jaw misalignment will occur.

Large scissors should cut four layers of gauze at the tip of the blade. Smaller scissors (<4 inches [10 cm] in overall length) should cut at least two gauze layers. Blades should be inspected for burs.

If a needle that is clamped in the jaws of a needle holder locked on the second ratchet tooth can be turned easily by hand, the instrument should be tagged for repair or replaced.

Finally, elevated heat temperatures weaken stress points and can actually change molecular structures of the metal. This change weakens and dulls instruments, resulting in their continual diminished performance. Be on the lookout for weakened stress points.

Preparing a set of instruments

Instruments made from differing alloys should be sterilized separately. Place all sharps (such as scissors, knives, skin hooks) individually so that they do not touch each other at the sharp areas during autoclaving. The tips of sharps can be protected with small corks. Cotton or gauze also can be used to protect some of the smaller instruments. Special trays are available to keep small instruments and microinstruments in place so that they cannot move during autoclaving or storage. An extra towel can be folded to a strip and wound around the critical areas of several cutting instruments in a set.

Make sure that all instruments are in an open position. Instruments autoclaved in a closed position (especially those with ratchet locking devices) may spring the box lock because of the increased tension during the heat and pressure in the autoclave. In cases of metal-to-metal contact in a closed instrument, such as near the tips and the ratchets, make sure that the steam reaches all these areas. Otherwise, the instruments may not be sterile.

Do not overload trays. Try to standardize with as few instruments as are commonly used in the particular procedure and keep all other instruments set up separately to be available as required. Overloading causes unnecessary handling and sterilization, which not only creates extra work but also shortens the life of the instrument.

Sterilization

Sterilization is the complete destruction of all microorganisms within or about an object. Articles are either *sterile* or *unsterile;* there is no middle ground. Essentially, sterilization is accomplished by subjecting all material to either physical or chemical treatment to destroy all microorganisms. Careful sterilization must be carried out not only to avoid infection of wounds but also to prevent the transmission of organisms from patient to patient. The bacterial spore is the most stubborn of all living organisms in its capacity to withstand destruction. Therefore standards of effectiveness of sterilization are based on the destruction of these bacterial spores.

The following methods are most commonly used in ophthalmology for sterilizing instruments and material:
1. Boiling
2. Dry heat (hot oven)
3. Moist heat (autoclave)
4. Chemical disinfectants (germicides, acetone, alcohol)
5. Gas
6. Radiation (ultraviolet, electron beam)

Boiling. Most microorganisms are destroyed by subjecting instruments to boiling water for 20 minutes. However, it may take several hours of boiling to kill some resistant spores and encapsulated bacteria. A timer should be available so that ineffective sterilization does not result from removing the instruments too early. Instruments with sharp points or blades are rarely boiled because this dulls the cutting edges. Some instruments rust after sterilization in boiling water if they are not properly dried, or if they are allowed to remain in the water. It is important to use distilled water because this prevents minerals from precipitating on the instruments and the walls of the sterilizer. It is recommended that the water sterilizer be emptied, washed, rinsed well, and dried thoroughly at the end of each day.

Dry heat (oven). Several types of dry heat ovens are available for sterilizing instruments. Run by electricity, these ovens provide a constant and controlled amount of heat to instruments, drapes, gowns, and gloves for a given time. Temperature should be maintained at 320° F (160° C) for 60 minutes. The disadvantage of this method is the long time required for the sterilization of instruments and packs (Fig. 33.8).

Moist heat (autoclave). The most common and practical form of sterilizing instruments is steam sterilization. The autoclave is designed to use steam under pressure to destroy microorganisms. Moist heat has a greater destructive effect on bacteria than heat alone (Fig. 33.9).

In autoclaving, the higher the temperature or pressure obtained, the shorter is the time required to sterilize. For instance, instruments under 15 pounds (6.8 kg) of pressure at 250° F (121° C) are effectively sterilized in 15 minutes. Under the same pressure at 270° F (132° C), they are effectively sterilized in 3 minutes.

The time of effective sterilization varies with the type of material being autoclaved. For example, cloth (gauze) takes longer to sterilize than steel (instruments). Autoclaving

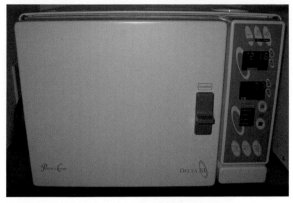
Fig. 33.9 Small autoclave.

may be used for a wide range of items of different materials, such as towels, sponges, rubber gloves, and masks. These items may be wrapped in special packages and they will remain sterile for some time after removal from the autoclave.

When ovens and autoclaves are loaded, it is important to prepare all the packs and to arrange the instruments in a way that will permit proper permeation of the materials by the moisture and heat. Crowding must be avoided. All oil and grease must be removed from instruments before autoclaving because steam does not penetrate through oil.

The autoclave has to be in good working order and operating perfectly in both steam and drying cycles. Commercially available autoclave tapes and chemical indicators may serve as controls to show that the autoclave is functioning properly.

Instruments loaded into the autoclave chamber should not be too cold because they can cause steam condensation and staining. In some instances, it may be advisable to heat the load (by using the drying cycle) to warm up the instruments before sterilization. This should be tried first whenever water stains are encountered after sterilization. Also it is important not to open the chamber immediately after sterilization, but rather to crack the door for a few minutes (7–10 minutes, as per manufacturers' recommendations) while the drying cycle is on. In any case, the instruments should come out bone dry, without any condensation moisture anywhere in the packs. To minimize steam staining, only distilled deionized water should be used in the autoclave. Also all autoclaves should be flushed according to manufacturers' time schedules and recommendations. Iron, sodium, calcium, magnesium, or copper in hard water can cause spotting, staining, or corrosion.

Chemical. Chemicals should be used when heat would dull the sharp cutting edges or would destroy the object to be sterilized (such as plastic). The chemicals that are

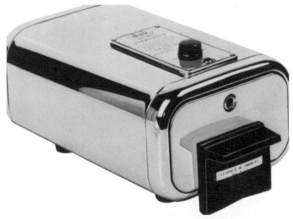
Fig. 33.8 Dry heat oven.

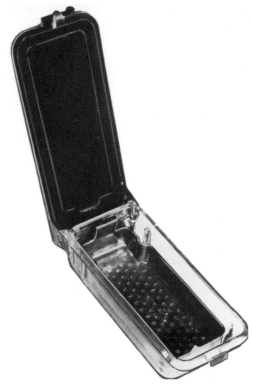

Fig. 33.10 Germicide and instrument container.

used on instruments and plastics are called *germicides.* (Chemicals that are used on living tissues are called *antiseptics.*) The process of chemical sterilization with germicides is commonly referred to as *cold sterilization* (Fig. 33.10).

Each autoclave has its own set of instructions. All instruments should be cleaned, and when lubricating instruments, be sure to wipe off excess lubricants. Check that all materials can be autoclaved. Examples of autoclavable organic materials are: nylon, polycarbonate, polypropylene, Teflon, acetal, polysulfone, polyetherimide, silicone rubber, and polyester. Examples of materials that cannot be autoclaved include polyethylene, styrene, cellulosics, polyvinyl chloride (PVC), acrylic (Plexiglas), latex, and neoprene.

Cold sterilization (germicidal solution bath). Contrary to popular opinion, cold sterilization is not better for instruments than steam sterilization. With cold sterilization, most professional offices leave the instrument in germicide for hours and even days at a time. Even though the germicides are only slightly corrosive, this extralong immersion takes its toll on the instrument surface. A short (20–30 minutes) steam exposure is much less corrosive and less dulling to sharp edges of scissors and knives than is long exposure to cold sterilization. Also some of the cold sterilization

solutions are either highly alkaline (high pH, >7) or highly caustic (low pH, <7) and can cause staining and corrosion when autoclaved after a germicidal bath. Make sure to rinse the instruments thoroughly after taking them out of the germicidal bath. Do not leave instruments in the following solutions for extended periods, because corrosion can result: aluminum, barium, calcium, ferrous or stannous chloride; phenol, Lysol or iodine; benzalkonium chloride (Zephiran); and any acid, mercury, or potassium solution.

The minimum time for chemical sterilization is 20 minutes. The pan in which the instruments are placed for sterilization should be padded with soft material to prevent the tips of the instruments from becoming damaged. Rust inhibitors are often added to some of the commercial germicides. The following germicides are commonly used: ethyl alcohol 70%, benzalkonium chloride (Zephiran), mercury cyanide solution (1:1000), formaldehyde germicides (Bard-Parker solution), cetrimonium bromide (Cetavlon), carbolic acid, aqueous nitromersol solution (Metaphen), phenol derivatives, alkaline glutaraldehyde, hydrochloride solution (sodium or calcium), benzyl ammonium chloride (Germiphene), and acetone (Table 33.3).

Acetone sterilization. Concentrated acetone is used by some practitioners for its rapid bactericidal effect. It has a track record of more than 50 years, is inexpensive and readily available, and evaporates rapidly at room temperature, thus eliminating residual activity. It is rapidly effective against bacteria, but it is only sporistatic (inhibits spores) rather than sporicidal (kills spores) against spores.

Acetone in 100% concentration may be used to disinfect instruments that have become contaminated in surgery. A 1-minute dip is sufficient for disinfection of minor surgical instruments for chalazia, foreign bodies, and eyelids. However, acetone does not kill some spores and may not be effective against the virus of serum hepatitis; it is not nearly as reliable as autoclaving. Acetone neither corrodes instruments nor damages sharp edges. It does not pass biologic tests for sterility, but it is a practical effective solution for minor nonintraocular surgical procedures.

Alcohol disinfection. Like acetone, alcohol is rapidly effective against vegetative bacteria and mycobacteria. Its action against fungi (30–60 minutes) is slower and virucidal activity is highly erratic. An ophthalmologist has to decide whether an item should be sterile or simply clean. If the item need only be clean, then the disinfection process of alcohol should destroy most microorganisms known to cause disease in that situation.

Gas and radiation. Ethylene oxide is an effective gas for sterilizing instruments and materials. It is useful in sterilizing articles that would be damaged by heat or by exposure to strong liquid disinfectants. It is the method of choice in sterilizing intraocular lens implants. Some of the advantages of gas sterilization are that it can be used on most

Table 33.3 Advantages and disadvantages of germicides

Germicide	Advantages	Disadvantages
Ethyl alcohol	Good bactericidal and virucidal activity in the presence of protein; reduced toxicity; not harmful to instruments, lenses, or plastics; inexpensive	No sporicidal activity
Benzalkonium chloride (Zephiran)	Controversial bactericidal activity; low toxicity	Reduced bactericidal activity against *Proteus* and *Pseudomonas* organisms; no sporicidal activity
Phenol derivatives (Staphene)	Good bactericidal activity	Poor sporicidal activity; toxic
Alkaline glutaraldehyde (Cidex)	Good sporicidal and bactericidal activity in presence of protein; rapidly effective but instruments should be soaked 3–10 hours and rinsed well; low toxicity; not harmful to lensed instruments	Three hours required to kill some spores; before product is effective, it must be activated with sodium bicarbonate
Benzyl ammonium chloride (Germiphene)	Rapid bactericidal activity with 30 seconds; no toxicity; not harmful to plastic, instruments, or rubber	Poor sporicidal activity

materials, can sterilize materials that cannot be sterilized by other means, is effective against all organisms, and achieves good penetration. The disadvantages of gas are that it is slow, costly, flammable, and toxic and it requires special equipment.

Electron beam irradiation may be applied to completely sealed articles, such as sutures.

Effectiveness. To test the efficacy of sterilization methods, one may attempt to culture organisms from the instruments after obtaining what is considered proper sterilization. If any organisms are cultured, the method and solution used must be reevaluated. In standard tests, specific organisms may be placed in the sterilizing apparatus and cultures analyzed to test effectiveness.

Sterile packs. Many microsurgical instruments and supplies are provided as disposables in sterile packs. Single-use instruments, such as blades, injection needles, trephines, and suture needles should conform to standards established and described in the manufacturer's promotional material.

A potential problem in shipping, storage, and use of sterile packs is the possibility of contamination or loss of sterility, or both. A sterile pack should contain an indicator to confirm maintained sterility and freedom from exposure to ambient air and possible contamination through cracks, tears, or perforations in packs sterilized by heat, ethylene oxide, or radiation.

Operating room microscope

Ophthalmic surgery has become microsurgery. The operating room microscope is the most important piece of equipment in ophthalmic surgery. Zeiss designed the first microscope so well that Zeiss operating microscope equipment is the kind most commonly used in operating rooms. Other brands, such as Mueller, Olympus, Weck, and Wild are also available throughout North America, with minor improvements over the more common Zeiss equipment. An advantage of Zeiss microscopes is that they are interchangeable with existing components and accessories.

The modern operating room microscope supplies the surgeon with illumination, magnification, and controlled positioning. Equipment is designed to minimize clutter and to be placed in the most accessible part of the operating room. Because of the magnification involved, a minimal amount of vibration is tolerated, and therefore heavy bases or ceiling mounts are required. A lightweight microscope beside the table stand is inconvenient and commonly causes troublesome vibration for the operating surgeon.

The first Zeiss microscope was the Omni One, developed in 1956. It has been improved and updated several times. Its microscope provides motorized zoom and focus capability in a short body, in addition to zoom capability that allows greater magnification and fine focusing adjustments. Also available is a movement attachment in two planes called

Self-evaluation questions

Q

True–false statements

Directions: Indicate whether the statement is true **(T)** or false **(F)**.

1. The ophthalmic assistant in a hospital setting is commonly a nurse. **T** or **F**
2. Blind or partially sighted individuals should take the assistant's arm, and follow. **T** or **F**
3. Preoperative orientation is not a function of the hospital ophthalmic assistant. **T** or **F**

Missing words

Directions: Write in the missing word in the following sentences:

4. An environment that is free of particles is called
   _____.
5. Sterilization of the operator's skin is called _____.
6. A technique of putting on gloves by not hand touching the cuffs of the gloves is called the _____ glove technique.

Choice-completion questions

Directions: Select the one best answer in each case.

7. Which is not an alarming immediate postoperative sign after cataract surgery?
   a. Blood in the anterior chamber.
   b. Severe pain.
   c. Photophobia.
   d. Pus in the anterior chamber.
   e. Prolapse of the iris.
8. Which is an incorrect postoperative instruction?
   a. Avoid heavy lifting.
   b. Avoid straining at bowel movement.
   c. Keep hands and face clean.
   d. Avoid car rides.
   e. Wear sunglasses outdoors.
9. Which is not an error in surgical technique?
   a. Splashing the surgical gown.
   b. Permitting hair to protrude from cap.
   c. Cleaning nails in scrub sink before scrubbing.
   d. Mask not covering the nose.
   e. Leaving skip spots while scrubbing.

Answers, notes, and explanations

A

1. **True**. Most often the nurse, when employed by a hospital or by an ophthalmologist, is the individual who assists in the care of eye patients. A nurse is usually the individual in the operating room who, by training and experience, can quickly learn the skills of assisting, aseptic technique, and microsurgery. At the bedside, the nurse can follow the progress of a patient, identify abnormal signs and symptoms, and report progress to the ophthalmologist. However, in many states someone who is not a nurse, but who is well trained in these functions, may accompany the ophthalmologist and assist with preoperative, operative, and postoperative care of the patients. In surgicenters, a trained layperson is taking on increasing importance in this role.

2. **True**. By taking the assistant's arm just below the elbow, the partially sighted individual will be protected from interfering objects in the pathway and will be able to anticipate directional changes. In this way, the person will feel more secure when walking. A blind person should never be steered. The assistant should engage in conversation and provide information on the patient's surroundings.

3. **False**. No matter how well the patient has been oriented to any particular surgery by the office personnel of the ophthalmologist, he or she is still apprehensive on the night before surgery. The evening before, the hospital

ophthalmic assistant should review the routines that will occur before the surgery and the convalescent care that may be required. The patient should be given necessary cautions that are routine at the hospital. The patient should be forewarned as to what to expect from the type of anesthetic to be given, be it local, intravenous, or general.

4. **Amoric**. Creating an amoric or particle-free environment is as important as creating a sterile environment for ocular surgery. Fine particles of dust, debris, or powder can be devastating if they enter the eye.

5. **Scrubbing**. The operator's skin may be rendered safe temporarily by vigorous scrubbing with a scrub brush soaked in antiseptic solution, although bacterial flora return to the skin rapidly (within minutes) and so the skin does not remain sterile. However, pathogenic microorganisms will be permanently destroyed. Thus although scrubbing does not produce sterility, it does produce a considerably decreased risk of transferring pathogenic organisms.

6. **Closed**. This is the most sterile way of putting on gloves. Here the hands enter the sleeves of the gown only down to the cuffs and then the gloves are grasped with the sterile gown cuffs until the hands enter the gloves. The purpose of this technique is to minimize bacterial recovery on the scrubbed hands from the outside of the glove.

Answers, notes, and explanations—Continued

7. **c. Photophobia**. In general, because of a traumatic iritis with cells on the anterior chamber, most eyes are light-sensitive after cataract surgery. A darkened room or sunglasses may be comforting for the first few days. A dilated pupil often contributes to the photophobia.

8. **d. Avoid car rides**. As long as the driver is careful to avoid bumps and jars, there is no reason why an individual cannot ride in a car, go for walks, or lead a reasonably normal life during the postoperative period. Today's modern suturing techniques avoid the one major complication of wound rupturing with iris prolapse that was seen in the past. However, excessive straining can raise thoracic pressure and, secondarily, the venous return. This may give rise to intraocular hemorrhage on relatively fragile vessels.

9. **c. Cleaning nails in scrub sink before scrubbing**. This is a correct and important part of achieving cleanliness before scrubbing. All of the other activities are serious breaks in surgical technique. For sterility and cleanliness, attention must be paid to three participants in the operation: (1) the operator and assistants, (2) the patient, and (3) the instruments, drapes, and surgical accessories that are used. All must be carefully cleaned and sterilized or disinfected.

Box 34.1 **Ways to avoid a lawsuit**

1. Ensure that you identify the correct patient and the correct side for any surgical procedure. Mark the procedure site preop and double-check before proceeding.
2. Establish good rapport with the patient. The patient who likes the physician and the environment where surgery is performed is less likely to sue. Some lawsuits are started because of the patient's vindictiveness, even if the physician is fault-free. A doctor whom the patient views as compassionate and understanding has already acquired some protection against legal actions.
3. Discharge the patient into the care of a competent adult, one who will take care of the patient at home. The name of this individual should be recorded on the chart.
4. Provide written, easy-to-understand directions for the follow-up care and return visits. These should be read and explained to the patient or relative and all questions answered.
5. Include in the list problems or symptoms that may arise at home and what to do if they occur.
6. Provide in the instructions some directions for obtaining an appropriate physician for medical problems. Telephone numbers of the physician, ophthalmologist, and a nearby hospital emergency room should be given.
7. Arrange for a nurse or assistant to telephone that evening or the next day to check on the patient's

condition if the situation warrants it, and record this on the chart.
8. Make operative notes immediately after surgery, not weeks or months later.
9. Instruct patients to leave valuables at home or arrange some system for safekeeping of the patient's valuables during surgery. Often lockers are provided.
10. Make sure that life-sustaining equipment is available and in good working order.
11. Be sure there is an adequate consent form that is well outlined to the patient. Good personal communication with the patient as to risks, benefits, and alternatives is highly valuable. An informed consent for major surgery is mandatory. These consent forms can range from a simple page or two to an elaborate 12-page document with video viewing and the patient's response questionnaire. Each physician determines his or her own comfort level. Appendix 3 contains the principles of informed consent.
12. Maintain good records in the office and the hospital. The quality and legibility of your records affect the quality of your practice. It is important to attach to the records a log of telephone advice. Cursory, sloppy, or nonexistent notes call the physician's credibility and standards of practice into question. The practitioner should initial all laboratory and x-ray reports before they are filed.

loss, and complications as a result of negligent surgery or follow-up (Box 34.1).

session. Providing written handouts also can be of some value (Box 34.4).

Preparation for admission

In preparation for admission to an ambulatory surgery center, each patient should have a careful medical evaluation by the ophthalmologist, family physician, or internist. A checklist should be made of such events as routine laboratory tests and electrocardiograms (Box 34.2). A complete eye workup should be performed. Intraocular lens measurements should be determined. If the power of the intraocular lens is beyond the range of stock maintained, then a correct dioptric power intraocular lens should be obtained from the manufacturer. An additional visit may be required for the patient to consult with the anesthesiologist, who can review the laboratory results and the workup of the family physician (Box 34.3).

All surgical patients should be given extensive education concerning their problem. Videotapes may be shown and visual aid instructions may be given. Every effort should be made to have the family present at the teaching

Admission for surgery

Each surgicenter has its own specific requirements for admission for cataract surgery. We arrange to have our patients report one hour before surgery to ensure adequate dilation of the pupil before the procedure. We apply name tags with the site of operation on each patient to avoid mistakes.

Vital signs are recorded. The patient is free to move around and sit with relatives. Preoperative intramuscular sedation may be given to the nervous patient. Local anesthesia is administered by way of topical drops. Rarely are peribulbar or retrobulbar injections given. Some surgeons prefer to give an injection of intravenous methohexital (methohexitone, Brevital) or sodium thiopental (thiopental, thiopental sodium, Sodium Pentothal, Trapanal) during this latter procedure to reduce any awareness of this injection. Either the Honan balloon or the super pinky may be used for compression. Some patients are given

Box 34.2 **Surgical checklist**

*Type of surgery; for example, secondary IOL
  *Site of surgery; for example, rt eye (or OD)
  CAT / IOL
  SECONDARY IOL
  OTHER _____
  OD / OS

_____
DATE OF SURGERY _____
**SPECIAL REQUESTS, for example, TYPE OF IOL, for
  example, toric, bifocal manufacture, power
PREOPERATIVE VISIT
_____ Preoperative booklet given
_____ Operative instructions given
_____ History and physical form given
_____ Laboratory tests arranged
_____ Appointment scheduled with Dr. _____
for _____
_____ A-scan scheduled for _____

_____ A-scan result: Lens style _____
Diameter _____
_____ Endothelial studies
_____ Financial planning
_____ Insurance
_____ Surgery scheduled: Date _____
PATIENT _____
ADDRESS _____
PHONE NO. _____
RELATIVE'S NAME _____
PHONE NO. _____
SURGERY DAY
_____ Operative consent reviewed and signed
_____ Premedication given
_____ Postoperative instructions given
_____ Postoperative appointment made for_____
_____ Responsible home person: _____
_____ Medication given
_____ Ultraviolet glasses given or ordered

Box 34.3 **Anesthetic questions**

The following questions have been designed for use by the Department of Anesthesiology. They are to be completed before your operation. Please answer each question carefully. Bring the completed form to the preadmittance laboratory.

Name _____
Address_____
Phone_____ Age_____ Sex_____
Health Card No._____

Answer ☑	Yes	No	Do not know
1. What is your approximate weight? _____ (pounds/kg)?			
2. Did you ever have trouble with your heart?	☐	☐	☐
3. Did you ever take any medicine or pills for your heart?	☐	☐	☐
4. Did you ever take any medicine or pills for your blood pressure?	☐	☐	☐
5. Did you ever have high or low blood pressure?	☐	☐	☐
6. Did you ever take any medicine or pills for your breathing?	☐	☐	☐
7. Did you ever have any trouble with your breathing?	☐	☐	☐
8. Did a doctor ever tell you had asthma?	☐	☐	☐
9. Do you take any medicine, pills, or injections of any type regularly while you are not in the hospital? If so, see Question 27	☐	☐	☐
10. Within the past year, have you taken any medicine for rheumatism, arthritis, or allergies?	☐	☐	☐
11. Have you taken a drug called cortisone or prednisone within the past year?	☐	☐	☐
12. Have you taken any tranquilizers or nerve pills within the past 2 weeks?	☐	☐	☐
13. Have you been pregnant within the past 3 months?	☐	☐	☐
14. Do you have any bleeding or bruising tendencies?	☐	☐	☐
15. Do you take pills for thinning your blood?	☐	☐	☐
16. Have you had a general anesthetic within the past 3 months?	☐	☐	☐

greater than with inpatient cataract surgery in hospitals. The patient's acceptance is, however, much greater with ambulatory surgery. Everywhere in the world, outpatient

cataract surgery has become the rule rather than the exception. Certified ASCs are as high in quality as major hospital operating rooms.

Questions for review and thought

1. List the significant advantages of ambulatory surgery.
2. List the possible disadvantages of ambulatory surgery.
3. Outline safety standards in a free-standing surgical facility.
4. What are the operative routines followed in your practice?
5. What are the preoperative testing routines before major surgery?
6. What medication, both ocular and systemic, is given before a cataract operation by your ophthalmologist?
7. What is the role of the ophthalmic medical assistant in the care of patients before and after cataract surgery?
8. What is the medicolegal responsibility of the ophthalmic assistant?

Self-evaluation questions Q

True–false statements

Directions: Indicate whether the statement is true (T) or false (F).

1. Operative notes must be detailed in a free-standing surgical facility. **T** or **F**
2. A consent form is required only in some major eye operations. **T** or **F**
3. Drugs and biologic agents can be administered only by a physician. **T** or **F**

Missing words

Directions: Write in the missing word(s) in the following sentences.

4. A _____ is used to record that all necessary preoperative and postoperative evaluations have been ordered.
5. The abbreviated form for medication given by injection in the muscle is called _____.
6. _____ is the Latin term for medication taken by mouth.

Choice-completion questions

Directions: Select the one best answer in each case.

7. Which is not true? Ambulatory cataract surgery may be performed in:
   a. a hospital-based facility.
   b. office treatment rooms.
   c. free-standing surgical centers.
   d. office surgical suites.
   e. hospital emergency operating rooms.
8. Which condition is least likely to be treated with ambulatory surgery?
   a. Cataract with intraocular lens (IOL).
   b. Orbital tumor.
   c. Strabismus surgery.
   d. Glaucoma surgery.
   e. Pterygium surgery.
9. Standards for an ambulatory surgical center involve a number of requirements. Which of the following is not required?
   a. A governing body responsible for policies.
   b. A mechanism for transfer to a hospital for emergencies.
   c. A mechanism for ongoing care.
   d. An attending nurse at all times.
   e. Maintenance of complete records.

Answers, notes, and explanations

A

1. **True**. The requirements for an ambulatory surgical center are as rigid as those of major hospital operating rooms. The details of the surgical procedure must be outlined in a standard operative report attached to the records.
2. **False**. All major surgery requires an informed consent form.
3. **False**. Drugs and biologic agents can be given orally or by eyedrops by allied health personnel who have been trained to do this. Intramuscular or subcutaneous injections must be given either by a physician or by someone licensed in the state to invade tissue. This may be a registered nurse.
4. **Surgical checklist**. Checklists are important to jog one's memory that all items necessary for preoperative and postoperative evaluations are available and the results tabulated. Such information as A-scan measurements may be critical when the time comes for surgery. A checklist is vital.
5. **IM**. The injection is given into the muscle mass.
6. **Per os**. When medication is given orally, it is often written per os, meaning through the mouth.
7. **b. Office treatment rooms**. Office treatment rooms usually do not have the sterility required for major surgery. They also are not adequately equipped for respiratory or cardiovascular emergencies that could occur.
8. **b. Orbital tumor**. Orbital tumors may result in bleeding postoperatively, which may require blood transfusions. There also is a danger that there could be an invasion of adjacent tissue or some unusual tumor found that requires more extensive dissection.
9. **d. An attending nurse at all times**. An attending nurse is not required at all times. Often the physician may supervise a great deal of the ambulatory surgery personally. The ophthalmic medical assistant can be trained to be responsible for a great deal of the patient's care.

and acoustic shock waves in tissue. This form of laser tissue destruction is known as *photodisruption* and can be accomplished by the Nd:YAG laser. The laser beam itself is invisible, having a wavelength of 1064 nm, and focusing is therefore accomplished by placing a red helium-neon laser in the beam path. The laser energy is "q switched" (quality switched) or "mode locked" and is delivered in a single pulse or train of pulses over an extremely short time interval of nanoseconds (q switched) or picoseconds (mode locked). The energy is supplied to the tissue so quickly that damage is produced by a microexplosion rather than by a heating effect, as in thermal photocoagulation.

It is critical that this laser be focused with extreme accuracy, with the minimum power and the minimum number of shots to achieve the desired effect. An appropriate contact lens is usually used because it forms part of the optical focusing system in the laser beam path. This improves accuracy and allows a higher power density, thus minimizing the total energy required to accomplish a given task, such as opening a posterior capsule after cataract surgery (Fig. 35.6). Vision can be improved immediately, as soon as the small opening is produced.

Patients with thick capsules or secondary cataracts occasionally may be treated with this form of laser surgery. Cyclitic membranes that form after trauma to the eye, surgery, or uveitis sometimes can be treated in this manner. High laser energies are usually required and generally, it is safer to use multiple treatment sessions. Iridotomies for the treatment of angle-closure glaucoma are accomplished with this form of laser application. Infrared laser systems that use short pulses are being evaluated in a number of clinical settings, including the production of a fistula as a filtering mechanism in the treatment of glaucoma. Most of these procedures can be carried out with use of a topical anesthetic, as in the case of thermal photocoagulation. Occasionally, however, local anesthesia is required.

Photochemical mechanism

When certain wavelengths of laser light interact with a photosensitizing agent, the absorbed light energy is converted into a highly reactive oxidative process that can bring about cell death. The therapeutic use of laser-induced photochemical damage in ophthalmology has been limited. Attempts have been made to treat cancer in the eye by shining red laser light at a photosensitizing agent known as *hematoporphyrin derivative*, which is preferentially localized in cancerous eye tissue. Cancer cell death has been achieved by this form of therapy. In the retina, photodynamic therapy (PDT) using verteporfin (Visudyne®) was approved for treatment of classic choroidal neovascular membranes (CNVMs) secondary to age-related macular degeneration (AMD), CNVM secondary to pathologic myopia, and presumed histoplasmosis syndrome. It was the treatment of choice before the introduction of anti-VEGF injections. Nevertheless, PDT is still used to treat chronic central serous chorioretinopathy, polypoidal choroidopathy vasculopathy (a variant of wet AMD) and vascular tumors (e.g., choroidal hemangioma). During the PDT, verteporfin is injected intravenously and accumulates slowly in the CNVM tissue. Fifteen minutes after the beginning of the injection, a nonthermal laser red laser (693 nm diode) is used to stimulate verteporfin causing the production of highly reactive short lived singlet oxygen and other reactive oxygen radicals. These lead to local damage to the endothelium with selective photothrombosis and temporary closure of the CNVM.

Photorefractive and phototherapeutic keratotomy

The development of short-wavelength lasers, called *excimer* (*exci*ted di*mer*) lasers, which can efficiently generate high-power ultraviolet light, has prompted the use of short-pulsed ultraviolet radiation for tissue destruction. Surgical modification of corneal refractive power occurs because this tissue possesses about two-thirds of the total refractive power of the phakic eye and is the only refractive surface once the lens is removed.

Pulsed 193-nm light is used to ablate a small amount of corneal stroma (5–100 microns) to induce corneal flattening or steepening in a spherical or cylindric manner.

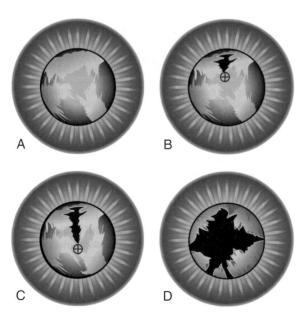

Fig. 35.6 Progressive opening of posterior capsule with Nd:YAG laser photodisruption. (From Steinert RF, Puliafito CA. *The Nd-YAG Laser In Ophthalmology: Principles and Clinical Applications of Photodisruption.* Philadelphia: Saunders; 1985.)

Outcomes have shown the procedure to be safe and with excellent refractive stability. Predictability for correction of myopia, hyperopia, and astigmatism often vary with the degree of refractive error correction required.

First-generation excimer lasers have large beams (6–7 mm) and very large diaphragms that expand or contract relatively slowly. Smoother ablations resulted with second-generation lasers by incorporating wobbling beams and less energy. Third-generation lasers are equipped with small scanning and tracking beams to assist patient fixation. These lasers also use less gas and require less optical maintenance but take longer to produce ablations because of smaller beam technology. Details of the clinical use of the excimer laser are found in Chapters 25, 35, 36 and 37.

Safety in the laser clinic

Everyday supermarket product-marking lasers, CD lasers (5 milliwatts [mW]), DVD players (10 mW), and DVD burners (100 mW) can produce vision damage if improperly used. Lasers used in surgical techniques (30,000–100,000 mW) have significant damage potential from direct or indirect exposure. Even low-mW class 2 lasers, such as those that are used as fixation or target devices, can damage vision. Variables, such as eye health, duration of exposure, and fixation time must be monitored carefully to avoid direct and indirect macular injury.

Safety features that protect the operator and patient from accidental laser exposure have been incorporated into most laser systems. Each product should be carefully scrutinized with these features in mind. It is difficult to formulate mandatory safety rules for an ophthalmic laser clinic because of lack of extensive clinical experience. It is possible, however, to suggest a list of precautions to be followed in the use of such an instrument:

1. Insist that all onlookers wear appropriate laser eye protection.
2. Keep all delivery optical equipment, including contact lenses, clean.
3. After extensive maintenance or unusual jolting of the instrumentation, check the laser beam alignment by firing the beam at a sample target; a sudden change in laser output for the same setting can indicate problems with the laser energy monitor.
4. Always use the lowest energy to accomplish the task.
5. In the case of Nd:YAG lasers, avoid procedures close to the retina and cease laser use if the plasma formation becomes sporadic, which implies malfunction or lowered energy output.
6. Position the patient to avoid accidental exposure, either directly or indirectly, to laser light.
7. Use appropriate signs or indicators to prevent direct viewing of the operating laser by a person entering the room.

Future applications of laser technology

As experience with laser energy increases in the field of ophthalmology, existing forms of therapy are undergoing revision and new treatments are emerging. Noninvasive ciliary body ablative procedures for glaucoma using frequency-doubled Nd:YAG and diode sources are being evaluated. Nd:YAG laser photodisruption of vitreous opacities and traction bands has been accomplished. Cataract degradation laser procedures may offer an alternative to ultrasound phacoemulsification in the quest for small-wound, low-energy cataract surgery. Excimer laser modification of corneal tissue continues to evolve as an effective method to modify refractive errors safely and consistently.

Finally, the introduction of a variety of laser-based imaging techniques used in optical coherence tomography (OCT), macular assessment devices, and wavelength technology is improving the clinician's diagnostic capabilities in managing a number of ocular conditions. The advance of automatic or preplanned laser delivery can minimize laser exposure time for patients and reduce operator treatment times and standardize treatments to increase energy delivery in a more precise way with less operator dependent factors.

Femtosecond laser technology has advanced the accuracy and refinement of tissue ablation in the anterior segment of the eye. The femtosecond laser used in ophthalmology uses near-infrared light applied with shorter pulses than Nd:YAG laser interaction. These ultrashort laser pulses disrupt very small fractions of tissue, which provides exceptional accuracy for clear corneal incisions, astigmatic correction, anterior capsulotomies, and lens fragmentation. With these laser systems, corneal dissection for flap formation in refractive procedures can be applied with greater safety, more consistency, and greater precision over shorter time intervals. Femtosecond laser technology also has advanced the potential for intraocular lens disruption in the continuing quest for minimally invasive cataract surgery. Technologies using laser applications, such as photoacoustic image capture are in their infancy, but promise further insight into more precise disease description.

As the future unfolds, we can look forward to further advances in laser applications in the field of ophthalmology that will bring novel diagnostic and treatment options to the management of ocular disease.

Questions for review and thought

1. What are the different types of lasers used in ophthalmology?
2. What are the indications for laser use?
3. What anatomic structures must the argon laser light pass through before being absorbed by the pigment epithelium of the retina?
4. What safety precautions should be in place when lasers are used?

Self-evaluation questions   **Q**

True–false statements

Directions: Indicate whether the statement is true **(T)** or false **(F)**.

1. Laser application to the eye requires the patient to undergo general anesthesia. **T** or **F**
2. The argon and krypton lasers work on the principle of thermal photocoagulation. **T** or **F**
3. The Nd:YAG laser works via the mechanism of photodisruption. **T** or **F**

Missing words

Directions: Write in the missing word(s) in the following sentences.

4. The letters of the word *laser* stand for _____.
5. The lasers that use ultraviolet radiation for tissue destruction are referred to as _____.
6. The letters of the word YAG stand for _____.

Choice-completion questions

Directions: Select the one best answer in each case.

7. Laser light is consistent with which of the following?
   a. Monochromatism
   b. Coherence
   c. Low divergence
   d. Brightness
   e. All of the above
8. Of the lasers, which has the shortest wavelength?
   a. Argon
   b. Krypton
   c. Nd:YAG
   d. Carbon dioxide
   e. Excimer
9. The argon laser is not used to:
   a. ablate ischemic retina in proliferative diabetic retinopathy.
   b. produce a full-thickness iris hole (iridotomy) in angle-closure glaucoma.
   c. create burns of the trabecular meshwork in patients with open-angle glaucoma.
   d. create a central opening in an opacified posterior capsule after cataract surgery.
   e. ablate ischemic retina in retinal vein occlusions.

Answers, notes, and explanations   **A**

1. **False**. Laser surgery can be performed under local anesthesia. If a specialized contact lens is used to focus the laser light, topical anesthesia is used. If the surgery involves coagulating the retina, for example, panphotocoagulation, then a retrobulbar block in addition to topical anesthesia will often make the patient more comfortable.
2. **True**. The light from argon and krypton lasers is absorbed by tissues, resulting in sufficient heat energy for the surrounding tissue to be coagulated.
3. **True**. Unlike the argon and krypton lasers, the Nd:YAG laser uses high energy and an extremely short period of light exposure, which results in vaporization of tissue.
4. **Light amplification by stimulated emission of radiation**.
5. **Excimer lasers**. Because the laser light has a wavelength less than 380 nm, this light will not penetrate to the back of the eye; it will be completely absorbed by the cornea and lens. For this reason, the laser can be used to produce fine cuts in the cornea to change the refractive error of the eye.

Answers, notes, and explanations—Continued

A

6. **Yttrium aluminum garnet**. These are the components (in addition to neodymium ions, an energy source that can excite the molecules and an optical feedback mechanism) that comprise the Nd:YAG laser.

7. **e. All of the above**. Lasers are composed of monochromatic light in that one or more specific wavelengths are characteristic of each type of laser medium. Coherence refers to the light waves traveling in perfect step. The low divergence means that, as light rays leave the laser cavity, they are nearly parallel. The brightness of laser light exceeds all known artificial and natural light sources.

8. **e. Excimer**. The excimer laser has the shortest wavelength (193 nm). The other lasers in increasing order of wavelength are argon (488 and 514.5 nm), krypton (568 and 647 nm), Nd:YAG (1064 nm), and carbon dioxide (10,600 nm).

9. **d. Create a central opening in an opacified posterior capsule after cataract surgery**. The Nd:YAG laser, unlike the argon, acts to vaporize tissue. For this reason, an opening in an opacified posterior capsule can be made. All the other answers are appropriate indications for use of the argon laser, which acts by photocoagulation.

Chapter | 36 |

Refractive surgery: today and the future

*Raymond M. Stein and Rebecca L. Stein**

Technologies and techniques continue to evolve in the correction of myopia, hyperopia, astigmatism, and presbyopia. Patients are increasingly interested in spectacle or contact lens independence. It is important to understand today's options for vision correction. This chapter provides an overview of this exciting area of clinical advancements and research.

With every surgical innovation, it is important to critically evaluate the outcomes and safety with long-term data. We need to be cautious with any new technology, as many refractive procedures have been abandoned because of lack of efficacy or late complications (Table 36.1).

Patients typically have high expectations with the available technology. They want their postoperative uncorrected visual acuity (UCVA) to be equal or greater to their preoperative best corrected visual acuity (BCVA). It is important to evaluate the patient and the ocular health to determine if they are good candidates for any refractive procedure. Preoperative findings will guide the surgeon in recommending specific refractive options (Table 36.2). To determine the preferred surgical option, we can differentiate higher-order aberrations of the cornea versus the lens. Advanced wavefront units allow measurement of total higher-order aberrations of the eye, which can be differentiated into those from the cornea versus the lens. In patients with significant higher-order aberrations of

---
* The content of this chapter is reproduced from Stein R, Stein R. Refractive surgery: today and the future. Ophthalmology Rounds. Department of Ophthalmology and Vision Sciences, Faculty of Medicine, University of Toronto. 2019.

the lens, a refractive lens exchange would be the treatment of choice to improve the overall quality of vision.

Laser vision correction

Laser-assisted in situ keratomileusis and photorefractive keratectomy

More than 35 million laser-assisted in situ keratomileusis (LASIK) and photorefractive keratotomy (PRK) procedures have been performed worldwide with reported improvement in outcomes and safety. Significant advances over the past 30 years in excimer laser technology include improved nomograms, flying spot lasers with smoother ablations, more accurate trackers, larger optical zones, aspheric curves, and customized treatments that reduce not only refractive errors but other optical aberrations of the eye.

PRK provides excellent outcomes similar to LASIK. Although some surgeons prefer PRK over LASIK because of the reduced risk of corneal ectasia, most offer LASIK first because of quicker postoperative healing. Surgeons typically recommend PRK when the cornea is thin, mildly irregular, or has evidence of epithelial basement membrane dystrophy. PRK may also be preferred if the patient has a narrow fissure that complicates flap creation or is at higher risk of flap subluxation because of factors, such as an occupation or sporting activity. PRK improves quality of day and night vision and maintenance of corneal clarity secondary to the use of larger optical zones, flying spot lasers that create a smoother ablation, adjunctive use of mitomycin C to reduce the risk of corneal haze, and custom treatments, such as topography- and wavefront-guided ablations and wavefront-optimized treatments. Custom ablation with PRK offers the same refractive results as small incision lenticule extraction (SMILE) but with fewer induced higher-order aberrations. Patients are relatively comfortable following

---

Table 36.1 Current and past refractive procedures

Refractive procedures	Myopia	Hyperopia
Current	• PRK • LASIK • SMILE • Phakic IOL • RLE	• PRK • LASIK • Phakic IOL • RLE
Past	• Keratomileusis • ALK • Epikeratophakia • Radial keratotomy • Corneal rings	• Epikeratophakia • Hexagonal keratotomy • Thermal keratoplasty • Lasso suture

ALK, Automated lamellar keratoplasty; *EDOF*, extended depth-of-focus; *IOL*, intraocular lens; *LASIK*, laser assisted in situ keratomileusis; *PRK*, photorefractive keratectomy; *RLE*, refractive lens exchange; *SMILE*, small incision lenticule extraction.
(From Stein R, Stein R. Refractive surgery: today and the future. Ophthalmology Rounds. Ophthalmology & Vision Sciences University of Toronto. https://www.bochner.com/wp-content/uploads/2019/03/Refractive_Surgery_Today_Future.pdf)

Table 36.2 Refractive options based on clinical findings

Clinical finding refractive options

- Thin cornea and/or high myopia
- PRK, phakic IOL

- High hyperopia (>3 D)
- RLE, phakic IOL

- Forme-fruste keratoconus, keratoconus, pellucid marginal
- PRK, topography-guided PRK, Intacs, phakic IOL, ± CXL degeneration, ectasia

- Lenticular changes
- RLE, early cataract surgery

- Higher-order lens aberrations
- RLE

- Predicted postoperative curvature <32 D or >50 D
- RLE, phakic IOL

- Presbyopia
- Monovision (with PRK, LASIK, SMILE), RLE, corneal inlay

- AMD or other forms of central vision loss
- Corneal photovitrification

AMD, Age-related macular degeneration; *CXL*, corneal cross-linking; *IOL*, intraocular lens; *LASIK*, laser-assisted in situ keratomileusis; *PRK*, photorefractive keratectomy; *RLE*, refractive lens exchange; *SMILE*, small incision lenticule extraction.
(From Stein R, Stein R. Refractive surgery: today and the future. Ophthalmology Rounds. Ophthalmology & Vision Sciences University of Toronto. https://www.bochner.com/wp-content/uploads/2019/03/Refractive_Surgery_Today_Future.pdf)

PRK with application of sterile ice to the surface of the cornea, bandage soft contact lenses, and nonsteroidal drops.

LASIK is among the most frequently performed and successful medical procedures. With proper preoperative screening, visual outcomes are excellent with a low complication rate. In North America, femtosecond lasers for creation of the corneal flap have generally replaced blade microkeratomes. Advances in femtosecond technology have shown predictable flap thickness and the ability to customize the diameter, location, hinge, and edge profile of the LASIK flap. In the rare event of suction loss with a femtosecond laser, the suction ring can be reapplied and the procedure completed. With suction loss using a mechanical microkeratome, the procedure is aborted and the patient must return a few months later for PRK.

In a large LASIK clinical review (97 papers; 67,893 eyes) from 2008 to 2015, 90.8% of eyes achieved a distance UCVA of 20/20 or more and 99.5% achieved 20/40 or more. The spherical equivalent refraction was within ± 0.50 D of target in 90.9% of eyes and within ± 1.00 D of target in 98.6%. These outcomes were superior to earlier reports, which reflect further advances in hardware and software of the lasers, surgical techniques, and improved patient selection. Loss of two or more lines of corrected distance visual acuity (CDVA) was 0.61%, less than one-half the number of eyes that had an increase in CDVA of two lines or more (1.45%). The more advanced treatments (topography- and wavefront-guided or wavefront-optimized) allowed for a UDVA of nearly a full line better than in eyes with conventional treatments. Most treatments in the review were for myopia and myopic astigmatism; hyperopic treatments represented 3% of cases. A 2-line or greater CDVA loss was more common in hyperopic than myopic treatments (2.13% vs. 0.95%); this may be related to more sensitive centration of the hyperopic treatment, which has been shown to be best centered on line of sight versus the center of the pupil. Hyperopic treatments are also associated with a greater risk of regression versus myopic treatments.

The most significant long-term complication of LASIK is corneal ectasia (incidence ~0.03%). The risk has been lowered by improved preoperative detection of formefruste keratoconus, keratoconus, and pellucid marginal degeneration with elevation tomography that detects elevation abnormalities on the anterior and posterior corneal surfaces. Other factors accounting for improved LASIK outcomes include avoidance of surgery on thin corneas or those with high myopia, creation of thinner corneal flaps, and leaving a thicker residual bed underneath the flap. The presently preferred treatment of corneal ectasia is with corneal crosslinking and possibly topography-guided PRK or an intracorneal ring to reduce irregular astigmatism. Early ectasia detection and treatment can limit corneal irregularity and provide better visual acuity.

Further research in tracking devices, torsional alignment, the ideal centration of ablations, an understanding of the biomechanical properties of the cornea, and medications or adjunctive procedures to modulate wound healing will enhance our outcomes and patient safety for all laser vision correction procedures.

Small incision lenticule extraction procedure

SMILE is a new method of intrastromal keratomileusis in which a femtosecond laser is used to create two cuts within the cornea and one small superficial cut. A lenticule is produced of a specific shape and thickness, and is pulled out mechanically through a 2 to 3 mm diameter corneal incision. SMILE is an alternative refractive procedure for the correction of myopia and myopic astigmatism. Recent studies have validated the efficacy and safety. Table 36.3 presents a comparison of LASIK, PRK, and SMILE.

SMILE is currently reserved for myopia and myopic astigmatism. Enhancement procedures tend to be with PRK,

Table 36.3 Comparison of photorefractive keratectomy, laser assisted in situ keratomileusis, and small incision lenticule extraction

	Photorefractive keratectomy	Laser-assisted in situ keratomileusis	Small incision lenticule extraction
Technique of Vision Correction			
Health Canada Approval	1990	1994	2015
Generation of equipment	5th Generation	5th Generation	1st Generation
Type of treatment	Laser photoablation	Laser photoablation	Laser photodisruption
Precision	0.12 µm/pulse	0.12 µm/pulse	2–3 µm/pulse
Smoothness of refractive correction	Smooth excimer ablation	Smooth excimer ablation	Femtosecond (rougher than excimer)

Continued

Table 36.3 Comparison of photorefractive keratectomy, laser assisted in situ keratomileusis, and small incision lenticule extraction—cont'd

	Photorefractive keratectomy	Laser-assisted in situ keratomileusis	Small incision lenticule extraction
Blade-free	Yes	Yes	Yes
Type of laser	Excimer	Femtosecond and excimer	Femtosecond
Myopic correction: Low (<3 D)	Yes	Yes	Difficult if thin lenticule
Higher (>3 D)	Yes	Yes	Yes
Myopic astigmatic correction	Yes	Yes	Yes difficult if spheroequivalent <3 D
Hyperopic correction	Yes	Yes	Future
Hyperopic astigmatic correction	Yes	Yes	Future
Topography-guided treatments	Yes	Yes	Future
Wavefront-guided treatments	Yes	Yes	Future
Optical centration adjustment	Yes	Yes	Future
Cyclotorsion adjustment	Yes	Yes	Future
Return of best UCVA	Slowest	Fastest	Slower than LASIK
Best UCVA	Superior (custom ablation)	Superior (custom ablation)	Good (noncustomized)
Higher-order aberrations	Less (custom ablation)	Less (custom ablation)	Highest (noncustomized)
Enhancements	Yes	Yes	More difficult
Dry eyes: <6 month >6 months	Increase (typically mild) Same	Increase (typically mild) Same	Increase (less than PRK or LASIK) Same
Risk of ectasia:	Lowest	Low	Greater (more tissue removed)
low myopia high myopia	Lowest	Low (similar to SMILE)	Low (similar to LASIK)

LASIK, Laser-assisted in situ keratomileusis; *PRK*, photorefractive keratectomy; *SMILE*, small incision lenticule extraction; *UCVA*, uncorrected visual acuity. (From Stein R, Stein R. Refractive surgery: today and the future. Ophthalmology Rounds. Ophthalmology & Vision Sciences University of Toronto. https://www.bochner.com/wp-content/uploads/2019/03/Refractive_Surgery_Today_Future.pdf)

although some recent evidence supports LASIK to correct residual refractive errors. Current limitations of first-generation SMILE versus LASIK include difficulty in performing low myopic corrections (<3 D) because of a thin and fragile lenticule, lack of effect on hyperopia or hyperopic astigmatism, inability to perform topography- or wavefront-guided treatment, less-smooth cuts with femtosecond laser than excimer, lack of optical centration adjustment when the suction device is placed on the eye, no cyclotorsion compensation, slower return of UCVA, and inferior improvement in best UCVA compared with custom treatments. Because the overlying cap in SMILE is adherent, there is

Extended depth-of-focus intraocular lenses

EDOF IOLs tend to produce less glare and halos or loss of contrast compared with multifocals. They provide good uncorrected distance and intermediate vision; however, near vision is better with multifocal implants. Surgeons using this type of lens tend to use a technique of micromonovision in which the EDOF IOL is placed in the dominant eye and the other eye is left mildly myopic to enhance reading.

Multifocal intraocular lenses

Among the most commonly used multifocal implants in Canada are the FineVision Trifocal (PhysIOL), PanOptix IOL (Alcon), and AT Lisa Trifocal (Zeiss). Glare and halos may occur especially in scotopic conditions; however, this tends to improve with time because of neuroadaptation. Trifocal implants provide better intermediate vision with fewer side effects by using diffraction and asymmetric light distribution. It is valuable to measure angle kappa preoperatively because patients with a large positive angle kappa may not be able to tolerate multifocals because of the difference in their line of sight and the center of the optic.

Segmented bifocal intraocular lenses

The rotationally asymmetric segmented bifocal IOLs with sector-shaped near vision provides two focus zones for distance or for reading. Implants in this category are the LENTIS Mplus and Mplus X (Oculentis), and SBL-3 (Lenstec). Similar to multifocal implants, the patients may have glare especially at night or in the presence of a residual refractive error. Refractions are more difficult, as patients will have refractive errors through the distance optic and the segmented bifocal.

Accommodative intraocular lenses

Accommodative IOLs have had limited success in providing satisfactory near vision. These lenses include the Crystalens AO (Bausch + Lomb), Tetraflex (Lenstec) and the dual-optic IOL, such as Synchrony (AMO).

Future accommodative IOLs in design or clinical study may offer patients the full range of vision without glare or halos, or quality of vision issues. The FluidVision IOL (PowerVision), currently in clinical trials, allows the quantity of fluid within the optic to increase or decrease, which changes the accommodative power (Fig. 36.2). With the accommodative response, fluid is displaced centrally into the lens, which expands the central membrane of the optic and facilitates near vision, with relaxation of the ciliary muscle, fluid returns to the periphery, and distance vision is created. The lens has been studied outside of North America with reports of accommodative amplitude of up

to 3 D to 4 D with 3 years of follow-up. The Sapphire IOL (ELENZA) uses nanotechnology and advanced electronics to adjust the focus of the implant in response to pupillary changes. Using artificial intelligence to differentiate between light stimulation and accommodation by sensing the speed and amplitude of the pupillary responses, the implant can provide quality of near vision.

A few sulcus-implanted accommodative IOLs are under clinical study. The DynaCurve IOL (NuLens) changes curvature in response to accommodation from a collapsed bag-zonular complex; this change activates a piston that induces a gel component to bulge and alter an anterior flexible membrane (Fig. 36.3). The optical power of the

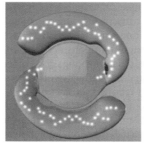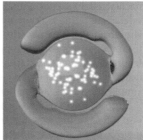

Fig. 36.2 FluidVision intraocular lens (PowerVision) is inserted in the capsular bag. Accommodative effort results in changes in optic power from fluid flow to the central portion of the lens, which increases the power of the lens to enhance near vision. Note: As of the time of publishing this edition, the FluidVision accommodating IOL is an investigational device and is not marketed or sold.

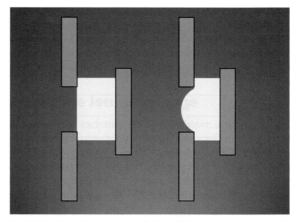

Fig. 36.3 Dyna-Curve intraocular lens (NuLens) is inserted in the ciliary sulcus with an intact capsular membrane. Accommodative effort pushes a gel centrally, which increases the optic power by bulging of an anterior flexible membrane to provide near vision. (From Stein R, Stein R. Refractive surgery: today and the future. Ophthalmology Rounds. Ophthalmology & Vision Sciences University of Toronto. https://www.bochner.com/wp-content/uploads/2019/03/Refractive_Surgery_Today_Future.pdf)

IOL will increase depending on the magnitude of the silicone bulge because of the contraction of the ciliary muscle. Early clinical studies improved near vision by up to 3.8 lines; however, 60% of eyes had significant capsular opacification that required a YAG capsulotomy. The Lumina lens (AkkoLens/Oculentis) is also implanted in the ciliary sulcus; it has two optical elements that move with ciliary muscle contraction, one on top of the other, producing accommodation. These elements provide a fixed optical power, with anterior element providing 5 D and the posterior providing 10 to 25 D. The lens can be inserted through a 2.8- to 3.0-mm incision. A 12-month clinical trial showed significantly enhanced near vision compared with a monofocal IOL and with similar contrast sensitivity.

Small-aperture intraocular lenses

Small-aperture IOLs can extend the depth of focus (Fig. 36.4). These IOLs are especially effective in patients with significant higher-order aberrations, such as those post-RK, keratoconus, or any other irregular corneal surface. The IC-8 IOL (AcuFocus) is a monofocal IOL similar to the Kamra corneal inlay that uses the pinhole design to enhance the depth of focus. It has a 1.36-mm central aperture and a surrounding opaque area of 3.23 mm. The IC-8 IOL is inserted into the capsular bag. Clinical results have shown good distance, intermediate, and near vision, especially when targeting up to –0.75 D of myopia. The XtraFocus Pinhole implant (Morcher) is a small-aperture sulcus implant of black acrylic with a central opening. This lens is inserted in the sulcus in pseudophakic eyes. It is especially effective in patients with unsatisfactory quality of vision despite lens implant surgery because of significant corneal aberrations.

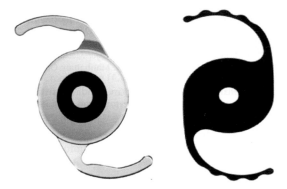

Fig. 36.4 Small-aperture intraocular lenses (IOLs) can extend the depth of focus and reduce higher-order aberrations by a small central clear area of the optic in which peripheral light is reduced. *Left*: IC-8 IOL (AcuFocus) for insertion in the capsular bag. *Right*: XtraFocus Pinhole implant (Morcher) for insertion in the ciliary sulcus. (MORCHER® GmbH, Germany).

Light-adjustable intraocular lenses

The light-adjustable IOL will be available in the future. This is a photosensitive silicone material that can be adjusted postoperatively with ultraviolet (UV) light to refine the outcome. After the standard IOL measurements and surgical procedure is performed, if the power of the IOL is not ideal then one can correct the sphere from –3.00 to +3.00 D or astigmatism up to 3 D to refine the patient's uncorrected vision. In addition, the UV light can be used to induce a change to reduce spherical aberration and potentially enhance reading vision.

Corrections of refractive errors in pseudophakes

Enhancing a patient's vision following lens implant surgery can be done by an IOL exchange, laser vision correction, or a secondary IOL in the sulcus. Rayner Sulcoflex IOLs can be custom-made to correct almost any refractive error. The lens has a 6.5 mm optic, a length of 14 mm, and is available in either monofocal or toric design. It has a concave posterior surface. Future trifocal implants will be inserted in the sulcus in pseudophakes. This will allow refinement of distance vision and improvement in both intermediate and near vision.

Corneal inlays

Corneal inlays have faced many challenges. Early inlays were associated with corneal opacification, vascularization, keratolysis, and decentration. The inlay must be thin, have a small diameter, allow adequate nutritional and fluid permeability, and inserted relatively deep in the cornea. The long-term success of inlays depends on biocompatibility and providing excellent refractive outcomes and quality of vision. The most commonly used implant today is the Kamra inlay, which is a small aperture inlay that enhances the depth of focus and is inserted deep in the cornea. Better outcomes are associated with insertion into a corneal pocket versus under a LASIK flap. The inlay is made of polyvinylidene fluoride. The reported clinical results have been highly variable, and many surgeons have abandoned the procedure because of either early or late complications. The Kamra inlay has a diameter of 3.8 mm, thickness of 5 μm, and a 1.6-mm central opening.

The Raindrop inlay is 2 mm in diameter and 25 m thick. Unlike the Kamra inlay, it induces central steeping to allow enhanced reading with pupillary constriction during accommodation. Although the early clinical results with the Raindrop were promising, a high percentage of patients developed a late reaction with corneal haze, necessitating

Diagnosis of keratoconus

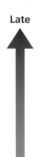

Late

- Corneal hydrops
- Munson's sign
- Apical scarring
- Vogt's striae
- Irregular keratometry mires
- Abdominal computerized topography
- High coma
- Epithelial thickness abnormalities

Early
- Posterior corneal curvature

Fig. 37.1 Clinical signs of keratoconus may be early or late in the disease process.

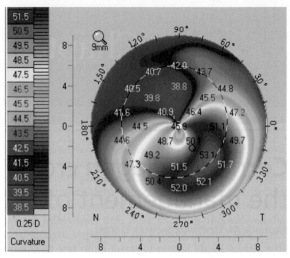

Fig. 37.2 Computerized videokeratography of keratoconus with inferior steepening.

in around half of keratoconic eyes. This ring is caused by deposition of the iron oxide hemosiderin within the corneal epithelium. Further progression can lead to breaks in Bowman's membrane, resulting in apical scarring. A break in Descemet's membrane results in rapid stromal and often epithelial edema, referred to as corneal hydrops. An advanced cone can create a V-shaped indentation in the lower eyelid when the patient's gaze is directed downward, known as Munson's sign. This finding, though a classic sign of the disease, tends not to be of primary diagnostic importance because it occurs late in the disease process.

Computerized topography and tomography

Sophisticated corneal imaging today allows for an early diagnosis of keratoconus. Computerized corneal topography can take the form of curvature analysis or with computerized tomography both curvature and elevation detection. Asymmetric astigmatism with inferior steepening is a typical topographic pattern (Fig. 37.2). Elevation imaging allows for the comparison of the anterior surface or posterior surface with a best-fit sphere. Changes to the posterior corneal curvature may represent the earliest clinical sign of keratoconus (Fig. 37.3). Corneas are typically thinner in keratoconus, and the finding of the thinnest spot on the cornea in the steepest region associated with posterior corneal elevation is characteristic for keratoconus. Clinical studies on the measurement of the thickness of the epithelium indicate that eyes with keratoconus typically have thinner epithelium overlying the cone and thicker at the base of the cone.

Etiology of keratoconus

The etiology of keratoconus remains unknown. Keratoconus likely arises from a number of factors: genetic, environmental, or cellular, any of which may form the trigger for the onset of the disease. A genetic predisposition to keratoconus has been observed, with the disease running in certain families, and incidences reported of concordance in identical twins. Most genetic studies agree on an autosomal dominant mode of inheritance. The condition is seen at a higher frequency in those with Down syndrome. Keratoconus also has been associated with atopic diseases, which include asthma, allergies, and eczema. There is support for the finding that excess eye rubbing contributes to the progression of keratoconus.

Pellucid marginal degeneration

Pellucid marginal degeneration (PMD) is a degenerative corneal ectatic disease that is often confused with keratoconus. It is characterized by thinning in the periphery of the cornea. The corneas typically have a normal thickness in the center. The inferior cornea exhibits a peripheral band of thinning. There is usually high against-the-rule astigmatism. Computerized topography shows a classic butterfly appearance. No known cause for the disease has been found. Like keratoconus, PMD represents a contraindication to LASIK and SMILE.

Keratoconus

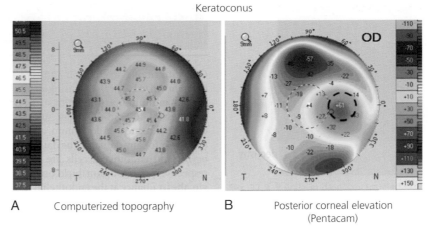

A   Computerized topography   B   Posterior corneal elevation
(Pentacam)

Fig. 37.3 (A) Computerized topography shows a relatively normal bowtie pattern of astigmatism. (B) However, posterior corneal elevation shows a focal area of bulging, characteristic of keratoconus.

Corneal ectasia following laser-assisted in situ keratomileusis or small incision lenticule extraction

Corneal ectasia is a rare, potentially devastating complication following LASIK or SMILE. Ectatic changes may occur as early as 1 week, but are usually delayed by many years. The actual incidence of ectasia is undetermined, although incidence rates of 0.04%, 0.2%, and 0.6% have been reported.

Risk factors for corneal ectasia include:

1. Abnormal preoperative topography as seen with keratoconus, pellucid marginal degeneration, or forme fruste keratoconus.
2. Low residual stromal bed (RSB) thickness is an important factor after LASIK or SMILE because tensile strength analysis indicates greater strength in the anterior 40% relative to the posterior 60% of stroma. LASIK or SMILE reduces corneal structural integrity; it is clear that a cut-off of 250 μm of the corneal bed does not absolutely discriminate development of ectasia; however, the risk of ectasia increases reciprocally relative to RSB thickness.
3. Young age may be a significant risk factor for ectasia in patients without other risk factors. One hypothesis is that some of these individuals would have developed delayed-onset forme fruste or keratoconus even without the LASIK or SMILE procedure.
4. Low preoperative corneal thickness is a factor along with the degree of myopia and RSB. RSB thickness is the most significant predictor of ectasia among them.

5. High myopia, especially greater than 10.00 diopters, is associated with a higher risk of ectasia. Despite this finding, post-LASIK and SMILE ectasia has been reported in patients with low refractive errors.

Other risk factors include eye rubbing, family history of keratoconus, refractive instability, and best corrected visual acuity (BCVA) of less than 20/20 preoperatively.

Development of corneal crosslinking

The derivation of the concept of CXL came from the recognition that diabetic individuals tend not to develop keratoconus because of natural crosslinking from high blood glucose levels and exposure to UV light. The basic research on CXL was conducted from 1993 to 1997 by Doctors Theo Seiler and Eberhard Spoerl in Germany. Research has shown that CXL increases corneal rigidity by 328%. New bonds are formed across adjacent collagen fibers to enhance the cornea's mechanical strength. The procedure has been effective in treating keratoconus, pellucid marginal degeneration, and ectasia following laser vision correction.

The idea of crosslinking is not new. The practice has been used since around 1940 in the field of material science in the conversion of silicone oil to rubber. Dentists have been using crosslinking for more than 25 years (Fig. 37.4). Natural crosslinking occurs as a normal aging change in connective tissues of the body. This may explain why the progression of keratoconus tends to slow down with age.

635

stromal edema to permit safe crosslinking. At the Bochner Eye Institute, we found that there is a 95% chance of inducing satisfactory swelling for corneas between 300 and 399 μm with hypotonic drops.

Clinical outcomes of corneal crosslinking

The first CXL treatments were performed in Europe in 1998. This is a relatively new treatment in North America since 2007. The success of CXL is based on the lack of progressive ectasia. In addition, often some corneal flattening occurs, with asymmetric changes often resulting in an improvement in best corrected spectacle visual acuity (BCSVA).

Wollensak et al. published their initial outcomes report on CXL in 2003, in 16 eyes of 15 patients with progressive keratoconus. A subsequent publication reported on 22 eyes of 24 patients with a follow-up time of between 3 months and 4 years. They reported that in all treated eyes, the progression of keratoconus was halted. In 70% of eyes, there was a regression with a mean reduction of the maximal keratometry readings by about 2.00 diopters and refractive error of approximately 1.00 diopter. Visual acuity improved slightly in 65% of eyes.

Since the initial study, there have been numerous studies reporting their results. The methodologies are variable and as such are not directly comparable; however, all reports demonstrated varying degrees of improvement in visual acuity and reduction in keratometry with a progressive trend of improvement in the duration of follow-up. The longest study to date by Raiskup-Wolf et al. reported their 7-year results in Germany. They reported a decrease in maximum keratometry of 2.7 diopters in year 1, 2.2 diopters at 2 years, and 4.8 diopters at 3 years. BCSVA improved by one line per year in 54% of patients in the first 3 years. Two patients had continued progression and had to undergo repeat crosslinking procedures.

In the only randomized prospective controlled clinical trial of collagen crosslinking in progressive keratoconus published to date, Wittig-Silva et al. reported on 66 eyes of 49 patients with documented progression of keratoconus. Interim analysis of treated eyes showed a flattening of the steepest simulated keratometry (K-max) by an average of 0.74 diopter at 3 months, 0.92 diopter at 6 months, and 1.45 diopters at 12 months. A trend toward improvement of BCSVA was also observed. In the control eyes, mean K-max steepened by 0.60 diopter after 3 months, 0.60 diopter after 6 months, and by 1.28 diopters after 12 months. BCSVA decreased by a logmar of 0.003 over 3 months, 0.056 over 6 months, and 0.12 over 12 months.

Complications following CXL are uncommon, but a few have been reported: herpes simplex virus (HSV) keratitis, sterile infiltrate, and a corneal ulcer, secondary to *Escherichia coli*.

At the Bochner Eye Institute, we reported on 12-month data of 30 consecutive eyes of 19 patients who had an average age of 34.4 years with a range of 17 to 44 years. There were 12 right eyes and 18 left eyes. All corneas were clear preoperatively. The minimum corneal thickness was 400 μm. Pachymetry data showed an average minimum corneal thickness of 461 μm (range 401–548 μm) and at the 3-month level the average thickness had gone down to 431 μm (range 337–514 μm). By 6 months, the average thickness increased to 441 μm and then at 9 to 12 months to 442 μm (Fig. 37.10). When we looked at the percentage of corneal thinning from preoperative average measurements, at 3 months there was a decrease in corneal thickness by 6.5%, at 6 months 4.3%, and at 9 to 12 months 4.1% (Fig. 37.11). There is significant variability in the degree of corneal thinning from patient to patient, and even in the same patient between the right and left eyes (Figs. 37.12 and 37.13). The average decrease in corneal curvature looking at the steepest diopter region of the cornea was 1.00 diopter at 12 months.

The change in the steepest power or average K does not provide all the important information when analyzing the

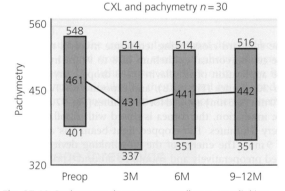

Fig. 37.10 Pachymetry decreases postcollagen crosslinking as the collagen fibers become more compact ($n=30$). *CXL*, Corneal crosslinking; *M*, months.

CXL and pachymetry $n=30$

% Corneal thinning from Preop

3M	6.5%
6M	4.3%
9–12M	4.1%

Fig. 37.11 Pachymetry changes over time postcollagen crosslinking: percentage thinning from preoperative measurement ($n=30$). *CXL*, Corneal crosslinking.

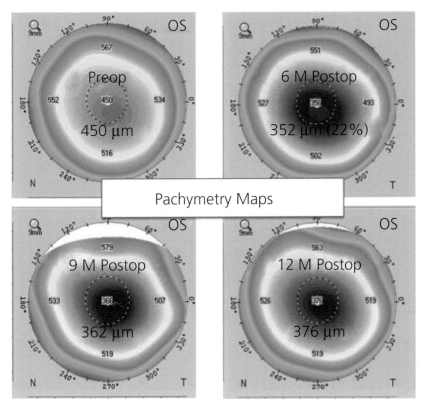

Fig. 37.12 Pachymetry postcollagen crosslinking changes at 6, 9, and 12 months (*M*).

effects from CXL. It is important to look at different maps to appreciate the change in curvature (Figs. 37.14 and 37.15). There is some mild postoperative corneal haze that peaks at 6 months and gradually decreases over time (Fig. 37.16). One of the most important clinical signs is the change in BCSVA (Fig. 37.17). In our series of 30 eyes, at 12 months postoperatively, 60% of eyes gained one or more lines of vision, 33.3% were the same, and 6.6% showed a one line decrease in BCSVA.

Following CXL, the epithelium becomes intact usually by 4 to 6 days. A pseudodendrite is typically seen, which is a normal healing response to any corneal abrasion. BCSVA may be worse during the first 1 to 2 months, as the epithelium undergoes remodeling that results in a thinner layer of cells over the cone and thicker over the base to reduce irregular astigmatism.

Post-laser-assisted in situ keratomileusis or small incision lenticule extraction ectasia

Post-LASIK or SMILE ectasia is a serious complication that rarely follows laser vision correction. Patients typically do well in terms of uncorrected visual acuity and best corrected visual acuity for years until ectasia develops. The topographic findings are similar to that of keratoconus. The biomechanical properties of the cornea have been weakened and this may be secondary to preoperative keratoconus, or minimal residual bed depth from the correction of high myopia, thin preoperative pachymetry, or a thicker flap than intended. The success rate of using CXL in ectasia cases has been reported and is the only current procedure to prevent progressive thinning and bulging (Fig. 37.18). These patients are the most motivated to see better without correction, which is why they underwent laser vision correction initially. Topography-guided PRK in combination with CXL offers the potential to improve BCVA. To enhance uncorrected acuity, an implantable contact lens inserted in the sulcus is an additional refractive option.

Topographically linked ablation

The use of a topography-guided photorefractive keratectomy (TG-PRK) is a valuable technique to reduce irregular

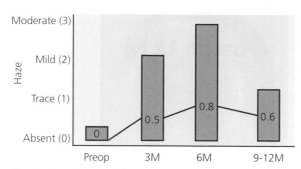

CXL and corneal haze n=30

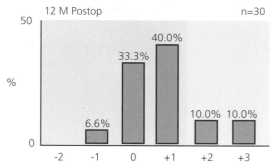

Line change in BCSVA

Fig. 37.16 Mild corneal haze is noted postcollagen crosslinking that peaks at 6 months then gradually decreases over time (*n* = 30). *M*, Months.

Fig. 37.17 Line change in best corrected spectacle visual acuity (BCSVA) postcollagen crosslinking. *M*, Months.

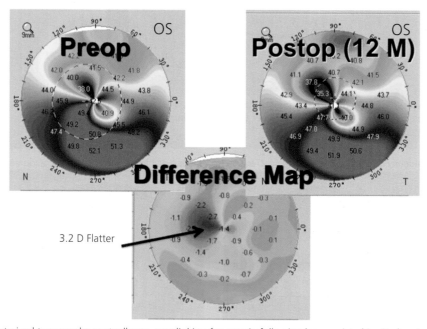

Fig. 37.18 Computerized topography postcollagen crosslinking for ectasia following laser-assisted in situ keratomileusis (LASIK). Difference map shows 3.2 diopter *(D)* of flattening. *M*, Months. (Courtesy Bochner Eye Institute, Toronto.)

rings are inserted, one suture is used to close the small corneal wound. The suture is typically removed in 6 to 8 weeks. The ring procedure offers the benefit of being reversible and potentially exchangeable because it involves no removal of tissue. Early studies on intrastromal corneal rings involved use of two segments to cause general flattening of the cornea. A later study reported that better results could be obtained for those cones located more to the periphery of the cornea by using a single ring segment. This leads to preferential flattening of the cone below, but also to steepening of the over-flat upper part of the cornea.

Potential future advances in corneal crosslinking

CXL is one of the most significant advances in the therapeutic treatment of keratoconus, pellucid marginal degeneration, and ectasia following LASIK. A great deal of research and clinical studies are ongoing to enhance outcomes. Can we direct the UVA light to specific areas of an abnormal cornea to improve outcomes? Although patients want their disease

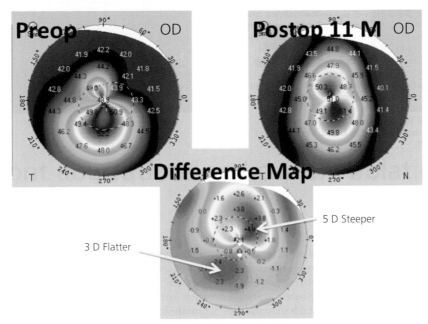

Fig. 37.19 Computerized topography postcollagen crosslinking and topographically linked ablation. Significant improvement in irregular astigmatism achieved by steepening superiorly and flattening inferiorly. (Courtesy Bochner Eye Institute, Toronto.)

process to be halted by CXL, they want their quality of vision to be enhanced. Further research will provide more answers.

Summary

Because CXL can prevent progressive disease, the earlier the disease stage when CXL is performed, the better is the final visual result. It is important for clinicians to make an early diagnosis of an ectatic disease and this is greatly aided by the use of computerized topography or tomography. If there is a family history of keratoconus, then corneal imaging would be helpful at an early age. If there is no family history of keratoconus, then a decrease in best corrected spectacle visual acuity, increasing astigmatism, or a scissors reflex on retinoscopy then keratoconus should be suspected and a topographic evaluation be performed. Today, the CXL procedure has been approved in most countries around the world and has become the standard of care for keratoconus, pellucid marginal degeneration, and ectasia following LASIK or SMILE to halt progression.

Further reading

Caporossi A, Mazzotta C, Baiocchi S, et al. Long-term results of riboflavin ultraviolet a corneal collagen cross- linking for keratoconus in Italy: the Siena eye cross study. *Am J Ophthalmol.* 2010;149(4):585–593.

Godefrooij DA, Gans R, Imhof SM, Wisse RP. Nationwide reduction in the number of corneal transplantations for keratoconus following the implementation of cross-linking. *Acta Ophthalmol.* 2016;94(7):675–678.

Hersh PS, Greenstein SA. Corneal crosslinking for keratoconus and corneal ectasia. In: *Foundations of Corneal Disease.* Cham: Springer; 2020:195–205.

Kanellopoulos AJ, Binder PS. Collagen cross-linking (CCL) with sequential topography-guided PRK: a temporizing alternative for keratoconus to penetrating keratoplasty. *Cornea.* 2007;26(7):891–895.

Kontadakis GA, Kankariya VP, Tsoulnaras K, Pallikaris AI, Plaka A, Kymionis GD. Long-term comparison of simultaneous topography-guided photorefractive keratectomy followed by corneal cross-linking versus corneal cross-linking alone. *Ophthalmology.* 2016;123(5):974–983.

expressed by refractive surgery patients. The postoperative lamentation of a patient who achieves a UCVA of 20/20 but maintains that the vision is not as good as preoperatively cannot be comprehended if a high-contrast chart is used as the only visual performance test. Low-contrast charts, by lowering letter contrast, increase the sensitivity of the visual acuity test, making it possible to detect more subtle changes in optical quality. Several studies have shown that low-contrast acuity is a more sensitive measure of changes in visual function after refractive surgery than is high-contrast acuity.

A further examination that improves the assessment of the postrefractive surgery eye is the contrast sensitivity test. If a custom ablation succeeds in reducing an eye's higher-order optical aberrations (in addition to eliminating the spherocylindric error), the outcome is likely to result in higher-contrast images, making it easier for the patient to drive at night or to perform other tasks in dim illumination.

Chapter | 39 |

Ophthalmic photography

Richard E. Hackel, Csaba L. Mártonyi, and Tim Steffens

In 1960 Novotny and Alvis performed the first successful fluorescein angiogram on a human being using black-and-white film. That event marked the advent of modern ophthalmic photography. Subsequent development of sophisticated instrumentation has made it possible to consistently produce precise documentation of subtle changes within the eye. Intravenous fluorescence angiography has contributed greatly to a better understanding of the posterior segment of the eye and continues to be of particular importance in the diagnosis and treatment of many of the diverse disease processes that affect it. Since 1976, endothelial specular photomicrography has made possible the documentation of the cell density of the posterior layer of the cornea of the living eye. Moreover, photography plays an indispensable role in many areas of research and teaching. With the techniques of optical coherence tomography (OCT), external photography, photo slit-lamp biomicrography, fundus photography, fluorescein and indocyanine green angiography, video recording, and endothelial specular photomicrography, ophthalmic photography today is a vital, well-established adjunct to ophthalmology.

The quality of digital imaging has improved dramatically and has replaced film. Very few clinics continue to use film; the discussion here is geared toward ophthalmic photography using digital imaging.

Although this chapter cannot cover the full scope of ophthalmic photography, it provides an introduction to its most practical applications and the essential concepts for understanding digital imaging. OCT has become a major diagnostic imaging tool in ophthalmology, but its use is not covered in this chapter (see Ch. 41).

Photographic terms

Even with the changeover to digital media, much of the basic film terminology still applies to ophthalmic photography. This chapter focuses on digital imaging and makes comparisons to film when helpful and appropriate.

Standard, handheld digital cameras have either fixed or interchangeable lenses. From there, they can be broken down into three basic types, based on their viewfinder configuration: single-lens reflex (SLR), those that use a liquid-crystal display (LCD) screen as a viewfinder, and the mirrorless reflex cameras that use an electronic viewfinder. Numerous lenses are available, and their important characteristics include focal length, lens speed, *depth of field*, and resolution. Exposure is determined with an exposure meter and fine-tuning since the mid-1980s, has evolved into a high-quality imaging standard. CMOS is a more recent challenger. Although far less expensive to produce than a CCD, it initially suffered from poor contrast and image noise. These problems have been resolved and the CMOS chip is now used in most cameras. The Foveon chip promises even more resolution and detail, but has been slow to enter the market.

Whichever chip is used, it is located in the camera at the same focal plane as film, known as the "film plane." Working in conjunction with the chip's ISO sensitivity, the shutter speed and lens aperture are adjusted according to the prevailing light levels.

Digital sensors chip comes in many sizes. Because the chips are expensive to produce, the manufacturers have tried to reduce cost by keeping the chip size small. Most digital SLR cameras are currently equipped with chips that are two-thirds the size of 35-mm film. Consequently, images produced on these digital cameras appear magnified compared with the same image on film. Because most fundus cameras are designed for 35-mm film, either a reducing lens is placed between the fundus camera and the digital camera back or a more expensive, larger chip is used.

Color balance

Unlike film, which needs to be matched for correct color temperature (daylight or tungsten), digital cameras correct for proper color balance by adjusting what is known as "white balance." Although this white balance can be set to automatically correct itself, it is sometimes preferable to set it to match the specific type of lighting environment.

All lighting sources have a color temperature, which is expressed in degrees Kelvin (K). Normal daylight, around midday, has a color temperature of approximately 5400 K. The light produced by an electronic flash has the same color temperature. Standard household lighting is often much warmer in color, and tungsten bulbs are approximately 3000 K. Fluorescent lighting and halogens all have their own color temperature, some cooler, some warmer. Whereas the human eye and brain constantly adapt to correct for these color imbalances, the camera must be told to adjust. Otherwise, a color balance setting for outdoor lighting will have a blue cast if that setting is used with indoor tungsten lights. A tungsten color balance setting used outdoors will look orange. Fortunately, most digital cameras can automatically adjust for color balance changes by constantly monitoring lighting conditions and self-adjusting using the "auto white balance" (AWB) setting. However, it is sometimes good to manually make this setting, especially if complex lighting conditions cannot be established with AWB.

Digital imaging software

The image on a 35-mm slide may be viewed by just placing it in front of a light source, such as a light box. To observe a digital image, the process is not as direct. Without a computer running compatible software, the image bits are meaningless. Imaging software is just as important as the hardware used to make it. With just basic software, one can look at a few images, but to manage thousands of images of hundreds of patients, a more sophisticated software program not only allows a more efficient review of these images, but also provides a system of image management that far exceeds the capabilities of film. There are a number of professional ophthalmic image and management programs available, and they all do a good job of taking, storing, and retrieving photographs.

Resolution

Among many other factors, the quality of a digital image is dependent on pixel resolution. The term *"pixels per inch"* (ppi) refers to the density of pixels in an image. *"Dots per inch"* (dpi) refers to the number of dots used by a printer to make a print based on the ppi of the image. In general, the higher the dpi, the finer is the detail in a print. However, how the dots are managed is just as important. A dye sublimation printer may have a low dpi rating, such as 300, but it uses heat to increase the tonal range of a print. Inkjet and laser printers use various algorithms to enhance performance beyond their dpi rating.

Image resolution is affected by many factors, including lens quality and exposure setting. Whereas different films have different resolving powers, digital imaging resolution is largely determined by the density of pixels. High resolution begins with a large number of pixels on an imaging chip. However, the amount of resolution actually needed is relative to how the image is used. Smaller images require fewer pixels than larger ones. Images displayed on a computer monitor require fewer pixels per inch than those displayed as a print.

File formats

Numerous imaging file formats accommodate different uses of images. The two main categories are uncompressed and compressed. An uncompressed file saves one pixel for every pixel. A commonly used uncompressed format is tagged image file format (TIFF). Image compression can be either lossless or lossy. *Lossless* compression reduces the file size by generalizing areas of common data. For instance, a large area of 100% black is stored with a more efficient description than repeating every pixel as black. *Lossy* compression takes more liberties with describing the data, but also enables more efficient storage and transporting of that data. Joint Photographic Experts Group (JPEG) is a common compression format that can be adjusted to various levels of compression. It is also widely recognized by most imaging programs and across Macintosh and Windows platforms, making it a format of choice when maximum versatility is required. Because there is some level of quality loss in JPEG, although slight to negligible at its "best" setting, it is best practice to work with an image in a lossless format until all corrections are made. As the final step, the image can be saved as a JPEG file. Readjusting images already in a JPEG file may introduce undesirable image artifact.

Many other file format types are available and are used by different camera manufacturers. It is important to know what these formats are to use these images outside that particular operating system.

Exposure

Exposure is the total volume of light that strikes the image sensor. It is the sum of light intensity and duration of exposure. Correct exposure is achieved through the balanced interaction of sensor, sensitivity, brightness of illumination, f-stop, and shutter speed.

With the use of available light, the shutter speed is used to control the duration of the exposure and the f-stop is used to regulate the intensity of the light striking the film. Each full f-stop setting (f8, f11, f16, and so on) and each shutter speed setting ($1/30$, $1/60$, and $1/125$ and so forth) affects the total exposure by a factor of two. For example, if the camera were set at a correct exposure of $1/60$ of a second at f11 and then the lens were opened to f8, twice as much light would reach the sensor and the image would be overexposed. Conversely, if the lens aperture were closed down to f16, only half the needed light would reach the sensor, and the image would be underexposed. Likewise, if the f-stop remained constant and the shutter speed varied, the same alteration in total exposure would result. By decreasing the shutter speed from $1/60$ to $1/30$ of a second, the exposure is doubled; by increasing the shutter speed from $1/60$ of a second to $1/125$ of a second, the exposure is halved. Correct settings therefore are vital to correct exposure. If either f-stop or shutter speed is off by just one setting, a serious overexposure or underexposure may result on the sensor.

Exposure meters

Whenever a light source other than a flash is used, the correct exposure can be determined with the light meter, which is built into most consumer digital cameras. For the best exposures, it is good to be familiar with how your camera's light meter reads the light in the viewfinder. If the light meter is allowed to respond to an area that is either much brighter or much darker than average, a proportionate underexposure or overexposure will result.

Flash illumination

With the use of electronic flash, the duration of the exposure is usually determined by the duration of the flash. Because most modern electronic flash units have a duration of approximately $1/1000$ of a second, the length of the exposure is $1/1000$ of a second. This very short, motion-stopping duration makes the electronic flash ideally suited for eye photography.

Because the duration of the exposure is now essentially beyond our control, correct exposure is achieved by regulating the intensity of the light, either at its source or when it passes through the lens, or both. In most cases, the intensity of the flash source itself need not be altered. In fact, it is desirable to have ample light to guarantee a good exposure at very high f-stops, thereby ensuring the greatest possible depth of field at close working distances.

Electronic flash sources have different amounts of light output, and exposure is greatly determined by the flash's distance from the subject. The farther the flash is away from the subject, the darker it gets, so either the camera's lens aperture must be adjusted or its ISO must be set higher.

The camera's shutter speed also must be set at the speed prescribed by the manufacturer to provide proper synchronization (maximum light output coincident with a fully open shutter). Shutter speeds that are too slow may allow extraneous ambient light to affect the exposure. Shutter speeds that are set faster than the shutter's synchronization result in partial or no pictures (Fig. 39.3).

External photography

A digital single-lens reflex (DSLR) camera with interchangeable lenses is recommended for external eye photography. The DSLR feature permits viewing and photography through the same lens system. Composition and sharp focus are thus made much simpler because the image being photographed is seen in the viewfinder exactly as it will appear on the sensor.

To achieve the necessary magnification, a macro lens (specially designed to permit focusing on very near objects) is recommended. Macro lenses for DSLR cameras are available from approximately 50 to 200 mm in focal length. The advantage of a longer (≥ 100 mm) focal length macro lens is that it permits a greater working distance between camera and subject and produces less perspective distortion. A good, practical magnification-to-working distance ratio can be achieved with the use of a 100-mm lens. Photography of an intraoperative procedure may dictate the use of a longer

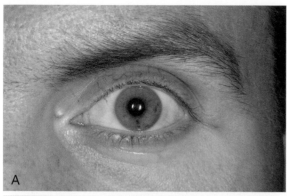

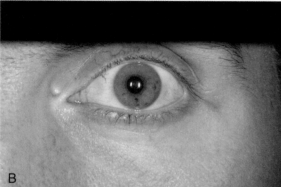

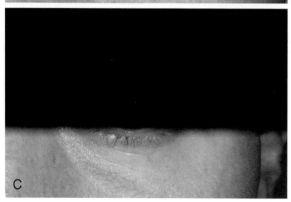

Fig. 39.3 The Nikon D100 camera can synchronize with an electronic flash up to a shutter speed of $^1/_{80}$ second (A). Increasing the speed to $^1/_{250}$ second results in partial exposure (B) and even less at the faster speed of $^1/_{500}$ (C).

focal length lens to provide a greater working distance-to-magnification ratio.

Using a DSLR with interchangeable lenses, a good choice is a 100-mm macro lens. The longer focal length provides the close focusing capability and comfortable working distance away from the patient that is needed in ophthalmology.

A fixed (noninterchangeable) lens camera may provide adequate working distance and magnification, but not all cameras have this capability. Before purchasing a new digital camera with a fixed lens, determine that it can focus closely on a single eye and that the flash functions at close distances.

Illumination

For illuminating external photographs, an electronic flash device is recommended. Problems created by rapid eye movements or blinking are eliminated by the extremely short duration of the flash. Many inexpensive flash units with automatic exposure control are available, eliminating the need to change f-stops while providing the ability to alter the distance between camera and subject over a given range. If such a flash is being contemplated, its ability to function in the automatic mode at such close distances must be ensured. Not all have that capability.

A flash source should always be positioned to provide even, diffuse illumination over the area being photographed. The bridge of the nose and prominent brows should not be allowed to cast a shadow onto the area of interest. When taking photographs of a single eye area, the light should be positioned on the patient's temporal side. For taking a two-eye view or full-face photograph, the light should be positioned directly above the lens. In some types of portrait photography, a ring flash is used to provide soft and even illumination. However, for close-ups of corneal pathology, the large ring of light reflex created by these flash units often obscures what is meant to be documented. The Nikon SB-29s (Fig. 39.4) is a convenient lens-mounted flash that uses two smaller flash tubes rather than a single large ring of light. The unit is mounted directly to the front of the lens and can be rotated and variously controlled for satisfactory illumination. The resulting photograph will show uniform illumination over the subject area, with shadows falling directly behind and below the patient. The use of a lens of a 100-mm focal length considerably lessens the problems arising with the use of sharply oblique illumination, which results from working at too close a range to the subject.

A suitable background should be provided. A simple solution is to obtain several large (30 × 40 inches [0.75 × 1 m]) matte boards available in a variety of colors. In general, a medium blue works well for most subjects.

Photo slit-lamp biomicrography

Many conditions affecting the anterior segment of the eye—especially the transparent cornea, anterior chamber, and lens—are of such a subtle nature that they defy detection

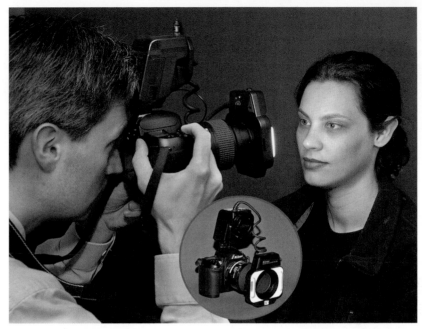

Fig. 39.4 The Nikon SB-29s flash unit mounts directly onto the front of a camera lens. It has two flash units on either side of the lens that can be controlled independently, as well as rotated. The flash is well situated for good illumination at close working distances, and the unavoidable specular reflection from the cornea is much smaller than with a ringlight flash.

by any means other than slit-lamp biomicroscopy. Because the adverse conditions occurring in these transparent or translucent structures are themselves commonly transparent, conventional, diffuse illumination is unsuitable for their visualization. Only the specialized capabilities of the slit-beam illuminator and high magnification of the slit-lamp biomicroscope provide an adequate view of subtle changes of interest to the ophthalmologist.

Fundamental to producing consistently useful photo slit-lamp documentation is thorough knowledge of the structures of the eye, the location and general appearance of the diverse conditions affecting the eye, and the basic forms of illumination and their application to these conditions. Basic illumination techniques include direct focal, tangential, direct, and indirect retroillumination from the iris; retroillumination from the fundus; transillumination; sclerotic scatter; proximal illumination; and Tyndall's phenomenon for aqueous cells and flare.

A slit-lamp biomicroscopic examination is a dynamic process. With the use of a narrow slit beam to provide optic sectioning, transparent structures, such as those in the cornea, can be examined in minute detail a small section at a time. The result is, in essence, a composite, mental image of the entire cornea. In slit-lamp photography, however, each photograph is restricted to a single moment of that examination. To overcome this limitation, some slit lamps are equipped with an additional diffuse illuminator. When

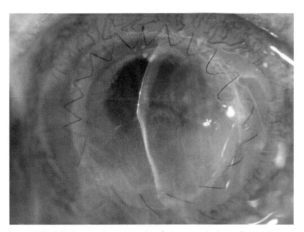

Fig. 39.5 Slit-lamp photograph of a corneal ulcer shown in diffuse, overall illumination with a superimposed narrow slit beam to demonstrate inferior corneal thinning. (From Mártonyi CL, Bahn CF, Meyer RF. *Clinical Slit Lamp Biomicroscopy and Photo Slit Lamp Biomicrography.* Ann Arbor, MI: Time One Ink; 1985.)

used in conjunction with the slit illuminator, the result can be a pleasingly illuminated image of the overall eye with a superimposed narrow slit beam to provide specific information about that section of the structure that it isolates (Fig. 39.5).

Whereas diffuse illumination causes some fine detail to become obscured through the scattering of light, it is useful to provide general, introductory photographs. With these as a basis, additional photographs can illuminate areas of more precise interest, further isolated through increased magnification. The result then is a series of images that leads the viewer through a logical progression from an overview to the subtlest detail. Fig. 39.6 shows some of the forms of illumination, along with recommended exposures as used on the Zeiss Standard photo slit lamp. For other photo slit lamps, exposures should be established by exposing test films based on the manufacturer's recommendations.

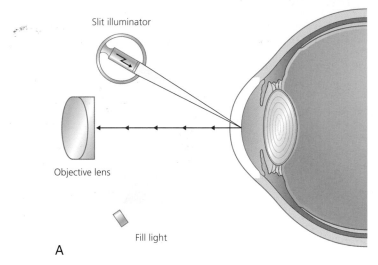

Fig. 39.6 (A) Optic sectioning with fill illumination. Overall, diffuse illumination (fill light) provides a view of the entire eye, and the superimposed direct focal illumination of the narrow slit beam provides specific information about the area that it isolates. Direct focal illumination in the form of a very narrow slit beam, without overall diffuse illumination, is the most selective, direct method of examining the structures of the eye.

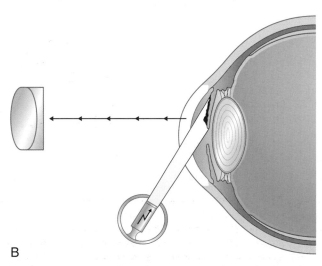

Fig. 39.6 (B) Tangential illumination. A moderate to wide slit beam is projected onto the area of interest at a sharply oblique angle to produce clearly defined highlights and shadow areas, greatly enhancing topographic detail.

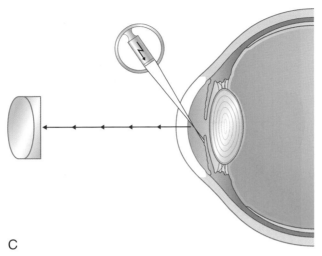

C

Fig. 39.6 (C) Pinpoint illumination. Pinpoint illumination, based on Tyndall's phenomenon, is used to visualize and photograph aqueous cells and flare. The smallest circle beam is directed through the anterior chamber at an oblique angle. If the aqueous is turbid with cells and protein, the small cone of light will be visible to a variable degree depending on the amount of abnormal material it contains, demonstrating anywhere from "one" to "four plus" aqueous cells or flare.

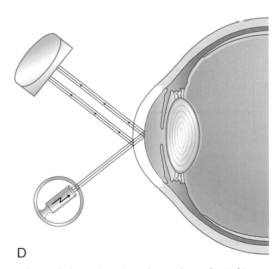

D

Fig. 39.6 (D) Specular reflection. A moderate slit beam is projected onto the surface of interest (the corneal endothelial surface in this example) and viewed at an angle from the perpendicular that is equal to the angle of incidence. An area of nonreflectance from normally flat, reflective surfaces indicates an abnormality.

Photo slit lamps may be film-based or digital. Desirable features include coaxial viewing (viewing and photography through the same lens system) and a flash source for both the slit and diffuse illuminators. Slit lamps not designed for photography may, on occasion, produce satisfactory photographs with the appropriate attachments. Of these attachments, electronic flash illumination is the most essential to provide the short exposures necessary to "freeze" eye movements. In addition, when camera backs with auto exposure are used on slit lamps not equipped with electronic flash within the slit illuminator, the metering system responds to the lightest portion of the image and underexposes most areas of interest illuminated by indirect methods. Electronic flash also provides the correct color temperature of light for daylight film. (Most tungsten bulbs used in slit-lamp biomicroscopes do not produce the exact

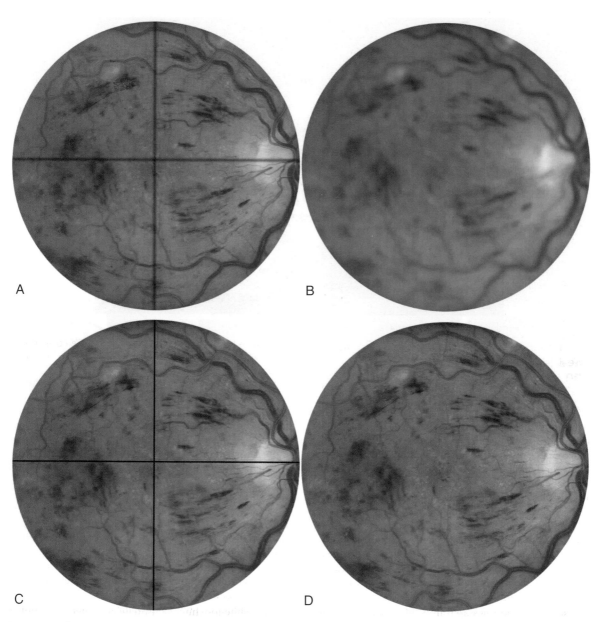

Fig. 39.11 A fundus image when viewed through the eyepiece of a fundus camera may look in focus, but if the eyepiece crosshairs are not in focus at the same time (A), the photographic results will be out of focus (B). Both the fundus image and the crosshair image must be in focus at the same time (C) to obtain a well-focused fundus photograph (D).

being photographed. Stereo photographs of the macula and disc can be taken at the same time. When a fundus "map" is required, following a routine sequence will aid in reconstruction of the photographic map after processing (Fig. 39.13). To achieve a view of other areas of the fundus, the patient's eye can be rotated by moving the

fixation target and moving the camera to stay lined up on the center of the dilated pupil.

When fundus photography is attempted for the first time, or when a new camera is being tried, careful documentation of exposures and procedures provides a baseline from which appropriate adjustments can be made.

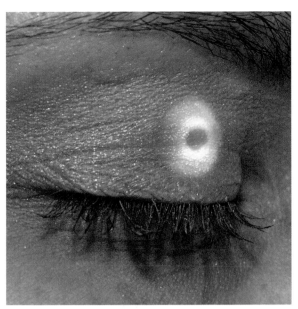

Fig. 39.12 Appearance of correctly focused image of viewing lamp filament on closed eyelid.

Stereo fundus photography

Sequential stereo fundus photography is achieved by aligning the camera initially as described, then moving it laterally from one side of the dilated pupil to the other, taking a photograph in each position to provide the three-dimensional (3D) effect. When crescents are encountered, the camera should continue in the direction of the crescent, which should cause it to disappear. If a crescent persists, the camera should be moved slightly back from the eye. By previewing the area to be photographed in stereo while moving the camera briskly between the two laterally displaced positions, the examiner can get an excellent appreciation for the elevation or depression of the structure or lesion being viewed. Optimum camera position for each side of the stereo pair can thus be appraised before making the actual exposures. The greater the stereo base (distance between the two camera positions), the greater is the 3D effect. Because stereo photography requires using the camera in a drastically off-center position, it may not be possible to eliminate all artifacts. At times, especially when the patient's pupil size is relatively small, stereo photography may involve a compromise to the quality of the individual frames. However, the two frames reinforce each other considerably, in addition to providing the 3D effect so vital to the evaluation of many disease entities. Whereas some cameras offer the option of a mechanical locking device to help establish a degree of stereo separation, its use is discouraged. Not only is it unreliable, given the wide disparity in pupil sizes, but it is also limiting when stereo photographs are required in the presence of ocular opacities. Under such circumstances, an unrestricted manual displacement technique will provide better results.

A wide range of fundus cameras is available: most are table-mounted and a few are handheld. Most systems offer two or three angles of view, usually from 20 to 50 degrees. Some older models have only one angle of view. Some specialized cameras using a contact lens arrangement are capable of photographing 180 degrees of the fundus in a single image. Handheld fundus cameras (Fig. 39.14) are useful for photographing children under anesthesia or other patients who are unable to sit at a table-mounted system. The handheld fundus camera can also serve as a helpful external camera.

Fluorescein angiography

For fluorescein angiography, a fundus camera must be equipped with a rapid-recycling, high-output power supply and an exciter and barrier filter combination. The exciter filter is placed in the path of the light and allows only a specific wavelength of blue light (~490 nm) to strike the fundus. When fluorescein is introduced into the circulation of the eye, the blue light excites the fluorescein molecules to a higher state of activity, causing them to emit a greenish yellow light of a higher wavelength (~520 nm), creating the fluorescence that we record. The barrier filter is positioned to filter out the blue exciter light and allow only the excited yellow-green light of actual fluorescence to strike the image sensor.

Modern filter combinations are so efficient that they permit the recording of true fluorescence only. Older filter combinations were less efficient and commonly produced a dim but discernible image of light structures within the eye (such as the optic nerve head) even without the injection of fluorescein. This level of exposure of light objects without fluorescein is generally referred to as *pseudofluorescence*. As a means of dealing with pseudofluorescence, a "control" photograph of the area to be documented should be taken. The exposure is made before the injection of fluorescein, with the exciter and barrier filters in place and the flash intensity set at the level for fluorescein angiography. When this procedure produces an image, it is generally indicative of filter failure, perhaps requiring filter replacement.

Before fluorescein angiography is undertaken, the patient is informed of the procedure and its implications, and consent is obtained. (Laws and regulations for obtaining consent vary among states and institutions.)

or with a microkeratome. OCT evaluation can demonstrate the exact depth of the inlay.

Corneal pathologies

The exact depth of corneal opacities can be measured with the OCT (Fig. 40.14). Using this information, the surgeon can then decide which surgical procedure would be best to enhance the patient's vision. With superficial opacities, a phototherapeutic keratectomy can be performed. With deeper opacities, a lamellar graft is usually the treatment of choice. OCT evaluation of corneas following surgical procedures, such as a corneal transplant (Fig. 40.15), can provide the surgeon with valuable information as to technique or complications.

Femtosecond laser cataract surgery

The majority of femtosecond lasers use OCT imaging of the anterior segment to guide surgical planning of many of the critical steps of the cataract operation. Detailed images are obtained of the cornea, iris, lens, and anterior vitreous. This information allows for surgical planning of the corneal wound incisions, arcuate relaxing incisions in the cornea for astigmatism, anterior capsulotomy, and fragmentation of the nucleus. OCT imaging allows the laser to be directed to the exact location and depth of the cornea and lens to enhance outcomes.

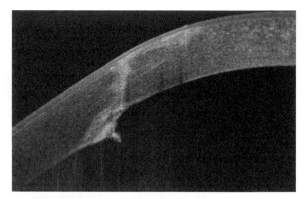

Fig. 40.15 Optical coherence tomography image of a penetrating keratoplasty.

Summary

OCT is a sophisticated cross-sectional imaging device that allows the clinician to make an accurate diagnosis of a variety of conditions of the anterior segment, retina, and optic disc. It also provides a great tool with repeat imaging to determine stability, improvement, or deterioration of an eye condition. This information allows the clinician to determine the success of treatment. If there is progressive disease, then further clinical steps need to be taken.

Chapter 41

Computerized corneal topography

A. Ghani Salim

Introduction and basics

Computerized corneal topography analysis is the measurement of the curvature of the corneal surface. This tool is based on the principles of keratometry and photokeratoscopy developed in 1880 by Placido. He placed a planar target with concentric alternating black-and-white rings in front of a patient's eye and then observed the shape of the rings in the virtual image of that target created from the reflection of the patient's anterior corneal surface. If the cornea is spherical, the rings appear circular and concentric. Deviations of the corneal shape appear as either distortions in shape or eccentricity of the rings.

Photokeratoscopy provides the user with only qualitative information about the curvature of the cornea, changes that accompany surgery, and progressive corneal abnormalities. The keratometer yields quantitative data, but only at four points. These points are located at approximately the 3-mm optical zone along two perpendicular meridians. One pair of points is aligned along the steepest axis of the corneal surface, with the second pair 90 degrees away. The keratometry has fundamental limitations in that it is able only to measure points along the annulus of the 3-mm optical zone.

With the capability of modern computers and software technology to qualify the data obtained from reflected Placido disc images, it has become feasible and practical to precisely analyze the radius of curvature (mm) and corresponding refractive power (diopter) on the corneal surface from inside the 1-mm optical zone to outside the 9- to 11-mm optical zone. This information is then translated into a complete color-coded map. The map is interpreted much like other topographic maps. These topographic maps provide the ability to monitor corneal curvature changes from the apex to the periphery.

There are a variety of corneal topographer systems available. Some use a back-lit conical dish as its Placido target; other systems use a cylindric light cone as the Placido target. With either a conical dish or a cylindric light cone, a Placido ring image is produced on the cornea.

The Orbscan IIz, Galilei, and Oculus Pentacam (Fig. 41.1) are the latest in the state-of-the art technologies for mapping the surfaces of the cornea and for anterior segment analysis. The Orbscan takes multiple cross-sectional scans of the cornea with an advanced Placido disc system and is able to analyze elevation and curvature measurements on both the anterior and posterior surfaces of the cornea, white-to-white measurement, anterior chamber depth, angle kappa, and corneal pachymetry values. Galilei analyzer merges two technologies, the rotating Scheimpflug and Placido technology, into one measurement, leading to accurate values of the posterior and anterior surfaces. The dual Scheimpflug approach offers accurate pachymetry readings and needs only to rotate 180 degrees. Pentacam is a rotating Scheimpflug camera that generates Scheimpflug images in three dimensions, with the dot matrix fine-meshed in the center as a result of the rotation. It takes a maximum of 2 seconds to generate a complete image of the anterior segment. Any eye movement is detected by a second camera and corrected in the process. The pachymetry and topography of the entire anterior and posterior surfaces of the cornea from limbus to limbus are calculated and depicted in Fig. 41.2. The analysis of the anterior eye segment includes calculation of the chamber angle, chamber volume, and

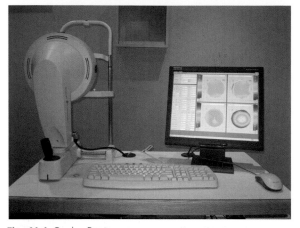

Fig. 41.1 Oculus Pentacam.

height. Images of the iris and anterior and posterior surfaces of the lens are also generated. The densitometry of the lens is automatically qualified. This chapter's focus is on the cornea.

Most corneal topography systems available today can generate various map displays. When performing computerized corneal topography for prerefractive surgery screening, diagnosis of a corneal pathology, or contact lens fitting, the most commonly used maps are discussed in the following.

Axial map or sagittal map

This is the most widely used and simplest of all topographic displays. It shows the curvature of the anterior surface of the cornea as a topographic map in diopteric values and measures it in an axial direction relative to the center.

Every map has a color scale. Cool colors, such as blue and green represent flatter areas of the cornea, whereas the warmer colors of orange and red represent steeper areas of the cornea. The analysis should include the keratometric values and should not be interpreted based on the colors alone.

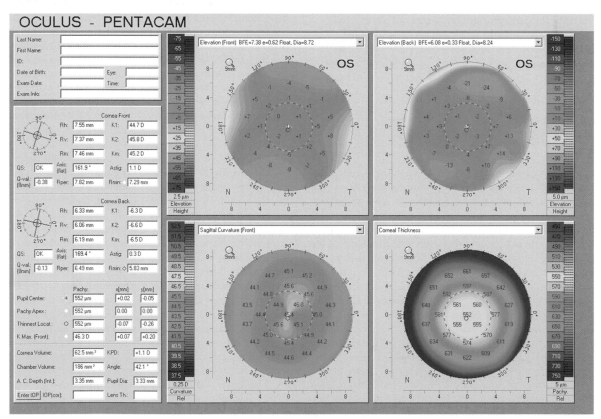

Fig. 41.2 Oculus Pentacam, normal four-map selectable showing *(top two images)* anterior and posterior elevation, *(lower left image)* corneal surface power, and *(lower right)* corneal thickness representation map.

Corneal irregularity measurement (CIM) and shape factor measurements are statistical indices that some topography units, such as Humphrey Atlas, provide on their axial map printout. The increase or decrease of these two over time indicates a change in the progress or healing of a condition. CIM values less than 0.5 indicate a normal-shaped cornea, and 1.0 or higher indicates corneal surface irregularities. Shape factor 0 to 0.3 is normal. Shape factor more than 1.0 indicates high irregularities (Fig. 41.3).

Elevation map

This is the difference in height between the measurements of the cornea and a reference shape called best fit. This value can be negative if the measurement is less than the reference and positive if it is greater than the reference. The reference shape could be a best-fit sphere, best fit ellipsoid, or a toric reference shape (Fig. 41.4).

Corneal thickness map

This describes corneal thickness measurements distributed across the cornea.

Other types of topography displays include tangential map, true net power, refractive map, keratometry map, multivue map (Fig. 41.5), differential map, photokeratoscopic view, profile view, and so on.

Clinical uses

Of all currently available technology, the corneal topography is the best to provide specific and detailed information about the curvature of the cornea. It offers an exact evaluation of the profile of the cornea and a better interpretation and control of some of the pathologic conditions that can occur and affect the cornea.

Variations that occur in corneal topography can be the result of the changes of the corneal stroma and epithelium. Tissue loss and scars cause a flattening of the area and increase the curvature of the cornea around the lesion. With thinning processes, such as keratoconus and pellucid marginal degeneration, thin tissues actually protrude and therefore the curvature of the cornea becomes greater.

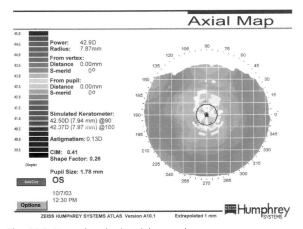

Fig. 41.3 Normal aspheric axial corneal map.

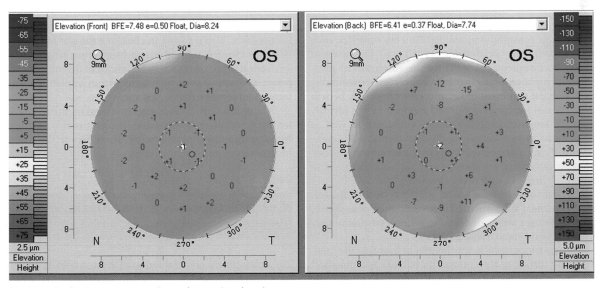

Fig. 41.4 Oculus Pentacam anterior and posterior elevation maps.

Although topography is important in achieving good visual outcomes, it is essential to ensure that the cornea is stable before performing any refractive procedure. Operating on an unstable cornea usually leads to disappointing visual outcomes.

Chronic hypoxia of the cornea and long-term wear of poorly fit contact lenses, particularly if the lens is decentered, cause changes in the contour of the cornea with resultant change in refraction. This reversible condition is referred to as corneal warpage (Figs. 41.8 and 41.9). This

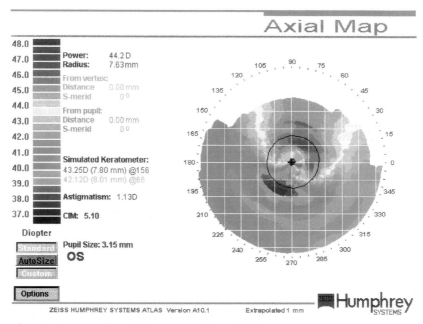

Fig. 41.8 Axial map of corneal warpage from rigid gas-permeable contact lenses.

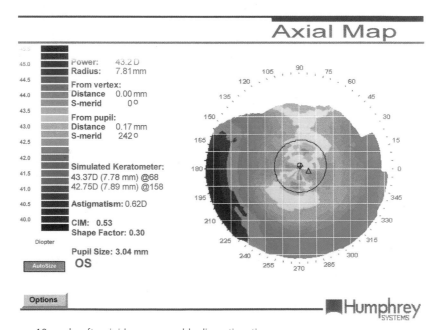

Fig. 41.9 The same eye 10 weeks after rigid gas-permeable discontinuation.

condition is not as prevalent today with rigid gas-permeable lenses as it was in the era of polymethyl methacrylate (PMMA) lenses. Therefore corneal topography is very useful in monitoring and evaluating the contact lens effect on the cornea for patients wearing contacts for a long time. Corneal refractive surgery is contraindicated until the warped area has reversed and refraction has become stable.

It is important to distinguish between corneal warpage induced by contact lenses and true keratoconus. Keratoconus is a red flag in refractive surgery, especially LASIK. Patients suspected of keratoconus are at greater risk of ectasia after LASIK. Even with advanced diagnostic tools and careful screening, the incidence of ectasia after LASIK could be as high as one in 2500 cases.

Corneal warpage is a reversible condition. It is important to distinguish between real corneal alterations and irregularities induced by contact lenses. A corneal pachymetry map shows no thinning at the warped area. Because differentiation may be difficult, the patient must abstain from wearing contact lenses until refraction and corneal topography are stable. Significant changes suggest that corneal warpage from contact lenses has not yet resolved. If contact lens wear is discontinued only a few days before the preoperative evaluation, the final refractive result may be unpredictable because the time for reestablishment of corneal stability after contact lens warpage may take days to months to occur. Stability can vary with soft lenses from minutes to 1 week or longer. One month is the minimum for discontinuation of rigid gas-permeable lenses, although it may take up to 6 months or longer before the cornea is stable. On a practical note, if serial refractions performed every 2 weeks show no change in refraction (<0.50 diopter) and computerized corneal topography is stable and appears normal, it is probably safe to proceed with laser surgery.

Topography is helpful in predicting outcomes. For example, patients achieve better visual results if their refractive astigmatic axis approximates their topographic axis. Theoretically, in these cases, PRK and LASIK that treat astigmatism can create a spherical cornea. These patients may achieve outstanding acuity levels as a result of the creation of a spherical cornea.

The preoperative identification of early or mild keratoconus is very important because lamellar refractive surgery is generally not indicated in these patients. Up until recently, irregular astigmatism could not be satisfactorily treated with the standard excimer laser treatments. Even if the myopia were reduced, any residual irregular astigmatism would require a rigid contact lens for correction. In addition, the correction of asymmetric astigmatism was difficult to treat with the older laser technologies because more laser pulses were required at the steeper quadrant compared with the meridian 180 away. Although keratoconus is still a contraindication for lamellar laser refractive surgery, such as LASIK, limited topography-guided and wavefront-guided customized PRK ablation has shown promise in reducing the irregular astigmatism and improving best corrected vision. The concern of treating unrecognized keratoconus patients is the potential for litigation if keratoconus is detected postoperatively and is thought to be caused by the laser procedure.

The newer topography systems, such as Orbscan IIz, Galilei analyzer, and Oculus Pentacam, provide true elevation and depression maps, as well as a map of pachymetry values. The measurement of the corneal thickness has important diagnostic and clinical implications in the planning of refractive surgeries, such LASIK and PRK and monitoring the progression of conditions, such as keratoconus or corneal edema. When the apex has been displaced inferiorly and is associated with the most prominent area of thinning, the surgeon can be confident of a keratoconus diagnosis.

Postoperative assessment of the cornea

In corneal laser refractive surgery, the excimer laser is used to reshape the cornea to correct myopia, hyperopia, and astigmatism. In cases of myopia, the center of the cornea is flattened (Fig. 41.10), and in hyperopia, it is steepened (Fig. 41.11). In cases of astigmatism, the steep axis is flattened and the flat axis is steepened. Corneal topography, along with other tests, qualifies and quantifies the changes induced by refractive surgery. It evaluates the centration of the ablated area and monitors the stability of the changes.

Ablation decentration (Fig. 41.12) relative to the entrance of pupil may produce increased glare and distortion from the edge of the ablation zone encountering the edge of the pupil. Patients with small pupils may be asymptomatic yet still have a slight or moderate decentration. Eccentric ablation zones always result in manifest refractive astigmatism.

Postoperative topography is helpful in assessing both symptomatic and asymptomatic patients. It provides feedback to the surgeon on the quality of the ablation and determines the changes, such as regression.

Corneal topography and cataract surgery

Clinical studies have demonstrated that posterior corneal astigmatism could be a factor in generating unexpected postoperative outcomes after cataract or refractive lens exchange surgeries. One of the new devices that measures total corneal astigmatism is the Cassini Corneal Shape Analyzer (Fig. 41.13). Reliable Purkinje imaging and precision ray tracing technologies are used to determine corneal shape and optical aberrations. Posterior and anterior data are calculated to provide surgeons with the total corneal power, as well as steep axis and magnitude of astigmatism (Fig. 41.14). Understanding the

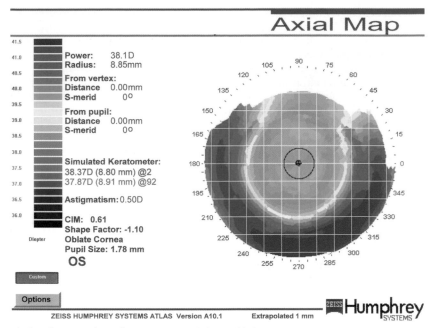

Fig. 41.10 Axial map of well-centered, small zone postmyopic laser ablation.

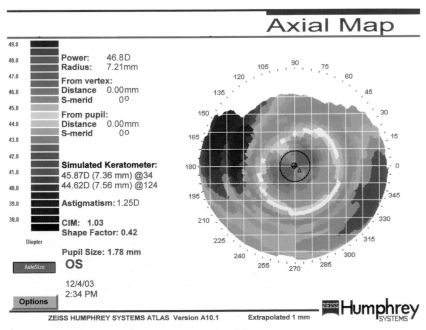

Fig. 41.11 Axial map of normal cornea posthyperopic laser ablation.

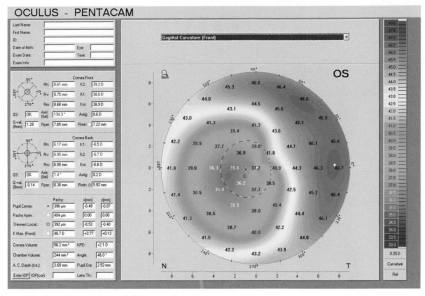

Fig. 41.12 Anterior sagittal curvature map of ablation decentration postmyopic laser vision correction.

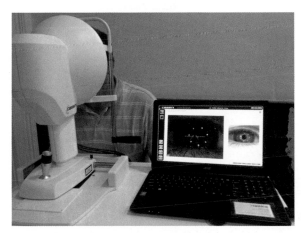

Fig. 41.13 Cassini Corneal Shape Analyzer.

relationship between the anterior and posterior of the cornea should help to provide a more customized planning approach to correcting astigmatism at the time of cataract surgery.

Corneal topography and contact lens fitting

Much of the success of a rigid contact lens fit is predicated on the delicate balance that exists between the anterior corneal surface and the posterior contact lens design. This interaction creates a number of bearing and clearance points that must be of appropriate location and pressure to maintain optimum lens dynamics and ocular health.

Of the more recent technologies to emerge, computerized corneal topography, has had the greatest commercial success and worldwide clinical acceptance.

Today, computerized corneal topographies have demonstrated their usefulness in quantifying the maps of normal eyes, as well as those involving corneal injuries, surgery, or disease. Color-coded maps have now become a universally accepted method of displaying corneal topography. Since the early 1990s, the instruments have been promoted as one of the better tools to aid in the fitting of rigid gas-permeable lenses, especially in patients with abnormal corneal topographies. Most of the current corneal topographers have software that has been installed to help in the contact lens fitting.

Keratoconus

Keratoconus is a bilateral, progressive disease of the cornea in which the cornea becomes conical and protrudes. The protruded area is usually the thinnest part of the cornea (Fig. 41.15). In the majority of cases, the cone is located in the inferior part of the cornea, but it can be found nasally, temporally, and even centrally. The ectatic part is about 3 to 6 mm in diameter.

Patients with advanced keratoconus (Fig. 41.16) showing clinical signs, such as an iron ring, corneal Descemet's

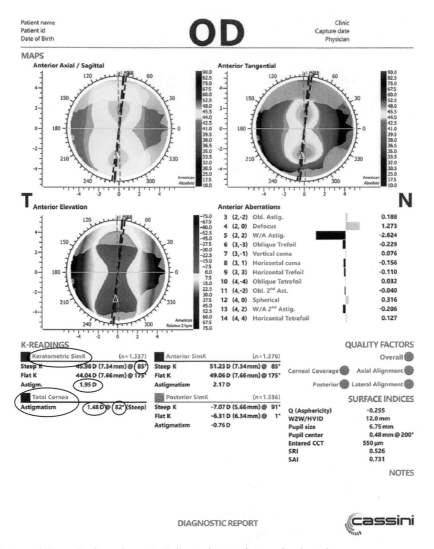

Fig. 41.14 Cassini Corneal Shape Analyzer shows 0.47 diopter less total corneal astigmatism.

folds, corneal scarring, or corneal hydrops do not require corneal topography to make the diagnosis. It is the patients who present with a clear cornea on slit lamp and less than 20/20 best corrected visual acuity that need corneal mapping.

The keratometry is helpful if corneal mires are irregular or distorted, and the cornea is relatively steep (>49.00 diopters). Also helpful in the diagnosis is the finding of scissoring of the retinoscopic reflex, less than 20/20 best corrected visual acuity, careful biomicroscopy to see an iron ring, and the changes in Descemet's membrane.

Today corneal topography is the gold standard for diagnosing all types of keratoconus including early and

asymptomatic (forme fruste keratoconus). Asymptomatic forme fruste keratoconus (Fig. 41.17) without affecting best corrected visual acuity can remain undiagnosed unless corneal topography is performed.

Corneal topography provides information on the location, size, and curvature of the cone apex and helps follow the progress of the disease. The typical findings of keratoconic corneal topography are irregular steepening of the cornea, decentered thinning (Fig. 41.18), inferior steepening of greater than two diopters compared with superior cornea (Fig. 41.19), elevation of the anterior surface of the cornea greater than 15 microns, and elevation of the posterior of the cornea greater than 20 microns (Fig. 41.20).

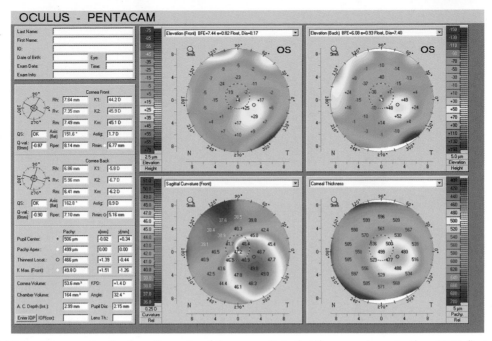

Fig. 41.15 Midkeratoconus extending from the center of the cornea. Note that the cornea is greater than 49.00 diopters steep at the apex of the cone.

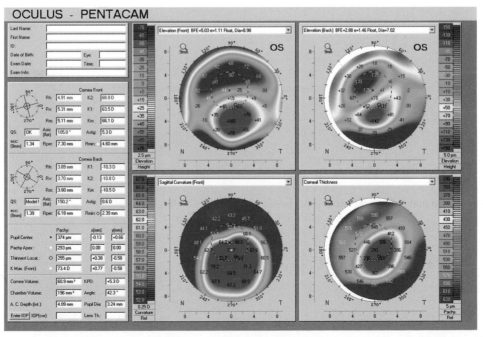

Fig. 41.16 Advanced keratoconus with the anterior elevation more than 100 microns, posterior elevation more than 140 microns, steepest *K* greater than 72.00 diopters, and the lowest corneal thickness less than 260 microns.

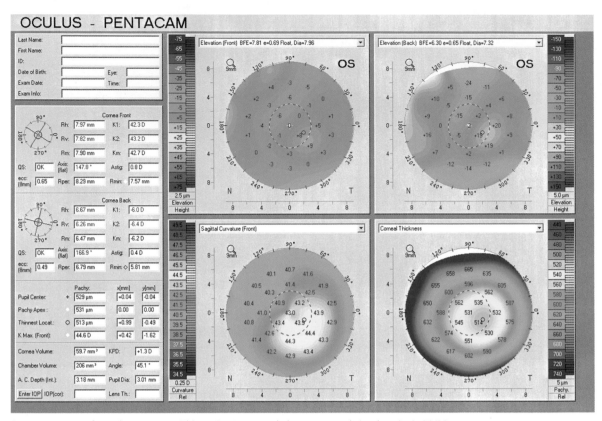

Fig. 41.17 Forme fruste keratoconus. This patient's spectacle best corrected visual acuity is 20/20.

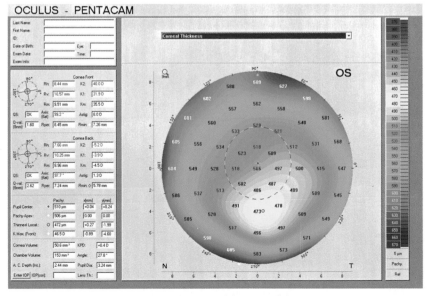

Fig. 41.18 Corneal thickness map in keratoconus. Note decentered thinning of the cornea.

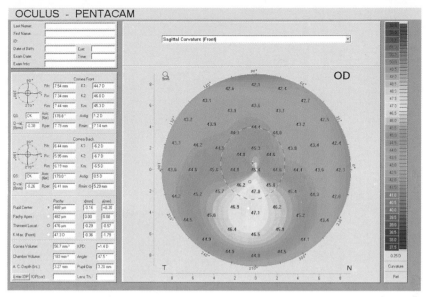

Fig. 41.19 Anterior sagittal map in keratoconus suspect. Note that the cornea is more than 2.00 diopters steeper inferiorly compared with the superior cornea.

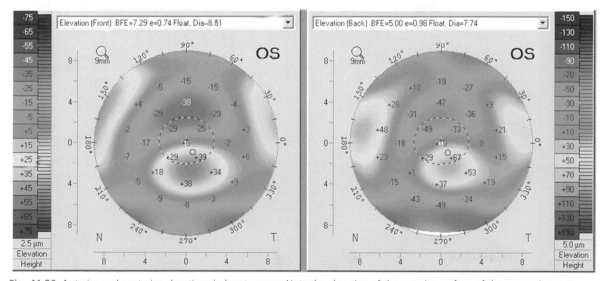

Fig. 41.20 Anterior and posterior elevations in keratoconus. Note the elevation of the anterior surface of the cornea is greater than 35 microns and elevation of the posterior of the cornea is greater than 60 microns.

The most difficult keratoconus to diagnose are the apical ones because of regularity and symmetry (Fig. 41.21). In these cases, one should look for keratometry readings and corneal pachymetry. Unexplained increased myopia and astigmatism, K higher than 49.00 diopters and corneal pachymetry less than 500 microns is suggestive of apical cone.

A new treatment for keratoconus that has shown great success is corneal CXL, a onetime application of riboflavin eyedrops to the eye. The riboflavin, when activated by illumination of ultraviolet A (UVA) light, augments the collagen crosslinking within the stroma and recovers some of the mechanical strength of the cornea. CXL has been shown

693

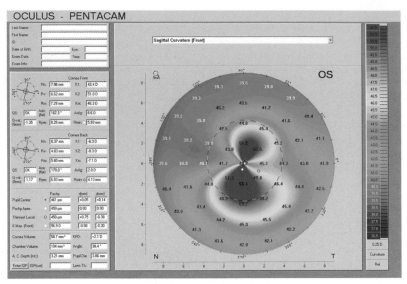

Fig. 41.21 Central apical keratoconus. Note that the center of the cornea is more than 50.00 diopters steep.

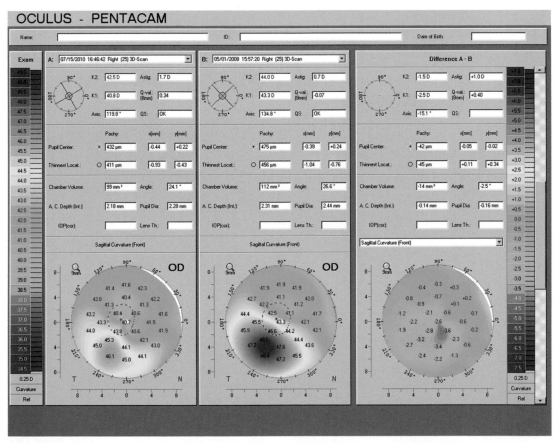

Fig. 41.22 Anterior sagittal curvature maps in keratoconus: *(left)* 2 years following corneal crosslinking, *(center)* pretreatment, and *(right)* difference map. Note that the cornea has flattened by more than 3.00 diopters in the difference map.

to slow or arrest and in some cases slightly reverse the progression of keratoconus (Fig. 41.22). After CXL, the patient can be fitted with contact lenses, or with limited customized topography-guided or wavefront-guided advanced surface laser ablation (LASIK is still a contraindication for diagnosed or suspected keratoconus). The goal of the treatment is to partially correct the refractive error and astigmatism, as well as to create a regular spherical surface on the cornea. This can be achieved by soft or rigid gas-permeable contact lenses in mild to moderate keratoconus and with rigid lenses or piggyback lenses in cases of advanced keratoconus. Sometimes surface ablation can help to flatten the cornea to fit with the contact lenses. When all attempts fail, corneal transplant is advised.

Summary

Computerized topography is an important tool for the anterior segment surgeon and contact lens fitter. It is an integral part of the pre- and postoperative evaluation of the cornea. The slit lamp and keratometry are not of great clinical value in assessing patients preoperatively for diagnosis of corneal warpage, keratoconus, and irregular astigmatism and postoperatively for those who complain of halos, glare, or monocular diplopia. Computerized corneal topography, however, often enables the clinician to make the correct diagnosis. It not only evaluates subjective complaints but also gives positive feedback to the surgeon about the size of the ablation, centration, regularity of the surface, development of ectasia, and progression of keratoconus. Some of these instruments directly input data into the laser computer (topography-guided customized laser ablation) so that laser pulses can be distributed to produce a more natural prolate cornea.

Corneal topography plays an important role in design and parameter calculation of contact lenses. Manufacturers are trying to design custom contact lenses that directly use corneal topography information. This would have exciting clinical implications for those patients who have been unable to wear contact lenses with comfort and substantially reduce the number of required visits to achieve adequate fitting in difficult cases.

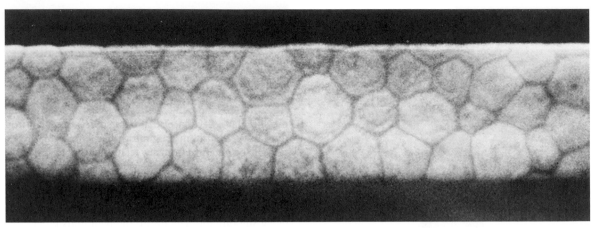

Fig. 42.3 Mosaic pattern of corneal endothelial cells.

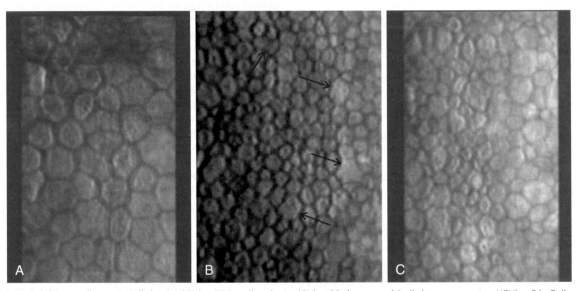

Fig. 42.4 (A) Low cell count: Cell density (CD) = 739, cell variance (CV) = 22, hexagonal (cell shape geometry; HEX) = 31. Cell density is low (CD = 739) and shows abnormal shape (HEX = 31%), but fairly equally enlarged (cell volume [CVL] = 22). Therefore the endothelium is fairly stable and the cornea still clear. (B) Cell coalescence. This image shows several cells going through the process of coalescence *(arrows)*, one mechanism of the wound-healing process. (C) Another example of high cell volume: CD = 2169, CVL = 51, HEX = 48. To avoid a sampling error, one must count all visible cells. More the better by Center Method (Semi manual). (Courtesy Konan Medical USA, Inc., Irvine, CA, USA.)

forehead-stabilizing bar. If the patient's forehead is allowed to move away from the camera, there is the risk of the patient moving abruptly forward and applying excessive pressure to the eye. The slight amount of pressure required for photography is no more than that needed to slightly flatten the cornea against the applanator surface. Contact microscopes help minimize the normal movements of the eye. Appropriate cleaning and disinfecting procedures should be followed between patients.

Noncontact microscopes may be extremely useful when direct contact with the patient's cornea is contraindicated.

The newer digital endothelial microscopes are of the noncontact type, and are easier to use than the older film-based contact models, which required touching the cornea. A digital display shows a sample image of the cells, from which the count can be made to determine cell density (see Fig. 42.2).

Chapter | **43** |

Diagnostic ultrasound

M. Bernadete Ayres

Ultrasound is an indispensable tool in medical imaging and plays an essential role in ophthalmologic diagnoses. It is the most critical imaging technique in eyes with opaque media. This chapter discusses the basic techniques of ultrasound examination and the technique of ultrasound biomicroscopy (UBM), which uses higher-frequency ultrasound to produce images of much higher resolution at or near the anterior chamber.

General considerations and conventional ultrasound diagnoses

Theoretic considerations

Mechanical waves and vibrations occur over a wide range of frequencies called the acoustic spectrum. This spectrum extends from the human audible range (20 Hz–20,000 Hz), with which we are all familiar, to the range of phonons (>1012 Hz) that comprise the vibrational states of matter. Ultrasonic waves exhibit frequencies above 20 kHz, which are inaudible.

The frequency most commonly used in ocular imaging is 10 MHz (Fig. 43.1A), which can provide an axial resolution of 100 μm. Recently, a 20 MHz probe has been introduced (Fig. 43.1B) allowing better detection of details at the posterior pole and orbit. Higher-frequency ultrasound using 50 MHz probe is now used to examine the anterior segment providing an axial resolution of 50 μm (Fig. 43.1C); however, the penalty to be paid is loss of penetration. All human tissues exhibit ultrasound attenuation coefficients that increase with frequency. The maximum penetration that can be achieved with a 10 MHz system is approximately 50 mm. For a 50 MHz system, penetration is only 5 mm.

Electrical impulses are converted to sound by a vibrating crystal (transducer). These sound waves are propagated through the tissues at various speeds and are reflected or scattered from interfaces between tissues of different acoustic impedance (a property related to the tissue density and the speed at which sound passes through it). After emitting a pulse, the transducer "waits" for the reflected waves (echoes) to return, strike the quartz crystal, and initiate the reverse process. The electrical impulses thus produced are electronically amplified and modified to produce the familiar A-scan and B-scan displays. The intensity of echoes displayed on the screen can be adjusting by the gain setting.

Two common types of ultrasound displays are used: the A-scan and the B-scan. The A-scan is a one-dimensional image in which are presented as vertical spikes from a baseline. The longer an impulse takes to return, the farther it is placed on the display. Time can be converted to distance if one knows the speed of sound in the tissue through which the sound is traveling. Each type of tissue has a characteristic speed at which the sound travels through it. The height of the spike on the graph relates to the intensity of the returned echo, which is proportional to the density of the tissue.

There are three types of A-scan used in ophthalmic ultrasound; biometric A-scan, standardized A-scan, and vector A-scan (Fig. 43.2). Biometric A-scan is most commonly used for axial eye length measurement. Cataract extractions are preceded by an A-scan examination to determine the

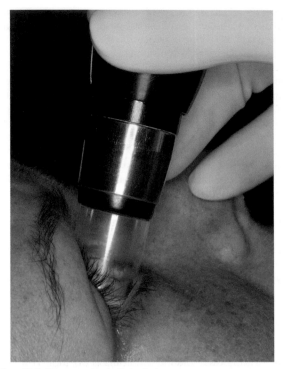

Fig. 43.6 B-scan water-bath technique.

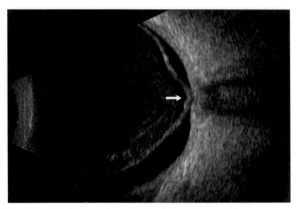

Fig. 43.8 Total, open funnel retinal detachment. Transverse B-scan view of a hyperreflective, continuous, slightly folded membrane with insertion into the optic disc (*arrow*).

with a classic A-scan display provides the most helpful information for diagnostics.

The most common problem encountered in routine cataract work is the patient with an opaque lens precluding a view of the fundus. While performing biometry on these patients, one should watch for any abnormal echoes between the lens echo and the echo from the retina. Artifacts can occur, but the presence of any persistent echo in this region should alert the examiner for the need for further assessment before surgery. A B-scan examination is indicated for any eye in which the posterior pole cannot be visualized.

Intraocular disease

Some typical ocular problems that can be diagnosed on B-scan examinations are discussed in the following paragraphs. It is important to remember that ultrasound is a nonspecific examination technique that can be used on any problem within the penetration range of the instrument.

Retinal detachment

Frequently, a major diagnostic question in an eye that we cannot see into is whether the retina is detached. The typical B-scan appearance of a total retinal detachment is that of a funnel-shaped, highly reflective, continuous membrane that inserts into the optic disc (Fig. 43.8). In case of localized retinal detachment, the retina may not extend to the optic disc.

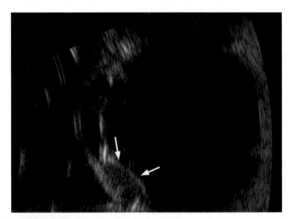

Fig. 43.7 Ciliary body tumor (*arrows*) imaged with water-bath technique.

Office biometry

It is possible to obtain useful diagnostic information from the biometry unit. This ability depends largely on the sophistication of the A-scan display. Machines with no display should be avoided because, in addition to the lack of diagnostic capabilities, it is impossible to monitor the accuracy of axial length readings. An ultrasound equipment

Choroidal detachment

Choroidal detachments have a typical appearance on B-scan ultrasound, shown as a thick, smooth, hyperreflective membrane. Choroidal detachment presents minimal or no aftermovement on kinetic examination. Because the choroid is tethered to the sclera at the exit of the vortex veins, large choroidal detachments appear as smooth lobular elevations that insert sharply in the posterior segment at a short distance from the optic nerve. Choroidal detachment and suprachoroidal hemorrhage represent two distinct entities. Choroidal detachment, also termed choroidal effusion, describe an abnormal collection of exudative fluid that expands the suprachoroidal space, which appears anechoic on B-scan (Fig. 43.9). Suprachoroidal hemorrhage is defined as blood within the suprachoroidal space, represented by typical opacities on B-scan (Fig. 43.10).

Intraocular tumors

Ultrasound is an indispensable tool for the diagnosis and follow-up of intraocular tumors. Differential diagnosis is

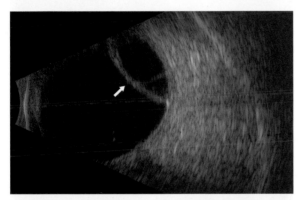

Fig. 43.9 Choroidal effusion. Longitudinal B-scan section shows a smooth, thick dome shaped membrane (*arrow*) with no optic disc insertion.

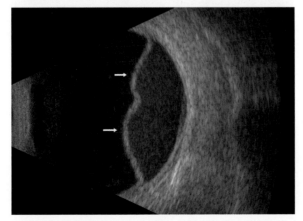

Fig. 43.10 Transverse view of a hemorrhagic choroidal detachment (*arrows*). Presence of dispersed pointlike opacities in the suprachoroidal space.

performed by reference to the shape of the tumor and the pattern of intratumor reflectivity, which can vary depending on the internal structure of the tumor.

Choroidal melanoma. Choroidal melanoma is the most common type of primary intraocular tumor. They are generally dome-shaped or collar button (mushroom)-shaped (Fig. 43.11) and have low to medium internal reflectivity. The collar button shape occurs when the tumor breaks through the Bruch's membrane, which is a dense barrier at the surface of the choroid.

The typical low to medium internal reflectivity of choroidal melanomas permits the echographic differentiation of this type of tumor from other choroidal lesions, such as choroidal nevus (Fig. 43.12) and choroidal hemangioma (Fig. 43.13), which exhibit high internal reflectivity.

Treatment of melanomas is based on the height and largest basal diameter measured with ultrasound examination. Follow-up measurements to determine growth are very important, and this is accomplished by imaging the greatest height of the tumor in both B-scan, transverse and radial sections using electronic calipers (Fig. 43.14). The tumor dimensions can also be assessed using the vector A-scan.

Retinoblastoma. Retinoblastoma is the most common intraocular malignancy afflicting children, with the highest incidence in patients less than 4 years old, and frequently presenting with leukocoria. Retinoblastoma is classically characterized by one or multiple nodular, white or cream masses often associated with increased vascularization (Fig. 43.15). The tumor can grow forward into the vitreous (endophytic) or beneath the retina (exophytic).

Often, retinoblastoma is highly calcified as a response to tissue damage or necrosis. Ultrasonography is indispensable in diagnosis of retinoblastoma, demonstrating a retinal mass with intralesional calcification (Fig. 43.16). The presence of intralesional calcium in retinoblastomas helps the echographic differentiation to other causes of leukocoria, such as congenital cataract, Coats' disease, persistent fetal vasculature, and ocular toxocariasis.

Orbital ultrasound

Ultrasound can penetrate most of the orbit and image problems, such as tumors behind the eye. However, there are limitations because ultrasound cannot penetrate the bony walls of the orbit, and imaging is difficult at the orbital apex. Computed tomography scans and magnetic resonance imaging are more commonly used for orbital imaging. Orbital ultrasound has the advantage of being a readily available, noninvasive technique that can be used as an adjunct to other imaging methods.

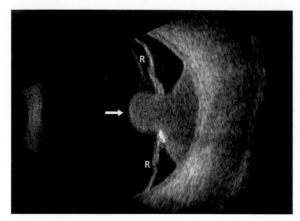

Fig. 43.11 Transverse view of a collar button choroidal melanoma (*arrow*) with associated exudative retinal detachment (R).

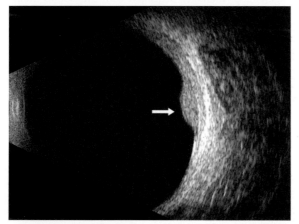

Fig. 43.12 Transverse B-scan of a slightly elevated, dome shaped choroidal nevus (*arrow*). Note the high internal reflectivity.

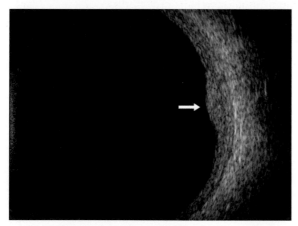

Fig. 43.13 Choroidal hemangioma. Transverse B-scan showing a hyperreflective fundus lesion with a shallow margins (*arrow*).

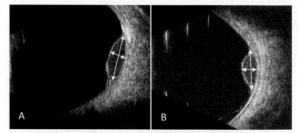

Fig. 43.14 Tumor height and base are measured using longitudinal (A) and transverse (B) ultrasound B-scan.

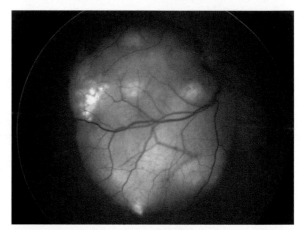

Fig. 43.15 Color fundus photography showing a large endophytic retinoblastoma.

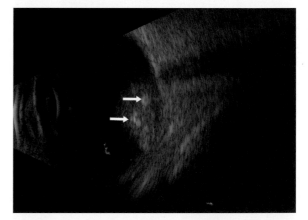

Fig. 43.16 Axial B-scan showing a retinoblastoma with mild intrinsic calcification (*arrows*).

Orbital cavernous hemangioma

Cavernous hemangioma is the most common vasculogenic lesion of the orbit. The classic symptom at presentation is slowly progressive and painless proptosis. On B-scan, cavernous hemangioma appears as a well outlined round or oval, intraconal lesion with smooth surface. The lesion is homogeneous, with medium-high to high internal reflectivity, and produces moderate to strong sound attenuation. Flattening of the globe, optic nerve, or muscle deviation can be observed in case of large masses (Fig. 43.17).

Orbital lymphoma

Lymphoproliferative lesions are the most common primary orbital tumor in older adults, and non-Hodgkin lymphoma accounts for the vast majority of this group. On B-scan examination, orbital lymphoma can be characterized as smooth, circumscribed or diffuse and ill-defined, usually extraconal mass with molding to the globe. The lesion is homogeneous, with low to medium internal reflectivity, and contains connective tissue septa (Fig. 43.18).

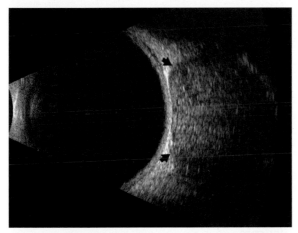

Fig. 43.17 Transverse B-scan of a large orbital cavernous hemangioma (*arrows*).

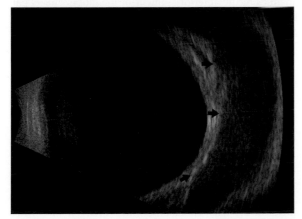

Fig. 43.18 Typical low reflective orbital lymphoma molding the eye (*arrows*).

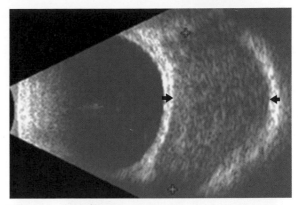

Fig. 43.19 Orbital rhabdomyosarcoma. B-scan displays well outlined, large medium reflective lesion (*arrows*).

Orbital rhabdomyosarcoma

Rhabdomyosarcoma is the most common primary orbital malignancy of childhood. Rhabdomyosarcoma is often presented with rapidly progressive proptosis and displacement of the eye over a period of days to weeks. On ultrasound images, rhabdomyosarcoma is typically a large, well outlined mass, indenting the globe, with a homogeneous internal structure with low to medium reflectivity. Bone destruction can be detected in advanced cases (Fig. 43.19).

Ultrasound biomicroscopy

UBM is a technique primarily used for imaging of the anterior segment. It was developed by Charles Pavlin, MD and F. Stuart Foster, PhD as a method to obtain cross-sections of the eye at microscopic resolution. The technology of UBM is based on a high-frequency transducer incorporated into a B-mode clinical scanner. Commercially available UBM units operate at 50 MHz, can produce a tissue resolution of approximately 50 μm, and penetrate 4 to 5 mm in the tissue.

Technique

The UBM examination technique is similar to the traditional B-scan ultrasound. Major differences include an oscillating probe without a covering, the use of a water bath, and the more refined movements required. The examination is done with the patient in a supine position. Topical anesthesia is applied to the eye. A specially designed-eyecup with methylcellulose (Fig. 43.20) or a ClearScan® probe cover filled with distilled water (Fig. 43.21) is used to separate the eyelids and create a water path standoff. During the examination, the acquisition of images is directly over the

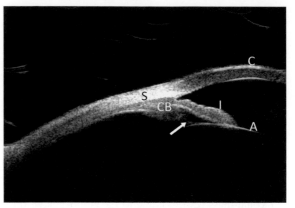

Fig. 43.22 Ultrasound biomicroscopy longitudinal view of a normal open angle. Cornea (*C*), iris (*I*), anterior lens capsule (*A*) ciliary body (*CB*), sclera (*S*) and zonule (*arrow*).

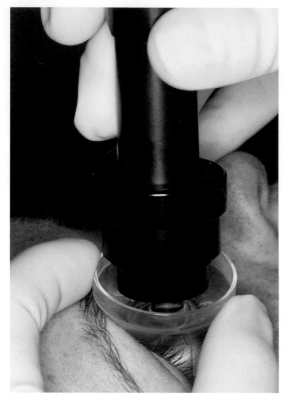

Fig. 43.20 Ultrasound biomicroscopy examination with a fluid-filled eyecup.

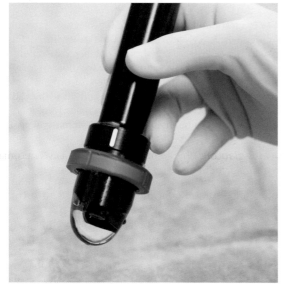

Fig. 43.21 Ultrasound biomicroscopy 50 MHz probe with probe cover.

anterior segment structure, scanning in axial, longitudinal, and transverse orientations. Fig. 43.22 shows normal anatomy of the angle in a longitudinal section.

Ultrasound biomicroscopy in ocular disease

Because UBM is a nonspecific imaging tool, it is suitable for examination of a large range of diseases that fall within the penetration limits of this technique. It is particularly benefecial when structural abnormalities are present in the anterior segment, that is, those conditions that produce rearrangement of the normal anatomy.

Glaucoma

Several types of glaucoma are caused by structural abnormalities of the anterior segment of the globe. This is particularly true of angle-closure glaucoma and infantile glaucoma. UBM is very useful to demonstrate the relationship between the peripheral iris, ciliary body, and trabecular meshwork.

Pupillary block. The most common etiology of angle-closure is pupillary block. In this case, the iris assumes a convex profile as a result of the differential pressure between the posterior and anterior chambers, pushing the iris forward and resulting in narrowing of the anterior chamber angle, which may result in iridotrabecular apposition and/or synechia (Fig. 43.23). The degree of iris–lens contact is relatively small in pupillary block, as the iris is lifted off the lens. The block is thus not related to the area of contact. The area of iris–lens contact becomes even smaller when the pupil dilates. A very common cause for referral for UBM is the patient in whom the angle does not open completely

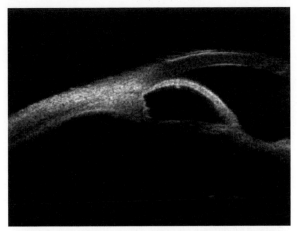

Fig. 43.23 Ultrasound biomicroscopy longitudinal view of anterior iris bowing and angle closure in pupillary block.

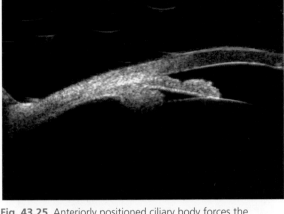

Fig. 43.25 Anteriorly positioned ciliary body forces the peripheral iris causing angle closure in plateau iris.

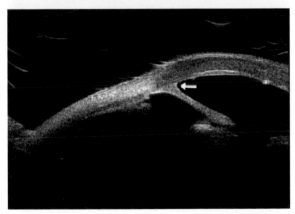

Fig. 43.24 Peripheral anterior synechiae (*arrow*) and diffuse corneal thickening (edema).

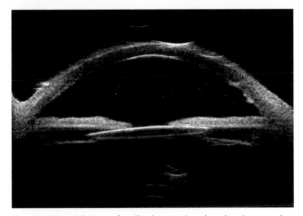

Fig. 43.26 Axial view of a tilted posterior chamber intraocular lens implant in contact with the posterior iris surface.

after iridotomy. The usual cause for this is an imperforate iridotomy, anterior synechiae, or plateau iris.

Anterior synechiae. Angle-closure by synechiae is illustrated in Fig. 43.24. Here, the iris takes an angular form instead of to the smooth curve in the case of a pupillary block. UBM can define the state of the angle behind synechiae.

Plateau iris. UBM has been used to elucidate the etiology of plateau iris configuration, which is characterized by flat central iris plane, a steep rise in iris root from the point of insertion, an anteriorly positioned ciliary body, absence of ciliary sulcus, large and long ciliary processes causing iridotrabecular contact impairing aqueous outflow (Fig. 43.25). In addition, the iris root is inserted anteriorly on the ciliary face, further crowding the anterior chamber angle. The axial anterior chamber is shallower in the plateau

iris than in the pupillary block. Plateau iris syndrome is characterized by persistent angle occludability in eyes with patent iridotomy. Pupillary block and plateau iris frequently coexist.

Uveitis-glaucoma-hyphema syndrome. Uveitis-glaucoma-hyphema syndrome is an infrequent but well-recognized complication of cataract surgery. It typically involves contact between a malpositioned intraocular lens implant (IOL) and the iris or ciliary body. A variable amount of anterior segment inflammation, pigment dispersion, hyphema, vitreous hemorrhage, and increased intraocular pressure may occur. The syndrome can be associated with anterior chamber IOL, sulcus fixated IOL and in-the-bag placed IOL. UBM can demonstrate the malpositioned IOL presenting contact between the haptics or optic and uveal tissue (Fig. 43.26), especially in areas inaccessible to slit-lamp examination.

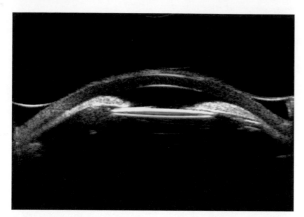

Fig. 43.27 Axial view of shallow anterior chamber and angle closure in malignant glaucoma.

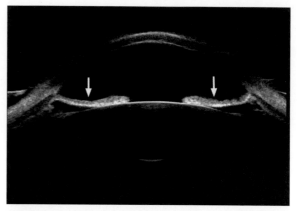

Fig. 43.28 Concave iris configuration (*arrows*) in pigmentary dispersion syndrome.

Supraciliary effusions and malignant glaucoma. In malignant glaucoma or aqueous misdirection syndrome, UBM shows an extremely shallow anterior chamber, occluded angle, and forward rotation of the ciliary body with or without fluid in supraciliary space (Fig. 43.27). It usually occurs during uneventful surgical procedures particularly in hyperopic eyes. Pavlin had found that most cases of malignant glaucoma have supraciliary effusions and anteriorly rotated ciliary processes. Effusions likely play a major role in the clinical manifestation of this condition.

Pigmentary dispersion syndrome. Pigmentary dispersion syndrome is characterized by loss of pigment from the iris, transillumination defects in the midperiphery of the iris and increased pigment deposition in the trabecular meshwork, which can lead to elevated intraocular pressure and subsequent glaucoma (pigmentary glaucoma). The concept of reverse pupillary block implies temporary reversal of the pressure differential in the anterior and posterior chambers, producing posterior bowing of the iris, which leads to iris–zonular friction with mechanical pigment loss. UBM has been used to confirm iris concavity seen in pigment dispersion syndrome/pigmentary glaucoma (Fig. 43.28).

UBM has shown that accommodation produces posterior iris bowing, which can be reversed by iridotomy.

Anterior segment tumors

Iris and ciliary body tumors. UBM is a very useful adjunct in the management of anterior segment tumors, providing great resolution of imaging lesion margins, internal structure, and accurate measurements. It is a preferred imaging method for the anterior segment to assess deeply pigmented lesions and ciliary body involvement. When observation is elected, lesions changes can be tracked with

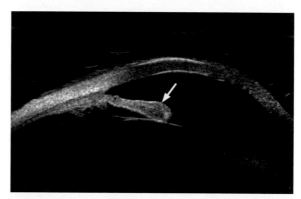

Fig. 43.29 Ultrasound biomicroscopy longitudinal view of all margins of a localized iris thickening in case of nevus (*arrow*).

greater precision. Where surgical intervention is indicated, information gained is helpful in planning the approach.

Iris nevi appear as minimally elevated iris stromal lesions with medium to high internal reflectivity and no disruption of the pigmented epithelium (Fig. 43.29). Conversely, ciliary body or iris melanomas are more elevated lesions, present low to medium internal reflectivity, and cause disruption of pigmented epithelium (Fig. 43.30).

Cystic lesions of the iris. There are two major categories of primary iris cysts, including stromal cysts and pigment epithelial cysts of the iris.

The usual clinical presentation of pigment epithelial cyst of the iris is a posterior elevation of the peripheral iris. The typical ultrasound biomicroscopic appearance of a thin-walled cyst with no internal reflectivity (Fig. 43.31) is diagnostic and essentially eliminates any question over whether a lesion is a cyst or a solid tumor.

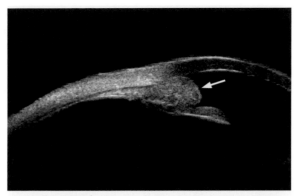

Fig. 43.30 Iridociliary melanoma. Ultrasound biomicroscopy shows an echodense, thick mass (*arrow*) involving the iris root and ciliary processes.

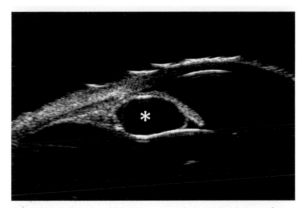

Fig. 43.31 Ultrasound biomicroscopy longitudinal view of a pigmented epithelium cyst (*asterisk*) at the iridociliary junction.

The stromal cyst has a characteristic clinical appearance with smooth and thick wall, echolucent mass on or within the iris stroma, occasionally with fluid-debris level (Fig. 43.32).

The zonule

In surgical planning for patients with clinically evident or suspicious zonulopathy, such as pseudoexfoliation syndrome, ocular trauma, Marfan syndrome, or advanced cataract, UBM is an effective method to detected missing zonules (Fig. 43.33), or identifying zonular stretch (Fig. 43.34). The examination is applied using longitudinal scans in all meridians over 360 degrees, moving the probe slightly to achieve maximal perpendicularity to the zonular fibers.

Scleral disease

UBM is a valuable diagnostic tool to differentiate the pathologies of the sclera, moreover the serial examinations

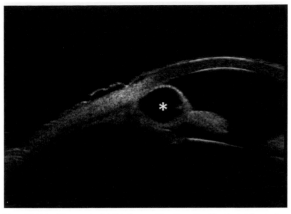

Fig. 43.32 Ultrasound biomicroscopy longitudinal section of a cyst (*asterisk*) of the iris stroma.

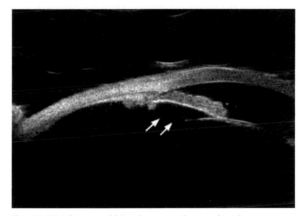

Fig. 43.33 Ultrasound biomicroscopy image showing an area of missing zonules (*arrows*).

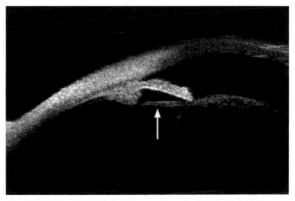

Fig. 43.34 Ultrasound biomicroscopy image showing zonular stretch (*arrow*).

Chapter | 44 |

Blind persons in the modern world

Harold A. Stein, Gwen K. Sterns, and Eleanor E. Faye

Blindness defined

The most widely accepted definition of blindness is central visual acuity of 20/200 or less in the better eye with a correcting lens, or whose visual acuity is better than 20/200 with a restricted central field of vision of no greater than 20 degrees.

Almost 1% of the U.S. population is blind and almost 2% of individuals have low vision. The leading cause among White Americans is age-related macular degeneration (54%), whereas cataracts and glaucoma lead the way among Black Americans (60%). Two-thirds of legally blind people have sight of various degrees. Some can distinguish only the difference between light and darkness, whereas others see vague shapes and patterns as if a thick fog were always in front of their eyes. Still others have peripheral sight and see the world around the edges of a blank or distorted area in the center of their vision (macula); they do not see the whole shape of anything if they look directly at it, but by shifting their eyes slightly to one side or up and down they see an image, although not with the detail of the normal macula. Others have no peripheral vision, but normal central vision.

In the visually impaired population, the degrees and different types of vision loss are almost as varied as the people themselves. It is estimated that among blind individuals in the United States and Canada, less than 10% are totally blind (with no light perception). Nonlegally blind but visually impaired individuals outnumber those who are legally blind. The Eye Diseases Prevalence Research Group concluded that approximately one in 28 Americans over the age of 40 years is affected by low vision or blindness, and that by 2020, the number of blind and low-vision persons in the United States will increase by 70% to 1.6 million. This study used data on blindness as defined by the World Health Organization (WHO) (<6/120 [<20/400]) and by the United States (<6/60 [<20/200]) and, for low vision, defined as vision in the better-seeing eye of less than 20/40.

A resolution adopted by the International Council of Ophthalmology, held in Sydney, Australia, April 2002, recommended to the world vision community the use of the following terminology to describe visual loss:

- Blindness. To be used only for total vision loss and for conditions in which individuals have to rely predominantly on vision substitution skills.
- Low vision. To be used for lesser degrees of vision loss, so individuals can be helped significantly by vision enhancement aids and devices.
- Visual impairment. To be used when the condition of vision loss is characterized by a loss of visual functions (such as visual acuity, visual field, etc.) at the organ level; many of these functions can be measured quantitatively.
- Functional vision. To be used to describe a person's ability to use vision in activities of daily living (ADL); presently, many of these activities can be described only qualitatively.

- Vision loss. To be used as a general term, including both total loss (blindness) and partial loss (low vision), characterized either on the basis of visual impairment or by a loss of functional vision.

Vision impairment and blindness are feared by most people throughout the world. Seventy percent of Americans older than age 45 years fear blindness more than losing a limb, needing a wheelchair, or deafness. When patients or families of affected patients hear the word "blindness," they think of loss of all vision, darkness, and gloom. Telling a patient or a parent of a child that he or she is losing vision should therefore be handled with sensitivity, knowledge, and hope. Options for rehabilitation for the patient must be introduced. The patient and family should be expected to grieve for their loss and we as professionals need to understand the grieving process and accept and support it. These families and patients must be given the opportunity to see there is hope for their independence and for attaining and maintaining meaningful lives, education, and jobs.

Partial sight and blindness

When patients are classified as legally blind, they have not always lost all of their visual function. In the United States, blindness is defined as reduction of central visual acuity to no more than 20/200 in the better eye with a correcting lens or limitation of the central field of vision to less than 20 degrees at its widest diameter. The WHO defines blindness as visual acuity less than 20/400. The definitions of blindness used by the WHO and the United States are intended as legal classifications and they do not necessarily convey important functional information. Most patients classified as legally blind can still distinguish between objects, can read with low-vision aids, and maintain their independence with visual aids and training; a smaller number can distinguish only the difference between light and darkness. Low vision is an impairment that cannot be corrected by medicine, surgery, or conventional aids and interferes with functional vision. Many people who are not legally blind are visually impaired and need low-vision rehabilitation.

Most people who are legally blind have some sight. However, it is inaccurate to label a visually impaired person as blind. An individual with sight can learn to use that residual vision in many ways, using a variety of optical devices and computerized reading machines. No one with sight is blind in the sense of having to use alternative nonvisual methods exclusively as the primary mode of functioning. For this reason, no one should be advised to learn to read Braille if he or she can read type, even though classified as legally blind. More than 90% of the legally blind children between 7 and 17 years of age attend regular school. Low-vision aids and computers make this possible.

Braille is probably useful when a person has profound loss of vision ($\leq$5/200) and cannot read type, or read fast enough, with a closed-circuit television (CCTV) or strong magnifier. If possible, children with profound vision loss should be taught print letters and numerals to aid visualization of text, even if they eventually have to switch to Braille.

Recent vision loss

In most instances, it is the ophthalmologist who is responsible for telling a person that he or she has a permanent loss of vision. Most authorities in the field of rehabilitation believe the person should be informed as early as possible once the diagnosis has been made. The sooner the disability is faced and accepted, the sooner the reality of vision rehabilitation can be accepted. The practice of prolonging hope of vision restoration not only impedes effective rehabilitation, but also delays facing reality.

Although it is important for the ophthalmologist to present the diagnosis in a candid and factual manner, it is just as essential for the practitioner to appreciate the emotional effect of such information. The doctor should provide a supportive environment in which the person is allowed time to ask questions, as well as be given information about community rehabilitation resources.

For most individuals, any loss of vision arouses an emotional response, usually fear of blindness. Depression is a normal response to becoming dependent and having to rely on others for help in basic living activities. Young adults fear loss of a job; older adults fear financial dependence, isolation, and loss of their friends and community.

Total blindness

Myriad repeated frustrations occur in the daily lives of the totally blind that accentuate the dependency of the condition. Maintaining a job and personal life becomes a feat in itself. The routines that the sighted do automatically and without thought must be deliberately learned, step by step, by the blind. For example, the blind person must learn how to eat all over again. If the portions on a plate are not placed in a certain location, the blind person must explore the plate with a fork to discover where the food is placed.

Simple tasks can arouse feelings of insecurity, fear, and anxiety, especially when they have to be performed in public. Blind people may be afraid of making mistakes and of being clumsy and awkward for fear that they will become an object of attention. It is these little things—such as eating out in public, combing the hair or shaving, putting on makeup, or setting down a glass of water without knocking it over—that the blind must be able to learn to do with confidence. One of the first decisions to be made is whether the person would be safer learning long-cane travel or whether a guide dog would be more compatible with the individual's temperament. Each method has its adherents, advantages, and disadvantages; it is a highly personal choice.

Totally blind people may choose to withdraw into a familiar and unchanging environment that can be controlled with their visual incapacity. If they withdraw, they will be safe from physical harm and public ridicule, but limited in thoughts and actions. The other extreme is to tackle the problem head on, that is, to ignore the disability and continue with life despite the inconveniences, dangers, and hardships, learning in a specialized agency or organization for the blind how best to adapt to life without sight. The most desirable reaction is one that balances the disability with new ability and redirects interests, skills, and strengths so that the visual need in selected activities is minimized. The physician can be supportive of this reorientation by referring the blind person to trained rehabilitation personnel who can transmit the new skills to help the individual move toward physical and psychologic adjustment.

Ophthalmic assistant's role

The ophthalmic assistant will encounter in his or her daily work individuals who have a variety of different vision impairments, including blindness. The assistant should be familiar with the methods used to provide orientation to those with visual disabilities and to facilitate their mobility.

On first meeting a blind person, one should introduce oneself. The assistant should always offer his or her arm to the blind person. With a hand lightly on the assistant's arm, the patient feels the body movement and, because the assistant is slightly in front, the patient will have a feeling of confidence with each step. To be propelled from behind can be most awkward and unnerving. The assistant should be sure to ask a blind person if he or she needs help because the need for assistance should not be assumed without question. When you reach the examination chair, tell the patient where the chair is and place his hand on the chair so that he can position himself properly. Naturalness, kindness, and inherent human respect result in the most successful relationships and avoid an overdose of assistance, which makes a handicap more noticeable and damages the value of the assistant's role.

The assistant should realize that he or she should go to the patient to escort the latter to the examination room, rather than expecting the patient to navigate the office alone. Also any paperwork to be completed by the patient should be handled by either the assistant or office personnel in a private setting. If a blind person has been guided to a place and is to be left alone, he or she should first be informed about the surroundings. It is also desirable, under such circumstances, to establish some position of safety and orientation, such as a table, chair, or wall, and to let the patient know if the door will be left open, so the person can call out for assistance if needed and be assured that someone will return shortly to check on the patient.

Because most patients with visual loss have normal hearing, medical personnel should avoid talking loudly to them. A patient with a visual impairment does not want to have his history discussed out loud in a waiting room any more than a sighted person would. You should not assume that the person accompanying the visually impaired patient is the one to whom questions of a sensitive nature should be directed. It is possible that this person is a neighbor or taxi driver and not someone with whom the patient wants to discuss private information. Visually impaired patients deserve the same courtesy as sighted patients.

The ophthalmic assistant should be aware of the thin line between giving someone assistance and making him or her feel helpless. Many blind people are quite proud of the many functions they can perform for themselves. They do not like having their disability emphasized and their dependency magnified. The assistant can ask the patient, in a quiet voice, if he or she can help him with this or that and let the patient make the decision about the degree of assistance wanted.

The ophthalmic assistant should avoid discussing with patients the status of their eyes, the state or federal assistance they can expect, or the details of the facilities available for them. Each of these areas should be handled by professionals trained in their fields. The assistant should also avoid giving false hope to patients by casually mentioning the miracles being achieved every day in the fight for sight.

Blind people should not be regarded as unimportant or incompetent. Patients should be asked questions directly, not through a second party. Conversation should never be allowed to flow around or through them as though they did not exist. They should be treated as individuals without sight, not as ones without insight.

The blind child

Congenitally blind children, unlike some of their adult counterparts, have no recollection of the visual world to assist them. Without this visual memory, blind children must learn about the world by being exposed to the environment and provided with the opportunity to explore it through other senses. Although parents know their child best, early intervention by child development specialists who have training in visual impairment can offer additional support to parents and assist them with encouraging their child's normal development. Other professionals who can offer support with the habilitation needs of blind children include orientation and mobility specialists and life skills instructors. These personnel are trained to assist blind children and their families with the development of daily living skills and the attainment of safe independent travel skills.

The young child who does not have a visual memory may have to be physically shown and encouraged to develop skills, such as creeping, walking, holding a spoon, and drinking from a cup. The blind child who has never seen these activities cannot rely on visual modeling as a learning tool. Parents of blind children must be patient and firm, allowing their child the opportunity to succeed by independently doing a task, as well as permitting the child to fail at times and learn from his or her mistakes.

It is important that some routine be established in the home to assist the blind child with understanding his or her environment. For example, it is easy for a totally blind child to confuse day with night; thus the routine of going to bed is important. Because bedtime is not accompanied by a change of light, a preliminary quiet period can be substituted. The blind child's language and concept development can be facilitated by bringing the child into direct association with the object or action while the appropriate words are being used. This helps the child to acquire a meaningful conceptual base.

Many congenitally blind children develop mannerisms, such as rocking, touching and rubbing their eyes, or waving their hands. These and other repetitive motions are known as blindisms. Early intervention with blind children focuses on trying to help the child prevent these blindisms from developing. Once blindisms are established, diminishing them may require persistent effort on the part of the blind person to correct them.

It is estimated that up to 60% of young blind infants and preschool children in North America have additional motor and cognitive disabilities. One reason for this is the greater ability of modern medicine to save low-birthweight infants. Although many of these infants may be perfectly normal, premature infants with very low birthweights (<750 g) tend to have a greater incidence of disability. Blind children with additional disabilities require either a transdisciplinary team approach or a special school to effectively meet their diverse and unique habilitation needs.

Although most blind children receive their education through local schools in an integrated educational setting, the totally blind child requires some form of educational support services to assist with meaningful learning in the integrated classroom. Residential schools for blind children still exist in some areas, thus allowing families and school placement personnel choices and options to best meet the educational needs of the individual child.

Braille

One form of written communication the blind child may use is Braille, a system of raised dots on paper read by touching them with the ends of the fingers (Fig. 44.1). Although

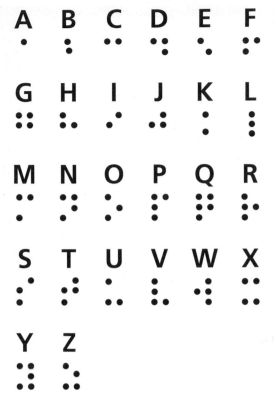

Fig. 44.1 Braille alphabet based on six-dot system.

modern technology presents blind children with more communication options, the importance of Braille has not diminished as a tool for literacy.

The Braille system was developed by Louis Braille, a blind student who in 1824 developed a six-dot raised code. The Braille alphabet consists of combinations of one or more raised dots in a six-dot square known as the Braille cell, which is three dots high and two dots wide. There are 63 possible combinations of dots; after the letters of the alphabet are arranged, the remaining signs are used for punctuation, music, codes, and mathematics. Braille can be written through the aid of a slate, a Braille writer, or a computer system using a Braille printer. To facilitate the development of later Braille skills, young children are introduced early to activities to assist with the development of tactile sensitivity, manual dexterity, and fine motor development. Later, the preschool blind child receives training and materials that focus on pre-Braille readiness skills. The reading and writing of Braille are taught to blind children in the early years, and Braille is still useful in spite of the advanced computer technology available for many simple labeling and writing tasks (Fig. 44.2). Some skilled Braille readers enjoy reading at night in the dark.

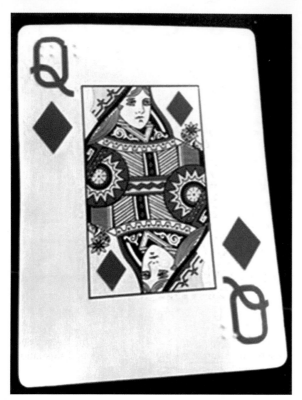

Fig. 44.2 Braille playing card.

Braille libraries are available from which the blind student can obtain books. To supply textbooks for blind students in higher education in Canada, the Canadian National Institute for the Blind has developed a large group of volunteers who have learned to write the Braille system and spend many hours each week transferring printed pages into Braille. In other countries, similar organizations provide this service. Many popular magazines, trade journals, and periodicals are available in Braille. There is still a place for Braille for blind people, although it is less prevalent than in the past century.

Blind children now have access to the latest development in written communication. The proliferation of communication technology has made it possible for blind students to gain access to print information by computer through synthesized speech, large print, or Braille access modes. The combined use of these devices makes possible a scenario in which blind students can access a print exercise through synthesized speech or Braille modes, respond to the exercise in their chosen medium of Braille, and then make a print copy of their answers for the sighted teacher and a Braille copy of the answers for their own files. The Americans with Disabilities Act makes it possible for visually disabled children to receive a good education.

Some blind people may find it difficult to read Braille in an efficient manner with their fingers. To help these individuals, the talking book was developed. Books are available on CD or as a digital download, and are referred to as a talking book. Some blind people do not like to be read to and do not enjoy talking books. They often say that the radio is their chief source of information and that they "listen" to television.

With the right support and appropriate early intervention for families, the capabilities of the blind child are limitless. Blind individuals today are independently employed successfully in an astounding variety of work roles. If society does not limit its expectations of the blind child, these children are capable of living fulfilling lives.

Ophthalmic assistant's role

The orientation of the blind child in an office or any situation is similar to that of an adult in that the assistant first introduces himself or herself to the child and family. With small children, the ophthalmic assistant can take their hand. With older children, the assistant can offer an arm, as for an adult. Children should be told in advance about the general geography of a room and the location of steps as they come to them. In the ophthalmologist's office, the assistant should lead the child to a chair, gently turn him or her, and, placing the child's hand on the arm of the chair, tell the child to sit on the chair at the side where the hand is placed. Again, the right and left sides should always be designated with reference to the position of the blind person. A blind child should be spoken to in a natural manner; these children are skilled in assessing people by the tone of their voice, just as a sighted child would assess a stranger by the person's facial expression.

Rehabilitation

Rehabilitation assists a totally blind person to acquire the practical skills to minimize the effects of disability and lead to independence and social competence.

Rehabilitation programs are often essential for working-age blind people to regain basic independent living skills that make possible further educational training or gainful employment. However, more than 70% of blind and visually impaired individuals are more than 65 years of age. For these individuals, prescribing low-vision aids and offering a rehabilitation program in daily living skills can contribute substantially to their quality of life and assist them with continuing to live in as independent an environment as possible.

Rehabilitation programs are usually staffed by a multidisciplinary team of professionals. The rehabilitation team assesses specific learning needs, develops a training program to meet these needs, and evaluates the blind person's progress in achieving established goals. Services include counseling, daily living skills instruction, orientation and mobility training, Braille and tape library services, sight enhancement services, and concept and sensory development, as well as the provision of consultation and educational information to caregivers, family members, and the general public.

Career development and employment

The goal of rehabilitation for working-age blind persons is competitive employment. Barriers faced by blind individuals seeking employment are related to educational background, skills, and attitudes.

In making an occupational choice, blind people must have information to make meaningful decisions. They need information about their own skills and interests, various occupations that they might find suitable, the technologic knowledge that would qualify them for the job, and how other blind persons have adapted various job tasks.

Occupations pursued by blind and visually impaired people cover the whole range of occupational categories, so there need be very few limits placed on their career aspirations. Obtaining the necessary information is still a problem for many blind and visually impaired persons. Expertise related to the disability and employment opportunities is often hard to find as mainstream employment services possess little knowledge of blindness and visual impairment. The specialized employment services for blind people are available from private organizations and from every state commission for the blind.

Prevailing public perceptions of the potential of blind people tend to influence employers' hiring practices. For this reason, the public education function of agencies for the blind is of critical importance. So too is the outreach function of specialized employment services for blind and visually impaired job seekers, in which employment counselors perform a marketing function on behalf of their clients.

The greatest single factor in increasing employment of blind individuals has been the emergence of information technology. Blindness is handicapping in terms of availability of information; thus access to information is of the utmost importance. Today, the prevocational education component of blind and visually impaired people, whether they are children or newly blinded adults, is in the field of electronic communications.

Vocations

Most rehabilitation programs place blind persons in a job within the sighted community. Job placements require, of course, that special safeguards be made available for the blind worker. It has been shown conclusively that the output of the blind worker in assembly work may be equal in both quantity and quality to that of sighted colleagues if the work is suitably chosen. However, only a limited number of industries have special facilities for the blind worker. Many workshops are run under the auspices of blind institutions and are geared to obviate the blind person's disability. Some blind people actually prefer working under these conditions because of the protections afforded them both physically and psychologically.

The active rehabilitation of blind people depends on many individual factors, such as aptitudes, skills, and training. The advancement of information technology has enabled the blind person access to the Internet and the ability to participate in many of the same things as their sighted peers. Blind people have gone on to attain advanced degrees and hold positions of management, law, social work, and economics. Many musicians are blind, and some have achieved a great measure of fame; pianist George Shearing is an excellent example.

Vocational teaching

The key figure in the rehabilitation of the blind is the rehabilitation teacher. These teachers, some who are blind themselves, are inspirational figures to an individual who has recently lost his or her sight and feels life is over. Such teachers understand very well the many small frustrations that accumulate daily and reduce the morale of the blind trainee. Their understanding of these frustrations and their own unwillingness to be defeated by such problems serve as an excellent example to individuals who have recently lost their sight. Rehabilitation teachers may teach Braille reading and computer skills. The function of the teacher is to show the newly blind person that skills still can be learned and acquired despite a handicap. The teacher is fundamentally a builder of confidence and self-esteem and one to open the minds of the blind person to the opportunities available.

Available aids

Many ingenious devices have been designed to assist the blind person to cope with everyday living. Among these devices are Braille or talking watches and clocks (Fig. 44.3). Braille watches typically have a spring catch that when pressed causes the watch glass to open, allowing the user to read the location of the raised hands on the Braille face of the watch. Talking watches announce the time aloud at the press of a button and many include auditory alarms. These watches are available in various designs, including both pocket and wrist types.

In addition, many computer-based technologic aids are available that provide audible access to information or Braille displays. Small portable devices, such as the Braille 'n Speak, which has a Braille input keyboard and speech output, allow the user to access a note taker, calculator, and

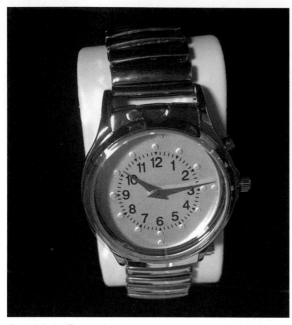

Fig. 44.3 Braille watch.

appointment book, all in a device that weighs less than 2 pounds (0.9 kg).

Kitchen aids available for the blind homemaker include microwave ovens with Braille timers and controls, liquid level indicators, and triangular pie cutters. There are self-threading needles that consist of a groove at the back of the needle before the actual eye of the needle. The thread is positioned into this groove and a small tug pulls the thread into the eye of the needle. Measurements can be made with a tape measure with inches or centimeters marked off in elevated markings.

Among the medical aids are talking thermometers that announce the temperature. For the blind diabetic patient, insulin needle guides enable the person to locate the center of the rubber cap over the insulin bottle. There are also tactile raised markings on the syringe itself to measure the amount of insulin drawn up.

Recreation is a vital part of everyone's life in today's modern world. Tactile games have been developed by the adaptation of standard games, such as bingo, chess, Scrabble, Monopoly, dominoes, and playing cards. For more vigorous exercise and recreation, blind individuals participate in all sports, including swimming, track, bowling, horseback riding, golf, hiking, and wrestling.

Questions for review and thought

1. In your area, what level of vision qualifies an individual to be considered as legally blind?
2. Imagine yourself having both eyes bandaged for 24 hours. Outline the inconvenience and problems you may be confronted with in your normal living.
3. Cover both eyes during a meal and try to cope with the problems of finding your silverware and eating.
4. What is the basis of the Braille system?
5. Name the agency or agencies in your area that help blind people.
6. What aids are available to help blind people?
7. Spend half a day touring your nearest agency for the blind and visually impaired. Outline your impressions and the facilities available.

Self-evaluation questions   Q

True–false statements

Directions: Indicate whether the statement is true (**T**) or false (**F**).

1. A legally blind person cannot read. **T** or **F**
2. The Braille system was developed by Louis Braille, a blind student who in 1824 developed a six-dot raised code. **T** or **F**
3. There is an association between blindness and mental retardation in the adult. **T** or **F**

Missing words

Directions: Write in the missing word(s) in the following sentences.

4. The mannerisms of blind children, such as rocking and rubbing their hands, are called _____.
5. Blindness is defined in the United States and Canada as vision of _____ or less in the best eye and a peripheral field no greater than _____.

Self-evaluation questions—Continued

Q

Choice-completion questions

Directions: Select the one best answer in each case.

6. The blind person can:
   a. ski.
   b. go to university and become a doctor.
   c. be employed, with better records for safety, productivity, and punctuality than for sighted counterparts.
   d. play golf.
   e. all of the above.
7. Braille should be taught:
   a. to every blind person.
   b. only to the young blind person.
   c. to a person recently blinded.
   d. only to those who cannot possibly read with visual aids.
   e. to people going blind.
8. In North America the leading cause(s) of blindness is (are):
   a. cataracts.
   b. corneal disease.
   c. retinal disease.
   d. diseases of the vitreous.
   e. diseases relating to dryness of the eyes.

Answers, notes, and explanations

 A

1. **False**. A legally blind person may have 20/200 vision and, with adequate visual aids and good lighting, can read normal-sized print. The ability to compensate depends on the person's drive, determination, and intelligence. The worst handicap a blind person has is acceptance of his or her blindness as a totally incapacitating event. Only 25% of blind people have no light perception and are truly blind.

2. **True**. The Braille cell is three dots high and two dots wide. Most popular books are available in Braille. Also many magazines, such as *Reader's Digest*, have a Braille edition. Textbooks in Braille are also available and blind students have graduated in medicine, law, accounting, and other demanding courses of study.

3. **False**. People who are blind may have macular degeneration, diabetes, or glaucoma, none of which is associated with mental deterioration. In developing countries, trachoma can cause blindness because of corneal scarring. Simple cataracts, undetected and untreated, are a common source of blindness. Whatever the cause, the blind person is commonly treated with pity, as though he or she not only cannot see but also cannot think properly.

4. **Blindisms**. These habit spasms are difficult to eradicate, but with trained help, they can be. They should be removed because such traits are an obvious stigma of a person's blindness.

5. **20/200, 20 degrees**. Blindness is not the absence of light perception; a person is considered blind only if unable to function in the ordinary world. With this definition, there are many legally blind people who neither consider

themselves blind, nor are they considered blind by others. In a sense, it is a state of mind.

6. **e. All of the above**. A protected environment is not needed for an ambitious, hardworking blind person. Blind people cannot fly a plane, drive a car, or play baseball. However, they can do many things at home, at work, or in sports without special assistance.

7. **d. Only to those who cannot possibly read with visual aids**. Although Braille has served the blind well for over 150 years (through Braille watches, typewriters, and so on), it does narrow the range of options for the blind. Only a small segment of the world's literature is turned into Braille symbols. The options for learning and promotion are far greater if the blind person can stay in the sighted world, even if it means a constant struggle. It is better to have a handicap than to be handicapped.

8. **c. Retinal disease**. Fortunately, cataracts and most forms of corneal disease can be treated surgically with great success. Diseases of the vitreous are usually secondary to retinal or ciliary body disorders. Whereas great advancement has been made in retinal disease, there are no replacement parts for a sick macula or optic nerve. When the macula is injured by disease or trauma, the effects are permanent. The optic nerve, the victim of such common disorders as temporal arteritis, glaucoma, and arteriosclerosis, cannot be helped once damaged. The retina and optic nerve play a major role in creating blindness simply because there is no therapy for these problems. Years ago, the same could be said for diseases of the cornea or lens.

Chapter | 45 |

Cardiopulmonary resuscitation

Joseph D. Freeman

CHAPTER CONTENTS

When a patient, family member, friend, or stranger stops breathing, his/her heart stops beating, or is found unresponsive, it can be one of the scariest situations of your career. However, this is also one of the times in which your knowledge and practice as a trained healthcare provider can make the difference between life and death. Basic life support (BLS) and cardiopulmonary resuscitation (CPR) is the skill set you will use to attempt to save the life of someone who otherwise would have no chance of survival. The rapid initiation and appropriate resuscitation of a person in sudden cardiac or respiratory arrest give that person the best hope of survival.

Cardiopulmonary resuscitation

How does cardiopulmonary resuscitation work?

For all of us to remain alive, our brains must have a constant flow of basic nutrients to function. One of the most important of these basic nutrients is oxygen. Oxygen is taken in from the air we breathe, absorbed into our blood through our lungs, and pumped by our hearts into our brains. If there is any significant interruption in this constant cycle of oxygenated blood flow to the brain, we die.

The heart is, in essence, a large muscle that pumps blood to the brain and all other parts of the body. As it is a muscle,

the heart also needs the nutrients found in blood so that it can have the energy to function. It gets these nutrients through the blood delivered by the coronary arteries, the arteries that run over the top of the heart and come directly off of the aorta, the central artery of the body.

Blood is able to store a certain amount of oxygen and other basic nutrients for a short amount of time. This is why we are able to hold our breath for short periods and do not have to be constantly eating food to remain alive.

In essence, CPR is attempting to re-create the function of the heart and lungs when they are not able to function on their own. This is why it is called cardiopulmonary resuscitation: *cardio-* (Latin/Greek: "heart"), *pulmo* (Latin/Greek: "lungs") *resuscitation* (Latin: "the act of reawakening something/someone"). By pushing down on someone's chest and breathing air into the lungs, you are re-creating the function of the heart and lungs in an attempt to get the blood's nutrients to the brain.

The first step of cardiopulmonary resuscitation: identify the need

How do you know if someone needs CPR? Identifying the need to start CPR can often be one of the hardest steps. A sense of shock and disbelief, in response to an event so out of the ordinary, often overwhelms the potential caregiver. However, rapid initiation of CPR leads to improved survival (the less time the brain is without the nutrients in blood, the better) and therefore is the most important step in CPR.

"Shake and shout" is the first step to establish if a person is responsive. If a person is responsive, he or she does not need CPR. If a person does not respond to attempts to be physically awoken (shaking a shoulder, pinching the arm, or doing something that would be uncomfortable for

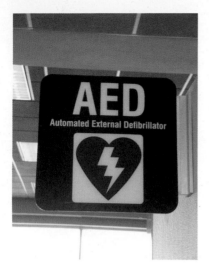

Fig. 45.1 A sign alerting the provider where an automated external defibrillator (*AED*) can be found.

a person but would not cause harm) and shouting loudly into the ear, then you need to call for help.

The second step of cardiopulmonary resuscitation: call for help and get an automated external defibrillator

A crucial step in starting CPR is obtaining help. If you are alone, yell for help. Call an ambulance immediately (phone 911 in the United States and Canada, 080 in Mexico, 999 in the UK, 112 in many countries in Europe), then try to find an automated external defibrillator (AED). An AED may be found in many public spaces designed for large groups of people (such as sport arenas, airports, large business offices), and is often marked by special signs (Fig. 45.1). If you are alone and do not have a mobile device, yell for help. If no one responds to your yells for help, your first priority is to call for an ambulance, even if this requires you to leave the patient temporarily. If you see an AED sign and can quickly get to it on your way back, obtain the AED. Otherwise, return immediately to the patient and check for breathing and a pulse.

The third step of cardiopulmonary resuscitation: check for breathing and a pulse

Check if the person is breathing. Look at the person's chest to see if it is rising and falling with breathing. Some people also find it useful to put their hand on the person's chest.

Look at the person's face to see if any air is coming in or out of the mouth or nose. To determine whether someone is breathing, observe if the mouth is open slightly or nostrils are expanding.

Common mistakes

Most people are able to recognize if someone is not breathing; however, distinguishing "agonal gasping" or "agonal breathing" from normal breathing can be hard. Agonal gasping is a movement that mimics breathing but does not actually get air into the lungs. It often occurs right before a person dies. Agonal gasping can take on several forms, the most common of which is gagging and irregular chest and mouth movements. Agonal gasping is not breathing and you must continue the CPR sequence.

At the same time as you are determining if the person is breathing, use no more than 10 seconds to check for a pulse. The most reliable parts on the body to find a pulse are the neck (for the carotid pulse, Fig. 45.2A), followed by the groin (for the femoral pulse, Fig. 45.2B), and then the wrist (for the radial pulse, Fig. 45.2C). If the patient has no pulse, begin chest compressions. If the patient does have a pulse but is not breathing or has agonal gasping, give one breath every 5 to 6 seconds for 2 minutes ("rescue breathing," see following text) and then recheck to see if the patient has a pulse. If there is a pulse but the person is still not breathing, or are having agonal gasping, continue rescue breathing. If there is no longer a pulse, begin chest compressions.

Hints

It can often be very difficult to feel a patient's pulse because of a multitude of factors (if the patient has a large amount of fat overlying the pulse, if the patient has a weak pulse because his or her heart is not functioning well, or if the pulse is irregular or very slow). There are several techniques you can use to feel for a pulse.

The first is to make sure that you are feeling in the correct location on the body. For the carotid pulse, begin at the midline of the neck and feel the hard tubular structure, the trachea or "windpipe." Slide your fingers to either side of it and into the slight nook or soft spot between the trachea and neck muscle (the sternocleidomastoid). There are two carotids, one on either side of the trachea. For the femoral pulse, find the hip bone (the anterior superior iliac spine, which is the hard bony point on top of the hip, not on the side of the hip) and go halfway across the hip toward the groin as a starting point. Move your fingers every few seconds to the right and left if you do not feel a pulse. For the radial pulse, mentally divide the back side of the wrist in half. Using the half of the wrist that is on the thumb side, mentally divide this area in half again. Put your fingers along this imaginary line.

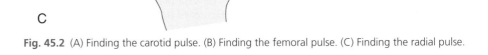

Fig. 45.2 (A) Finding the carotid pulse. (B) Finding the femoral pulse. (C) Finding the radial pulse.

For all pulse checks, use two fingers (your index and middle finger) and the most sensitive area of your finger (this is the very tip of your finger just underneath your fingernail). If there are multiple people, have at least two people check for pulses simultaneously (carotid and femoral or carotid and radial if the patient is clothed).

If you still do not feel a pulse, if you are unsure that you are checking the correct spot, or if you think the patient has a pulse but you are unable to feel it, you must start chest compressions. If the patient really does have a pulse and you are unable to feel it, chest compressions will not stop a heart from beating. If the patient does not have a pulse, then you have taken the correct step by starting chest compressions immediately.

The fourth and most critical step of cardiopulmonary resuscitation: perform chest compressions

Of all the steps you do as part of CPR, early and correctly performed chest compressions are the most critical to saving a patient's life. These are done as a cycle: 30 chest compressions followed by two breaths, done for 2 minutes, then 10 seconds to feel for a pulse. If there is no pulse, continue the cycle of 30 chest compressions followed by two breaths, done for 2 minutes, before checking for a pulse again. If two rescuers are available, one person should do chest compressions and the other person should perform the rescue breaths (Fig. 45.3), as well as help the person

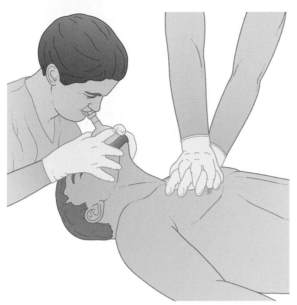

Fig. 45.3 Two-rescuer cardiopulmonary resuscitation with one person performing chest compressions and the other performing rescue breathing.

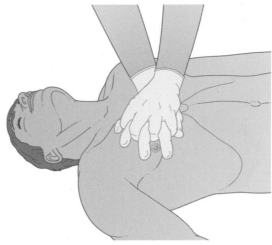

Fig. 45.4 Hand positioning for effective chest compressions.

doing the chest compressions to count and provide feedback when needed ("go faster," "push deeper," "let the chest recoil").

How to perform chest compressions

Performing chest compressions can be exhausting. However, fast and deep chest compressions are critical to saving a patient's life. High-quality chest compressions should have all of the following elements: between 100 and 120 compressions per minute, pushing down between 2 and 2.5 inches (5–6 cm) into the chest, letting the chest wall recoil all the way so that it comes back to its normal starting position between each chest compression, and having as few interruptions or pauses in chest compressions as possible.

Tips

Correct positioning allows for effective chest compressions, as well as preventing the rescuer from getting exhausted too early in the resuscitation. Pushing down on the middle of the chest (above the xiphoid process, where the soft abdomen meets the hard chest wall in the middle of the body), have one hand on top of the other and use the heel of your hand to push down hard in the middle of the chest (Fig. 45.4). Keep your elbows just slightly bent and your back straight. Instead of using your shoulder, back, and arm

muscles to push down on the chest, have the motion start near your lower back from your waist. Performing CPR by using your waist will make you feel hot and sweaty, but allows for more muscle endurance so that you can perform effective CPR longer. Have your chest leaning over the patient so you can use the weight of your chest pushing down on your arms. This will increase the strength of your chest compressions while decreasing the amount of energy your muscles are using to further increase your endurance (Fig. 45.5).

One of the most common mistakes in performing chest compressions is going too slowly. You should be doing at least 100 chest compressions per minute, although no faster than 120 chest compressions per minute, as long as you are performing them effectively. To avoid going too slowly, either have someone count for you or frequently ask yourself if you can go faster. To be effective, however, compressions must be between 2 and 2.5 inches deep and allow for full chest recoil.

Sometimes, especially in the case of older adult patients, chest compressions break the ribs. When doing chest compressions, broken ribs have a crunching, clicking, or popping sensation. If you feel this, continue CPR without any interruptions or pauses. Although it is not ideal to break ribs, it is better to have broken ribs and be alive than be dead without broken ribs.

If you have multiple trained people available during CPR, use them: performing CPR is exhausting. Switch out the person performing chest compressions often. Do this with minimal amounts of pauses in chest compressions by having the next person to perform get into position with arms ready. Place yourself right next to and in parallel to the person currently performing chest compressions and

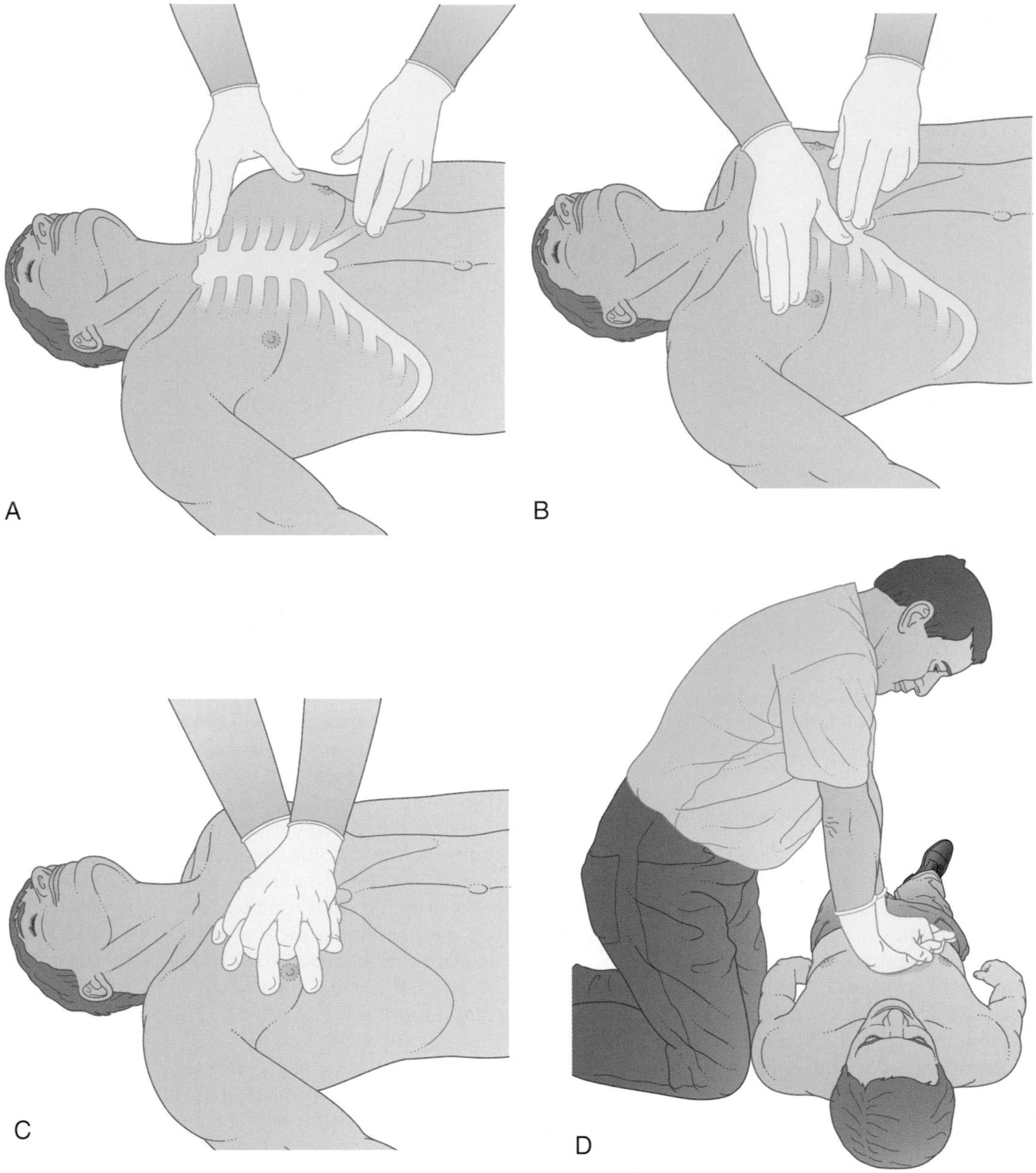

Fig. 45.5 Proper body positioning for effective chest compressions. (A) Find the correct hand position by feeling the soft belly. (B) Move up the belly until you feel the hard chest wall and xiphoid process. (C) Place the heel of your hand at this spot on the chest wall, then place your other hand on top with fingers interlaced. (D) Proper body positioning.

count down to switch so that it happens smoothly and without pauses. One provider can check the pulse while the other performs chest compressions. Well-performed chest compressions should result in one pulse per chest compression.

How it works

The concept behind chest compressions explains why appropriate compression depth and allowing for recoil are so important. By pushing down on a patient's chest, you are

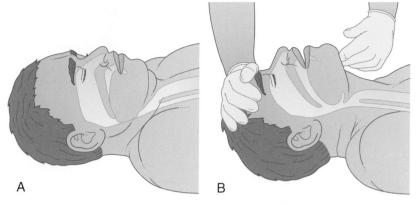

Fig. 45.6 (A) Airway in need of proper positioning. (B) Head tilt–chin lift for proper airway positioning.

creating a pressure within the chest cavity that causes the blood in the heart to go forward toward the brain. Pushing down hard enough provides the appropriate amount of pressure necessary to allow for the blood to move forward. During the temporary pause in a chest compression, the chest is able to recoil, causing a negative "sucking" pressure within the chest that allows blood to fill up the heart, as well as to flow through the coronary arteries, giving the heart much needed oxygen and nutrients.

Rescue breathing

Rescue breathing becomes more important the longer CPR continues before a patient's heart starts beating and he or she begins breathing spontaneously. The oxygen that is stored in the blood is used up by the brain and other parts of the body and needs to be replenished.

Effective rescue breathing first requires proper positioning of the airway (the mouth, throat, and windpipe). This can be done through the head tilt–chin lift maneuver (Fig. 45.6). Place one hand on the back of the head and the other hand underneath the chin. Push with both hands (down with the hand that is on the back of the head, up with the hand underneath the chin) so that the patient's head moves upward. It will seem as if he or she is trying to look up toward the forehead. This movement, called extension, straightens out the larynx and trachea and locks down the tongue into the floor of the mouth. This way air can pass smoothly from the mouth into the lungs. Using the hand that was on the back of the head to hold the head in place in extension, breathe one full breath into the patient's mouth over the course of 1 second (mouth-to-mouth resuscitation, Fig. 45.7). Breathe enough to see the patient's chest rise. Let the air come out of the chest fully and then repeat one more full breath: a total of two rescue breaths. Then immediately return to chest compressions. When performing

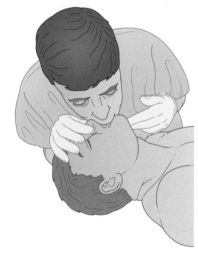

Fig. 45.7 Mouth-to-mouth resuscitation.

rescue breathing as part of CPR, it should be done in cycles of 30 chest compressions to two rescue breaths.

Hints

When performing mouth-to-mouth resuscitation, you should first feel a small amount of resistance to your breath as the chest starts to rise. This will be followed by easier and smoother air flow. If you meet resistance (you try to blow hard but you are unable to move any air and your cheeks puff out), try to reposition the patient's head. Repeat the same technique you used to position the head the first time (one hand behind the head, the other hand underneath the chin and move the head as if the patient is looking upward).

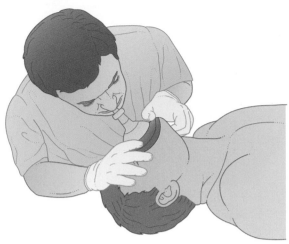

Fig. 45.8 Proper use of one type of protective mouth barrier.

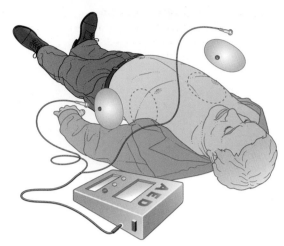

Fig. 45.9 An example of an automated external defibrillator.

If you try mouth-to-mouth resuscitation again and still are unable to blow air into the patient's mouth, consider the possibility that the patient has a foreign body in the airway (see following text). If when looking at the airway you see a large amount of blood or vomit in the mouth, attempt to clear it out of the airway. Put the patient on his or her side and with gloved hands, suction (if available) or scoop out the material. Do not put your hand into the patient's mouth unless you are sure he or she is unconscious and unresponsive and will not bite your hand. If at all possible, always use some form of protective mouth barrier (Fig. 45.8) when performing mouth-to-mouth resuscitation, for your own safety.

The automated external defibrillator

It is important to use the AED as soon as it arrives (Fig. 45.9). There are several different companies that manufacture AEDs, and they look and work slightly differently. However, all of them work using the same basic principle and components. First, look for the directions located on top of the AED or inside the large panel, if present. Follow the instructions. This typically involves placing a large conducting pad on the chest and one on the back or side of the chest, connecting the wires from the pads to the AED (if they are not already connected), turning on the AED, letting the AED analyze the rhythm, and then following the prompts to initiate an electric shock to the heart or continue CPR. Some AEDs have an audio voice and some have a small computer screen with text. Some AEDs use the terms "shockable rhythm" (you need to initiate an electric shock) and "nonshockable rhythm" (you need to continue chest compressions immediately).

When using an AED, it is important to minimize the amount of time the patient is without chest compressions. If the AED tells you to initiate a shock or if it automatically initiates a shock, resume chest compressions immediately after the shock has been delivered. Use the cycle of 30 chest compressions and two rescue breaths for 2 minutes before performing a 10-second pulse check. If the AED says that no shock needs to be delivered (a nonshockable rhythm), immediately continue 30 chest compressions and two rescue breath cycles for 2 minutes before performing a 10-second pulse check.

How automated external defibrillators work

To understand how an AED works, you first need to understand how the heart coordinates itself to make a large muscle contraction to forcefully pump blood through the body. The pacemaker of the heart (the sinoatrial node) uses chemicals to create electricity that travels down electric highways in the heart. This causes the heart muscles to contract in a fast, consistent, and organized fashion. Sometimes this electric rhythm can become disrupted, either through certain chemicals that are out of proportion in the body or because of damage to the heart. Two of these types of abnormal electric rhythms—ventricular fibrillation and pulseless ventricular tachycardia—are "nonperfusing" (the heart is not pumping blood effectively through the body) shockable rhythms. By causing a large external electric shock to the heart through an AED, it is possible that the external electrical shock will reset the heart's abnormal electrical rhythm back to a normal "perfusing" rhythm. It should also be noted that during the delivery of a shock by the AED, people helping with the resuscitation should not touch the patient so that they will not accidentally get shocked themselves. That being said, it is extremely rare to get shocked even if touching the patient. Care should be taken to minimize all interruptions in chest compressions.

Special situations

Children

The previous sequence and techniques for CPR are the same for a child found to be unresponsive, not breathing, or with agonal gasps except for the following seven exceptions:

1. If the child is found unresponsive and not breathing or with agonal gasps, but with a pulse, perform rescue breathing with one breath every 3 seconds (vs. every 5–6 seconds in adults).

2. If during the initial pulse check the child has no pulse or if during the second pulse check (after a cycle of rescue breathing has been given) the pulse is slower than 60 beats per minute, start chest compressions (different than adults). Chest compressions are also done in cycles. If the child's pulse rate becomes greater than 60 beats per minute, go back to rescue breathing. Check the pulse every 2 minutes to determine whether it has started to go slower than 60 beats per minute and if you need to resume chest compressions.

3. If you are the only person able to perform the resuscitation, perform chest compressions in cycles of 30 compressions and two rescue breaths. If there is at least one other person who can help, perform chest compressions in cycles of 15 compressions and two rescue breaths (different than adults).

4. If you are the only person able to perform the resuscitation and do not know when the child was last seen breathing normally (an unwitnessed arrest), you should perform 2 minutes of cycles of 30 compressions and two rescue breaths immediately, then yell for help or temporarily leave the child to call an ambulance (vs. immediately call for an ambulance with both adults and children in witnessed arrests).

5. The depth of chest compressions is different in infants (children <1 year old) versus adults. In infants, push down the chest about one-third of the way, or 1.5 inches (4 cm). In children greater than 1 year old, push down the same amount as you would for an adult (2 inches, or 5 cm).

6. The hand position for infant or small child chest compressions is also done differently than with larger children and adults. In infants, if you are the only person available, perform chest compressions by pushing down on the chest, between the nipples, with your index and middle fingers (Fig. 45.10).

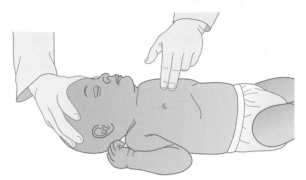

Fig. 45.10 Two-fingered chest compressions for single-rescuer chest compressions in infants.

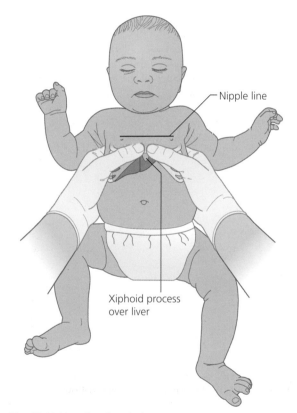

Nipple line

Xiphoid process over liver

Fig. 45.11 Two-thumb technique.

7. If there is more than one person available to help with the resuscitation, perform chest compressions by encircling the infant's chest between your hands and using your thumbs to push down on the chest between the nipples (Fig. 45.11). In small children, you may choose to use the heel of just one hand to perform chest compressions (Fig. 45.12).

Hint

A child's airway anatomy is slightly different than that of an adult (Fig. 45.13). In proportion to their body, children's heads are much bigger and therefore cause the head to flex (looking down instead of looking up) when they are lying flat. Be sure to use the head tilt–chin lift technique to fully extend the head (looking upward) so the larynx and trachea become a straight tube for air to easily pass (Fig. 45.14). If it is still difficult to breathe air into the child's mouth despite repositioning, look for a foreign body in the airway. Because a child's head is large, chest compressions may be difficult to perform effectively. If this occurs, try placing a small towel underneath the child's shoulders for support.

Airway foreign body

If the throat becomes blocked by a foreign body (most often a piece of food in adults, and food or a toy in children), it can stop oxygen from entering the lungs and getting into the blood. This can quickly cause the brain and heart to stop functioning from lack of oxygen, and lead to death. Suspect that the airway is blocked by a foreign body if witnesses said that the patient was choking before becoming unconscious, or if despite positioning and repositioning the head and airway you are unable to blow breaths into the mouth. If the patient is unconscious and unresponsive, lay him or her on the floor, face up, put one hand on top of the other and, with the heel of the bottom hand, push hard and fast on the belly button angling toward the head several times. This is called the Heimlich maneuver. You will usually need to straddle the patient with your legs to get into the proper position if the patient is on the floor.

Next, open the mouth by holding the head and pushing down on the chin, and look at the back of the throat to see if there is any foreign body. If there is, use a finger to scoop

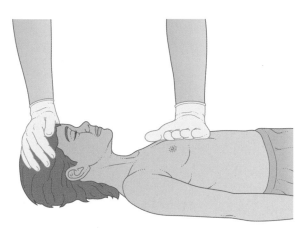

Fig. 45.12 One-handed chest compressions in small children.

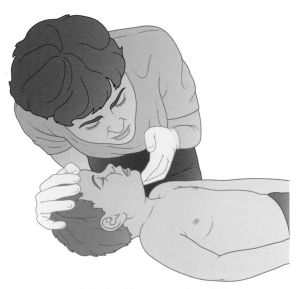

Fig. 45.14 Head tilt–chin lift maneuver in a child.

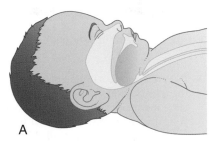
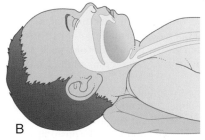

Fig. 45.13 (A) A large head in proportion to the body causes a child's head to be flexed forward. (B) Repositioning the airway using a small towel underneath the child's shoulders may help.

it out (Fig. 45.15). Do this only if you are sure that the patient is unconscious and unresponsive or else he or she may bite down on your finger. If you are unsure, you may use any type of safe instrument to remove the foreign body. If you see no airway foreign body, reposition the head again by extending the head and attempt to breathe air into the patient's mouth. If air will still not go in, attempt several chest compressions just as you would in performing CPR.

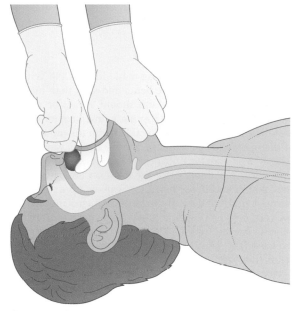

Fig. 45.15 Finger sweep.

Continue this cycle of alternating abdominal thrusts and chest compressions and checking the airway for a foreign body with pauses for pulse checks, until an ambulance arrives. Begin CPR if no pulse is present.

The Heimlich maneuver is performed differently in children, infants, and pregnant women. In infants, five back blows followed by five chest thrusts should be done in sequence (Fig. 45.16), repeated as necessary. In children, five abdominal thrusts should be performed in quick succession followed by checking the airway to see if the foreign body has been dislodged. If no foreign body is seen, attempt two rescue breaths after repositioning the airway. In pregnant women, no abdominal thrusts should be performed so as not to hurt the baby. Instead, only chest compressions should be performed.

Trauma and motor vehicle accidents

BLS care in the setting of trauma is performed in the same manner as in nontrauma cases, with a few important exceptions. A common cause of severe injury or death from trauma is in the setting of motor vehicle accidents. If you witness a motor vehicle accident in which you think someone may be seriously hurt or dying, your first priority is to call an ambulance. Once this is done, your second priority is to assess for scene safety. You must be sure that you and other noninjured bystanders do not sustain injuries during the rescue and resuscitation efforts. If on the road, make sure that all traffic has stopped, especially if on a freeway with other vehicles traveling at high speeds. Rescuers have been seriously hurt and killed when hit by cars while attempting to help accident victims. If the scene is safe, approach the vehicle, telling the patient that you are there to help and ask

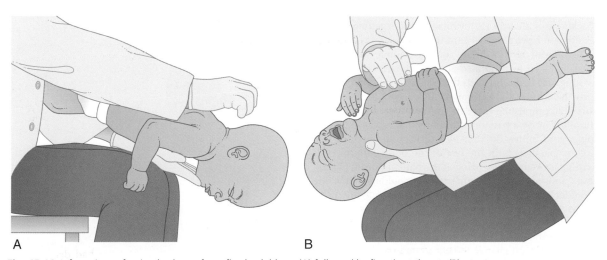

A   B

Fig. 45.16 Infant airway foreign body: perform five back blows (A) followed by five chest thrusts (B).

if he or she is hurt. If possible, tell the patient to turn off the car's engine. If the patient does not talk back to you, assess as you would an unresponsive patient. Check the patient's breathing and pulse, and initiate CPR if indicated. If there is any evidence or concern that the patient may have hurt the neck or back, do all tasks, including CPR, with cervical spine precautions (see following text).

The most common cause of death from trauma is bleeding. Blood carries the necessary nutrients that the brain and heart need to survive. If through a serious injury a patient loses too much blood, there will be no way for the necessary nutrients to reach these vital organs. Thus it is important to control bleeding. This is most easily accomplished by covering the site of bleeding and pushing down hard until the blood clots and stops actively bleeding. In an emergency situation when medical supplies are not available, balled up clothing works well to stop bleeding. If the patient is awake and responsive, this step can be done immediately. If the patient is not responsive and requires CPR, begin it immediately and have another person control bleeding by covering the site and applying direct pressure.

Cervical spine injury

In the case of a serious trauma victim, it is best to assume that the patient has sustained a cervical spine injury until proven otherwise. The brain controls the function and sensation of the rest of the body through nerves. The vast majority of these nerves leave the brain through the bottom of the skull, forming the spinal cord. The spinal cord travels down the spine and branches off to innervate various parts of the body. The spine vertebrae, or backbones, protect the spinal cord from damage. If any of these bones become broken, the spinal cord is at risk of becoming injured, potentially resulting in permanent neurologic disability. In patients who have undergone trauma, the cervical spine (backbone of the neck) is the most at risk of getting broken, resulting in cervical spinal cord injury.

To prevent further injury after a trauma, precautions must be taken to minimize all neck movements, such as twisting and bending. Keep the neck in a neutral position with the head looking straight ahead and neck relaxed. This is accomplished through "in-line immobilization." If you must move a patient with a possible cervical spine or spinal cord injury, do your best to keep the neck in line (e.g., in parallel) with the rest of the body. Minimize all twisting movements by being at the patient's head, placing your hands along the patient's upper shoulders (above the shoulder blades), and using your forearms to lightly press against the patient's head. When the upper body moves, the neck and head will move in the same direction, trying to prevent further neck injury.

One important change to CPR in trauma victims is that you do not perform the head tilt–chin lift maneuver to check the airway. This moves the neck and could cause further injury. Instead, use the jaw thrust method. There are two ways to perform a jaw thrust, depending on whether you are standing at the patient's head or chest. If you are at the patient's head, use both your palms to cup the side of the head and your fingers to grab the angle of the jaw and pull upward, causing just the lower jaw to move up without causing the head or neck to move. If you are at the patient's chest, use your palms and fingers to grab the side of the patient's head and your thumbs under the angle of the jaw and push upward, again causing the lower jaw to move up without moving the head or neck.

Bag-mask ventilation

You might have access to a bag-mask during CPR. Ventilations given by bag-mask are better and safer than mouth-to-mouth rescue breathing and should always be used if available. To properly use a bag-mask, the most important technique is to create a good seal between the mouthpiece of the mask and the patient's mouth. In this way, no air escapes. If you are the only person who is available to help with rescue breathing, place the mask on the patient, use your thumb and index finger to create a "C" that pushes the mask firmly and evenly across the patient's mouth, and use your middle, ring, and pinky (little) fingers along the patient's jaw line, pulling the patient's lower jaw up toward the mask (Fig. 45.17). Use your other hand to squeeze the ventilation bag.

If two people are able to help with rescue breathing, one person uses one hand on each side of the mask and jaw in the same way that you would hold the mask and pull up

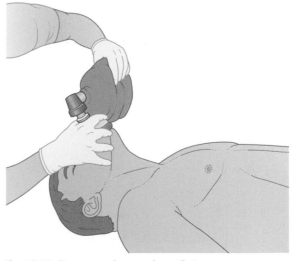

Fig. 45.17 One-person bag-mask ventilation.

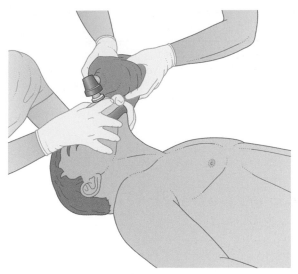

Fig. 45.18 Two-person bag-mask ventilation.

Advanced cardiac life support/ advanced airways

If you have interest in learning more about resuscitation, consider taking a course in advanced cardiac life support (ACLS) or an advanced airway course. In ACLS, you will learn further resuscitation management. Topics covered include giving the patient very strong drugs that work directly on the heart and blood vessels, as well as what to do in other life-threatening situations. In an advanced airway course, you can learn how to use nasopharyngeal airways. These are soft rubber tubes pushed down the nose that go to the back of the throat and help air reach the lungs. You will also learn about oropharyngeal airways: hard rubber devices that go into the mouth and down the back of the throat to help air reach the lungs. Endotracheal intubation uses a special instrument called a laryngoscope to look directly into the back of the throat so as to place a tube into the windpipe to deliver air directly into the lungs. Courses are also available in pediatric advanced life support, neonatal resuscitation program, and advanced trauma life support, among others.

on the jaw as if you were by yourself (Fig. 45.18). The other person squeezes the ventilation bag. Squeeze the ventilation bag just enough to see the chest rise each time to give the correct amount of air.

Hints

If you have difficulty getting the chest to rise with bag-mask ventilation, first check to make sure that you have a good mask seal. Listen carefully: if you hear air escaping out the side of the mask, make sure that the mask fits correctly, covering only the nose and mouth. If you do have a good mask fit, then try to reposition the neck with the head tilt–chin lift or the jaw thrust technique, again pulling up on the jaw to open the throat and windpipe as much as possible.

Final thoughts

Seeing someone suddenly become unresponsive or finding an unresponsive person can be a frightening experience as a healthcare provider. Thankfully, these situations are rare. However, this can make performing CPR correctly very difficult because you will have little practice. It is important to periodically review the CPR guidelines and techniques so when the unexpected situation occurs, the skills you have practiced will come naturally. The quick initiation of CPR with minimal interruptions in fast and deep chest compressions will give someone the best chance of survival. When the situation arises, take a deep breath, try to remain calm, and trust yourself to quickly start CPR.

Questions for review and thought

1. In what cases should you start CPR?
2. Outline your procedure for performing one-person CPR.
3. What are the differences between one-person and two-person CPR?

4. What are the various procedures to deal with obstructed airways?

Self-evaluation questions   Q

True–false statements

Directions: Indicate whether the statement is true **(T)** or false **(F)**.

1. In an adult patient found unresponsive but with irregular gasps, you do not need to start the CPR sequence. **T** or **F**
2. The most common cause of death in trauma is as a result of spinal cord injury. **T** or **F**
3. If after an initial cycle of CPR a child remains unresponsive, is still not breathing but has a heart rate of 50 beats per minute, chest compressions should be started immediately. **T** or **F**

Missing words

Directions: write in the missing word(s) in the following sentences:

4. The _____ maneuver should be used to open the airway in a patient with a potential cervical spine injury.
5. If at all possible, use a _____ when performing mouth-to-mouth resuscitation.
6. The _____ pulse, followed by the _____ pulse and then _____ pulse are the most reliable locations to feel for a pulse.

Choice-completion questions

Directions: Select the one best answer in each case.

7. When seeing a motor vehicle injury in which you are concerned about serious injury, the most important first step is to:
   a. assess scene safety.
   b. call an ambulance.
   c. assess if the patient is responsive.
   d. perform in-line stabilization of the cervical spine.
   e. turn off the damaged car's engine.
8. If you are alone and come upon a child who had an unwitnessed arrest and is found to be unresponsive or not breathing without a pulse, the first step is to:
   a. call an ambulance.
   b. reposition the airway.
   c. perform 2 minutes of 30 chest compressions and two rescue breath cycles.
   d. search for an AED.
   e. perform the Heimlich maneuver.
9. Effective chest compressions should:
   a. be at least 100 compressions per minute.
   b. have the chest pushed down at least 2 inches (5 cm) in an adult.
   c. allow the chest wall to fully recoil after each chest compression.
   d. have all attempts made to have the minimal amount of interruptions or pauses in chest compressions.
   e. all the above.
10. The correct algorithm of adult chest compressions is:
    a. cycles of 30 chest compressions and two rescue breaths for 2 minutes followed by a 10-second pulse check.
    b. cycles of 15 chest compressions and two rescue breaths for 2 minutes if you have another provider to help you with the CPR.
    c. one cycle of 30 chest compressions and two rescue breaths followed by a 10-second pulse check.
    d. if an AED is available and the patient has a shockable rhythm, a 10-second pulse check should be performed after a shock and before starting cycles of 30 chest compressions and two rescue breaths for 2 minutes.
    e. if an AED is available and the patient has a shockable rhythm, continuous cycles of 30 chest compressions and two rescue breaths should be performed without any interruptions for pulse checks.

Answers, notes, and explanations   A

1. **False**. If the patient is unresponsive and has irregular gasps (agonal gasping), you need to continue the CPR sequence. Call for an ambulance and perform a pulse check to see if chest compressions need to be initiated. Although agonal gasping can take on several forms, the most common is irregular, ineffective, short, loud air movements in the mouth that do not reach the lungs.
2. **False**. Although spinal cord injury is a common and potentially serious injury, bleeding is the most common cause of death from trauma. It should be addressed by trying to stop the bleeding with direct pressure early in resuscitation.
3. **True**. In children, chest compressions should be immediately started if there is no pulse or if the pulse is less than 60 beats per minute after a cycle of rescue breathing.
4. **Jaw thrust**. If near the patient's head, place both palms along the head and use your fingers to pull the jaw upward. If near the patient's chest, place your fingers along both sides of the head and use your thumbs to

Answers, notes, and explanations—Continued   A

push the jaw upward. It is important to minimize all neck movement during this maneuver.

5. **Mouth barrier**. Unfortunately, mouth barriers are rarely available outside a hospital scenario. If available, they should always be used for your safety.

6. **Carotid, femoral, radial**. It can be hard to feel a pulse in a high-stress situation and within the required amount of time (10 seconds) before chest compressions should be started or resumed. If available, it is always best to have multiple providers feeling for a pulse simultaneously.

7. **b. Call an ambulance**. Once this is done, assess if the scene is safe. If you get injured while trying to help, there will now be one more injured person that requires care. Once these two steps are done, begin your CPR assessment by seeing if the patient is responsive.

8. **c. Perform 2 minutes of 30 chest compressions and two rescue breath cycles**. Contrary to an adult found unresponsive, not breathing, and without a pulse, a child in the same condition should immediately have 2 minutes of cycles of 30 chest compressions and two rescue breaths, if you are by yourself. Then an ambulance should be called. If there are multiple providers, one provider should call for an ambulance and look for an AED, while other providers perform cycles of 15 chest compressions and two rescue breaths for 2 minutes.

9. **e. All of the above**. Quality chest compressions will contain each one of these elements. Early initiation and minimal interruptions in chest compressions have the greatest effect when attempting to save the life of a person whose heart has stopped beating.

10. **a. Cycles of 30 chest compressions and two rescue breaths for 2 minutes, followed by a 10-second pulse check**. This is the correct CPR algorithm for an adult. The correct CPR algorithm in children, if you have another provider, is cycles of 15 chest compressions and two rescue breaths for 2 minutes. If an AED is available and the patient has a shockable rhythm, after the shock is delivered, cycles of 30 chest compressions and two rescue breaths for 2 minutes should be initiated immediately without first assessing for a pulse after the shock. However, you should assess for a pulse at the end of the 2-minute cycle of CPR.

Gradually, it was realized that there were many people with myopia who needed daily spectacle wear. This necessitated fixed lens positioning in front of the eyes and resulted in production of various models of iron, brass, and precious metals and later, in the United States, frames of buffalo horn. Most lenses were round, but they were available in oval shape in horn frames.

Single lenses and monocles

Next to the classic spectacles, the single lens was the most common alternative for many years. The lens could be positioned directly over the eye by hand or other methods. Interestingly, many of these lenses were concave for myopia. In 1585 William Bourne listed such glasses as perspective glasses. About this time, public wearing of spectacles was either frowned upon or forbidden, so single lenses, although difficult to wear, were an alternative. Shortly thereafter, in England, wearing glasses became stylish. Glasses were thought of as jewelry and were worn on a chain around the neck. Because of their ornamental status, they were completed by goldsmiths rather than by opticians.

The common man carried a single lens mounted in a grooved copper wire. Mass-produced versions, such as the lorgnon made in Nuremberg (Fig. 46.9) were priced for the average person.

Another form of the single lens is the so-called monocle worn by the British King Charles II. This version was held in front of the eye by compression from the musculus orbicularis. The edge of the frame was rounded and often grooved to improve wearing retention (Fig. 46.10). Small loops were often attached to the frame to help keep the lens in place. To achieve greater distance between the eye and the lens and to increase comfort, an additional ring, a so-called gallery, was attached to offset the lens frame from the lids.

Fig. 46.9 Monovision lens in copper frame, Nuremberg, 1680.

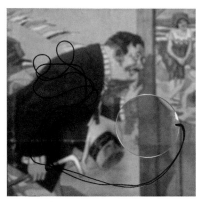

Fig. 46.10 Model of a monocle, about 1870.

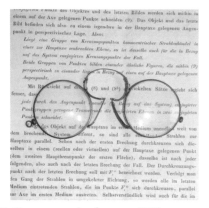

Fig. 46.11 Pince-nez made of copper, 1860.

In 1727 Baron von Stosch appeared in public wearing a monocle. This had an effect on style-conscious people, who immediately adopted this form of eyewear. Scientists warned about the health-related dangers of such wear but this did not halt its use. The monocle increased in popularity for most of the ensuing two centuries, usually among the upper classes and especially military officers.

Spring spectacle frames

These frames were common in various countries including England into the 18th century. An example was the invention of a variety of elastic metal nose clamps (Fig. 46.11). Lenses were framed with metal, wood, horn, or leather. Later the entire apparatus including the metal hoops and nose clamps were made of the same metal, which enabled mass production of less expensive spectacles. These

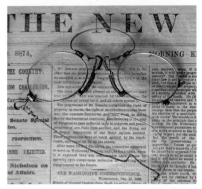

Fig. 46.12 Golden pince-nez with chain, 1860, Chicago, USA.

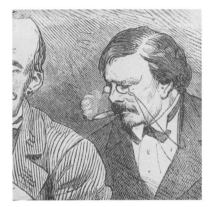

Fig. 46.13 Pince-nez with cord, 1890.

so-called spring frames were the forerunners of the *pince-nez* (Fig. 46.12). The French physician Joseph Bressy published a patent in 1825 for small, thin steel plates that held the frame on the nose with more or less comfort. Wearing oval lenses became common. Small nosepieces or patches lessened the uncomfortable pressure on the nose. An attached cord prevented the glasses from being dislodged onto the ground or secured them when they were not needed (Fig. 46.13).

The variations in form were large. One type used a vertical construction to spread the glasses, while another permitted adjustment of the interpupillary distance by moving the glasses along a horizontal axis, necessary in the correction of astigmatism with toric lenses.

For more than 100 years, until the time of World War I, the primary method for visual correction required glasses to be held in place by being clamped to the bridge of the nose. This eyewear became a symbol of position and of intelligence because the main wearers were merchants or teachers. Military officers wore the monocle because other forms of visual aids were officially forbidden when on parade.

Temple pieces and curved earpieces

In 1890 frames with sidebars, called *temple pieces*, were produced, some with curved portions that extended behind the ears. These additions provided a more secure fit on the head. The earpieces were present on the earliest form of temple pieces (Fig. 46.14) and gave spectacles the configuration they have today. Extension of the sidebars behind the ears became common at the start of the 20th century and provided an improved fit.

Lorgnettes

The *lorgnette* (Fig. 46.15) evolved from the scissor spectacle; in 1770 George Adam introduced a glass case that could be used to store them. In 1800 the lorgnette was the most frequently used form of glasses and was produced in

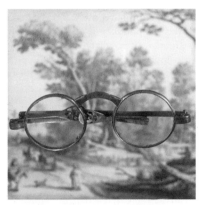

Fig. 46.14 Early temple spectacle, brass frame, 1760.

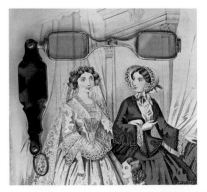

Fig. 46.15 Spring glass or lorgnette, horn, about 1850, Paris.

a multitude of variations. M. Lepage improved the mechanism in 1818 so the connections between the lenses permitted it to be folded. Pressure on a button released the glasses from the case.

The lorgnette was the typical eyewear of the bourgeoisie and was prized by prominent women, who often carried it as jewelry. Finally, by the onset of the last century, this style was converted into spectacles with curved earpieces.

Early glasses were used to correct for presbyopia and had a range of powers between +1.00 and +4.00 diopters. With the awareness of other refractive errors and the knowledge that minus lenses could correct myopia, spectacles were developed for distant vision. These improvements brought the need to enable sharp vision at both near and far distance with one pair of glasses. The problem was solved with the invention in 1785 that joined two lenses of different refractive powers, or bifocals. The inventor was the American statesman and scientist Benjamin Franklin. John Hawkins improved the system in 1827 with the development of the trifocal lens.

It is astounding that before 1800, no one was aware that the human cornea has two major refractive zones, one vertical and the other horizontal. The English physicist and physician Thomas Young first reported this, but correction for astigmatism was not possible until 1825 when the Scottish astronomer George Airey created the first astigmatic lens for daily wear. In 1850 the first industrially produced lens containing a cylinder was manufactured by the best-known glass factory of the time, which was located in Rathenow. This commercial availability enabled correction of astigmatism in the general population.

The onset of the 19th century saw the use of biconcave or biconvex lenses. In a series of experiments, the English physician William Wollaston showed how the sharpness of vision can be improved when the refractive capabilities of lenses are better used; for example, in 1804 he reported that acuity can be increased when the concave surface of the lens faces the eye. Johannes Kepler had reported this principle in 1611 with the use of polished meniscal lenses. However, it was not until 1904 that the Danish ophthalmologist Hans Tscherning reported that the refractive benefit could be optimized by the use of so-called periscopic spectacle lenses.

It is amazing that the use of curved earpieces is only 100 years old and that it was not until 1906 that Moritz von Rohr of Zeiss Oberkochen developed the so-called punctal glass to eliminate peripheral visual images.

Goggles and sunglasses

Glasses have uses other than correcting visual anomalies, such as preventing injury from particulate matter or from

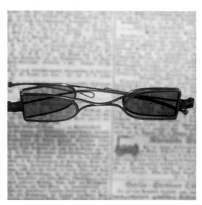

Fig. 46.16 Sunglasses, blue tinted, 1750.

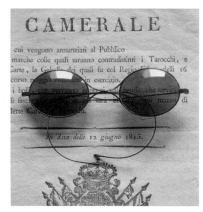

Fig. 46.17 Sunglasses without refraction, blue, 1815.

glare. Pliny reported that Roman nobles viewed through a polished emerald for protection. In the 16th century spectacles were first tinted; this prompted scientific discussions regarding which color provided not only the most wearing comfort but also the greatest protection to the eye. The color of the oldest goggles was either yellow or blue (Figs. 46.16 and 46.17), whereas Chinese glasses were tinted gray or yellow.

In 1885 the French ophthalmologist Fieusal was the first to connect glare sensitivity to a range of short-wave light and to recommend light absorption in this short-wave region. In 1912 the Swiss ophthalmologist Vogt reported that absorption of infrared radiation led to eye damage. In the following years, the glass industry developed absorbing lenses that filtered out dangerous light radiation, permitting only harmless rays to impinge on the eye. Currently, more sunglasses than glasses for visual anomalies are worn.

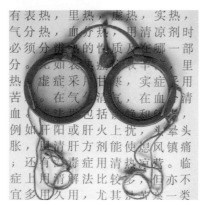

Fig. 46.18 Chinese reading glasses, 1690.

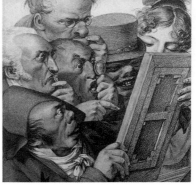

Fig. 46.19 The upper class; French color print of 1875.

Glasses in the Far East

Glasses are a classic, typical, and essential item in Asian culture. Although it may be assumed that glasses have been part of the culture for many years, there are no accounts in contemporary Chinese literature or encyclopedias indicating this. It is reasoned that Venetian merchants, including Marco Polo, introduced spectacles to the Chinese Empire. It is sure that during the 16th century, glasses were imported because there is no record of any local manufacturing. The earliest Chinese-made spectacles had lenses of rock salt or quartz (Fig. 46.18) instead of glass. Also, they were made not so much to correct refractive anomalies but to indicate the high social position of the wearer. The configuration of spectacles copied those manufactured in Europe. In the early 20th century Chinese spectacles were made with curved earpieces.

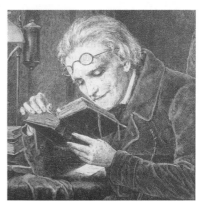

Fig. 46.20 Modern spectacle for myopia, 1920.

Summary

The history of spectacles is the history of scientific progress; it is an integral part of our culture (Figs. 46.19 and 46.20).

Spectacles have enabled millions of people with visual problems to take part in daily life and to acquire an education. From their beginning as a reading lens made of the gemstone beryl, glasses have improved to include multifocal lenses, contact lenses, and implants into the living eye.

Further reading

Corson R. *Fashions in Eyeglasses From the 14th Century to the Present Day*. London: Peter Owen; 1967.

Court TH, von Rohr M. On the development of spectacles in London from the end of the 17th century. *Trans Opt Soc*. 1929;30:1–12.

Emsley HH, Percival AS. Percival and best form lenses. *Man Opt*. 1963;17:21–23.

Hardy WE. An outline history of British spectacle making from 1629 onwards. *Man Opt*. 1966;151:677–684.

McConnel JW. The history of spectacle lens correction in Germany. *Man Opt*. 1967;20:260–270.

Poulet W. *Atlas on the History of Spectacles*. Bonn/Bad Godesberg, Germany: Wayenborgh; 1978.

Rosen E. Did Roger Bacon invent eyeglasses? *Arch Int Hist Soc*. 1954;7:32–41.

Roth HW. *A Contribution to the History of Contact Lenses*. Bonn/Bad Godesberg, Germany: Wayenborgh; 1978.

as the world turned. He is said to have wished that he "had been born blind to experience sight suddenly: to see the world naively, as pure shape and color." He actually did experience temporary blindness at the age of 27 years, which was attributed to worries about his wife, Camille, who was about to give birth to his son, Jean.

As he entered his 66th year, Monet became aware of changes in his vision, although bilateral cataracts were not diagnosed until 4 years later. He consulted with several ophthalmologists but was advised to defer surgery. Although the cataract in his right eye was almost mature and the eye virtually useless, he was deathly afraid of surgery. His close friend, the diplomat Georges Clemenceau, had been a physician and helped to provide both medical advice and a shoulder to lean on. Although Clemenceau assured Monet that his sight could be restored through surgery, Monet remained opposed to an operation. By 1918, then 78 years old, Monet reported:

> I no longer perceived colors with the same intensity.
> I no longer painted light with the same accuracy.
> Reds appeared muddy to me, pinks insipid and the
> intermediate or lower tones escaped me....
>
> At first I tried to be stubborn. How many times,
> near the little bridge where we are now, have I
> stayed for hours under the harshest sun, sitting on
> my campstool, in the shade of my parasol, forcing
> myself to resume my interrupted task and recapture
> the freshness that had disappeared from my palette!
> Wasted efforts. What I painted was more and more
> dark, more and more like an "old picture," and when
> the attempt was over and I compared it to former
> works, I would be seized by a frantic rage and slash
> all my canvases with a penknife.

Subtle differences in color became difficult to distinguish, although vivid colors were still visible against a dark background, and the bright noonday sun forced him to abandon painting at midday. Aware of his problems differentiating colors, he arranged his paints according to their labels, in a set sequence, on his palette. Acknowledging that he was unable to select colors appropriately, he destroyed a number of canvases. By now, his cataracts had become brunescent and were affecting his color perception by filtering out blue, violet, and some shades of green. His paintings reflected his vision and became increasingly hazy and more red, yellow, and brown (Figs. 47.2 and 47.3).

Although Monet had agreed to produce 19 large water lily panels that the French government would place in the Orangerie Museum in Paris, he felt, by 1922, that he would be unable to complete the project. In a letter, he lamented:

> I wished to profit from what little (remained of) my
> vision to bring certain of my decorations to completion.

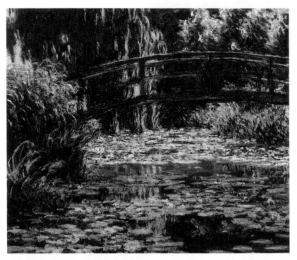

Fig. 47.2 Claude Monet: *Water Lily Garden*, 1900. (From Marmor MF, Ravin JG. *The Eye of the Artist*. St Louis: Mosby; 1997. Mr. and Mrs. Larned Coburn Memorial Collection. Reproduction, The Art Institute of Chicago.)

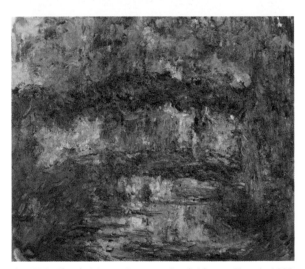

Fig. 47.3 Claude Monet: *Japanese Footbridge at Giverny*, 1923. (From Marmor MF, Ravin JG. *The Eye of the Artist*. St Louis: Mosby; 1997. Musée Marmottan, Paris. Bridgeman Art Library.)

> And I was gravely mistaken. For in the end, I had
> to admit that I was ruining them, that I was no
> longer capable of making something of beauty. And I
> destroyed several of my panels. Today I am almost blind
> and I have to renounce my work completely.

By September 1922, Monet's vision had decreased to light perception with projection OD and 20/200 OS. Yet he continued to resist surgery. An attempt was made to enhance the vision in his left eye by dilating the pupil with eucatropine hydrochloride, a mydriatic used at that time, so he could see around the opacity. For a brief period of time, it seemed to help. Monet wrote to his ophthalmologist:

It is all simply marvelous. I have not seen so well for a long time.... The drops have permitted me to paint good things rather than the bad paintings which I had persisted in making when seeing nothing but fog.

Within a month, however, he realized the futility of his strategy to circumvent surgery and agonized over the inevitable procedure. He wrote to Clemenceau about his torment and nightmares. At the time, cataract surgery was a complex procedure. Monet knew of others, including the American Impressionist Mary Cassatt and the French caricaturist Honore Daumier, who had undergone unsuccessful cataract extractions and he became increasingly despondent. Finally, in January 1923, in response to the strong urging of Georges Clemenceau, who reminded him of his agreement with the French government to complete the water lily panels, Monet underwent an extracapsular cataract extraction, which had been preceded by an iridectomy the month before. The only anesthetic available was cocaine and the surgeon probably used no sutures or perhaps just one.

Monet found it difficult to adapt to the postsurgical regimen of lying in total darkness, both eyes bandaged shut, flat on his back (with no pillow), his head between sandbags to prevent movement and with no nourishment except bouillon and lime tea, for 10 days. The only time light entered his eyes during this period was when the bandages were removed from his right eye every hour or two to instill eyedrops. Monet had to be forcibly restrained from tearing off his bandages and expressed a preference for being blind rather than having his eyes covered. He was attended by a guardian at night, not only to make sure he did not move but also to engage in conversation because lack of contact with the outside world could cause delirium or psychotic behavior. Three weeks after surgery, he was given a pair of temporary cataract glasses and began his "adjustment" to the aphakic world.

As anticipated by his ophthalmologist, the posterior capsule opacified, necessitating still another surgical procedure. Severe depression set in. He wrote to his surgeon, Dr. Charles Coutela:

I am absolutely discouraged and as much as I read, not without effort, 15 to 20 pages per day, outdoors from a distance, I cannot see anything with or without glasses (with the right eye). And for 2 days, black spots have bothered me.

Remember that it has been 6 months since the first operation, 5 since I left the clinic and 4 that I have been wearing glasses. It has taken me 4 or 5 weeks to get used to my new vision. Six months that I would have been able to work if you had told me the truth.

It is to my chagrin that I regret having had this fatal operation. Pardon me for speaking so frankly and let me tell you that it is criminal to have put me in this situation.

Dr. Coutela noted Monet's "profound discouragement and despair" and related that "Monet saw himself as blind forever and, completely demoralized, refused to leave his bed." The secondary membrane was removed at Monet's home in Giverny in July 1923, after which he was able to achieve vision of about 20/30 in his right eye with a prescription of + 10.00 + 4.00 × 90. Unfortunately, because he refused to have the cataract in his left eye removed, he was unable to use his eyes together. The brunescent cataract in his left eye caused him to experience a marked difference in color perception between the two eyes. The colors seen with his left eye were muddied by the cataract; with his right eye, the lost blues and violets returned with a vengeance. He painted his house, as seen from the rose garden, through the mature cataract in his left eye (Fig. 47.4) and the aphakic (probably uncorrected) vision in his right (Fig. 47.5).

Monet found it difficult to adjust to aphakic spectacles. He was bothered by the abnormal curvature of objects

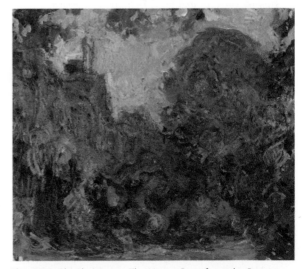

Fig. 47.4 Claude Monet: *The House Seen from the Rose Garden*, 1923. (From Marmor MF, Ravin JG. *The Eye of the Artist*. St Louis: Mosby; 1997. Musée Marmottan, Paris. Bridgeman Art Library.)

Fig. 47.5 Claude Monet: *The Artist's House Seen from the Rose Garden*, 1923. (From Marmor MF, Ravin JG. *The Eye of the Artist*. St Louis: Mosby; 1997. Musée Marmottan, Paris. Bridgeman Art Library.)

caused by the high-plus astigmatic lens for his right eye and had difficulty walking with his glasses. He expressed his disappointment in a letter to Dr. Coutela:

> *I have just received them (new glasses) today but I am absolutely desolated for, in spite of all my good will, I feel that if I take a step, I will fall on the ground. For near and far everything is deformed, doubled and it has become intolerable to see. To persist seems dangerous to me.*

And to Clemenceau, he wrote:

> *I'm doing exercises and can read easily but the distortion and exaggerated colors that I see are quite terrifying. As for going for a walk in these spectacles, it's out of the question for the moment anyway and if I was condemned to see nature as I see it now, I'd prefer to be blind and keep my memories of the beauties I've always seen.*

Clemenceau urged him to have surgery on the second eye but he responded:

> *I absolutely refuse, for the moment at least, to have the operation done to my left eye. … You can have no idea of the state I'm in as regards my sight and the alteration of colors…so unless I find a painter, of whatever kind, who's had the operation and can*

tell me that he can see the same colors he did before, I won't allow it.

Aphakic glasses, even today with corrected curve lenses, have a great deal of aberration; they create a ring scotoma that restricts the wearer's peripheral vision and induce magnification of 1.5% to 2% per diopter of correction, making it impossible for patients who have had surgery in only one eye to use their eyes together. Monet had to block his unoperated left eye with a piece of paper or, in a later pair of glasses, what appears to be an occluder lens. He had separate glasses for near and distance rather than bifocals, and experienced far greater distortion, as well as spherical and chromatic aberration, than a wearer of contemporary aphakic spectacles would today. The high magnification and high astigmatic correction contributed to his depression and his refusal to have surgery on the contralateral eye. A pair of his aphakic spectacles on display at the Musée Marmottan in Paris reads: OD + 14.00 + 7.00 × 90; OS plano. He complained of overwhelming blue and yellow vision and expressed his desolation to Dr. Coutela:

> *For months I have worked with obstinacy, without achieving anything good. I am destroying everything that is mediocre. Is it my age? Is it defective vision? Both certainly, but vision particularly. You have given me back the sight of black on white, to read and write and I cannot be too grateful for that but I am certain that the vision of (this) painter…is lost and all is for nothing.*
>
> *I am telling you this confidentially. I hide it as much as possible but I am terribly sad and discouraged. Life is a torture for me.*

Eventually, Monet was fitted with a Zeiss aphakic spectacle lens, which had a wider field of vision. He continued to complain about colors:

> *I see blue; I no longer see red or yellow. This annoys me terribly because I know that these colors exist, because I know that on my palette there is some red, some yellow, a special green and a certain violet.… It's filthy, it's disgusting, I see nothing but blue. …*

Relief was finally achieved and a more normal perception of blue obtained with glasses that were tinted yellow-green, allowing him to better adapt to his aphakic vision. He still experienced dramatic mood swings that are evidenced in letters he wrote in the final years of his life:

> *I am more certain than ever that a painter's eyesight can never be recovered. When a singer loses his voice he retires; the painter who has undergone an*

operation of the cataract must renounce painting and this is what I have been incapable of.

But a few months later, in a letter to Dr. Coutela, he wrote:

I am very happy to inform you that I have recovered my true vision and that nearly at a single stroke. I am happily seeing everything again and I am working with ardor.

Monet continued to paint until his death, at age 86 years, from lung cancer and chronic obstructive pulmonary disease, retouching and completing his water lily series, which can be seen today at the Orangerie in Paris.

Vincent van Gogh (1853–1890)

Vincent Willem van Gogh was born into a Dutch family of preachers a year to the day after his stillborn brother and given the same name as the firstborn son. Although he studied for the ministry and tried his hand at teaching, he gradually drifted into a troubled and tragic life as an artist.

Many theories have been put forth in an attempt to explain his mental illness, bizarre behavior, and artistic technique. As an adult, particularly during the last 2 years of his life, he experienced periods during which he appeared to be perfectly normal and lucid, interspersed with episodes of severe mental disturbances. His mental illness has been attributed to epilepsy, bipolar illness, schizophrenia, Ménière disease, and chemical toxicity. More recently, the possibility of porphyria, a genetic disease caused by an enzyme deficiency and manifested by symptoms that include abdominal pain and neurologic and psychiatric disturbances, has been proposed as the cause of his bizarre behavior because others in his family also exhibited symptoms of insanity. However, dark urine is characteristic of porphyria, and scholars have found no references to this in his letters, nor has any other medical documentation been uncovered.

How can we envision van Gogh's vision? Did his paintings reflect an abnormality of vision? Trevor-Roper hazards a guess that van Gogh was short-sighted, based on the fact that his paintings are best viewed within a short radius; the subjects in his paintings are placed at an unusually close range; and that he had a "childhood habit of walking with half-shut eyes, hunched shoulders, looking at his feet, and being a duffer (incompetent) at ball games." Ravin and Marmor, however, report that in May of 1890, van Gogh's vision was informally tested by Dr. Paul Ferdinand Gachet, a homeopathic physician, amateur artist, and rather eccentric individual himself. Gachet was entrusted with van Gogh's care after van Gogh left the mental institution in Provence, where he had admitted himself after cutting off part of his left ear. Van Gogh was intrigued by an eye chart hanging on the wall of Gachet's country home in Auvers-sur-Oise, north of Paris. On reading the letters on the chart and also being tested for color vision with the materials that Gachet used to test railroad workers, he was found to have excellent visual acuity and normal color vision. In spite of these findings, many questions have been raised about his style and use of color, particularly during the last 2 or 3 years of his life.

Van Gogh's halos

The colored halos and swirls in the sky in *Starry Night* (Fig. 47.6), perhaps van Gogh's most well-known painting, and similar waviness and halos in some of his other works, have been the subject of much analysis. In *Starry Night*, the moon and sun are superimposed, stars magnified and surrounded by halos, and the sky filled with swirling nebulae. Some think that the painting resulted from a dramatic revelation that he experienced during a vivid hallucination. Others have entertained the possibility that the colored halos were indicative of an attack of angle-closure glaucoma, although there is no reference to the nausea, intense pain, and severe clouding of vision that accompany an angle-closure glaucoma attack in any of his letters, most of which have been preserved. Perhaps, as used by previous artists symbolically in religious paintings, the aura in the sky represented his "sentimental attachment to stars from his youth…when he felt a need for religion, he went out at night and painted them."

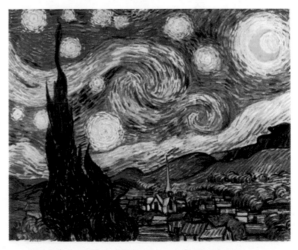

Fig. 47.6 Vincent van Gogh: *Starry Night*, 1889. (From Mühlberger R. *The Unseen Van Gogh*. Chesterfield, MA: Chameleon Books; 1998. Museum of Modern Art, New York, NY.)

Xanthopsia

Even more fascinating is van Gogh's preoccupation with the color yellow. In many of his paintings, not only the scene itself but also the flesh of his characters have a yellowish cast (Figs. 47.7 and 47.8). Was this a result of a conscious choice of yellow pigments or was the yellow vision caused by xanthopsia? If, indeed, he was experiencing xanthopsia, was it caused by substance abuse or chemical toxicity?

In March 1889, in a letter to his brother, art dealer Theo van Gogh, he wrote:

> *M. Rey (a physician) says that instead of eating enough and at regular times, I was keeping myself going by coffee and alcohol. I admit all that but it is true all the same that to attain the high yellow note that I attained last summer, I really had to be pretty well strung up.*

By July he appeared to have given up alcohol and wrote to Theo:

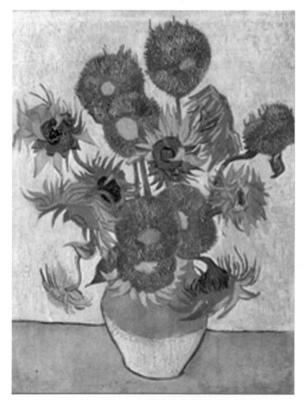

Fig. 47.7 Vincent van Gogh: *Still Life With Fourteen Sunflowers*, 1889. (From Mühlberger R. *The Unseen Van Gogh*. Chesterfield, MA: Chameleon Books; 1998. Van Gogh Museum, Amsterdam, The Netherlands.)

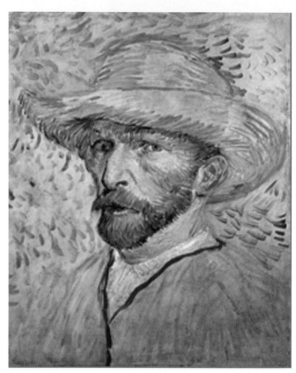

Fig. 47.8 Vincent van Gogh: *Self-Portrait With Straw Hat*, 1889. (From Mühlberger R. *The Unseen Van Gogh*. Chesterfield, MA: Chameleon Books; 1998. Van Gogh Museum, Amsterdam, The Netherlands.)

> *I drank in the past because I did not know how to do otherwise. Anyway, I don't care in the least!!! Very deliberate sobriety—it's true—leads nevertheless to a state of being in which thought, if you have any, moves more readily. In short it is a difference like painting in grey or in colors. I am going in fact to paint more in grey.*

While van Gogh was hospitalized in Arles after cutting off part of his ear, he was diagnosed with a seizure disorder by a psychiatric intern. Today, we think of digitalis as a medication used for patients with heart abnormalities. In van Gogh's day, the drug was also used to treat seizure disorders, and digitalis toxicity was a known cause of yellow vision. No evidence has ever surfaced to indicate that van Gogh's seizures were ever treated with digitalis, but some interesting theories have been put forward.

The eccentric Dr. Gachet, responsible for the care of van Gogh in Auvers, "was known as Dr. Saffron because he dyed his hair yellow." Van Gogh was much aware of Gachet's unconventional demeanor and wrote to Theo:

> *I have seen Dr. Gachet, who made the impression on me of being rather eccentric but his experiences as*

a doctor must keep him balanced while fighting the nervous trouble from which he certainly seems to be suffering at least as seriously as I.

Digitalis was also a homeopathic remedy used, among other things, for managing "melancholic thoughts, hypochondria, mental illness, headache, nausea, vomiting, pain in the eyes, swelling of the eyelids, tearing, and inflammation of the eyes" and Gachet was a homeopathic practitioner. He has been accused of overdosing van Gogh with digitalis and mismanaging his care. Yet Gachet was said to understand the physiologic dangers of digitalis and its potential for problems. He also felt that van Gogh's mental illness, which he diagnosed as manic depression (which would explain the periods of lucidity that alternated with periods of mania and melancholy), was not treatable at that time with medication.

There are substances other than digitalis that can cause yellow vision, one of them being santonin, which was used at that time as a preventive medicine and antibacterial agent to treat intestinal parasites. Van Gogh was known to have digestive problems and may have been treated with santonin for them. He was thought to have abnormal cravings (pica) for camphor, thujone, and turpentine, which are chemically similar to santonin. He might have ingested santonin to relieve the pica. He was also an insomniac and known to use large doses of camphor as a sleep remedy, often drank absinthe, a potent alcoholic beverage that contained thujone, and was reported by the artist Paul Signac to express the desire to consume a large amount of turpentine.

Although there is much support for the hypothesis that van Gogh's xanthopsia was chemically induced, other evidence fails to substantiate the findings. Van Gogh often experimented with color. In a letter he wrote:

Monticelli was a painter who painted the south all in yellow, orange and sulfur colors. Most painters do not see these colors because they are not really experts in color.

And in 1885, he argued:

Suppose I have to paint an autumn landscape, trees with yellow leaves. All right—when I conceive it as a symphony in yellow, what does it matter if the fundamental color of yellow is the same as that of the leaves or not?

And Gauguin commented:

Oh yes, he loved yellow, this good Vincent, this painter from Holland—those glimmers of sunlight rekindled his soul that abhorred the fog, that needed the warmth.

The collection of van Gogh's letters contains numerous passages dealing with his experimentation with other colors and he studied the basic color triangle, complementary colors, color harmonies, and color contrasts. The truth remains a mystery.

Fame came to van Gogh only after his death. On July 27, 1890, at the age of 37 years, he could no longer bear his loneliness and torments. He shot himself with a revolver in the fields through which he had often wandered and painted, and although mortally wounded and in excruciating pain, struggled back to his room at the inn. He died 2 days later, in his brother Theo's arms. Although only one of his paintings was sold during his lifetime, he always felt that fame would be achieved after his death. He had written:

Just as we take the train to get to Tarascon or Rouen, we take death to reach a star. One thing absolutely true in this reasoning is that we cannot get to a star while we are alive, any more than we can take a train when we are dead.

Edgar Degas (1834–1917)

When we hear the name Degas we often visualize ballet dancers in motion, soft, hazy pastel renditions, smudges of flesh coloring across a featureless face, off-center focal points. Were these deliberate stylistic schemes, or were they related in some way to a disturbance in his vision? Examination of Degas' early works of art reveals finely detailed facial features and central focal points. His medium of choice in the early years was oil on canvas, and his color vision appeared to be normal.

We have learned from Degas' letters and accounts from his contemporaries that he began to experience progressive loss of vision at an early age and, by the time he was 36 years old and a member of the National Guard during the Franco-Prussian war, he was unable to see a rifle target with his right eye. He attributed this loss of vision to exposure to extreme weather conditions that he experienced during his service as a sentinel at the time of the siege of Paris. Later, he blamed it on a "cold in the eye" that he developed at the age of 19 years when forced to live in a garret after his father cut off his allowance. He was bothered by bright sunlight and cold weather, blaming them for his eye weakness, and, unlike his fellow Impressionists, abandoned open-air painting for the comfort of cafés, dance studios, opera houses, offices, and other indoor venues.

During a trip to New Orleans in 1873, Degas complained of the strong Louisiana sunlight. He also became acquainted with his first cousin, Estelle, who had become his sister-in-law. By the time she was 25 years, little vision

749

remained in her left eye and, within 7 years, she became blind in both eyes. Like Degas, her loss of vision was progressive, affected just one eye initially and ultimately resulted in bilateral loss of vision. The trip to New Orleans increased Degas' anxiety about his own vision and he began to realize that he, too, probably had a progressive, incurable eye condition, which at that time was simply referred to as *ophthalmia*. After his return, he wrote to fellow artist, James Tissot, that he expected to remain in the ranks of the infirm until he passed into the ranks of the blind.

As his vision deteriorated, he described a blind spot in the center of his field of vision and spoke of his difficulty in trying to see around this blind spot when he was drawing or painting. He described painting as "an exercise of circumvention." He experienced a loss of central vision in both eyes during the next 2 decades, which, today, would classify him as legally blind. Eventually, he lost the ability to differentiate colors and needed assistance to identify them. The softness of his early works evolved into coarser compositions with more intense colors. When he became resigned to the reality that there was no hope for his eye condition to improve, he looked for solace and help from the sisters of a religious order and began exploring other media. Pastels replaced oils. Faces lost their features. Focal points moved to the periphery (Fig. 47.9), with few details in the center. He turned to sculpture (Fig. 47.10) because he was able to use his sense of touch, and he experimented with photography.

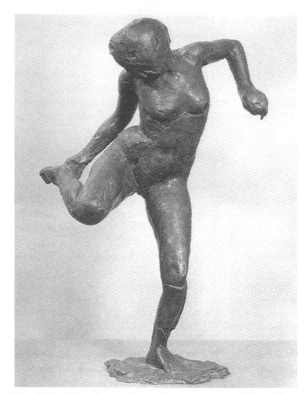

Fig. 47.10 Edgar Degas: *Dancer Looking at Sole of the Right Foot*. (From Marmor MF, Ravin JG. *The Eye of the Artist*. St Louis: Mosby; 1997. Musée Marmottan, Paris. Bridgeman Art Library.)

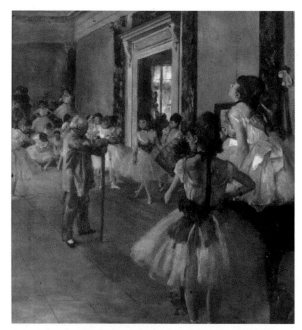

Fig. 47.9 Edgar Degas: *La Classe de Danse*, vers 1873–76. Musée D'Orsay, Paris.

Degas' medical records have been lost, but his symptoms have received much attention from contemporary ophthalmologists. Some of his glasses are in the possession of the Musée d'Orsay in Paris. They include neutral gray plano pince-nez glasses, which block out 85% of incoming light; deep blue-tinted pince-nez glasses with a small correction for myopic astigmatism; deeply tinted regular spectacles with a −1.50 sphere correction OU; and an unusual pair of spectacles with an occluder lens for the right eye and a stenopeic slit at 160 degrees for his left, which aligned with his astigmatic axis. This was meant to reduce dispersion of light, but Degas found the spectacles useless and embarrassing to wear. Trevor-Roper assumed that the stenopeic slit was used to improve vision that was affected by irregular astigmatism, but stenopeic slits were also used for other eye conditions, particularly for reducing glare.

Degas' condition was referred to as *chorioretinitis*, a catch-all term used in the 19th century for a broad spectrum of retinal diseases, and some analysts suggested that he might have had uveitis or corneal disease. Present knowledge points to a form of macular degeneration, certainly not age-related, and possibly familial. Retinal disease would also explain his extreme sensitivity to light and progressive loss of color perception. Because blue cone deficiencies are associated with central retinal disease, this might explain the prevalence of red and limited use of blue as his vision loss increased, as well as his use of more intense colors.

Did Degas eventually become totally blind? In photographs taken late in life, his eyes appear to be orthophoric, which would indicate that he retained at least some peripheral vision and was thus able to attain peripheral fusion. It has also been pointed out that if the right eye was totally blind, he would not have needed an occluder lens in his glasses.

What Degas might have created if he had retained good vision throughout his life will never be known, but the masterworks that he did produce have not only contributed to the annals of art but also enabled the medical community to analyze and interpret the path from his eye, to his brain, to his canvas.

Camille Pissarro (1830–1903)

The French Impressionist movement was profoundly influenced by a West Indian-born Sephardic Jew of Portuguese Marrano descent, Camille Pissarro, who, with Claude Monet, is regarded as a cofounder of Impressionism. Educated in France and returning there at the age of 25 years to establish a long and prolific career, his wisdom, integrity, and benevolence made his fellow artists turn to him for comfort and advice and earned him the title of "Père Pissarro."

Pissarro's early years in France were spent in the Île de France, just north of Paris, where he painted under open skies, applying Impressionist techniques to the everyday scenes around him—village streets, country meadows, landscapes with peasants, farmers, strollers, fruit gatherers, fragments of rural life. He was characterized as myopic, with scarring from corneal ulcers that dated back to childhood, making his personal world a constant Impressionist panorama.

As the sixth decade of his life drew to a close, he developed a chronic inflammation of his right nasolacrimal duct. A firm believer in homeopathic medicine and one who regarded conventional medicine with mistrust ever since the death of his friend, the artist Edouard Manet, he located an ophthalmologist, Dr. Daniel Parenteau, who was an advocate of homeopathic therapy. Initially, he was advised that the problem was not serious and that rest would bring recovery, but recurrent inflammation, necessitating a probing, revealed a bony obstruction. Pissarro described his visit to Dr. Parenteau:

After having skillfully probed the lacrimal canal, he told me there was a growth of bone that was

obstructing the canal's passage: generally one forces the passage but he told me that it is absolutely dangerous. The consequences are disastrous....Here is what he advised me: To take a homeopathic medicine [Aurum] to reconstitute the covering of the bone, which is bare and let the tissues heal themselves; it will take at least 6 months. But precautions must be taken—avoid wind, dust, wash the eye with boric acid immediately. All that is hardly easy for a painter who has to face the elements.

The inflamed passages eventually had to be incised and drained to obtain relief. Recurrent abscesses developed and, with each episode, Pissarro was forced to protect the eye from the elements with a patch. The homeopathic medication failed to prevent abscess formation and Pissarro, unable to paint, returned to Paris for additional therapy, this time with injections of silver nitrate.

Right now Parenteau (who was not averse to using conventional medical treatment when necessary) is giving me injections of silver nitrate (to close off the abnormal passageways that had been created by probing) while waiting for another abscess to form. When that happens and the eye is sufficiently inflamed, he will perform the slight operation necessary [to drain the abscess]. So the thing is only deferred. I will probably now not suffer from abscesses so constantly, thus I will be able to do a little work. Besides, I am getting used to the idea of working with just one eye, which is certainly better than none.

Pissarro consulted with other ophthalmologists and received conflicting advice that ranged from destruction of the lacrimal sac, which could cause constant tearing, to attempting to locate the passage through the bone to the nose, the only two ways of treating dacryocystitis that were available in France at the time. Complications of probing included the creation of false passages, cellulitis, and further scarring. Afraid of surgery, Pissarro decided to remain a patient of Parenteau. Large doses of quinine were prescribed as preventive medicine, but recurrences erupted from time to time. He described his treatment to his son, Lucien, in a letter dated 1897:

I am afraid of complications for my eye. I have gone daily for a dozen days to Parenteau, who has been cauterizing me and has been putting an astringent on the veins of the eye...Parenteau gave me silver nitrate drops to put in the eye and on the lids. This is hardly easy. Every morning there is more pus in the eye, so that I dare not venture a trip. Your mother

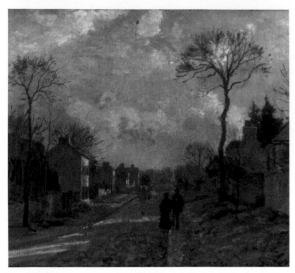

Fig. 47.11 Camille Pissarro: *La Route de Louveciennes*, 1872. Musée d'Orsay, Paris.

advised me not to leave (to see his son, Titi, who was dying of tuberculosis in London).

Abandoning the woods and fields of the Île de France (Fig. 47.11) for the comfort and safety of an indoor environment, Pissarro moved his paints and easel indoors and set them up in front of windows. There, he could paint without cold, wind, and dust, and, looking out, he created cityscapes that are now considered to be some of his finest works. It was not until 1904, a year after Pissarro's death, that an Italian surgeon, Toti, published a paper on his procedure, dacryocystorhinostomy, which opened the door to modern lacrimal surgery. One mystery remains: if, as Trevor-Roper claims, Pissarro was myopic, why is he wearing half-glasses, pushed slightly down on his nose, in several of his self-portraits (Fig. 47.12)?

Mary Cassatt (1844–1926)

Mary Cassatt, the most well-known American Impressionist, spent most of her life in France, developing friendships with her French contemporaries and exhibiting at four of the eight Impressionist shows. Unlike her French counterparts, she eschewed landscapes and chose predominantly indoor settings of mothers and children. Her paintings also differed from theirs in technique, her brushstrokes being smooth rather than coarse and broken (Figs. 47.13 and 47.14).

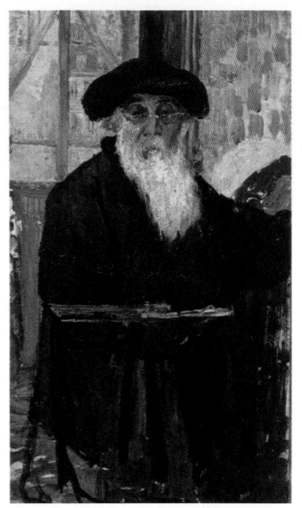

Fig. 47.12 Camille Pissarro: *Self-Portrait*, 1898. (From Marmor MF, Ravin JG. *The Eye of the Artist*. St Louis: Mosby; 1997.)

Cassatt began to experience difficulty with her vision around 1900, although cataracts were not diagnosed until she was 68 years, in 1912. She had also been diagnosed with diabetes and, because insulin was not available until the 1920s, bizarre methods of treatment were attempted. Radium was the miracle discovery of the early 20th century and was being used to treat diabetes and even cataracts. In a letter dated December 14, 1911, while undergoing treatment for her diabetes, Cassatt wrote:

I am at the doctor's taking inhalations of radium.
This is the eighth day and I am suffering very much,
which it seems would prove that it is doing me good,
that it will be a success provided I can stand it.

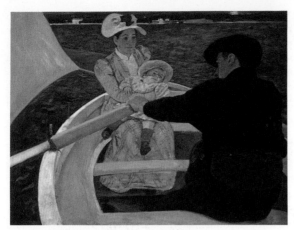

Fig. 47.13 Mary Cassatt: *The Boating Party*. (From Marmor MF, Ravin JG. *The Eye of the Artist*. St Louis: Mosby; 1997.)

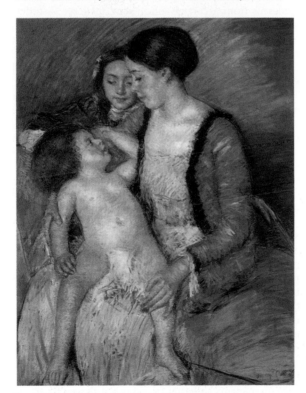

Fig. 47.14 Mary Cassatt: *Young Mother, Daughter and Baby*. (From Marmor MF, Ravin JG. *The Eye of the Artist*. St Louis: Mosby; 1997. Memorial Art Gallery of the University of Rochester. Marion Stratton Gould, Fund.)

There is no mention about Cassatt being treated with radium for her cataracts, but a 1920 article in the *American Journal of Ophthalmology*, titled "Radium for Cataract," reported that:

Of the 31 patients under observation, 84.3% showed a change for the better. In the cases that showed a marked improvement, the opacities were definitely thinned out; one of these, a very early nuclear cataract, disappeared entirely, leaving no trace of the opacities. Radium is of proven value in the treatment of incipient cataracts.'

Another article, "The Technic of Radium Application in Cataracts," was published in 1920 in the *American Journal of Roentgenology* and concluded that "the application of radium is harmless to the normal tissues of the eye." The dangers of radium were yet to be discovered. In fact, Marie Curie, the discoverer of radium, developed cataracts herself and had to undergo surgery in both eyes.

As Cassatt's cataracts progressed, her brushstrokes became coarser and thicker, her colors harsher, her paintings less delicate. By 1913, she wrote:

My eyes, which have always been my strong point, are troubling me. If I only was sure of a good oculist but Dr. Whitman is again away. I don't know for how long.

And later that year:

My oculist has turned out terribly. I have conjunctivitis, an inflammation of the eyelids. He said it was nothing, that I had good sight, one eye very good, the other not so good but not very bad. Then when I saw him again, change of front. Wants to keep me here 2 months and try experiments on the poorer eye, trained nurse to assist at the operation twice a week! Dr. Whitman was horrified. He told me plainly it was to make money…one goes for a little simple advice and to be tested for glasses and they see a chance of making money and do not hesitate to rush making you blind! My theory is that they get so hardened with vivisection that human suffering is nothing to them.

Cassatt underwent cataract surgery in her right eye in 1917. On December 28, 1917, she wrote:

Operating on my right eye before the cataract was ripe is the last drop. …The sight of that eye is inferior but I still saw a good deal in spite of the cataract. Now I see scarcely at all.

Following the extracapsular extraction, the capsule opacified, necessitating additional surgery the following year. Cassatt wrote:

The secondary cataract is covering the right eye which was operated on in October and no doubt it can be removed in the fall. The operation, which was made in October and followed by so long a treatment, was a complete failure and ought not to have been attempted, if only it has not injured what there was of sight in that eye! The cataract over the left eye, which is the eye in which depends my hope of future sight, is not nearly ripe or I could not write this to you....

A month later, she wrote:

My sight is getting dimmer every day. I find writing tires my eyes. I look forward with horror to utter darkness and then an operation which may end in as great a failure as the last one.

The cataract in her left eye was removed in October of 1919 and was probably an intracapsular extraction. Afterward, Cassatt wrote:

The operation was a very daring one as the cataract was not ripe but he (Dr. Louis Borsch, an American ophthalmologist married to a French woman) staked his reputation on the result. He is the only man in Paris capable of doing such an operation and I am told few anywhere in the US....

Results were poor and she wrote:

I am old and so blind that I don't feel up to much...I see less with the eye that was operated in October than I did with the one with the secondary cataract in it! ...I think the state of my eyes will, I hope, shorten my life.

And a 1921 letter reads:

Last May I had an operation upon my best eye. The operation was very successful and the oculist promised me I should paint again but a hidden abscess in an apparently sound tooth caused a violent inflammation and I have not yet recovered from it. Nor has the sight of the eye returned.

And finally:

I have had a very serious operation for cataract several weeks ago and have my eye still bandaged and can see very indifferently with the other eye which is my poor eye. I shall not be able to use my eyes, nor be allowed glasses for several months to come, after that my oculist promises great results. I do not allow myself such sanguine hopes.

As Cassatt's vision diminished, she turned from oils to pastels, using broad strokes on large sheets of paper. The delicacy of her earlier works and her careful color choices disappeared with her dimming sight. By 1915, her days as an artist had ended and by 1918, she could no longer read. Although she lived until 1926, the same year Monet died, her diabetes and cataracts cut short her career and deprived her of the work she loved.

Summary

The artists we have discussed represent only the tip of the iceberg. Other artists showed signs of color deficiencies or presbyopia; some had symptoms indicative of syphilis and various genetic and neurologic diseases. Unfortunately, the absence of medical records or other documentation precludes us from accurately diagnosing their eye disorders and they remain only conjecture. The works of many artists were profoundly influenced by their eye conditions, a great many of which are treatable today.

The eye diseases of the Impressionists were managed with treatments that seem primitive and even barbaric. Today, three of the four major causes of visual loss in older adults are treatable: simple outpatient, minimally invasive surgery with the implantation of intraocular lenses enables us to quickly restore normal vision to patients with cataracts. They no longer have to wait until their vision is severely impaired before undergoing the procedure. Lens implants enable them to maintain binocular vision when only one eye is involved. They no longer have to endure prolonged recuperation periods and adapt to a highly magnified, distorted world. If their postoperative vision becomes hazy owing to opacification of the lens capsule, a painless yttrium aluminum garnet (YAG) laser capsulotomy can restore clarity in a few minutes. Insulin and oral medications have helped those with diabetes control their blood sugar and prolong their lives. Diabetic retinopathy can be treated with argon lasers and vitrectomy. Glaucoma can be treated medically and/or surgically. Macular degeneration, though, still remains a challenge and we are currently unable to restore normal color perception to those with color deficiencies or cure a number of retinal problems and genetic eye conditions.

Many patients suffering from mental illnesses respond well to modern psychotherapy and treatment with psychotropic drugs. Seizure disorders can be controlled. The wearing of glasses has become accepted not only as a means of vision correction, but also as a fashion accessory; contact lenses or refractive surgery can correct vision invisibly. Progressive multifocals have replaced conventional bifocals or separate glasses for near and distance. Patency of the lacrimal system can be safely established and modern antibiotics are available to treat dacryocystitis and other infections.

Would these acclaimed artists have achieved the same degree of achievement, recognition, and renown if modern medical and surgical procedures had been available to treat their pathology? If they lived in current times, would the Impressionist movement have even occurred? And if it had, would they be, as they were in the latter half of the 19th century, shunned by traditional artists and art patrons?

Dedication

This chapter is dedicated to Michael F. Marmor, MD, and James G. Ravin, MD, whose book *The Eye of the Artist* served as my major resource and my inspiration.

Further reading

Marmor MF, Ravin JG. *The Eye of the Artist*. St Louis: Mosby; 1997.

Metzger R, Walther IF. *Van Gogh*. Koln, Germany: Taschen; 1998.

Ravin JG. Monet's cataracts. *JAMA*. 1985;254(3):396.

Ravin JG, Kenyon CA. Degas' loss of vision: evidence for a diagnosis of retinal disease. *Surv Ophthalmol*. 1994;39(1):57.

Seitz W. Monet and abstract painting. In: Stucky CF, ed. *Monet: A Retrospective*. New York: Hugh Lauter Levin Associates;; 1985.

Trevor-Roper P. *The World Through Blunted Sight*. London: Souvenir Press; 1997.

Chapter | **48** |

Allied health personnel in ophthalmology

Rod A. Morgan

The technology of medical science expands significantly every year and these changes lead to a more complex clinical practice. The Western world, principally involved in the technical and social evolution of healthcare provision in recent years, expects these improvements to be included in their routine eye care. Simultaneously, worldwide clinical opportunities are expanding because of economic and social growth in previously underprivileged societies as healthcare services improve. As a result, the opportunities for work in the health field continue to grow significantly as medical services are being organized and modernized. Such developments have led to the need for highly skilled personnel to use instruments developed to analyze the technology. The field of ophthalmic medical assistance has grown to keep up with these advances.

Highly trained assistants now routinely use complex instruments to assist the ophthalmologist in providing a higher quality of care to a greater number of patients. Office operations have also become more involved requiring staff with more complex management skills.

The first clinical program for ophthalmic medical assistants (OMAs) was established in England's London Moorfields Eye Hospital in 1929 for service and training in strabismus,[1] rapidly leading to the formation of the British Orthoptic Council in 1934 to monitor training and certify orthoptists. Since that time, the development of allied health training in ophthalmology has developed in many countries and clinical fields of ophthalmology. Application of these developments has been slower where education and financial opportunities are limited, but have shown strong growth in recent years.

Evolution of training and service requirements of allied health personnel

Canadian and American standards for OMAs will illustrate what is now developing in countries all over the world as their health organizations mature.

Canadian and American ophthalmology (*medicine*) and optometry (*functional eye care*) developed separately before direct government regulation of healthcare quality became standard. In modern times, these two groups work as allies, with separate authority in providing health care. In other countries, vision specialists work together as teams under a direct authority and local government relations.

Visual eye care personnel have become defined by their educational background. Thus ophthalmologists and their assistants are referred to as *ophthalmic medical personnel (OMP)*. Personnel working in other visual fields, not under the direction of ophthalmology, are referred to as *allied health personnel (AHP)*. Optometry and ophthalmic registered nurses are AHP in Canada and the United States as they are independent of medicine and have authority over their allied personnel.

Other ophthalmic medical personnel specialties have independent educational and certification status because science formalized their organizations before government regulation linked their science to the medical authority, even though they currently work within the authority of medical science. *Orthoptics* and *ophthalmic medical photography* are two examples, directing their own education and certification. The Joint Commission on Allied Health Personnel in Ophthalmology (JCAHPO),[2] after its foundation in 1969, came to coordinate the education and provide certification of the newly developing technical fields within ophthalmology.

As JCAHPO grew it became involved in the education and certification developments in other parts of the world, developing international educational programs and certification standards to reflect scientific advances applicable to the developing world. The international involvement of JCAHPO became significant in the early 21st century and led to its reincorporation into the International Joint Commission of Allied Health Personnel in Ophthalmology (IJCAHPO) in 2018. The "International Care Curriculum for Ophthalmic Assistants" and "Value Report" available at IJCAHPO relate to this growth. The JCAHPO corporate name is still in use to serve the *JCAHPO Research Fund*, which is active in provision of scholarships and awards to achieving OMP.[3]

Advancements have lead OMA programs to include administration and business issues, as well as the scientific fields of optics, eye movements, contact lenses, surgical science, physics applications of x-ray, ultrasound and nuclear magnetic resonance, genetics and microbiology.

Divisions of ophthalmic medical personnel developing under the International Joint Commission of Allied Health Personnel in Ophthalmology

Business and administration

Office management and business relations involve several skill levels from relating to patient service and office procedures in smaller offices to office management of all business affairs in multipractitioner larger clinics (Fig. 48.1).

Clinical evaluation and testing

Generalized ophthalmic assistant

This multitasking role involves administrative functions (patient appointments, greeting, chart preparation, filing, and billing) and clinical functions (history taking, visual acuity, measuring glasses, eye pressure, and basic eye movements; Fig. 48.2).

Specialized ophthalmic assistant

Continuing scientific development in specialized eye care requires highly technical OMP to aid in diagnosis and management of special eye problems. Cataract, refractive, glaucoma, retinal, pediatric ophthalmology, and specialized

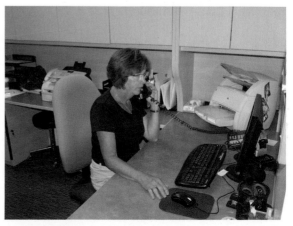

Fig. 48.1 Office administrator, manager.

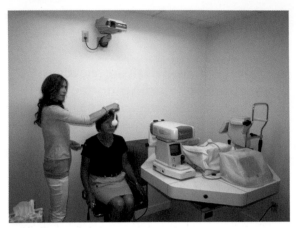

Fig. 48.2 The assistant completes vision testing.

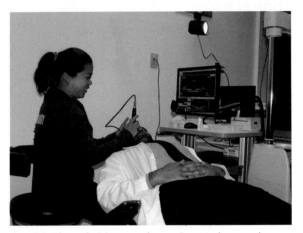

Fig. 48.3 The technician completes a B-scan ultrasound.

surgical fields are rapidly developing new equipment for analysis of special visual issues. Most patients who have major vision problems require services that involve several assistants (Figs. 48.3).

Education of ophthalmic medical personnel

Personal characteristics essential for success as an OMA includes working with people and dealing with visual health problems, a curious scientific nature, responsible and analytical thinking, multitasking ability and a desire to

solve problems. It is estimated that about 125,000 people work as allied health personnel in ophthalmology in North America. The majority of these assistants are "generalized" OMAs and require a high school diploma to enter a career in an ophthalmology office where they perform office procedures and clinical services.

Ophthalmic medical technicians and technologists are trained in more complex technical services. Large clinics and specialized eye services use several highly specialized technicians and management personnel to provide these services. Assistants interested in these fields attend formal training programs involving schools, colleges and universities, usually involving 6 months to 2 years. Financial support for their education is available through a wide variety of sources, including the JCAHPO Research Foundation.

Therefore ophthalmic medical personnel have been directed by the needs of society, the ophthalmologist, and personal interests and skills to become formally educated and certified in highly specialized areas. Current medical standards are required for all of the ophthalmic staff and are provided by the process of organized education and certification. There are currently about 30,000 IJCAHPO certificants.

Certification and training levels for ophthalmic medical personnel

Certification standards are developed to meet community requirements. Personnel with certification offer a standard level of skill to their employers and can use that standard anywhere the certification is accepted, allowing competitive employment opportunities to those who are qualified. IJCAHPO has developed the following programs for OMP certification:

The certified ophthalmic assistant

Informal training is usual for the certified ophthalmic assistant (COA). An ophthalmologist can support an interested employee to complete an accredited, independent home study course or distant learning program, which generally leads to the basic certification level of COA.

Certified ophthalmic technician and certified ophthalmic medical technologist

Formal training is required for the more senior levels of certification: certified ophthalmic technician (COT) and certified ophthalmic medical technologist (COMT). Subspecialty requirements reflecting advancing skills and certification in selected areas of vision care are also available under IJCAHPO.

International *Core Certificates* are certified at COA, COT, and COMT levels. Details of eligibility and requirements for these certificants and special program registrations are available at IJCAHPO.

Subspecialty certification fields for ophthalmic medical personnel in the International Joint Commission of Allied Health Personnel in Ophthalmology

Corporate certified ophthalmic assistants

Corporate employees are taught the relating essential technical knowledge in both ophthalmology and industry.

Certified diagnostic ophthalmic sonographer

Ophthalmic sonographers complete accurate ocular sonograms using high frequency sound waves to produce two-dimensional B-scan images of the eye. This method is mostly applied to cataract surgery.

Ophthalmic scribe certification examination

American standards of medical records for patient histories, physical, and all essential patient information are met.

Ophthalmic surgical assistant

Working with the ophthalmic surgeon, the OSA understands procedures and instrumentation necessary to assist in ophthalmic surgical suites. OSAs work under the authority of the ophthalmologist and supervising personnel, generally an ophthalmic surgical registered nurse.

Registered ophthalmic ultrasound biometrist

Ophthalmic sonographers complete three-dimensional ultrasound images of the eye and orbit in the study of intraocular and orbital disease. There are currently about 30,000 IJCAHPO certificants.

Ophthalmic medical personnel allied with the International Joint Commission of Allied Health Personnel in Ophthalmology

Ophthalmic photographers

An ophthalmic photographer takes film and digital photographs of eye and orbital tissues using a variety of single frame or motion picture images and often with the use of drugs to highlight tissue detail. Internet technology transmits images to allows the photographer to work independently from the ophthalmologist. The Ophthalmic Photographers' Society educates and certifies ophthalmic photographers in North America.

Orthoptists

Eye movements, and related visual functions, are used to identify problems within the visual system. These include strabismus (squint), lazy eye (amblyopia), double vision, and loss of binocular vision. As eye movement problems are commonest in children, orthoptics is a specialty field of pediatric ophthalmology but is also associated with many eye and systemic diseases later in life. Canadian and American Orthoptic Councils certify their orthoptists.

Independent allied health personnel in visual science

Ophthalmic operating room registered nurses

The nursing profession educates and certifies under national and regional authority in Canada and the United States. Thus ophthalmic operating room registered nurses (OORNs), specially trained in ophthalmic surgery, work independently with surgeons under hospital and government authority.

Opticians

Opticians work as *technical opticians* who manufacture and repair spectacle and contact lens, and *dispensing opticians* who fit these optical devices to patient and professional service needs. Contact lens manufacturing and fitting are often entirely separate from the field of spectacles. Ophthalmology participates in regulatory and management levels in this field.

The International Joint Commission of Allied Health Personnel in Ophthalmology certification process

IJCAHPO certification is issued for 3 years and requires employment and continuing educational standards to be met before recertification at that time. Certification requires meeting skill-level standards through education, examination, and continuing education. The higher the level of certificant standard held, the higher the level of education and technical skills that must be developed and maintained. Appropriate educational credits relate to the level of certification and are available through IJCAHPO. Recertification is required every 3 years.

To maintain certification, educational events are regularly held under IJCAHPO auspices or authority. Many are held in association with ophthalmology educational meetings. Distance learning is now a significant program through EyeCareCE (TM), an on-demand e-learning website series involving live, online instructors and a broad range of topics with current medical standards being taught. In addition, a wide range of tools and resources on EyeCareMarketplace (TM) provides the physical materials appropriate to continuing education. Other accredited providers are also able to offer educational credits with reciprocal agreements. Full details of these matters are available from IJCAHPO.

Table 48.1 International Joint Commission on Allied Health Personnel in ophthalmology governance structure: organizations and councilors, 2020

Regular council representatives 17	Internet web address
American Academy of Ophthalmology (1)	www.aao.org
American Association for Pediatric Ophthalmology and Strabismus (1)	www.aapos.org
American Glaucoma Society (1)	www.glaucomaweb.org
American Ophthalmological Society (1)	www.aosonline.org
American Society of Cataract & Refractive Surgery with American Society of Ophthalmic Administrators (1)	www.ascrs.org www.asoa.org
American Society of Retinal Specialists (1)	www.asrs.org
Association of Technical Personnel in Ophthalmology (2)	www.atpo.org
Association of University Professors in Ophthalmology (1)	www.ophthalworld.com
Association of Veterans Affairs Ophthalmologists (1)	www.avao.org
Canadian Ophthalmological Society (1)	www.eyesite.ca
Canadian Society of Ophthalmic Medical Personnel (2)	www.cos-sco.ca/csomp
Consortium of Ophthalmic Training Programs (1)	www.cotpedu.org
North-American Neuro-Ophthalmology Society (1)	www.neuroeye.com
Contact Lens Association of Ophthalmologists (1)	www.clao.org
Society of Military Ophthalmologists (1)	www.mcg.edu/eyes
Affiliated organizational council representatives number	
American Association of Certified Orthoptists (1)	www.orthoptics.org
American Orthoptic Council (1)	www.orthoptics.org
Ophthalmic Photographers' Society (1)	www.opsweb.org
Philippine Academy of Ophthalmology (1)	www.pao.org.ph
The Canadian Orthoptic Society (1)	www.tcos.ca
Pan-American Association of Ophthalmology (1)	www.paao.org

The educational and certification history of the International Joint Commission of Allied Health Personnel in Ophthalmology

In 1969 six American professional medical organizations created JCAHPO and shortly after membership with the Canadian Ophthalmological Society (COS) made it international. Today 21 ophthalmic professional organizations are members of IJCAHPO, comprising Canadian and American Societies, the Pan-American Association of Ophthalmology, and the Philippine Academy of Ophthalmology. Councilors of these societies govern the operations through a Board of Directors. Table 48.1 lists these societies.

National organization of ophthalmic training and certification programs

In Canada, education and accreditation is regulated by provincial authority. National medical organizations, such as the Canadian Ophthalmological Society, share major responsibilities with provincial authority-granting bodies to accredit ophthalmic training programs. In the United States, accreditation authority rests with the Federal Secretary of Education. Subordinate bodies direct educational and certification issues based upon medical and other groupings. The International Council of Accreditation authorizes the centers of ophthalmic medical education based upon standards sponsored, and maintained, by four organizations: Association of Technical Personnel in Ophthalmology, IJCAHPO, Consortium of Ophthalmic Training Programs, and the Canadian Society of Ophthalmic Medical Personnel.

Other countries are developing their own educational, certification and accreditation standards. As nations are ready for structured organization, IJCAHPO is well positioned to offer organization assistance and direct involvement in the development of standards of quality medical eye care. An IJCAHPO reference guide: "A Framework for Allied Ophthalmic Training Programs" is available to aid in the development of such ophthalmic assistance programs.

National and international ophthalmologic societies

As nations develop their health programs, IJCAHPO is capable of aiding in the establishment of standards that regulate OMAs.

Table 48.2 Some international and English-speaking allied ophthalmic personnel societies outside Canada and the United States of America

Organization	Website
British and Irish Orthoptics Society	www.orthoptics.org.uk
International Council of Ophthalmology (327 international links)	www.icoph.org
International Orthoptic Association (links to orthoptic societies)	www.internationalorthoptics.org
Orthoptics Australia	www.orthoptics.org.au
Pan-American Association of Ophthalmology (21 Trans-American links)	www.paao.org
Royal Australian and New Zealand College of Ophthalmologists	www.ranzco.edu

For those wishing to explore these organizations and the development of OMAs in these regions, web services are currently the easiest way to find links that identify regional developments. Table 48.2 is a guide in this direction. The International Council of Ophthalmology currently lists 327 ophthalmic societies. The Pan-American Ophthalmological Society lists 21 member countries in North and South America.

The future of allied health personnel in ophthalmology

Ophthalmologic science continues to show significant advances which are being developed to evaluate visual pathology in clinical practice. Education and certification relating to these interesting fields offers a strong, and growing, market for ophthalmic medical personnel.

References

1. Lyle TK, Wayber KC. *Lyle and Jackson's Practical Orthoptics in the Treatment of Squint.* 5th ed. London: HK Lewis & Co; 1967.
2. IJCAHPO. 2025 Woodlane Drive, St. Paul, MN, USA 55125-2995, toll free 001-800-284-3937. www.ijcahpo.org.
3. The JCAHPO Research Foundation. https://www.ijcahpo.org/foundation.

AOP use evidence-based practices and the application of technology to optimize patient outcomes to prevent and manage patients' diseases. Thus, the scope of allied ophthalmic health covers the individual, the family, and the community. Their scope of practice includes the use of protocols across all healthcare delivery sites including, but not limited to, the hospital, the clinic, and the physician's office. They enter acquired clinical data and dictated information from the physician into paper or electronic medical records. These activities are supported by education, research, and administration.

AOP in countries other than Canada and the United States may have a scope of practice that looks very different. Some countries may combine AOP job roles and responsibilities. For example, in parts of Africa and the South Pacific, it is common for an ophthalmic nurse to have job tasks that are both surgical and clinical. AOP scope of practice as outlined will most certainly evolve, and most likely expand, as ophthalmic technology changes.[5]

Changing scope of practice

With rapid changes occurring in the delivery of health care, ophthalmology practices know the importance of being as efficient as possible, and to constantly reassess processes to create improvements in how a clinic functions. As a result, sets of principles, such as "Lean management" and "Six Sigma" are being more commonly employed to improve process within clinics.[6,7]

These processes reduce time wasting steps, to improve the use of resources and decrease expenses, while attempting to improve overall patient care results and patient satisfaction.[8] Six Sigma is a metrics driven system to reduce medical errors and eliminate defects in how care is delivered. Lean management, conversely, is more focused on eliminating waste and making practices more efficient over time. Both concepts attempt to improve healthcare delivery by improving the value of patient visits, and decreasing overall waste.[7] Through practice analysis, AOP can aid in reducing waiting times for patients, decreasing patient idle time, improving patient examination and surgical flow, minimizing required clinic inventory to prevent waste and expense, eliminating process and system failures that can lead to medical mistakes and misdiagnosis, and improving the use of medical records.[9]

These types of changes to clinic flow and processes have become especially important with the COVID-19 pandemic because clinics have significantly changed in how ophthalmology care is delivered. Examples where AOP can assist in adapting to rapid changes include maintaining proper cleaning of examination rooms and equipment, proper physical distancing of patients within the clinic flow, appropriate ordering and use of personal protective equipment (PPE). AOP input is crucial to initiating

such rapid change, while guaranteeing the success and sustainability of these significant changes in ophthalmology care delivery.

Direct AOP input into quality eyecare delivery is in the relatively new burgeoning telemedicine field in ophthalmology.[10] Telemedicine techniques are slowly becoming accepted in ophthalmology, especially as computer technology has improved.[10] The use of telemedicine and AOP for coordinating retinopathy of prematurity (ROP) evaluations with RetCam images is a good example of how AOP are being successfully integrated into telemedicine techniques.[11] Again, as a result of the COVID-19 pandemic, telemedicine has been pushed rapidly to the forefront in an effort to effectively deal with patient care delivery in this new environment.[12] AOP have already demonstrated they are extremely effective in telemedicine by gathering scheduling information for patients, history taking, measuring visual acuity, and some basic examination gathering, all through the virtual domain, as well as patient education and scribe tasks for physicians during patient virtual visits. AOP have an important role in the time-consuming information gathering, thus allowing the ophthalmologist to deal directly and more efficiently with patient diagnosis and treatment.

Licensure and certification

Licensure and certification are two processes that govern scope of practice in the medical profession. Licensure is defined and understood as having been granted authority or legal permission to practice as regulated by federal, state, or provincial governmental agencies. Certification denotes that a person is recognized by the private sector as having achieved standards set by the profession. Certification is generally granted by an independent organization but may also be mandated by a government regulation. For example, AOP, such as ophthalmic nurses, are licensed as well as certified. Registration is another term that recognizes government regulation of AOP.

Most AOP are not licensed by government agencies but may be voluntarily certified, based on their knowledge and skill levels, to perform delegated tasks and procedures. The International Joint Commission on Allied Health Personnel in Ophthalmology (IJCAHPO) certifies AOP at three core levels: ophthalmic assistant, ophthalmic technician, and ophthalmic medical technologist. The IJCAHPO is an internationally recognized, accredited organization by the National Commission of Certifying Agencies. Certificates of completion and microcredentials are also recognition that AOP have obtained specific knowledge and skill levels in particular areas. The Ophthalmic Photographers' Society (OPS), American Orthoptic Council (AOC), Canadian Orthoptic Council (COC), National Contact Lens Examiners (NCLE), and American Board of Opticianry (ABO) are other examples of organizations that certify their respective cadres.

AOP certified at one of IJCAHPO's three core certification levels may perform similar duties. However, AOP with higher levels of certification are expected to perform the tasks at an advanced level of expertise, and to exercise considerable technical clinical judgment as they perform these tasks.[13] This applies both in the clinic and virtually.

Certification establishes national and global standards on AOP tasks performed. These standards are based on statistically valid, reliable data collected through research studies of job incumbents, employers, and ophthalmologists. This extensive research provides data on the importance of tasks, the frequency that tasks are performed, and the task difficulty level. Certification examinations test the knowledge and skills needed for minimal competency on these tasks by job descriptions and used by ophthalmic practices to grade the level of AOP status obtained.

Patient information and privacy practices

There is a complicated balance between patient privacy, and healthcare providers' need to use and disclose medical information. Health information may be disclosed to law enforcement agencies and public health agencies as required by law. In most countries, national privacy standards regulate patient health information rights. These include the right to:

- Request restrictions on the use and disclosure of health information
- Receive confidential communication concerning the patient's medical condition and treatment
- Inspect and copy health data and information
- Amend and/or submit corrections to health information
- Receive an accounting of how and to whom health information has been disclosed
- Receive a printed copy of the privacy practice of the healthcare provider

AOP, as part of the healthcare provider team, are required to maintain the privacy of the patient's protected health information and to provide the patient with notice of the privacy practices of the provider. Notices typically address the uses and disclosure of health information and what may be used by staff members or disclosed to other healthcare professionals for the purpose of evaluating the patient's health, diagnosing medical conditions, providing treatment and insurers for payment. The patient's health information may be used to support the day-to-day activities and practice management of the provider.

Insurance risk and malpractice

AOP should always ascertain that they are insured under the umbrella of their employer's medical malpractice policies. In addition, they should seek expressed, written indemnification from their employers for all activities performed, within the scope and capacity delineated by their supervisors and employers.

Ethics and scope of practice

The hierarchy of values and standards of conduct for the medical profession and all allied healthcare workers, become the code of conduct and ethical guidelines for AOP. AOP require an excellent understanding of medical ethics to serve the best interests of both the patient and the practice. The ophthalmologist who allows AOP to treat patients without adequate supervision compromises the licensing standards set by the government and erodes the standards of patient care. The eye care team must never neglect patient safety in the pursuit of efficiency for the practice.

Summary

Major shifts in health care are driven by rapidly advancing technology, by the pressure on lawmakers for open access to medical systems, by telemedicine, and by the desire to cut healthcare costs. These issues become even more important in times of crisis, such as the recent COVID-19 pandemic. New laws are often supported by third-party payers to save money, reduce premiums, and reimburse nonphysicians' services at a lower rate.

In this changing environment, ophthalmologist's shifting of tasks and delegation of responsibility and authority to the eye care team will progressively increase to prevent overworking the ophthalmologist, to increase the practice's efficiency, to manage the costs of eye care to the public, third-party payers, and government requirements. As important physician extenders, AOP are a critical part of the eye care team in providing quality patient care.

Table 51.1 Certified ophthalmic assistant, certified ophthalmic technician, certified ophthalmic medical technologist examination content areas

Content areas	Certified ophthalmic assistant	Certified ophthalmic technician	Certified ophthalmic medical technologist
Number of Examination Questions	200	200	190
Examination Length	180 minutes	180 minutes	180 minutes
Examination content areas	**Percent of examination**		
Patient Evaluation			
History and Documentation	5%	3%	3%
Visual Assessment	6%	7%	3%
Visual Field Testing	4%	3%	6%
Pupil Assessment	3%	4%	3%
Tonometry	4%	4%	2%
Keratometry	2%	3%	2%
Ocular Motility Testing	4%	6%	12%
Lensometry	3%	3%	4%
Refraction, Retinoscopy, and Refinement	5%	5%	6%
Biometry	3%	5%	3%
Supplemental Testing	3%	2%	6%
Assisting with interventions and procedures			
Microbiology	3%	3%	2%
Pharmacology	3%	3%	4%
Surgical Assisting	4%	6%	4%
Ophthalmic Patient Services and Education	14%	12%	8%
General Medical Knowledge	14%	5%	4%
Corrective lenses			
Optics and Spectacles	2%	5%	2%
Contact Lenses	2%	5%	7%
Imaging			
Ophthalmic Imaging	5%	7%	9%
Photography and Videography	5%	6%	8%
Office and clinical skills			
Equipment Maintenance and Repair	2%	1%	1%
Medical Ethics, Legal and Regulatory Issues	4%	2%	1%

Note that percentages indicate the amount of content area covered for each examination level. Used with permission by the International Joint Commission on Allied Health Personnel in Ophthalmology, Inc. (2019–2020).

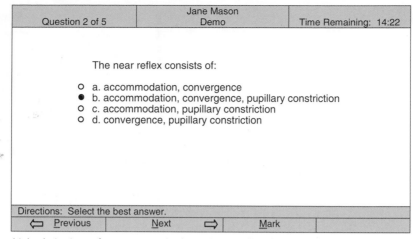

Fig. 51.1 Sample multiple-choice items from computerized examination. (Used with permission of the Joint Commission on Allied Health Personnel in Ophthalmology, Inc.)

Online virtual proctoring is a technology advancement that will become more common and standardized.

IJCAHPO certification examinations test content-specific and most often in a multiple-choice format (Fig. 51.1). Practice examinations provide candidates the opportunity to become familiar with computer testing and the examination. Upon test completion, many certification agencies provide immediate performance feedback with unofficial pass/fail test results with automated scoring. Box 51.1 gives sample certified ophthalmic assistant (COA) examination test items (answers are in Box 51.2).

Skill-based examinations

The certification process may include knowledge-based examinations and test the candidate's ophthalmic skills and abilities with a skills-based examination. IJCAHPO, the American Orthoptic Council, and the Canadian Orthoptic Society conduct skill-based examinations. IJCAHPO's COA examination is a knowledge-based multiple-choice examination. IJCAHPO's advanced certifications require both a knowledge-based examination and a skill-based test: certified ophthalmic technician (COT) skills test and the certified ophthalmic medical technologist (COMT) performance test.

Skill-based examinations evaluate specific skills and abilities performed in a clinical setting. Some skill-based examinations may include the examinee performing standardized tasks and processes while being observed, timed, and rated by evaluators. IJCAHPO skill-based examinations are administered using a computer-based skills format. IJCAHPO's COT skill evaluation and the COMT

Box 51.1 Sample certified ophthalmic assistant examination test items[a]

1. A patient's history of pain and low vision could be attributed to
   A. acute glaucoma.
   B. strabismus.
   C. stroke.
   D. subconjunctival hemorrhage.
2. What is a probable cause of blurred distance vision that is improved by squinting?
   A. Esotropia.
   B. Glaucoma.
   C. Uncorrected presbyopia.
   D. Uncorrected myopia.
3. Visual acuity of 6/12 is equivalent to
   A. 20/20.
   B. 20/30.
   C. 20/40.
   D. 20/50.
4. Schirmer testing is frequently used for a patient who is considering
   A. contact lenses.
   B. cataract surgery.
   C. new spectacles.
   D. muscle recession.
5. The three-color receptors found in cones are
   A. blue, green, and yellow.
   B. red, green, and blue.
   C. red, green, and yellow.
   D. red, yellow, and blue.

[a]Sample certified ophthalmic assistant (COA) questions used with permission of the International Joint Commission on Allied Health Personnel in Ophthalmology, Inc. (IJCAHPO).

Box 51.2 **Answers**

1. A
2. D
3. C
4. A
5. B

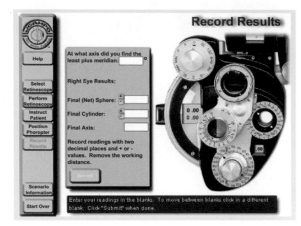

Fig. 51.2 Certified ophthalmic technician skill evaluation tutorial: lensometers. (Used with permission of the Joint Commission on Allied Health Personnel in Ophthalmology, Inc.)

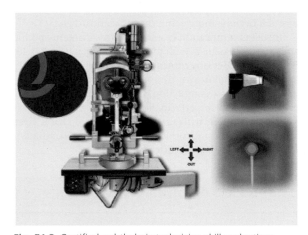

Fig. 51.3 Certified ophthalmic technician skill evaluation: tonometry patient examination. (Used with permission of the Joint Commission on Allied Health Personnel in Ophthalmology, Inc.)

performance test use innovative computer-based simulations specifically designed to evaluate the required advanced levels of competency, knowledge, and skills. The COT skill evaluation consists of seven skills: keratometry, tonometry, ocular motility, lensometry, visual fields, retinoscopy, and refinement. The COMT performance test evaluates the candidate's abilities in ocular motility, advanced lensometry, fundus photography and fluorescein phases, versions and ductions, and the evaluation of pupil function.

Candidates are provided a tutorial and training material for use in test preparation. Tutorials give candidates confidence in learning how the computer and simulated equipment functions, practice by using the dials and controls, as well as the mouse and keyboard, on simulated equipment, and becoming familiar with the examination format. Fig. 51.2 is a computer screen image showing dials and controls of the retinoscopy examination from the COT skill evaluation tutorial.

IJCAHPO's skills examinations include a real patient case-based scenario that an ophthalmic technician would encounter in clinical practice. The candidate's performance is based on performing the skill correctly and obtaining an accurate reading of the final result. Fig. 51.3 represents the tonometer examination from the COT skill evaluation. Computer-based skill examinations have certain advantages over evaluations performed with live patients, primarily providing greater standardization and consistency in the evaluation of procedures.

Value of certified allied ophthalmic personnel

Certified allied ophthalmic personnel are valued members of the eye care team. The contribution that they offer to employers include increasing practice efficiency, patient satisfaction, and ophthalmologist productivity.[1] "There are several reasons that certification leads to greater practice productivity and more desirable employee AOP attributes. The first and most obvious is that certification is intended to distinguish those who have mastered the technical skills that are important in clinical situations. Additionally, to pass the certification examinations, AOP must show many of the attributes that are desirable in the workplace, such as diligence, intelligence, and time management."[2]

A candidate's decision to become voluntarily certified exhibits pride in the profession, the desire to be recognized for IJCAHPO certification content mastery, and commitment to quality patient care. "The impact of AOP certification on patient care is significant; healthcare professionals are able to focus on delivering higher quality care when supported by certified AOP."[1]

Studies by Astle et al. in Canada, and Woodworth et al. in the United States, document that certified AOP enhance most practice productivity measures. As a result, higher

Table 51.2 Canadian certificates' top reasons for achieving International Joint Commission on Allied Health Personnel in Ophthalmology certification

Top reasons	Percent responding
Personal challenge and achievement	79%
Increased skills	71%
Increased marketability	62%
Respect from peers	48%
Increased responsibility autonomy	45%
Better compensation	41%
Respect from patients	40%

wages were associated with certification of AOP. Astle et al. found that in four measures certified AOP contributed more than noncertified AOP: doctor productivity was increased, number of patients seen per hour increased, the practices documented improved trouble-shooting rapport, and improved triage screening.[1] When AOP were surveyed on reasons for achieving certification, most cited an increase in personal challenges and achievement, work skills, marketability, and respect from their peers (Table 51.2).[1] Other reasons included increased responsibility and autonomy, improved compensation, and more respect from patients.[1] Studies have shown that employers prefer to hire certified AOP and healthcare personnel over noncertified healthcare personnel.[1-4]

Career advancement

Credentialing and career ladder opportunities for the ophthalmic assistant start with IJCAHPO's three core certifications COA, COT, and COMT. Ophthalmic careers may advance with specialty certifications, such as the ophthalmic surgical assisting–surgical technician (OSA-ST), registered ophthalmic ultrasound biometrist (ROUB), and the certified diagnostic ophthalmic sonographer (CDOS). These additional certifications may offer career opportunities leading to other eye care credentials.

As specialty certifications evolve, IJCAHPO is developing competency-based digital "microcredentials," indicating demonstrated competency/mastery in a specific skill or set of skills. Successful completion of a microcredential examination provides a digital microcertification that certificants can add to their resume to showcase the specialty skill.

Summary

Allied ophthalmic personnel are in high demand and certified AOP are an asset to the ophthalmologist and their patients. Certification by examination remains a primary method to assess learning and competency in many healthcare professions. Comprehensive and advanced examination preparation are essential in reducing test anxiety, improving performance, and successfully passing the examination.[5] Certification guarantees process and content standardization, enhanced objectivity in measurement, and improved overall test quality, all of which ultimately enhances the profession of ophthalmic assisting which leads to candidate competency. Well-trained, certified AOP are a necessity for the modern-day ophthalmic practice.

References

1. Castle W, El-Defrawy S, LaRoche GR, Lafontaine M, Anderson L, Dukes A, et al. Survey on allied health personnel in Canadian ophthalmology: the scalpel for change. *Can J Ophthalmol*. 2011;40(1).
2. Woodworth K, Dashiki P, Ehlers W, Paucal D, Anderson L, Thompson N. A comparative study of the impact of certified and noncertified ophthalmic medical personnel on practice quality and productivity. *Eye Contact Lens*. 2008;34(1):28–34.
3. Fights SD. Reap the benefits of certification. *Am J Nurs*. 2012;112(1):10–11.
4. Stromsburg MF, Niebuhr B, Prevost S, et al. More than a title. *Nurs Manag*. 2005;36(5):36–46.
5. International Joint Commission on Allied Health Personnel in Ophthalmology. Criteria for Certification and Recertification Handbook, 2019; and Preparing for the IJCAHPO Certified Ophthalmic Assistant (COA), Certified Ophthalmic Technician (COT), and Certified Ophthalmic Medical Technologist (COMT) publications. 2020.

Chapter 52

The development of allied ophthalmic personnel in North America and worldwide

William F. Astle and Lynn D. Anderson

Introduction and history

Ophthalmic assistants are essential members of the ophthalmologist-led eye care team (Fig. 50.1).[1] In an informal way, ophthalmic assistants have functioned for as long as there have been ophthalmic offices.

Although the ophthalmologist authorizes and always directs activities in his or her professional capacity, the ophthalmologist relies on the ophthalmic assistant to serve as a liaison between the doctor and the patient. The ophthalmic assistant's function and role may be broad as well as specialized. Assistants are well-skilled and specially trained to aid ophthalmologists in delivering high quality patient care.

Until the late 1950s, ophthalmic assistants were an unorganized and uncertified group of individuals who assisted ophthalmologists in their day-to-day technical activities. Ophthalmologists provided a major role as mentor to the ophthalmic assistant. Training standards and efficiency varied greatly and depended heavily on the talents of the individual assistant, and the teaching ability of the supervising ophthalmologist. Ophthalmic assistants have been allied to ophthalmologists in offices and hospitals. No credentialing was required.

Formal academic programs, rather than on-the-job training, have been established in Canadian and American universities and colleges during this time, and official textbooks have been written that have been accepted, indeed welcomed, by both the Canadian and American ophthalmologic associations.

In 1962 in the province of Ontario, Canada, the government began requesting formal information regarding manpower and service to patients. Governments were being pressured to legislate that ophthalmologists perform only surgery, and nonmedical practitioners perform medical work and refractions. Ophthalmology leaders explained to the government that although there were many more optometrists than ophthalmic surgeons, an ophthalmologist had available a large resource in allied groups of ophthalmic assistants available to deliver eye care. The ophthalmologists performed surveys which found at that time, in Ontario, that there were at least two or three ophthalmic assistants to every ophthalmologist in practice. These assistants were formed into an organized group to aid in eye care delivery, which was the beginning of the formalization of the role for ophthalmic technicians.

In the early 1960s in Ontario, Drs. Harold Stein and Bernard Slatt organized instructional short courses and provided credit for examination for existing ophthalmic personnel. Drs. William Hunter and Stein formed an association of ophthalmic assistants to provide recognition of their special skill set, with membership certificates and pins. This eventually developed into the Canadian Society of Ophthalmic Personnel (CSOMP), which was a forerunner of similar societies, such as the Association of Technical Personnel in Ophthalmology (ATPO).

Along with Ms. Debra Kaplan, in the late 1960s, formal training courses were started at the Centennial College of Applied Arts, Scarborough, Ontario, Canada. The course ran daytime for 6 weeks. After graduating 35 ophthalmic assistants from this intensive course, they encountered difficulty in finding employment with ophthalmologists for the technical graduates. Consequently, the training program was shifted to evenings and only granted admission to ophthalmic assistants who were already employed by an ophthalmologist. This evening educational program, held once weekly, has continued in Toronto since 1965, and has been highly successful.

Centennial College in Toronto, and the Southern Alberta Institute of Technology (SAIT) in Calgary, Alberta started a home study course for ophthalmic assistants working for ophthalmologists across Canada. The course updated their skills; a graduate was given a "certificate of completion", but there was no formal licensing required or other academic qualification.

In 1968 Dr. Bernard Sakler of Cincinnati asked Dr. Stein to present at the American Association of Ophthalmology (AAO) annual meeting. Dr. Stein presented on Canada's development of allied health personnel's training programs. His statistics demonstrated that there were many ophthalmologists and ophthalmic assistants sufficient to service the eye care needs of the Ontario's population.

The AAO accepted this concept and began a program similar to Ontario. Drs. Slatt and Stein were asked by the AAO to begin a home study course for technicians, which advertised across the United States to upgrade the skills of ophthalmic assistants in offices. Dr. Stein eventually became the chairman of the House of Delegates for the AAO. Under the executive director at the time, Mr. Larry Zupan, this ophthalmic assistant home study course was a landmark success for the AAO. Eventually, the American Academy of Ophthalmology adopted the American Association of Ophthalmology as their council, with delegates from across the United States.

Concurrently with these events, Drs. Slatt and Stein coauthored the first clinical textbook for allied health personnel in ophthalmology, entitled *The Ophthalmic Assistant*, published by the CV Mosby Company, in 1968. It is now in its 11th edition and is accepted worldwide as a standard for ophthalmic technician education.

In 1968 Drs. Hugh Monahan and Peter Evans, established the Joint Commission on Allied Health Personnel in Ophthalmology (JCAHPO) with three delegates from each of the major ophthalmology organizations and the American Medical Association in Canada and the United States being represented. JCAHPO developed examinations and certification for a more senior level called the ophthalmic technician and the ophthalmic medical technologist. JCAHPO's annual continuing education program became the largest and leading nonacademic education program to train ophthalmic assistants, technicians, and medical technologists.

Nature of the work

In North America, the main role of the ophthalmic assistant is to help the ophthalmologist in patient care. The assistant is responsible for taking the patient's history and conducting the preliminary patient eye examination, for maintaining sterile equipment in the office, and assisting in minor surgical duties. Another key role is to provide patient education.

The ophthalmic assistant performs many diagnostic technical tests, including assessing vision, visual fields, pupillary assessment, keratometry, ocular motility, pachymetry, biometry, and tonometry. In North America, the ophthalmic assistant also performs the automated or subjective refraction examination to determine best optical correction for the patient. The ophthalmic assistant does not write the prescription for the uncorrected refractive error to prescribe eyeglasses. This preliminary refraction is then typically followed up by the ophthalmologist who uses clinical judgment to determine the best prescription for the patient. Imaging has also become an important test performed by technicians. The technician performs diagnostic testing procedures including topography, specular microscopy, wavefront analysis, ultrasound (B-Scan and ultrasound biomicroscopy), optical coherence tomography (OCT) and OCT-angiography (OCT-A), and fundus imaging and fluorescein angiography.

The assistant's role includes working with patients on preventive measures in dealing with eye problems, low vision with older patients, electronic medical records (EMR) and scribing for the ophthalmologist, rehabilitation of partially sighted adults, community volunteer work for vision and glaucoma screening programs, and international mission trips to serve the blind.

To ensure competency in ophthalmic assisting skills, IJCAHPO conducts certification examination on the core and specialty skills. There are currently 70,000 certified and noncertified ophthalmic assistants/technicians in North America. Canada and the U.S. ophthalmologists recognize these accredited certifications as milestones in the competencies and careers of allied ophthalmic personnel (AOP). Canada and the U.S. do not require licensing of ophthalmic allied personnel.

Two important studies by Astle et al. in Canada, and Woodworth et al. in the United States, showed that North American ophthalmologists highly value their certified ophthalmic assistants.[2,3] Approximately 80% of these ophthalmologists indicated that certified ophthalmic assistants/technicians enhance practice productivity measures more than noncertified ophthalmic assistants (Fig. 52.1).[2]

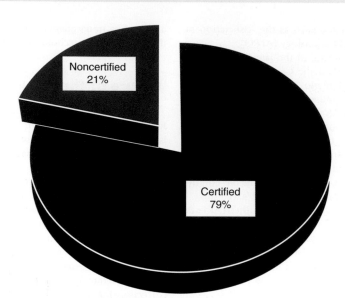

Fig. 52.1 Ophthalmologists study: certified allied ophthalmic personnel (AOP) add more value to their practice than noncertified AOP.

Astle et al. found that certified AOP contributed more than noncertified AOP in four measures: increased doctor productivity, increased number of patients seen per hour, improved trouble-shooting rapport, and improved triage screening.

Future of ophthalmic assisting

Since 1980, Flaxman et al. refreshed the Global Vision Database to review the most prevalent worldwide causes for visual impairment and blindness.[4] They reviewed 288 studies, representing close to 4 million participants, contributing data from 98 countries. The World Health Organization (WHO) published in 2019 the leading cause of moderate to severe visual impairment were uncorrected refractive errors (123.7 million)[5] which had not been recognized as major causes of world visual impairment and blindness until recently.

As a result of these findings, the first World Congress on Refractive Error and Service Development was held in Durban, South Africa in March 2007, to discuss the need identified to diagnose and treat uncorrected refractive errors worldwide. Over 650 delegates attended representing eye care professionals, researchers, governments, civil society, nongovernmental organizations (NGOs), universities, institutions, eye care professionals and industry from all over the world, and included a representative from JCAHPO. The meeting was hosted by the International Center for Eyecare Education (ICEE), with representation from the World Health Organization (WHO), the International Agency for the Prevention of Blindness (IAPB), the World Council of Optometry (WCO), the International Council of Ophthalmology (ICO). Concluding the meeting, a landmark document was published, the "Durban Declaration on Refractive Error and Service Development." Ophthalmic technical support would become a key element to successfully dealing with the worldwide scourge of uncorrected refractive errors, one of the most common causes of visual impairment and blindness.

Related to these issues, international eye care agencies were recognizing the need for standardized education and certification of ophthalmic technicians worldwide. As a result of continued International requests for help, JCAHPO continued to expand educational and certification efforts worldwide. In 2009 in recognition of the need for well-trained ophthalmic technicians worldwide, the JCAHPO transitioned to become the International Joint Commission on Allied Health Personnel in Ophthalmology (IJCAHPO) with official registration in 2018. There are now over 31,000 IJCAHPO certificants in 45 countries with over 52 formalized educational programs and certification agreements. These expansions will provide sustainable support to standardize ophthalmic technical training and improve eye care delivery worldwide.

Throughout the world, the terms used to describe ophthalmic technicians have been varied and inconsistent in use. In 2013 the WHO made a concerted effort to label the cadre of ophthalmic technicians in a consistent way. As a result, the term allied ophthalmic personnel is now the accepted term for this group. Quoting directly from the WHO global action plan published in 2013[6]:

Allied Ophthalmic Personnel may be characterized by different educational requirements, legislation and practice regulations, skills, and scope of practice between countries and even within a given country....AOP comprise opticians, ophthalmic nurses, orthoptists, ophthalmic and optometric assistants, ophthalmic and optometric technicians, vision therapists, ocularists, ophthalmic photographer/imagers, and ophthalmic administrators.

Based on the Durban Declaration, IJCAHPO, ICO, IAPB, and other non-governmental organization (NGO) representatives interested in supporting the education and certification of AOP worldwide met in Cambridge, United Kingdom in 2015. The "Cambridge Declaration" was dedicated to ensuring the high-quality capacity development of eye care teams and maintenance of well-skilled AOP globally. The Cambridge Declaration acknowledged that the new way of viewing successful eye care delivery worldwide is through the concept of the Ophthalmologist-led eye care team (see Fig. 52.1), which comprises cadres of eye care personnel broken down that includes: ophthalmologists, optometrist, and allied ophthalmic personnel. The declaration recognizes that successful community eye care health includes all stakeholders working together with appropriate levels of training and skill. The declaration recognizes that AOP are committed members of eye care teams in every country of the world, and play an essential role in delivering high quality, efficient, comprehensive eye services, inclusive of all persons, and in achieving Universal Eye Health. There is now more formal recognition worldwide that AOP are an essential member of the eye care team, and standardized education and certification of AOP at the same level worldwide, is essential to the sustainability and growth of universal global eye care.

Conclusion

In North America, the ophthalmologist profession and governments have long-time embraced and recognized the AOP workforce as a valid and legitimate profession. Canadian and U.S. governments, such as the U.S. Bureau of Labor, have established national occupational classification codes to recognize this ophthalmic workforce that also helped create educational and career pathways.

The worldwide need for skilled, consistently trained AOP is crucial and constantly growing to deal with the ever-increasing burden of visual impairments and treatable blindness. Regardless of continent, region or country, there remains a critical shortage of well trained, certified AOP in North America, as well as globally.[7] This is especially true with the more recently identified needs for treating visual impairment and blindness caused by uncorrected refractive errors, which requires a large cadre of AOP to deal with the sheer numbers of people affected internationally. In addition, ongoing success will also require the help of all cadres of eye care professionals, to effectively deal with the increasing numbers of patients with eye disease.

It is important that AOP worldwide can access high quality, sustainable capacity development. All ophthalmic organizations involved in eye care delivery need to seek government recognition of AOP, and gain sustainable provision for AOP education, certification, posttraining support, deployment, and ongoing professional development. There must be ongoing recognition, advocacy, resources, and funding for the education of AOP, and for the individuals who train AOP. Organizations like IJCAHPO and other NGSs need to collect and share best practices for AOP as technology advances and changes. Training materials, train-the-trainer guides, and assessment tools are crucial to ensure that AOP have access to high quality training programs worldwide.

Increasing the number of highly skilled AOP globally is crucial to the goals outlined in this chapter. In our post COVID-19 world, this is an exceptional time for AOP to be part of the global eye care team, and AOP are now even more essential to long term sustainable success in dealing with treatable visual impairments and blinding eye disease worldwide.

References

1. International Joint Commission on Allied Health Personnel in Ophthalmology, Inc. Ophthalmologists-Led Eye Care Team. Presentation. IJCAHPO. 2018.
2. Astle W, El-Defrawy S, LaRoche G, et al. Survey on allied health personnel in Canadian ophthalmology: the scalpel for change. *Can J Ophthalmol.* 2011;46(1):28–24.
3. Woodworth K, Donshik P, Ehlers W, Pucel D, Anderson L, Thompson N. A comparative study of the impact of certified and noncertified ophthalmic medical personnel on practice quality and productivity. *Eye Contact Lens.* 2008;34(1):28–24.
4. Flaxman S, Bourne R, Resnikoff S, et al. Global causes of blindness and distance vision impairment 1990–2020: a systemic review and meta-analysis. *Lancet Glob Health.* 2017;5(12):e1221–1234.
5. World Health Organization. World report on vision. (2019).
6. World Health Organization. WHO universal eye health: a global action plan 2014–2019 (2013).
7. Astle W, Simms C, Anderson L. A workforce in crisis: a case study to expand allied ophthalmic personnel. *Can J Ophthalmol.* 2016;51(4):288–293.

Chapter | 53 |

Ophthalmic assisting in the international community and in the prevention of blindness

Peter Y. Evans, Victoria M. Sheffield, and Lynn D. Anderson

Introduction

Across the globe, the ophthalmic team is seen as critical to improving quality of and access to quality eye care services. The purpose of this chapter is to highlight the varying types of allied ophthalmic personnel (AOP),[a] an inclusive term defined by the World Health Organization (WHO) to encompass the many varied titles and responsibilities of AOP in different countries. As countries develop their own AOP, they increasingly are looking at the North American experience, particularly with regard to planning and organization. Therefore this short historical review of the United States experience is provided.

The 1960s was a turbulent decade for the United States politically. At the same time, positive achievements were made in the area of civil rights and socioeconomic benefits. Specifically, the introduction of Medicare and Medicaid made it possible for patients to access health care including eye care and particularly cataract surgery because it would now be covered by insurance.

In anticipation of significant increases in the number of patients seeking care, government and academic health planners met early to discuss challenges and explore solutions. Funds were made available by the government to drastically enlarge medical school classes and in ophthalmology, new residency positions were created. At that time, eye patients had to wait 3 to 5 months for an appointment and the ophthalmologist's time with each patient became shorter and shorter. It was clear that increasing the number of eye care providers and creating efficiencies was critical, but how to do it in a short period of time? The idea of AOP was identified, but they needed to be reliable and well trained.

In 1963 after 2 years of preparation and under the direction of Dr. Peter Evans, the first full-time 2-year training program for ophthalmic medical personnel (OMP) in the United States was established at the Georgetown University Medical Center in Washington, DC. Soon similar programs followed in university departments across the United States and in Canada. It became clear that not only could more patients see their ophthalmologist in a timely fashion, but that a greater number of important but often time-consuming diagnostic tests could be provided for which the

---

[a]In 2015 the World Health Organization in its Cambridge Declaration stated "The definition of allied ophthalmic personnel may be characterized by different educational requirements, legislation and practice regulations, skills and scope of practice between countries and even within a given country. Typically, allied ophthalmic personnel comprise opticians, ophthalmic nurses, orthoptists, ophthalmic and optometric assistants, ophthalmic and optometric technicians, vision therapists, ocularists, ophthalmic photographer/imagers, and ophthalmic administrators."

ophthalmologist simply did not have the time to perform. The original time-saving motive had actually resulted in a significant improvement to the quality of ophthalmic patient care.

Many ophthalmologists, especially those establishing training programs, felt there was an urgent need for standardization of training, comparable or uniform examinations, and clear definitions of different levels of expertise: in short, for quality control. In 1969 the Joint Commission on Allied Health Personnel in Ophthalmology (JCAHPO) was established and has since enjoyed the support of all North American ophthalmologic and allied health organizations (see also Chapter 52).

JCAHPO established an organization to accredit ophthalmic assistant (OA) and technician training programs and to certify personnel at these levels. In the early 1980s, an additional category of OMP was added to the OA and Ophthalmic Technician levels which was the Ophthalmic Medical Technologist which had increased levels of training and examinations. In 2017 JCAHPO became the International Joint Commission on Allied Health Personnel (IJCAHPO). The Commission on Accreditation of Ophthalmic Medical Programs (CoA-OMP) was under the U.S. Commission on Accreditation of Allied Health Education Programs (CAAHEP). CoA-OMP became independent of CAAHEP in the mid-2000s. In 2018 CoA-OMP became the International Council of Accreditation (ICA) and accredits ophthalmic training programs in Canada, the United States and globally.

At the last census in 2010, the American Medical Association stated there were approximately 23,861 ophthalmologists in the United States (pop. 309.4 million) reflecting a ratio of one ophthalmologist per 12,967 people, an entirely adequate ratio, not considering some regional maldistributions. It is estimated that U.S. ophthalmologists are supported by well over 45,000 AOP, not including administrative and other staff. More than 27,200 AOP are certified and recertified every 3 years. Typically, certified AOP earn good salaries with very good job satisfaction. In addition, more than 818 AOP (2020) are now certified in Canada and in other countries where the IJCAHPO certification examination is administered.

These figures are dramatically different in other areas of the world, especially low to middle-income countries (LMICs). In sub-Saharan Africa, the average is just one ophthalmologist per one million population. With most ophthalmologists being located in urban areas and most of the population living in rural areas, this ratio is smaller in urban areas and wider in rural settings when considering access to care. Blinding diseases, such as trachoma and onchocerciasis, almost never seen in developed countries, still exist in LMICs. In 2015 the Vision Loss Expert Group (VLEG) estimated the prevalence of visual impairment globally at 253 million including 36 million who are blind. Approximately 89% of these live in LMICs and 55%

are women. Another 1.1 billion have near vision impairment simply because of the lack of reading glasses.[1] In the 1950s initiatives were developed by WHO and nongovernmental organizations (NGOs), to address the inequities in these countries, many of which were still under colonial rule. European and American NGOs, often with funding from their own government agencies, were founded for the express purpose of preventing blindness and restoring sight in LMICs. The WHO works specifically with national governments on policy and public health initiatives to combat disease, and also with a number of NGOs including those focusing on eye health. Most of the leading international eye health NGOs along with academic institutions and corporations are members of the International Agency for the Prevention of Blindness (IAPB; www.iapb.org), a global advocacy organization working in official relations with WHO and supporting global initiatives to reduce vision impairment.

With unoperated cataract being responsible for as much as 47% of the world's blindness caused by disease, NGOs including IJCAHPO helped develop national eye health services, provide treatment and surgery, and train ophthalmologists and AOP. Today, most LMICs have their own ophthalmic infrastructure with qualified ophthalmologists and AOP, but the numbers are not adequate to meet the needs of their populations.

Many projects supporting eye health in LMICs are implemented by international NGOs in collaboration with local NGOs, government Ministries of Health, and the ophthalmic community. National governments recognize the need for ophthalmologists and AOP in creating ophthalmic teams to provide efficient, quality eye care. IJCAHPO and ICA work collaboratively with governments, NGOs, and local ophthalmologists to implement an international AOP curriculum, and establish certification and accreditation standards for the workforce and ophthalmic training programs respectively.

VISION 2020: The Right to Sight

Launched by IAPB and WHO in 1999, this ambitious global initiative aimed to eliminate avoidable (preventable and treatable) blindness by the year 2020. WHO passed three resolutions on the elimination of avoidable blindness (2003, 2006 and 2009) and in May 2009 at the World Health Assembly, passed WHA66.4 "Towards universal eye health: a global action plan 2014–2019" demonstrating WHO's commitment to eliminating visual impairment and giving eye health stakeholders a powerful advocacy tool.

This chapter describes regional challenges and training approaches. Much of the information has been provided by NGOs, ophthalmologists, and AOP working in these countries.

The IAPB's Vision Atlas is an excellent online source for eye global eye disease data, the leading causes of eye disease by region, human resource availability, and other important data around blindness and visual impairment—https://www.iapb.org/learn/vision-atlas/. The Vision Atlas is updated annually with data from the Vision Loss Expert Group—https://www.iapb.org/learn/vision-atlas/about/contributors/vleg/.

Latin America and the Caribbean

In most regions of the world, the work of AOP is driven by the need to reach more patients needing eye care. IAPB's Vision Atlas estimates a prevalence of vision impairment (blindness and low vision combined) of between 1.98% and 3.92% in the Latin America region and 2.6% in the Caribbean. Unoperated cataract is responsible for 42.46% to 43.44% in Latin America and 41.62% in the Caribbean.

The Ophthalmology Society of the West Indies (OSWI) has taken a leadership role in training AOP at the OA level by supporting an annual training program conducted during the OSWI annual meeting. OSWI and IJCAHPO collaborate in conducting a 4 to 5 day program with the students who have studied throughout the year, taking IJCAHPO's certification examination as the capstone event.

Brazil

The largest country of South America representing 50% of the entire continent, Brazil also has the region's largest population of 212.6 million.[2] With 21,063 ophthalmologists,[3] the ratio of ophthalmologist per population is 1:10,000. The ophthalmology residency training is similar to that of the United States. However, the urban versus rural maldistribution of ophthalmologists is even more pronounced than in most other countries in the region. More than 95% of all eye care services are located in urban areas with large swaths of Brazil and its Amazon regions isolated from modern health and eye care.

Originally, only orthoptists were trained in formal courses. In 1988 Professor Newton Kara-José at the University of Campinas in Sao Paulo started a training program for OAs which has continued without interruption. Four times a year, a full-time 2-month course is offered to 10 high school graduates, 90% of them women. There also are a number of short, 1 to 3 day courses offered by professional societies, the University of Campinas, and during ophthalmic meetings (20–30 per year). Therefore, very few of the estimated 6000 to 7000 AOP in Brazil have had any formal training. The upper income limit for AOP is equivalent to approximately U.S. $8000 annually.

The leading causes of blindness in Brazil are similar to most countries: cataract, uncorrected refractive error (URE), glaucoma, and diabetic retinopathy. Most important in children are infantile cataract, uncorrected refractive error (URE), toxoplasmic retinitis, and retinopathy of prematurity. Since 1999, as a result of collaborative efforts between the Ministry of Health and the Brazilian Council of Ophthalmology, cataract surgery has dramatically increased from under 70,000 per year to more than 300,000 per year.

Despite a few notable exceptions, most ophthalmologists in Brazil still need to be convinced of the advantages to them and to the public of formal training of AOP. The situation is similar in other countries in the region. Kara-José notes that ophthalmic societies are strongly opposed to training of allied eye health personnel because of a perceived threat of these people working independently without ophthalmic supervision.

Guatemala

Located in Central America, Guatemala has a population of 17,915,568[4] and 96 ophthalmologists[5] for a ratio of 1:186,621 with most ophthalmologists located in urban areas. There are no formal training programs in Guatemala except for ophthalmologists. AOP are trained within eye units and hospitals for specific skills. Visualiza located in Guatemala City with its satellite Vincent Pescatore Eye Hospital in the Peten reached only by air, uses ophthalmic nurses, OAs, operating room (OR) nurses, optical shop dispensers, and equipment technicians (angiograms, optical coherence tomography), as well as patient counselors and outreach coordinators. Visualiza has developed courses to improve skills of existing ophthalmic technicians, OR nurses, and counselors for their own facilities as well as others in the country.

Haiti

Haiti, the poorest country in the Western Hemisphere, has a population of 11.4 million with 1.23 million living in the capital Port-au-Prince.[6] Haiti is mountainous and has very poor electrical service, mostly from aging generators. Although improved, the estimated prevalence of blindness is 1.2%. Cataract is responsible for approximately 50% with glaucoma responsible for approximately 30% of blindness. Blinding malnutrition from vitamin A deficiency can still be found, and diabetic retinopathy is common.

There are 65 ophthalmologists in Haiti,[7] nearly all in urban areas. In the 1980s NGOs began supporting sporadic training of OAs for 1 year who were deployed throughout the country. With new eye clinics and hospitals being established outside the capital, access to eye care has improved but is still limited with some parts of the country having no eye care services at all.

The estimated number of AOP in Haiti is 100 with an average monthly salary of less than U.S. $200. Most AOP work in eye centers outside the capital where they receive on-the-job training. Political unrest is still a challenge and the devastating earthquake of 2010 destroyed infrastructure including at the university's Department of Ophthalmology. The Haitian National Committee for the Prevention of Blindness (CNPC) coordinates with international and national NGOs and donors to strengthen eye health services in the country.

Peru

Peru counts 222 ophthalmologists[8] for its population of almost 33 million (2020)[9] for a ratio of 1:149,000 and again, they are located in urban areas. A large geographic part of Peru is in the Amazon. The government hospital in Peru's Amazonian capital Iquitos has an eye unit and a new eye hospital has been built by the Peruvian NGO Clinica Divino Nino Jesus with support from international NGOs These. are the only eye care services accessible to Peru's Amazonian population who cannot reach the rest of Peru except by rivers or by air. Although the National Eye Institute in the capital Lima conducted ophthalmic training courses for nurses and auxiliary personnel from 1979 to 1995, there are at this time no similar programs in Peru. Challenges are a lack of direct supervision after the trained personnel returned to their original sites, little continuing education or evaluation of their activities, and often AOP were reassigned to duties outside of eye care for which they had been trained.

Today in Peru, AOP are trained in the eye hospitals where they work. The government requires that those being hired and trained as AOP must be either 5-year university trained nurses (equivalent to Registered Nurse) with a sixth year of training in rural/public health, or a 3-year trained Technical Nurse (equivalent to Practical Nurse). They are trained at their hospitals to perform specific skills, such as measurement of visual acuity, visual fields, and autorefraction, and university-trained nurses usually have supervisory positions in clinics and ORs.

Puerto Rico

Although Puerto Rico is part of the United States, it had very few U.S.-graduated ophthalmologists in the 1950s. The first ophthalmology residency program was established in 1954 at the University of Puerto Rico by Professor Guillermo Picó. In 1961 the International Eye Foundation (IEF) helped establish the first Basic Science Course in Spanish for ophthalmologists and is attended annually by ophthalmologists from throughout the Latin America region.

In 1972 there was one ophthalmologist per 42,000 population. Because a more ideal ratio was felt to be unattainable, planning began for an ophthalmic technician training program at the university's Department of Ophthalmology. This became a 2-year undergraduate degree program with the first year in general education and the second in ophthalmic technology. It was officially accredited at the ophthalmic technician level by ICA and students take the IJCAHPO certification examination. Today, the program is rated highly with students coming from throughout Latin America.

The population of Puerto Rico in 2018 was 3.2 million[10] reflecting a significant decline after Hurricanes Maria and Irma. With 120 ophthalmologists,[11] also a decline after the hurricanes, the ratio of 1:26,600 is much improved but would be better had it not been for the destructive hurricanes and their aftermath. There are approximately 300 ophthalmic technician graduates, mostly women, working under the direct supervision of ophthalmologists, usually in urban areas. The value of AOP has resulted in more patients being seen by an ophthalmologist at a lower cost. Uniformly, the community benefits are an increase in the number and quality of ophthalmic services. The remuneration of AOP in Puerto Rico is comparable to that of other mid-level health workers and nurses in the country.

Sub-Saharan Africa

Until the end of World War II, only four countries in this second largest continent of the world were independent nations: Egypt, Ethiopia, Liberia, and South Africa. During the following turbulent decades, almost 40 former African colonies gained independence from their European rulers (Great Britain, France, Belgium, Germany, and Portugal). The continent is divided geographically between Arab North Africa and sub-Saharan Africa with their own cultural, social, economic, and language differences.

Many sub-Saharan African countries experience civil strife, terrorism, and epidemic health problems, such as malnutrition, malaria, human immunodeficiency virus (HIV)/acquired immunodeficiency syndrome (AIDS), and outbreaks of diseases, such as Ebola. National governments, WHO and international donor budgets focus, rightly, on diseases causing mortality leaving per capita spending on eye health insufficient compared to the need. The training and utilization of AOP in Africa has been critical with AOP often serving as the backbone of public eye health services.

Notation: Egypt and Cameroon

The Magrabi Foundation based in Egypt has taken a leadership role in expanding AOP in the Eastern Mediterranean and African regions where the need is significant. The Magrabi Foundation is funding two important programs to train OAs and technicians; one in Cairo, Egypt and the second in Yaoundé, Cameroon. The programs follow the International Core Curriculum for Ophthalmic Assisting and have embraced the ICA accreditation standards to ensure quality measures. Both programs implement IJCAHPO's certification program by using the certification as a graduation examination. Most AOP are employed by NGO managed eye hospitals and paid according to each hospital's wage structure.

Kenya

On the East African coast of the Indian Ocean astride the equator, Kenya's population is 53.8 million[12] and two-thirds of the population live in rural areas.

Kenya's Ministry of Health reports 115 ophthalmologists in the country of which 60 are located in the capital Nairobi[13] reflecting an ophthalmologist per population ratio of 1:468,000, far below the WHO's recommended 1:250,000.

The leading causes of blindness in Kenya are cataract, corneal blindness caused by trachoma, and glaucoma. The first group of ophthalmology residents graduated from the University of Nairobi School of Medicine in 1981 after 3 years of training. To supplement the need for more qualified medical personnel, Kenya's government began training medical assistants in the Kenya Medical Training College. The program recruited high school students and trained them for 3 years in clinical medicine to become clinical officers (COs). A CO could then specialize for another year to attain a diploma as CO in pediatrics, orthopedics, and so on.

In 1956 during British colonial times, it was recognized that the severe undersupply of ophthalmologists could not be changed in the foreseeable future. Kenya's government with administrative support from the Kenya Society for the Blind established the Kenya Ophthalmic Programme (KOP).[14] The first cadre of Clinical Officers trained in ophthalmology (OCOs) were trained for 1 year and recognized as a separate cadre within the Ministry of Health and paid by the government at a higher rate than general COs thanks to advocacy to make sure OCOs would not leave service for better pay elsewhere. They were deployed to a network of over 70 government and NGO static and outreach service delivery points throughout the country, often working independently. They provide comprehensive eye care, referrals for surgery, outreach services, and participate in community education for prevention of blindness. In 1993 OCOs could train for an additional year as OCO Cataract Surgeons (OCO/CS) performing intracapsular cataract extraction (ICCE) and then extracapsular cataract extraction (ECCE)/intraocular lens (IOL) under supervision of an ophthalmologist.

The official acceptance of primary eye care (PEC) as an element of primary health care (PHC) in 1996 led to a work overload for OCOs. In the 1990s the need for formal training of other cadres of AOP became evident, such as community eye care workers, OAs, ophthalmic nurses, ophthalmic scrub nurses, and nursing assistants. With the advent of the IAPB/WHO "VISION 2020: The Right to

Sight" targets, childhood blindness became a priority and special training for low-vision therapists was accepted by the government.

Nurses have been the backbone of healthcare services in East Africa. The Kenya Nursing Council (KNC) has evolved in its recognition of nursing and Nurse Assistant (NA) training.

In 2003 a 1-year university diploma course was established specifically for ophthalmic nurses with financial support from international NGOs.[15] Their training and job description aimed to avoid duplicating the responsibilities of OCOs and concentrate on health promotion, management of eye units and eye camps, and the operating room.

Training of OAs began at the Kikuyu Eye Unit near Nairobi with support from the German-based NGO Christoffel Blindenmission (CBM). The aim was to give the necessary skills to the OA to screen, diagnose, prescribe for common eye infections, and to know when and where to refer patients with serious eye problems. OAs could be deployed to primary or secondary government or mission hospitals.

The 3-month course covers basic ophthalmology with an emphasis on eye conditions, such as trachoma, practical procedures related to administering medications, and preoperative patient preparation, as well as postoperative care after surgery, especially for patients in rural areas who are operated by a visiting surgical team. OAs working in areas with endemic trachoma are taught how to perform bilamellar eyelid surgery for trichiasis. An OA training program was established by Dr. Kiage in Kisii, western Kenya, which implements IJCAHPO's certification program.

Malawi

Malawi is a small, landlocked country in southern Africa, one of 16 member states of the Southern African Development Community (SADC).[16] Malawi has a population of 17 million people, 87% of whom live in rural areas. There 12 ophthalmologists in the country equate to 1.4 ophthalmologists per million people.[17] Fortunately, Malawi is a very small country and patients can usually reach ophthalmic services in Blantyre in the south, Lilongwe in the center of the country, and Mzuzu in the north by public transport.

The major causes of blindness are cataract, trachoma, and glaucoma. Blinding malnutrition from vitamin A deficiency can still be found, especially in the arid south. In 1980 the International Eye Foundation (IEF) established the first OA Training Program in Malawi which ended in 1997 as trainees preferred the OCO training described later. In 1983 the SADC Ophthalmic Training Center was established at the Malawi College of Health Sciences in Lilongwe, with financial and human resources support from the British-based SightSavers International (SSI). It is run by the Ministry of Health and Population and its specific objective is to create trained mid-level eye health personnel equipped with the knowledge, attitudes, and skills to prevent and cure eye diseases.

Training in Malawi has evolved. There is a 3-year OCO training program awarding a diploma in clinical medicine and training approximately 30 OCOs per year. There is an 18-month "Cat. Surgeon" (nonphysician) training program for OCOs to perform cataract surgery and external ocular surgery awarding an advanced diploma and training approximately 10 per year. These "Cat. Surgeons" work in SADC countries and Kenya. Malawi's ophthalmic nurses were actually general nurses who took an OMA course receiving a certificate but were not trained formally as ophthalmic nurses. Botswana and South Africa have postgraduate ophthalmic nurse courses with Botswana basing its course on Malawi's OCO curriculum.

Malawi now has a 4-year degree course for optometrists and an 18-month optometric technician course, each training approximately 20 per year. A key challenge is the lack of continuing education because of lack of funds for trainee costs and for international trainers.

Mali

The Institut d'Ophtalmologie Tropical de l'Afrique (IOTA) originates from the former Trachoma Institute transferred from Dakar, Senegal to Bamako, Mali in 1953. In 1960 IOTA joined the Organisation De Coopération Et De Coordination Pour La Lutte Contre Les Grandes Endémies (OCCGE), an intercountry network of research and training institutions. In 2000 at the termination of OCCGE, IOTA was transferred to the Malian authorities and became a specialized national public hospital. In 2006 IOTA became a University-affiliated Teaching Hospital (Centre Hospitalier Universitaire CHU-IOTA).

Being a tertiary level facility, CHU-IOTA has four essential functions: (1) research, (2) specialized eye care, (3) training and education, and (4) provision of technical support and expertise in eye care, training, research, and prevention of blindness to Francophone countries in Africa.

Annual services provided include 100,000 outpatient visits, 6000 ocular surgeries, 7000 specialized eye examinations, and 1000 laser treatments (yttrium aluminum garnet [YAG] and Argon). Academic and clinical staff include 24 senior specialists in ophthalmology, optometry, and anesthesiology including academic subspecialists (professors and lecturers), and consultants. IOTA's research capacity includes, on average, 10 research studies per year.

CHU-ITOA's training capacity includes 10 ophthalmology residents per year in a 4-year training program; 10 ophthalmic nurses (Technicien Spécialisé en Ophtalmologie) per year in a 2-year training program; 10 optometrists per year in a 3-year training program; and eight opticians per year in a 6-month training program. In addition, IOTA provides Continuous Professional Development and additional training on an ongoing basis for eye care professionals from Francophone Africa, as well as surgical training supported by fully equipped wet and dry labs.

Since 1991, IOTA has trained 267 ophthalmologists, 487 ophthalmic nurses, 66 optometrists at the bachelor level, 163 optical technicians, and 30 ophthalmic nurses who received specialized training in special ocular examinations.[18]

Nigeria

Nigeria has the largest population in Africa at 206,139,589[19] and reports 300 ophthalmologists,[20] many being subspecialists. The ophthalmologist to population ratio is 1:687,000. Nigeria's ophthalmic nurses are trained in the Nigerian Teaching Hospitals, optometrists are university trained, and opticians are trained on the job. Hospitals take high school graduates for 6-week courses for OAs and ophthalmic technicians at the National Eye Centre in Kaduna established by Prof. Adenike Abiose. There is a constant need to train and retrain to retain staff but lack of funding is a challenge.

Tanzania

There are 27 ophthalmologists in Tanzania[21] with a population of 59.7 million[22] people yielding an ophthalmologist per population ratio of 1:2.2 million with most located in urban areas. The leading causes of blindness are cataract and corneal disease from trachoma.

Although known and described for thousands of years, trachoma had been studied particularly in Egypt in the 19th century and became known as the "Egyptian [eye] disease." The *chlamydia* infection is endemic, highly contagious, and usually bilateral, affecting especially women and children in arid areas. Trachoma causes conjunctival inflammation under the upper eyelids leading to scarring, entropion, and trichiasis over time. Trichiasis causes corneal opacification and blindness. This preventable cause of blindness is a major focus for community eye workers and OAs who can jointly enact the WHO's SAFE strategy to prevent trachoma—Surgery, Antibiotics, Facial cleanliness, Environmental hygiene. The trained OCO can perform eyelid surgery to remove the scarring, relieve entropion, and eliminate trichiasis (Fig. 53.1). The critical activities revolve around providing antibiotic ointment to treat early, infectious trachoma and teaching community members about the importance of face washing and environmental hygiene to reduce fly populations that spread the disease. Tanzania has paramedical ophthalmologists, ophthalmic nurses, and OAs similar to Kenya. They are trained by either government or NGO-supported programs and work in government facilities or NGO or mission eye units (Fig. 53.2).

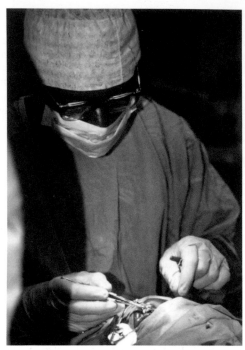

Fig. 53.1 Ophthalmic clinical officer performing lid surgery in Malawi. (Courtesy International Eye Foundation.)

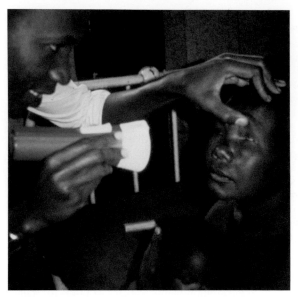

Fig. 53.2 Ophthalmic nurse examines with flashlight in Tanzania where only D-cell batteries are readily available in rural areas. (Courtesy International Eye Foundation.)

Uganda

The population of Uganda is 45.7 million[23] with 37 ophthalmologists[24] yielding an ophthalmologist per population ratio of 1:1.2 million with most in urban areas. Uganda, like Kenya and Tanzania, trains ophthalmologists at the tertiary level; OCO at the secondary/district level; nurses, midwives and other health workers for the primary level; and community health workers (volunteers) for the village health teams to provide health services at the household level.

Since 1989, Uganda Registered Nurses can undergo a 1-year diploma in ophthalmology to qualify as an OCO. OCOs refer patients with complicated problems to ophthalmologists and those requiring refraction to optometrists. They review patients after operations, perform extraocular surgery, such as lid surgery for trichiasis, assist surgeons in the OR, and conduct outreach to schools, rural communities, and remote health facilities. OCOs also can train as Cataract Surgeons (OCOCS), and there is a National Association of Ophthalmic Clinical Officer and Cataract Surgeons (NAOCOCS) that addresses coordination, governance, and social concerns of OCOs. The association organizes annual continuing professional education development workshops. OCOs are represented at the National

Prevention of Blindness Committee and its technical arm at the Ministry of Health.[25]

North Africa and the Middle East

In general, the countries of North Africa enjoy somewhat better ophthalmologist-to-population ratios than those in sub-Saharan Africa with the exception of the Republic of South Africa.

Egypt

Egypt has a population of 102,125,693[26] and counts 400 ophthalmologists[27] reflecting an ophthalmologist per population ratio of 1:255,300 with most located in urban areas, especially Cairo and Alexandra. The Magrabi Eye Hospital in Cairo hosts a training in scrub and recovery nursing for 4-year university degree nurses, and a 2-year course for institute trained clinical assistants. Four-year optometrists are trained at the Institute for Optics and Technology, which also has a 2-year course for opticians. The Magrabi Eye Hospital trains technical nurses and opticians as Low Vision Aids Assistants on the job. Two-year Technical Health Institute graduates can be trained as OAs and at Magrabi as Ophthalmic Technicians. This course follows the International Core

Curriculum for Ophthalmic Assisting and has embraced the ICA accreditation standards to ensure quality measures. It implements IJCAHPO's certification program by using the certification as a graduation examination.

Tunisia

Tunisia's population is 11,805,813[28] with 200 ophthalmologists[29] reflecting an ophthalmologist per population ratio of 1:59,000 with most being in the capital Tunis. There are registered nurses and OR technicians working in ophthalmology. There are no optometrists in Tunisia. AOP are trained on the job and work in the government and private sectors. Some benefit from training in France as Tunisia is a Francophone country. Many leave for employment in the Gulf countries for better salaries.

South-East Asia

Bangladesh

Bangladesh has a population of 164,519,918[30] and 610 ophthalmologists[31] for an ophthalmologist per population ratio of 1:270,000. Much of Bangladesh is under water and people live in densely populated regions with the eye hospitals and ophthalmologists mainly located in the capital Dhaka and the southern city of Chittagong.

Several institutions conduct training courses for ophthalmic nurses. In 1979 the private Chittagong Eye Infirmary and Training Complex and Institute of Community Ophthalmology established by the Bangladesh National Society for the Blind, an NGO, and directed by Prof. Rabiul Husain, embarked on a comprehensive program of training not only ophthalmologists but also OAs. Professor Frank Billson with an Australian team and Brenda Down from London helped develop a special workforce in eye health care. After 2 years of training, the doctors achieve a Diploma of Community Ophthalmology from the University of Chittagong. Their training has a strong focus on community-based ophthalmic conditions and their management. The skills of the OAs are critical in the ORs where they perform instrument sterilization, equipment storage, and assistance at surgery, as well as providing postoperative care for cataract patients, clinic outpatients, school eye health programs, and community disease screenings, including the important Under-5-Clinics for the detection and prevention of blinding malnutrition (vitamin A deficiency). An exchange program with Australia for Bangladeshi AOP provides frontline management training and skills.

Of special importance for the rural, underserved population of Bangladesh is the concept of primary eye care as an integral component of the primary healthcare system. Traditional healers, the Ayurveda, although originally based on ancient religious health beliefs, are medically untrained practitioners who are usually seen first for any illness including ocular conditions. They have the confidence of their communities. But because of their lack of knowledge, they were also often found to prescribe harmful medicines, sometimes leading to blindness. In a forceful move to overcome this situation, primary eye care centers were set up in rural communities, where AOP assume the dual role of providing needed treatment to patients, as well as teaching and training traditional healers in proper primary eye care activities, a unique model of skills transfer.

India

Since gaining independence from Great Britain in 1947, the population had more than tripled by the end of the 20th century. The population of India is 1.4 billion[32] with over 15,000 ophthalmologists[33] for an estimated ophthalmologist per population ratio of 1:93,300. Much of India is rural and people have difficulty reaching the major cities and towns for ophthalmic care. They depend on outreach services provided by many NGO eye hospitals.

The National Blindness and Visually Impaired Survey conducted in 2019[34] showed that the estimated prevalence of blindness in India has been reduced by approximately 47% in the last 12 years while unoperated cataract remains the leading cause of blindness. According to the Union Health Minister Harsh Vardhan, the estimated blindness prevalence rate was reduced to 0.36% from 1% in 2006 to 2007 (the last survey). The survey noted that 92.9% of the blindness was arising from avoidable causes.

A great deal of credit for these achievements goes to the visionary leaders who established programs to train AOP and to increase services for the poor, especially cataract surgery. Services for the poor were financially supported by the government, initially from a loan by the World Bank and now through a government-sponsored insurance scheme enabling the eye health sector to reach more and more patients than ever before.

There are many excellent AOP training programs among the 80 in the country. Three outstanding programs are at the Aravind Eye Care System (AECS) founded by the late Dr. G. Venkataswamy in Madurai, the LV Prasad Eye Institute (LVPEI) founded by Dr. G.N. Rao in Hyderabad, and the Dr. Shroff's Charity Eye Hospital founded in 1904 in Delhi. All three are tertiary eye hospitals with multiple satellite hospitals, the full complement of subspecialties, as well as ophthalmology residency and fellowship training programs. They train AOP and use many of them in their own centers. Aravind's Aurolab produces ophthalmic equipment, instruments and supplies including high quality, low-cost IOLs and viscoelastic. Aurolab uses AOP throughout its facility.

Many eye hospitals offer training courses for optometrists, ophthalmic nurses, ophthalmic technicians, opticians, clinical assistants, ophthalmic and optometric dispensers, outreach coordinators, and healthcare managers.

The Aravind Eye Care System and the L.V. Prasad Eye Institute share the distinction of being considered international model programs for blindness prevention and AOP training (Fig. 53.3). Both have research centers, satellite hospitals and vision centers around their respective states, and strong outreach programs for rural eye care. Their sophisticated training programs for all levels of the eye care team include multilevel ophthalmic assisting and vision care technicians. Students complete their ophthalmic assisting program by sitting for IJCAHPO's certification examinations.

Nepal

Nepal's population is 29 million[35] with 201 ophthalmologists[36] for a ratio of 1:144,200. Nepal's government, health agencies and hospitals recognize AOP including optometrists, refractionists, opticians, and OAs who work in vision centers. Some are trained in Nepal at the Tilganga Eye Institute in Kathmandu and the Lumbini Eye Institute in Siddharthanagar near the India border whilst some also go to India for specialized training.

Pakistan

Pakistan has approximately 1860 ophthalmologists with a population of more than 212 million (2012) reflecting an ophthalmologist per population ratio of 1:114,000. The Pakistan Institute of Community Ophthalmology (PICO) and the Comprehensive Health and Education Forum International (CHEF International), both in Peshawar, have worked together to provide quality healthcare and educational opportunities to the underprivileged population. In the late 2000s, they established ophthalmic training programs in five universities across Pakistan. The educational program was developed to provide three levels of ophthalmic education and training in the universities: OA, technician, and medical technologist. The universities initiated the IJCAHPO certification examination as a final examination criteria. Specialized training courses also are offered for ultrasound biometrists and ophthalmic photographers.

Western Pacific

China

He University is an example of the evolving eye health system in China. Established in 1999 by Prof. Wei He at the He University in Shenyang, China encompasses six disciplines: Medicine, Natural Science, Engineering, Management, Literature, and Art. Also, 22 undergraduate majors are offered that range from Clinical Medicine, Nursing, Medical Imageology, Medical Imaging Technology, Hearing and Speech Rehabilitation, to Optometry and Ophthalmology, as well as six Higher Vocational Education programs including Medical Cosmetology, Rehabilitation Technology, Midwifery Studies, Optometry, and Nursing. China has had few mid-level personnel training programs, and He University is a leader in establishing a multilevel eye-care team training program. They are in the process of establishing two levels of ophthalmic education programs for OAs and technicians. He Eye Institute entered into an alliance agreement with IJCAHPO to establish an education and certification center for mid-level personnel.

Fiji

The Pacific Eye Institute (PEI) and the Fred Hollows Foundation, an NGO, work together to provide an OA education program at PEI in Fiji. PEI collaborates with the National University's College of Medicine, Nursing and Health Sciences to offer postgraduate courses and provides professional development and support to graduates and eye care workers. PEI also collaborates with IJCAHPO to offer the International Core Curriculum for Ophthalmic Assisting for OAs, ophthalmic technicians, and ophthalmic surgical assistants (OSA). The IJCAHPO certification examinations for OA, ophthalmic technician, and OSA are the capstone examination.

Marshall Islands

There is one ophthalmologist in the Marshall Islands which has a population of 59,146.[37] That ophthalmologist is training an ophthalmic technician and there are no other AOP in the country. The Marshall Island's ophthalmologist trained in India.

Micronesia, Federated States of

There is one ophthalmologist in the Federated States of Micronesia which has a population of 548,311.[38] That ophthalmologist is training an ophthalmic technician and there are no other AOP in the country. The ophthalmologist trained in Fiji & New Zealand.

Myanmar

According to the 2019 Myanmar Ophthalmological Society census, there are 443 ophthalmologists in Myanmar with about 80 residents in training. With Myanmar's population

AOP TRAINING PROGRAMME: ARAVIND EYE CARE SYSTEM

COURSE STRUCTURE
Total Duration: Two Years

Orientation & Basic Training
(common to all streams)
3 months

↓

Basic theory & Basic skills
(specific to course stream)
9 months

↓

Advanced theory
Advanced skills
Supervised practice
(specific to course stream)
12 months

AOP CAREER PLAN:

Placement: All AOP graduates are employed within the Aravind Eye Hospital network.

Vision Centre Technician: Clinical AOP staff with over 2 years of work experience and additional training are eligible to be posted as vision centre technicians.

Leadership role: AOP with 3 years of work experience are eligible to be considered for the position of supervisors, tutors, coordinators or managers.

COURSE STREAMS:

AOP trainees are recruited and inducted into one of the following course streams. They are trained specifically for a specific role in the eye hospital.

- Outpatient assistant
- Refractionist
- Inpatient assistant
- Operation theatre assistant
- Medical Records assistant
- Counsellor
- Pharmacy assistant
- Opticals sales assistant
- Optical technician
- Housekeeper
- Laboratory assistant
- Stores assistant
- Instrument maintenance assistant

Fig. 53.3 Structure of Aravind Eye Care System training program. (Courtesy Aravind Eye Care System.)

of 54,370,216,[39] the ophthalmologist per population ratio is 1:122,732.

Except for optometrists and ophthalmic nurses, there are no other AOP in Myanmar. There is a prerequisite to graduate from a science background to become an optometrist, followed by work in the health department, then 2 years of training. The NGO Sight for All also has a training program for optometry which takes place 1 week per month over the course of a year. After graduation, ophthalmic nurses in Myanmar are placed in different hospitals across the country. After their service, they can take the examination for specialty training which lasts 9 months.

Singapore

The Singapore National Eye Centre (SNEC) is the designated national center for Ophthalmology within the public sector healthcare network. SNEC spearheads and coordinates the provision of specialized ophthalmologic services with an emphasis on quality education and research. Since its opening in 1990, SNEC has achieved rapid growth and currently manages an annual workload of 250,000 outpatient visits, 14,000 major eye surgeries, and 13,000 laser procedures.

Ten subspecialties in Cataract, Cataract and Comprehensive Ophthalmology, Corneal and External Eye Disease, Glaucoma, Neuro-Ophthalmology, Oculoplastic and Aesthetic Eyeplastic, Paediatric Ophthalmology and Strabismus, Refractive Surgery, Ocular Inflammation and Immunology, and Vitreo-Retina have been established to provide a full range of subspecialty ophthalmology services at the tertiary level.

Thousands of ophthalmologists from neighboring countries and beyond have participated in SNEC's annual teaching courses and international meetings. To advance ophthalmic science and service, and to increase opportunities for professional interactions and collaboration, SNEC also fostered strategic links with leading ophthalmic institutions around the world. SNEC also embarked on training of AOP for local and regional needs. Its AOP course, the Duke NUS—SNEC Basic Certificate for OAs and technicians was accredited by IJCAHPO in 2014 and reaccredited in early 2017. SNEC provides IJCAHPO's core and subspecialty certification examinations and aims to be a regional center of excellence in training the eye care workforce.

Thailand

Thailand has 1700 registered ophthalmologists for its population of 69,799,987[40] for an ophthalmologist per population ratio of 1:41,000. AOP in hospital clinics include registered nurses, certificate of practical nurses, nurse aids, and technicians. Optometrists also are needed in some hospitals.

Registered nurses train for 4 years, practical nurses for one year, and nurse aids for 6 months. The training program for optometrists is 6 years. Optometrist training is new and available only in two universities that do not include any of the five largest universities of Thailand. For technicians, there is a 4-year training program for medical technology which is not specific to ophthalmology. However, hospitals mostly accept technicians who graduate in any science and medical technology.

Australia: special note

In a country that constitutes an entire continent, one might reasonably expect a large population. However, it numbers only 25,470,472 million[41] with the population skirting the east and west coasts. Professor Frank Billson, a senior educator with a strong commitment to the training and use of OAs stated:

The importance of the role of ophthalmic assistants in extending the arms of the ophthalmologists, particularly in developing countries, cannot be overemphasized. Still today, much can be achieved through training as an apprentice. How much, depends on the skills and willingness and generosity of spirit of the teacher or mentor. Ophthalmic assistants range from nurses with ophthalmic training to orthoptists and ophthalmic paramedics. Skill transfer can also occur to traditional medical healers. In developed countries, senior ophthalmologists may occasionally choose to reduce their activities to those of assistants.

Australia is similar to other developed countries except for its Aboriginal and Torres Strait Islander peoples who are unique. The late Prof. Fred Hollows and Prof. Hugh Taylor used their bully pulpits as Commanders of the Order of Australia to highlight the tremendous needs of these ancient peoples and the need to train eye health workers from their midst because of both their language and cultural understanding, and ownership of their own health programs which ensures full participation. Aboriginal and Torres Strait Islander health workers receive skills transfer so that they may participate in screening, particularly in outback areas. The majority of screening, however, is performed by optometrists and the federal government gives them a rebate for screening.

Where cross training has occurred, the Aboriginal and Torres Strait Islander eye health workers also take digital fundus photos for the recording of diabetic retinopathy (Fig. 53.4), and they form an important interface with the general practitioners in the remote rural areas of middle Australia who value the photographic records and the increased understanding of their patients' problems.

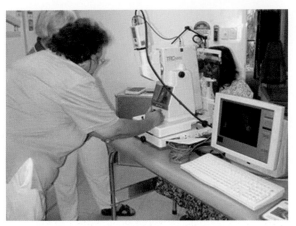

Fig. 53.4 Aboriginal eye health worker, Dot Butler, taking digital fundus photos in the screening for diabetic retinopathy in Australia. (Courtesy Frank Billson, MD.)

Aboriginal and Torres Strait Islander peoples are trained in the Northern Territory and in New South Wales.

Summary

The evolution of the profession of AOP differs around the world. It is important to acknowledge the profound effect of global and local prevention of blindness programs, especially in LMICs, and the role that AOP play. Specifically, the human resource and blinding disease targets set by WHO and IAPB in the VISION2020: The Right to Sight initiative have reshaped the training, deployment, and daily tasks of AOP not to mention the advocacy and legislation to support the training and employment of AOP in many countries.

Over the years, quite a few of the JCAHPO-certified AOP (OMP) have been motivated to serve as instructors or in other capacities in places of great need, especially in Africa and Asia. And in 2009, JCAHPO's long-standing interest in worldwide ophthalmic assisting led to the official creation of IJCAHPO, the International JCAHPO. The languages, methods, diseases, and certainly the job descriptions may be different, but the common cause remains the same for all AOP throughout the world: their patients' right to sight.

In Remembrance

Peter Y. Evans, M.D. passed away on December 18, 2020, 1 day before his 95th birthday. He was born in Tokyo, Japan and grew up in Germany and Austria. He graduated from the University of Innsbruck Medical School and completed his ophthalmology residency at the University of Innsbruck and the University of Frankfurt/Main. In 1959 he accepted a teaching position at Georgetown University Hospital in Washington, DC. He was instrumental in elevating the Division of Ophthalmology under the Department of Surgery to an independent Department of Ophthalmology where he served as Professor and Chairman from 1969 to 1983 and Professor *Emeritus* until 1992. Peter Evans was an educator at heart finding nothing more rewarding than teaching residents to become outstanding ophthalmologists. He saw the need to formally train paramedical ophthalmic personnel and in 1963, established the world's first 2-year training program for allied ophthalmic personnel at Georgetown University's School of Medicine. As a Founding Commissioner of the Joint Commission on Allied Health Personnel in Ophthalmology (JCAHPO), he served as its President (1980–1981) and Executive Vice President (1981–1995). JCAHPO honored him with their "Commissioner Statesmanship Award" in 1988 and "Special Decade Award" in 1997 among his many distinguished awards. He was dedicated to the development of Allied Ophthalmic Personnel globally and will forever be remembered as a founder of the allied ophthalmic profession.

Acknowledgments

The authors are grateful to the following for their contributions to this chapter: Prof. Dupe Ademola-Popoola, MBBS (Lagos 1991), FMCOphth(2001), FWACS(2001) Nigeria; Carlos Arieta, MD, Brazil; Nermine El-Bahtimy, DHCHM, Egypt; Prof. Seydou BAKAYOKO, Mali; Prof. Frank Billson, AO, MBBS(Melb) DMedSc(Melb) FRANZCO FRACS FRCS FACS, Australia; Mitchell V. Brinks, MD, MPH, USA; Milagros Colon de Lopez, RN, Puerto Rico; Prof. Francisco Contreras, MD, Peru; Prof. Allen Foster, UK; Prof. Paul Foster, UK; Suzanne Gilbert, PhD, MPH; Prof. Wei He, China; Brigitte Hudicourt, MD, Haiti; Khumbo Kalua, PhD, MSc, DLSHTM, MMed MBBS, Malawi; Jefitha Karimurio, MD, Kenya; Dr. Dan Kiage, Kenya; Ing. Alberto LAZO Legua, Peru; Prof. Amel Ouertani, Tunisia; Howard Pyle, JD, USA; Serge Resnikoff, MD, PhD, Switzerland; Luis Serrano, MD, Puerto Rico; Dr. Ahmed Trabelsi, Tunisia; Arq. Juan Francisco Yee, Guatemala.

References

1. IAPB Vision Atlas, First Edition, 2017. atlas.iapb.org.
2. Worldometer. https://www.worldometers.info/demographics/brazil-demographics/.
3. International Council of Ophthalmology, Brazilian Council of Ophthalmology. http://www.icoph.org/advancing_leadership/ophthalmologic_societies/society_detail/001A00000085c5GIAQ/Brazilian-Council-of-Ophthalmology.html.
4. Worldometer. https://www.worldometers.info/demographics/guatemala-demographics/.
5. Guatemalan Association of Ophthalmology. http://oftalmologosdeguatemala.org/directorio_lista.asp?clc=328&di=25.
6. Worldometer. https://www.worldometers.info/demographics/haiti-demographics/.
7. International Council of Ophthalmology, Haitian Society of Ophthalmology. http://www.icoph.org/advancing_leadership/ophthalmologic_societies/society_detail/001A00000085c5aIAA/Haitian-Society-of-Ophthalmology.html.
8. International Council of Ophthalmology, Peruvian Society of Ophthalmology. http://www.icoph.org/advancing_leadership/ophthalmologic_societies/society_detail/001A00000085c66IAA/Peruvian-Society-of-Ophthalmology.html.
9. Worldometer. https://www.worldometers.info/demographics/peru-demographics/.
10. Pew Research Center, July 2019. https://www.pewresearch.org/fact-tank/2019/07/26/puerto-rico-population-2018/.
11. International Council of Ophthalmology, Haitian Society of Ophthalmology. http://www.icoph.org/advancing_leadership/ophthalmologic_societies/society_detail/001A00000085cd8IAA/Puerto-Rican-Ophthalmology-Society.html.
12. Worldometer. https://www.worldometers.info/demographics/kenya-demographics/.
13. Universal Health 2030. http://universalhealth2030.org/2016/10/26/kenyauneven-distribution-eye-specialists-aggravates-kenyas-blindness-plight/.
14. Karimurio J, African Programme: Kenya, Community Eye Health Journal, International Centre for Eye Health, London, 2000. https://www.ncbi.nlm.nih.gov/pmc/articles/PMC1705981/.
15. National Nurses Association of Kenya. https://www.nnak.or.ke/ophthalmic-chapter/.
16. Southern African Development Community. https://www.sadc.int/about-sadc/.
17. Kalua K. How to create a balanced eye team: an example from Malawi. *Comm Eye Health J*. 2018;31:102.
18. Personal communication from Dr. BAKAYOKO Seydou, 21 May 2020.
19. Worldometer. https://www.worldometers.info/demographics/nigeria-demographics/.
20. Ophthalmological Society of Nigeria. http://www.icoph.org/advancing_leadership/ophthalmologic_societies/society_detail/001A00000085c60IAA/Ophthalmological-Society-of-Nigeria.html.
21. International Council of Ophthalmology. http://www.icoph.org/ophthalmologists-worldwide.html.
22. Worldometer. https://www.worldometers.info/demographics/tanzania-demographics/.
23. Worldometer. https://www.worldometers.info/demographics/uganda-demographics/.
24. International Council of Ophthalmology. http://www.icoph.org/ophthalmologists-worldwide.html.
25. Kaggwa G. Ophthalmic Clinical Officers: developments in Uganda. Comm Eye Health Journal, International Centre for Eye Health, London, 2014. https://www.ncbi.nlm.nih.gov/pmc/articles/PMC4194849/.
26. Worldometer. https://www.worldometers.info/world-population/egypt-population/.
27. Egyptian Ophthalmological Society. http://www.icoph.org/advancing_leadership/ophthalmologic_societies/society_detail/001A00000085c5QIAQ/Egyptian-Ophthalmological-Society.html.
28. Worldometer. https://www.worldometers.info/world-population/tunisia-population/.
29. International Council of Ophthalmology. http://www.icoph.org/advancing_leadership/ophthalmologic_societies/society_detail/001A00000085cdJIAQ/Tunisian-Ophthalmological-Society.html.
30. Wordometer. https://www.worldometers.info/world-population/bangladesh-population/.
31. International Council of Ophthalmology. http://www.icoph.org/advancing_leadership/ophthalmologic_societies/society_detail/001A00000085c5DIAQ/Ophthalmological-Society-of-Bangladesh.html.
32. Worldometer. https://www.worldometers.info/demographics/india-demographics/.
33. International Council of Ophthalmology. http://www.icoph.org/ophthalmologists-worldwide.html.
34. https://www.livemint.com/news/india/estimates-of-blindness-reduced-by-47-in-12-years-govt-survey-11570733865393.html.
35. Worldometer. https://www.worldometers.info/world-population/nepal-population/.
36. Nepal Fact Sheet, Seva Foundation 2018. http://www.seva.org/pdf/Seva_Country_Fact_Sheets_Nepal.pdf.
37. Worldometer. https://www.worldometers.info/world-population/marshall-islands-population/.
38. Worldometer. https://www.worldometers.info/world-population/micronesia-population/.
39. Worldometer. https://www.worldometers.info/world-population/myanmar-population/.
40. Worldometer. https://www.worldometers.info/demographics/thailand-demographics/.
41. World Population Review. https://worldpopulationreview.com/countries/australia-population/.

Chapter | 54 |

Eye banking

Jeremy Shuman and Lisa Buckland

Introduction

What is eye banking and why is it relevant to *me*, the ophthalmic assistant?

Ophthalmic clinics will see patients with cornea disease. Some of those patients may require a cornea transplant to treat the diseased cornea. Other eye surgeries also require ocular tissue for transplant (glaucoma shunt patch, enucleation, and others). The eye bank provides corneas and other ocular tissue to surgery centers for transplantation (Fig. 54.1).

Around the world, there are tens of millions requiring a cornea transplant.[1-3] In more developed countries, the prevalence is very low and transplant rate is very high,[2] with nearly everyone being treated as needed. Whereas in low and middle-income countries, the incidence and prevalence is very high; there are patients who remain untreated for multiple structural reasons (cost, access, infrastructure, training, funding, etc.).[1] In these cases, many patients in the clinic may be evaluated and diagnosed, but will not be treated to effectively restore sight in that eye.

For those able to be treated with a cornea transplant, the eye bank provides the cornea. This comprises 99% of the activity of an eye bank. Some eye banks also provide other ocular tissues. For glaucoma shunt surgeries, the eye bank provides a piece of sclera or cornea to cover the outer end of the tube. For enucleations, the eye bank provides a whole sclera as a globe-shaped envelope for a prosthesis. Because corneas are the primary focus of eye banking, this chapter will be focused on cornea donation and transplantation.

The eye bank

The eye bank serves as a community resource and a link between the person who donates their eye or cornea (the donor), and the surgeon who transplants it into the patient needing a transplant (the recipient). Some organs and tissues can be donated from living donors (blood donation or kidney donation), however most donations of organs and tissues only can occur after death (heart, lung, bone, etc.). Like the latter, eye donation can only occur after death. Once an individual passes away, they can be considered for eye donation. The surgical recovery and preservation of the cornea must occur soon after death. The eye bank manages the identification of potential donors, screening for eligibility of donation, surgical recovery, processing, testing for infectious diseases, and distribution to surgery—thus forming the link between the donor and the surgeon (and the surgeon is the link between the eye bank and the recipient).

The eye bank is uniquely specialized to cover all these key activities from death of the donor to distribution of donor's cornea to the surgeon; the eye bank must maintain key relationships with community organizations for each step of the process.

For example, many potential donors pass away in hospitals. The hospital must provide the eye bank technician

Once a cornea arrives at a surgery center, it must remain at a suitable storage temperature to maintain cell viability. The suitable temperature depends on the method used (and will be clearly labeled as such). Freezing will destroy living cells; freezing is only appropriate in special circumstances and if so, will be clearly labeled as such. Usually, corneas are transplanted within 24 hours of arrival.

Finances/sustainability

Because of the potential for misuse, human organ and tissue donation must have safeguards to ensure ethical stewardship of the donated gift. One way to do that is through regulatory oversight, and the other is through financial incentives (or disincentives). The sale of human organs and tissues is illegal worldwide, and clear ethical guidelines support this.[10] The financial structure of the eye bank can encourage ethical stewardship of the gift by disincentivizing profits. The overwhelming majority of eye banks are nonprofit, and many are subsidiary programs within larger nonprofits, public educational systems (universities), or government agencies. This structure removes personal incentives to profit from eye banking.

Although the incentives for profiteering are reduced, there remains a need for financial sustainability, to keep the organization viable and financially healthy. Most eye banks charge a service fee to cover the costs of their services, including everything from employees' salaries and facility costs, to the donor's laboratory blood test for infectious disease and the cornea storage solution, and shipping or delivery charges to transport the cornea from the eye bank to the hospital operating room.

Facility

Surprisingly, an eye bank serving a modest city of 1 million population, only needs a few rooms (laboratory space, office space, supply/storage space). The largest eye banks, serving worldwide usually have multiple facilities for recovery, and one facility for centralized tissue processing and distribution. The more services provided, the more space and specialized equipment or rooms required. Many leading eye banks now have operating rooms for in-house aseptic tissue processing and preparation procedures.

Management and Staff

Specially-trained staff perform various duties. There are specialists for each part of the process: to approach the deceased families for consent for donation, screen for medical contraindications, surgically recover the cornea from the cadaver, evaluate the corneas via microscope, surgically process the corneas into various graft types, medically approve the donor for transplant, match each cornea with a patient, oversee quality and regulatory affairs, liaise with donor hospitals, and various other functions. All training occurs at the eye bank. There is standardization available for eye bank technicians in the United States—a certification examination similar in concept to the Ophthalmic Assistant certification. The eye bank technician certification examination is taken after training is complete and technicians are already working independently. In the United States, career paths have opportunity for growth. Many organization's CEOs began their careers as technicians.

Eye bank associations and medical standards

The field of eye banking is relatively small, which makes international connections ever more important. Worldwide, there are several eye bank associations that have related purposes, although all are different. The EBAA (www.restoresight.org) is the longest-standing eye bank association, with a rich history of technician and surgeon (or vendor and customer) collaboration toward a common goal (Fig. 54.6). This association independently sets medical standards, provides eye bank accreditation, provides technician certification, lobbies government, promotes donation, tracks surgical activity and outcomes, and supports scientific progress. Most eye bank associations have similar aspirations and are regionally located around the world.

Eye Bank Associations worldwide include (Fig. 54.7):

EBAA (www.restoresight.org)
European Eye Bank Association (www.eeba.eu)
Association of Eye Banks of Asia (eyebankingasia.org)
Eye Bank Association of Australia and New Zealand (www.ebaanz.org)
Pan American Association of Eye Banks (www.apaboeyebanks.org) and (www.apabo.org.br)
Eye Bank Association of India (www.ebai.org)
Global Alliance of Eye Bank Associations (www.gaeba.org)

Medical regulations are also created by government entities. Many countries have a transplant agency within or associated with the Ministry of Health. In the United States, the FDA sets the rules, regulations, and performs on-site facility inspections. The regulation is published in the Code of Federal Regulations, titled 21 CFR 1271 (www.ecfr.gov). These rules and regulations are coordinated with the EBAA Medical Standards to create a cohesive rules environment.

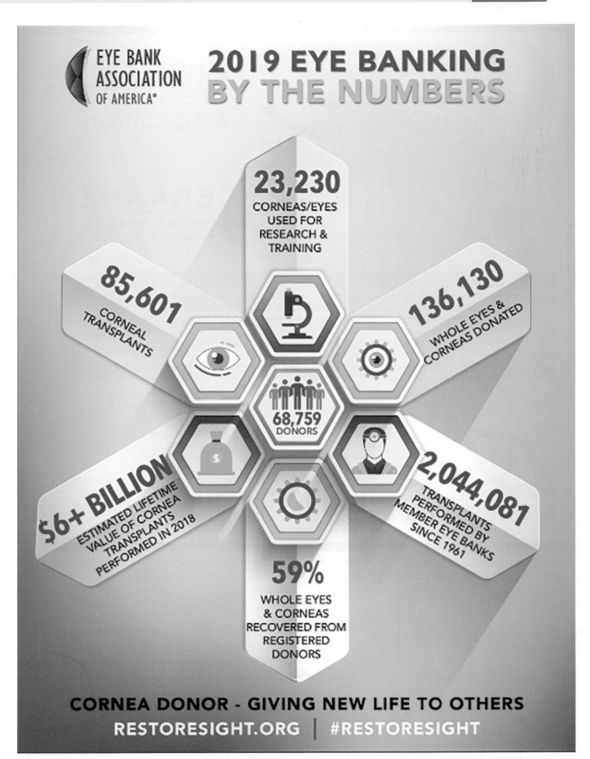

Fig. 54.6 Eye Bank Association of America statistical summary graphic. (Courtesy Eye Bank Association America.)

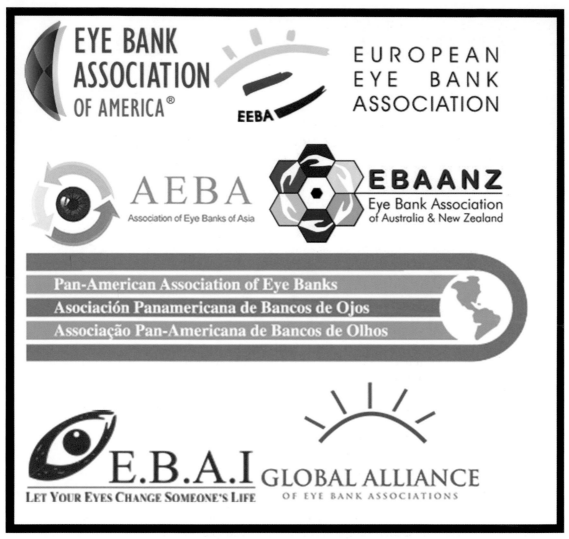

Fig. 54.7 Eye Bank Association Logos. (Courtesy Eye Bank Association of America, European Eye Bank Association, Association of Eye Banks of Asia, Eye Bank Association of Australia and New Zealand, Pan-American Association of Eye Banks, Eye Bank Association of India, and Global Alliance of Eye Bank Associations.)

Ethics and guiding principles

The World Health Organization (WHO) publishes guiding principles regarding human cell, tissue, and organ transplantation. The guiding principles outline the absolute basic requirements for ethical and safe donation and transplantation. A few are listed here:

- Organs may be removed from deceased if there is legal consent obtained, and no known objection by the donor

- Those involved in death of the potential donor should not be directly involved in donation from that individual or transplantation of those organs or tissues
- No payment or reward to the donors next-of-kin
- No sale or purchase of organs, or access to organs, but reasonable costs may be reimbursed for donation and processing
- Allocation of organs and tissues should be by clinical criteria and ethical norms (not financial considerations)
- Tissue should be safe and efficacious for transplant

The principles can be read in full as published by WHO in WHA63.22 (www.who.int/transplantation). These are also a basis, in part, to The Barcelona Principles published by the Global Alliance of Eye Bank Associations (www.gaeba.org/publications)—which is a global bioethical frame-work and agreement on the use of ocular donations. This is specific to eye banking and developed in agreement with eye banking and ophthalmic organizations worldwide. With a similar theme, this agreement provides more fidelity and relevance to eye banking, including principles such as:

- Support sight restoration for recipients: encourage development of new technologies
- Promote fair, equitable, and transparent allocation (urgent and severe cases get corneas first)
- Uphold the integrity of the custodian's profession (good stewardship of the gift)
- Develop services to promote ethical management, traceability, and utility (prevent fraud)
- Recognize and address potential ethical, legal, and clinical implications of cross-border activities

These and many other public debates, guiding principles, and publications inform the worldwide community of eye banking on appropriate policies and program management.

References

1. Oliva MS, Schottman T, Gulati M. Turning the tide of corneal blindness. *Indian J Ophthalmol*. 2012;60(5):423–427.
2. Gain P, Jullienne R, He Z, et al. Global survey of corneal transplantation and eye banking. *JAMA Ophthalmol*. 2016;134(2):167–173.
3. World report on vision. World Health Organization Web site. https://www.who.int/publications/i/item/9789241516570. Accessed June 24, 2021.
4. Hoffman N, Wittmershaus I, Michaelis R, et al. Pre-prepared corneal grafts for facilitated descemet membrane endothelial keratoplasty (DMEK)-controlled and standardized manufacturing in the eye bank may lead to reduced re-DMEK rates. *Int J Eye Bank*. 2018;6(3):1–6.
5. Doughman DJ, Roger CC. Eye banking in the 21st century: How far have we come? Are we prepared for what's ahead? *Int J Eye Bank*. 2012;1(1):1–15.
6. Wang X, Jin L, Wang J, et al. Attitudes and knowledge concerning corneal donation in a population-based sample of urban Chinese adults. *Cornea*. 2016;35(10):1362–1367.
7. Religion and Organ Donation. Heath Resources & Service Administration Web site. https://www.organdonor.gov/about/donors/religion.html. Accessed June 24, 2021.
8. Bruzzone P. Religious aspects of organ transplantation. *Transplant Proc*. 2008;40(4):1064–1067.
9. Lass JH, Sugar A, Benetz BA, et al. Endothelial cell density to predict endothelial graft failure after penetrating keratoplasty. *Arch Ophthalmol*. 2010;128(1):63–69.
10. World Health Organization. WHO guiding principles on human cell, tissue, and organ transplantation. May 2010. https://www.who.int/transplantation/Guiding_PrinciplesTransplantation_WHA63.22en.pdf. Accessed June 28, 2021.

Websites

- Eye Bank Association of America: www.restoresight.org.
- European Eye Bank Association: www.eeba.eu.
- Association of Eye Banks of Asia: eyebankingasia.org.
- Eye Bank Association of Australia and New Zealand: www.ebaanz.org.
- Pan American Association of Eye Banks: www.apaboeyebanks.org and www.apabo.org.br.
- Eye Bank Association of India: www.ebai.org.
- Global Alliance of Eye Bank Associations: www.gaeba.org.

Continued

Q

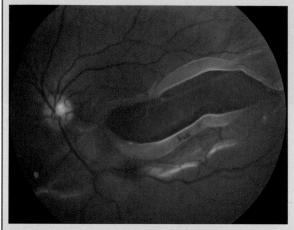

Fig. 55.11 Question 11 What is your diagnosis?

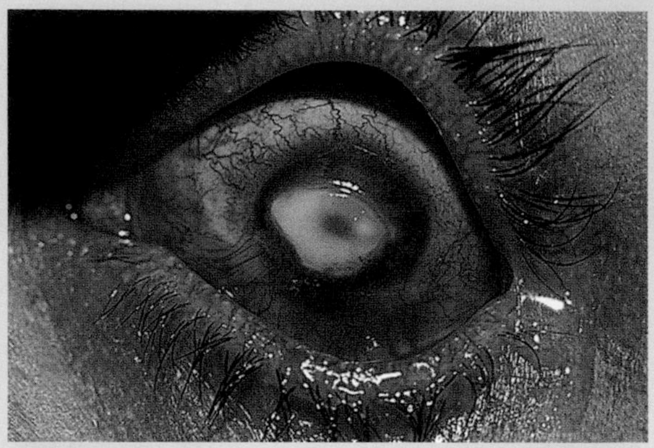

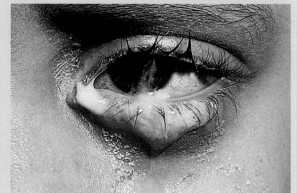

Fig. 55.14 Question 14 What is your diagnosis?

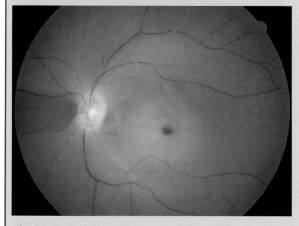

Fig. 55.12 Question 12 What is your diagnosis?

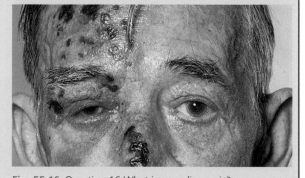

Fig. 55.15 Question 15 What is your diagnosis?

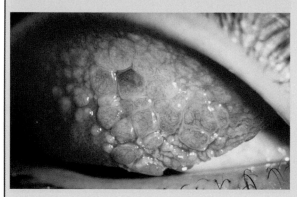

Fig. 55.13 Question 13 What is your diagnosis?

Fig. 55.16 Question 16 What is your diagnosis?

Continued Q

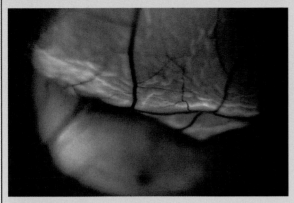

Fig. 55.17 Question 17 What is your diagnosis?

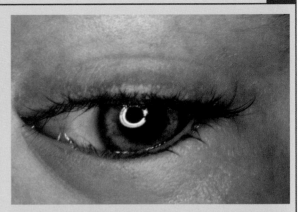

Fig. 55.20 Question 20 What is your diagnosis?

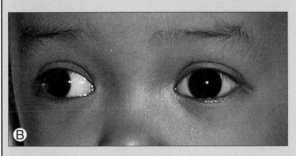

Fig. 55.18 Question 18 What is your diagnosis?

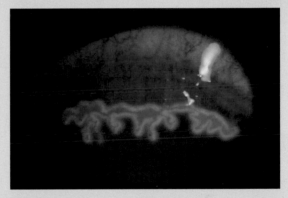

Fig. 55.21 Question 21 What is your diagnosis?

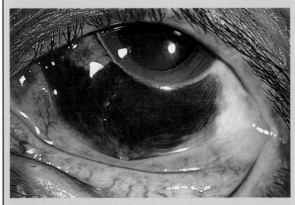

Fig. 55.19 Question 19 What is your diagnosis?

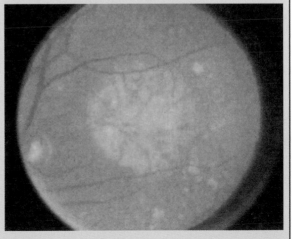

Fig. 55.22 Question 22 What is your diagnosis?

Continued

Q

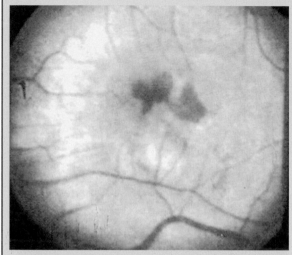

Fig. 55.23 Question 23 What is your diagnosis?

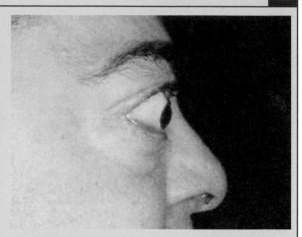

Fig. 55.25 Question 25 What is your diagnosis?

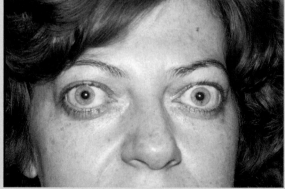

Fig. 55.26 Question 26 What is your diagnosis?

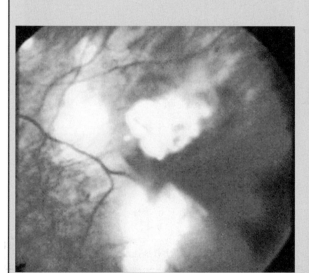

Fig. 55.24 Question 24 What is your diagnosis?

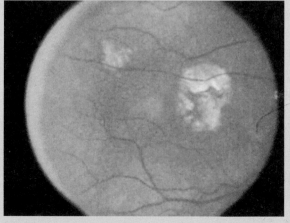

Fig. 55.27 Question 27 What is your diagnosis?

Continued

Q

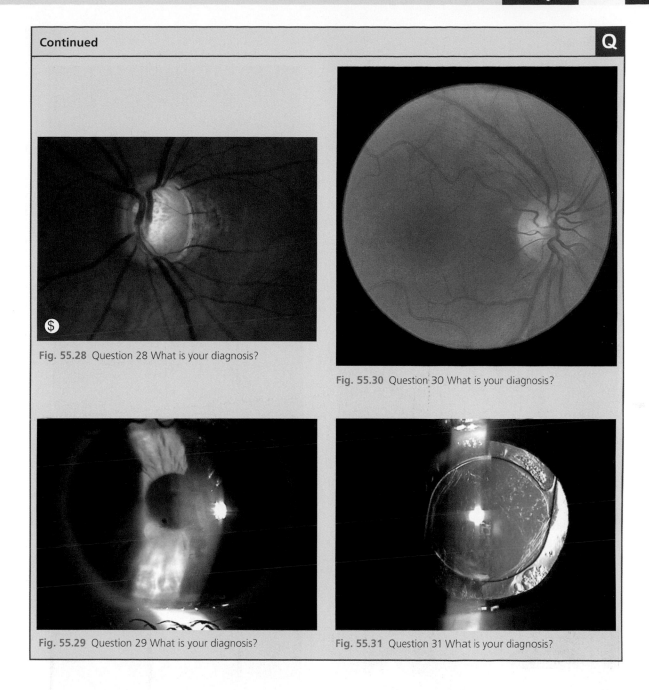

Fig. 55.28 Question 28 What is your diagnosis?

Fig. 55.30 Question 30 What is your diagnosis?

Fig. 55.29 Question 29 What is your diagnosis?

Fig. 55.31 Question 31 What is your diagnosis?

Continued Q

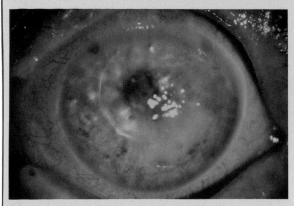

Fig. 55.32 Question 32 What is your diagnosis?

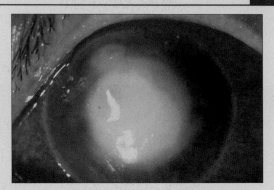

Fig. 55.35 Question 35 What is your diagnosis?

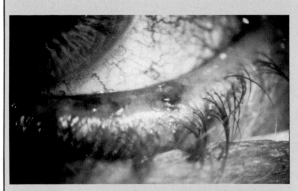

Fig. 55.33 Question 33 What is your diagnosis?

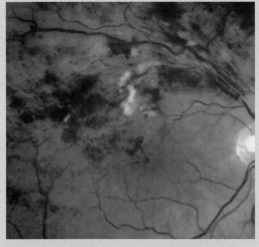

Fig. 55.36 Question 36 What is your diagnosis?

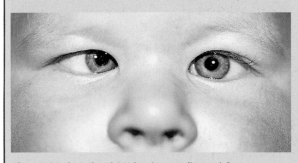

Fig. 55.34 Question 34 What is your diagnosis?

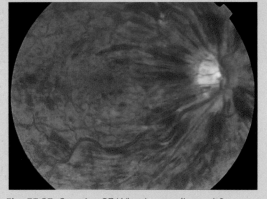

Fig. 55.37 Question 37 What is your diagnosis?

Answers

A

1. Dacryocystitis
2. Hyperthyroidism
3. Corneal ulcer with hypopyon
4. Advanced keratoconus
5. Arcus senilis
6. Acute bacterial conjunctivitis
7. Traumatic cataract
8. Corneal abrasion
9. Acid burn of the cornea
10. Central retinal vein occlusion
11. Retinal tear with associated retinal detachment
12. Retinal artery occlusion
13. Vernal conjunctivitis
14. Corneal ulcer caused by *Acanthamoeba*
15. Conjunctivitis
16. Herpes zoster
17. Retinal detachment
18. Strabismus—exotropia
19. Subconjunctival hemorrhage
20. Entropion
21. Dendritic patter of herpes simplex keratitis on the cornea
22. Macular degeneration
23. Choroideremia
24. Retinoblastoma
25. Thyroid exophthalmos
26. Exophthalmos in Graves disease
27. Histoplasmosis
28. Glaucoma optic atrophy
29. Corneal edema
30. Cystoid macular edema
31. Capsular opacification
32. Pseudophakic bullous keratopathy
33. Blepharitis
34. Infantile esotropia
35. Corneal ulcer
36. Branch vein occlusion
37. Central vein occlusion

References to Figures

Fig. 55.2 From Spalton D, Hitchings R, Hunter P. *Atlas of Clinical Ophthalmology*. 3rd ed. St Louis: Mosby; 2004, with permission.

Fig. 55.10 From Kanski J, Bowling B. *Clinical Ophthalmology: a Systematic Approach*. 7th ed. Edinburgh: Saunders; 2011, with permission.

Fig. 55.11 From Kanski J, Bowling B. *Clinical Ophthalmology: a Systematic Approach*. 7th ed. Edinburgh: Saunders; 2011, with permission.

Fig. 55.12 From Kanski J, Bowling B. *Clinical Ophthalmology: a Systematic Approach*. 7th ed. Edinburgh: Saunders; 2011, with permission.

Fig. 55.16 From Spalton D, Hitchings R, Hunter P. *Atlas of Clinical Ophthalmology*. 3rd ed. St Louis: Mosby; 2004, with permission.

Fig. 55.18 From Yankoff M, Duker JS. *Ophthalmology*, 5th ed. Edinburgh: Elsevier; 2019, with permission.

Fig. 55.20 From Kanski J, Bowling B. *Clinical Ophthalmology: a Systematic Approach*. 7th ed. Edinburgh: Saunders; 2011, with permission.

Fig. 55.21 From Yankoff M, Duker JS. *Ophthalmology*, 5th ed. Edinburgh: Elsevier; 2019, with permission.

Fig. 55.28 From Bowling B. *Kranski's Clinical Ophthalmology: a Systemic Approach*, 8th ed. Edinburgh: Elsevier; 2016, with permission.

Fig. 55.30 From Spalton D, Hitchings R, Hunter P. *Atlas of Clinical Ophthalmology*. 3rd ed. St Louis: Mosby; 2004, with permission.

Fig. 55.34 From Kanski J. *Clinical Ophthalmology: a Systematic Approach*. 5th ed. Burlington, MA: Butterworth-Heinemann; 2003, with permission.

Fig. 55.35 From Yankoff M, Duker JS. *Ophthalmology*, 5th ed. Edinburgh: Elsevier; 2019, with permission.

Fig. 55.36 From Kanski J, Bowling B. *Clinical Ophthalmology—a Systematic Approach*. 7th ed. Edinburgh: Saunders; 2011, with permission.

Fig. 55.37 From Kanski J, Bowling B. *Clinical Ophthalmology—a Systematic Approach*. 7th ed. Edinburgh: Saunders; 2011, with permission.

Glossary*

3 and 9 o'clock staining erosion of the cornea at the 3 and 9 o'clock positions; seen commonly in rigid lenses.

A-scan an ultrasound technique to determine the axial length of the eye to calculate the intraocular lens power required.Abbe number an indication of optical quality. Number is inversely proportional to the chromic dispersion of a specific lens material. Crown glass is 59.

abduct to turn away from the midline.

abductor a muscle that rotates the eye away from the midline (e.g., lateral rectus).

aberrant deviating from the usual course.

ablation removal of tissue as occurs with the excimer laser on the cornea for refractive changes.

abrasion rubbing off of the superficial layer.

abscess localized area of inflammation.

AC/A accommodative convergence/accommodation ratio; expressed as the ratio between convergence caused by accommodation (in prism diopters) and the accommodation (in diopters).

accommodation adjustment by the eye for seeing at different distances, accomplished by changing the shape of the crystalline lens through action of the ciliary muscle.

achloropsia color blindness to green.

achromatic lens a lens that neutralizes dispersion without interfering with refraction.

acuity clearness; visual acuity is measured by the smallest object that can be seen at a certain distance.

add the total dioptric power added to a distance prescription to supplement accommodation for reading.

adductor a muscle that exerts force toward the midline (e.g., medial rectus).

adenovirus a virus comprising a large group of different serotypes. Types 3, 7, 8, 11, and 19 are those most commonly associated with eye infections. Types 8 and 19 are associated with epidemic keratoconjunctivitis (EKC) and types 3 and 7 with pharyngoconjunctival fever (PCF).

Adie's pupil a tonic pupil with sluggish response to light, accommodation, and convergence.

adnexa oculi accessory structures of the eye, such as the lacrimal apparatus and the eyelids.

adoptive optics devices and methods to custom correct high-order aberrations. These include special spectacles, contact lenses, intraocular lenses, and refractive surgery.

afterimage image of an object that persists when the lids are closed.

AIDS (acquired immunodeficiency syndrome) a viral infection characterized by a compromised immune system.

akinesia absence of motor function.

albinism hereditary loss of pigment in the eye, skin, and hair; usually associated with lowered visual acuity, nystagmus, and light sensitivity.

alexia inability to read words previously known even though visual perception is clear.

allied ophthalmic personnel (AOP) skilled professionals, qualified by didactic and clinical ophthalmic training, who perform ophthalmic procedures under the direction of a licensed ophthalmologist. The World Health Organization has established definitions of the eye care workforce cadres and their levels with AOP including ophthalmic assistants, technicians, and medical technologists. This AOP definition was adopted by the Cambridge Declaration for Global Recognition, in a collaboration of the International Joint Commission on Allied Health Personnel in Ophthalmology, Agency for the Prevention of Blindness, and the International Council of Ophthalmology.

amaurosis partial or total blindness from any cause.

amaurosis fugax temporary blindness.

amblyopia loss of vision without any apparent disease of the eye.

amblyopia ex anopsia loss of vision from disuse of the eye, usually a result of uncorrected refractive errors.

ametropia a refractive error in which the eye, when in a state of rest, does not focus the image of an object on the retina; includes hyperopia, myopia, and astigmatism. *See* refractive error.

Amsler's grid a chart with horizontal and vertical lines for testing macular distortion.

---

*Attention is directed to the companion texts for a more complete set of reference dictionaries: Stein HA, Slatt, BJ, Stein RM. *Ophthalmic Terminology: Speller and Vocabulary Builder*. 3rd ed. St Louis: Mosby; 1992 and Stein HA, Stein RM, Freeman MI, Massare JS. *Ophthalmic Dictionary and Vocabulary Builder—for Eye Care Professionals*. 4th ed. New Delhi: Jaypee-Highlights Medical Publishers; 2011. Also adopted from Stein HA, Slatt BJ, Stein RM, Freeman MI. *Fitting Guide for Rigid and Soft Lenses: A Practical Approach*. 4th ed. St Louis: Mosby; 2002.

angiography outlining of the lumen of the blood vessel by injection of material that can be visualized by x-ray film or the eye.

angioma a tumor consisting of blood vessels.

angle kappa the difference between the direction of gaze and the apparent direction in which the eye points; this normal structural feature may cause a false interpretation of strabismus.

aniridia congenital absence of the iris.

aniseikonia a condition in which the ocular image of an object as seen by one eye differs so much in size or shape from that seen by the other eye that the two images cannot be fused into a single impression.

anisocoria inequality of the pupils in diameter.

ankyloblepharon adhesion of upper and lower eyelids.

annulus ring-shaped structure.

anomaly departure from the normal.

anophthalmia absence of a true eyeball.

anterior chamber space in the front of the eye, bounded in front by the cornea and behind by the iris; filled with aqueous humor.

anterior chamber angle angle between the iris and the cornea that contains the trabecula and through which the aqueous flows out of the eye.

anterior segment referring to the front part of the eye.

antibody a specific substance produced by the body in the presence of an antigen

antigen any substance that when introduced in the body incites formation of an antibody.

antihistamine substance that acts against the action of histamine.

aphakia absence of the lens of the eye.

aphasia loss of power of expression either by speech or by writing.

applanation flattening of the cornea in measurement of the intraocular pressure.

aqueous humor clear, watery fluid that fills the anterior and posterior chambers within the front part of the eye.

arcuate scotoma characteristically arc-shaped area of blindness in the field of vision; caused by interruption of a nerve fiber bundle in the retina; most often seen in glaucoma.

arcus senilia grayish white ring in the periphery of the cornea.

Argyll Robertson pupil a pupil characterized by nonreaction to direct and consensual light but normal contraction for accommodation and convergence.

argyrosis gray discoloration of the skin and conjunctiva caused by deposition of silver salts; occurs with either systemic intake of a silver compound or topical application.

arteriography visualization of blood vessels by injection of material that can be seen by x-ray film or naked eyes.

arteriosclerosis thickening and loss of contractibility of an artery, usually associated with old age.

artifact that which is altered.

asepsis absence of microorganisms.

asteroid resembling a star.

asteroid hyalitis round or disc-like bodies (calcium soaps) in the vitreous; they do not impair vision.

asthenopia eye fatigue caused by tiring of the internal and/or external muscles.

astigmatism a refractive error that prevents the light rays from coming to a single focus on the retina because of different degrees of refraction in the various meridians of the eye.

astigmatism, "against-the-rule" condition in which the steepest corneal meridian is in the horizontal (180-degree) plane.

astigmatism, irregular astigmatism caused by an irregularly shaped cornea (arising from a condition, such as scarring or keratoconus). Irregular astigmatism is not correctable by cylinders.

astigmatism, oblique regular astigmatism in which the principal meridians are other than 90 and 180 degrees.

astigmatism, regular astigmatism that is correctable by cylinders (there are two retinal focal points in regular astigmatism).

astigmatism, residual astigmatism remaining after the corneal astigmatism has been neutralized. In general, residual astigmatism is *lenticular*, resulting from the eye's crystalline lens having a toric surface.

astigmatism, "with-the-rule" condition in which the steepest corneal meridian is in the vertical (90-degree) plane.

atrophy wasting or decrease of a tissue because of faulty nutrition or loss of nerve supply.

atropine an alkaloid that produces mydriasis and cycloplegia.

attenuation narrowing of a vessel

automated lamellar keratoplasty (ALK) a surgical procedure in which the patient's own anterior cornea is removed with a microkeratome. The removed cornea is reshaped in a flattened state and the anterior layer is replaced on the patient's cornea.

B-scan an ultrasonic technique to provide a two-dimensional cross-section of the eye and orbital tissue.

bacteriocide a chemical that disinfects and kills pathogenic organisms.

ballasted lens a contact lens that has a cross-sectional shape with a heavier base so that it orients inferiorly when the lens is worn.

bandage lens a contact lens that is used over the cornea to protect the cornea from external influences and permit healing of underlying pathology.

bar reader an appliance that provides for the placement of an opaque septum, or bar, between the printed page and the reader's eyes so as to occlude different areas of the page for each of the eyes. Used for diagnosis and training of simultaneous binocular vision.

Barr body sex-linked inactive X chromosome.

base curve the curvature of the central part of the posterior surface of a lens. Base curve is expressed in millimeters of radius of curvature or in diopters. Also referred to as *central posterior curve*.

819

bear tracks of the retina congenital pigmentation deposits on the retina.

bedewing cornea an edematous condition of the epithelium of the cornea characterized by irregular reflection from a multitude of droplets when the cornea is viewed with the slit lamp.

belladonna the plant *Atropa belladonna*, from the leaves and roots of which may be obtained the poisonous alkaloid precursors of various medically useful narcotics, chief among which is atropine.

benign tumor nonmalignant growth.

biconcave lens lens having a concave surface on both faces.

biconvex lens lens having a convex surface on both faces.

bifocal lens a lens with two areas for viewing, each with its own focal power.

binocular vision ability to use the two eyes simultaneously to focus on the same object and to fuse the two images into a single image that gives a correct interpretation of its solidity and its position in space.

biomicroscopy microscopic examination of the cornea, anterior chamber lens, and posterior chamber contents with a slit-lamp microscope. The magnification is approximately × 10 to × 50.

Bjerrum's scotoma a half ring-like visual field defect arising from the disc and extending around fixation.

Bjerrum's screen a tangent screen.

blennorrhea a mucoid discharge from various parts of the body, including the external eye, caused by an inflammatory process.

blepharitis inflammation of the margins of the eyelids.

blepharochalasis excessive relaxation of eyelid skin caused by loss of elasticity.

blepharoclonus exaggerated form of reflex blinking.

blepharoconjunctivitis inflammation of the eyelid and conjunctiva.

blepharophimosis a condition in which the palpebral aperture is abnormally small.

blepharoplasty plastic surgery of the eyelid.

blepharoptosis drooping of the upper eyelid.

blepharospasm excessive winking; tonic or clonic spasm of the orbicularis oculi muscle.

blind spot the natural blind area of the retina where the optic nerve enters the eye.

blindness in the United States, usually defined as central visual acuity of 20/200 or less in the better eye after correction, or visual acuity of more than 20/200 if there is a field defect, in which the widest diameter of the visual field subtends an angle distance no greater than 20 degrees (some states include up to 30 degrees).

blue sclera thin altered sclera.

Bowman's membrane a layer of condensed stromal tissue that separates the epithelium from the stroma proper.

breakup time (BUT) tear film breakup time: the time it takes for dry spots to form on the cornea when the eye is kept in the staring position. Normal range is 10 to 30 seconds; less than 10 seconds indicates a pathologic condition.

bulbar pertaining to the globe.

buphthalmos enlargement of the eyeball, resulting usually from congenital (infantile) glaucoma.

C, CC (sum correction) with correction; that is, wearing prescribed lenses.

canal of Schlemm *see* Schlemm's canal.

canaliculus passageway for drainage of tears from eyes to tear sac.

candle unit of luminous intensity in the photometric system.

canthotomy surgical procedure for lengthening the opening between the eyelids.

canthus the angle at either end of the slit between the eyelids; specified as outer, or temporal, and inner, or nasal.

caruncle, lacrimal a pink fleshy or relatively isolated skin located in the medial canthus area adjacent to the plica semilunaris.

cataract a condition in which the crystalline lens of the eye or its capsule, or both, becomes opaque, with consequent loss of visual acuity.

central visual acuity ability of the eye to perceive in the direct line of vision.

chalazion inflammatory enlargement of a meibomian gland of the eyelid.

chamber, anterior *see* anterior chamber.

chemosis severe edema of the conjunctiva.

chiasm, optic *see* optic chiasm.

chorioretinitis inflammation of the choroid and retina.

choroid vascular, intermediate coat that furnishes nourishment to the other parts of the eyeball.

choroiditis inflammation of the choroids.

cilia (plural), cilium (singular) eyelashes.

ciliary body portion of the vascular coat between the iris and the choroid; consists of ciliary processes and the ciliary muscle.

ciliary processes finger-like projections from the ciliary body that produce aqueous humor and provide attachment for the zonules.

Coats disease a chronic exudative retinopathy, occurring between the retina and the choroid.

coloboma congenital cleft caused by the failure of the eye to complete growth in the part affected.

color deficiency diminished ability to perceive differences in color; usually reds and greens, rarely blues and yellows.

colorimeter a color-matching device used to designate an unknown colored stimulus by matching it with a known colored stimulus.

colors, complementary two colors that when mixed produce a neutral color when mixed in correct proportions.

colors, primary set of colors (red, yellow, blue) from which all other color sensations can be produced.

commotio retinae an edematous condition of the retina caused by trauma to an eye.

computerized corneal topography a computer-assisted diagnostic technique that creates a three-dimensional color-coded map of the surface curvature of the cornea, as well as a cross-sectional corneal profile. The information gained is used in fitting contact lenses, recognizing irregular corneal conditions that are difficult to detect with most conventional testing, and planning laser vision correction.

concave lens a lens having the power to diverge rays of light; also known as *diverging, reducing, negative, myopic,* or *minus lens,* denoted by the − sign.

cones and rods two kinds of cells that form a layer of the retina and act as light-receiving media. Cones are concerned with visual acuity and color discrimination, rods are used for motion and vision at low degrees of illumination (night vision).

conformer a device placed in the socket after enucleation or evisceration of an eyeball to preserve the shape of the fornices.

conjunctiva mucous membrane that lines the eyelids and covers the front part of the eyeball.

conjunctivitis inflammation of the mucous membrane lining of the eyelid and/or eyeball.

conjunctivitis, giant papillary *see* giant papillary conjunctivitis.

consensual contraction of one pupil when light is directed into the fellow eye.

consensual light reflex constriction of the opposite pupil when a beam of light is directed into the pupil of an eye.

contact lens refers to any lens that is placed on the surface of the cornea and sclera, either for *optical* purposes (improvement of visual acuity) or for *therapeutic* purposes (treatment of eye disorders).

conventional replacement contact lens a contact lens that does not have a specific replacement schedule. Conventional replacement lenses are sometimes referred to as "traditional," "durable," or "reusable" replacement lenses.

convergence process of directing the visual axes of the two eyes to a near point, with the result that the pupils of the two eyes are closer together.

convex lens a lens having the power to converge rays of light and to bring them to a focus; also known as *converging, magnifying, hyperopic,* or *plus lens,* denoted by the + sign.

cornea clear, transparent portion of the outer coat of the eyeball, forming the covering of the aqueous chamber.

corneal collagen crosslinking (CXL) a treatment for keratoconus and corneal ectasia after previous refractive surgery that uses the photosensitizer riboflavin (vitamin B_2) which when exposed to longer-wavelength ultraviolet light (370 nm UVA [ultraviolet A radiation]) induces chemical reactions in corneal stroma that result in the formation of covalent bonds between the corneal collagen molecules, fibers, and microfibrils.

corneal endothelium the innermost layer of the cornea, consisting of a single layer of cells.

corneal epithelium the outermost layer of the cornea.

corneal graft operation to restore vision by replacing a section of opaque cornea.

corneal stroma multiple sheets of collagen in the center of the cornea, which make up 90% of its thickness.

cross cylinder a lens used to measure the power and axis of an astigmatic refractive error. The cross cylinder consists of a plus and a minus cylinder set at right angles to each other with the handle set midway between the two cylinders.

crystalline lens a transparent colorless body suspended in the front part of the eyeball, between the aqueous and the vitreous, the function of which is to bring the rays of light to focus on the retina.

cup-to-disc ratio (C/D) a disc that has become cupped, usually with glaucoma, with 0.9 being the most severe.

custom ablation wavefront-guided laser treatment used to treat high-order visual aberrations allowing customized refractive surgical procedures for an individual's unique visual requirements.

cyclitis inflammation of the ciliary body.

cyclodialysis an operation to reduce the intraocular pressure by forming a pathway for fluid to drain from the anterior chamber to the space between the choroid and sclera.

cycloplegic a drug that temporarily puts the ciliary muscle at rest and dilates the pupil; often used to ascertain the error of refraction.

cylindric lens a segment of a cylinder, the refractive power of which varies in different medians, used in the correction of astigmatism.

cyst a sac containing fluid.

cystinosis disease in which ocular manifestations occur as dispersed crystals causing refractile opacities in the cornea and conjunctiva.

dacryocystectomy operation to remove the tear duct sac.

dacryocystitis inflammation of the lacrimal sac.

dacryocystogram an x-ray photograph of the lacrimal apparatus of the eye, made visible by radiopaque dyes.

dacryocystorhinostomy an operation to create a new tear duct for drainage of tears directly into the nose.

daily disposable contact lens a disposable contact lens designed for a single 1-day use. A new lens is inserted each morning and discarded before sleep the same day. The lens is not cleaned or reused, nor does the wearer sleep with the lens in place.

daily wear contact lens wear in which the lenses are inserted each morning and removed each night before sleep.

dark adaptation ability of the retina and pupil to adjust to a dim light.

decompression, orbital surgical relief of pressure behind the eyeball, as in endocrine exophthalmos, by the removal of bone from the orbit.

degeneration deterioration of an organ or a tissue, resulting in diminished vitality, either by chemical change or by infiltration of abnormal matter. In the eye, cystic degeneration of the macula is a localized macular degeneration, resulting in edema and the formation of cystic spaces in the central area of the retina, which lead to macular depression or to a complete macular hole.

dendritic keratitis fern-like projection on the cornea from herpes simplex.

depth perception ability to perceive the solidity of objects and their relative position in space; also called *stereoscopic vision*.

dermatoconjunctivitis inflammation of the skin and the palpebral conjunctiva near the eyelid margin.

dermoid congenital tumor seen as a raised yellowish lesion.

Descemet's membrane corneal layer separating the stroma from the endothelium.

detached retina complete or partial separation of retina from choroid.

dial, astigmatic a chart or pattern used for determining the presence and amount of astigmatism.

distichiasis lashes growing from openings of meibomian glands.

diopter unit of measurement of strength or refractive power of a lens.

diplopia seeing of one object as two.

direct light reflex contraction of the pupil in the presence of a beam of light with the eye gazing at a distant object. The room illumination should be dim.

disinfection physical or chemical procedures that kill common pathogenic organisms but may permit some nonpathogenic organisms to survive.

disposable contact lens a hydrogel contact lens designed to be discarded on removal from the eye.

distometer a caliper used to measure vertex distance, which is the distance from the cornea of the patient's eye to the back surface of the lens inserted in the trial frame, phoropter, or glass.

distortion aberration of rays of light.

DK a measure of the *oxygen permeability* of a given contact lens material. D is the diffusion coefficient for oxygen movement in the material and K is the solubility constant of oxygen in the material.

DK/L the DK value of a lens material divided by the central thickness (L) of a specific lens of that material. DK/L is known as the *oxygen transmissibility* of the lens.

-duction a stem word used with a prefix to describe the turning or rotation of the eyeball (abduction, turning out; adduction, turning in; deorsumduction, turning down; sursumduction, turning up).

dyslexia difficulty in reading, either in recognition of letters or interpretation, in spite of good vision in each eye.

dystrophy abnormal or defective development; degeneration.

Early Treatment Diabetic Retinopathy Study (ETDRS) acuity testing chart a special chart that incorporates specific design criteria to make it more accurate than the Snellen or Sloan acuity test charts. The designs include same number of letters (five) per row, equal spacing of the rows on a log scale, equal spacing of the letters on a log scale, and individual rows balanced for letter difficulty.

ecchymosis discoloration of skin caused by extravasation of blood into tissues after injury.

ectropion an eversion, or turning outward, of the eyelid.

electronic health records (EHRs) healthcare records that provide the ability for electronic exchange of patient data from practice setting to practice setting.

electronic medical records (EMRs) a system of computerized information, similar to a paper-based chart, that contains a wide range of patient data including patient demographics, medical history, medications, allergies, immunizations, vital signs, physical examination findings, laboratory tests, radiologic images, photos, prescriptions, and billing and insurance information.

electroretinogram a recording of the cornea–retinal potential.

emmetropia refractive condition of the normal eye; when the eye is at rest, the image of distant objects is brought to a focus on the retina.

endophthalmitis inflammation of most of the internal tissues of the eyeball.

enophthalmos backward displacement of the globe.

entropion turning inward of the eyelid.

enucleation complete surgical removal of the eyeball.

eosinophil a form of white blood cells containing cytoplasmic granules that are stained by the dye eosin. They are present in increased numbers with allergic reactions and some parasitic conditions and decrease with steroid therapy.

epiphora excessive tearing causing an overflow onto the face.

episclera a loose structure of fibrous and elastic tissue on the outer surface of the sclera. It contains a large number of blood vessels, in contrast to the sclera, which contains none.

episcleritis inflammation in the tissues overlying the sclera.

equivalent oxygen performance (EOP) an in vivo measurement of how much total oxygen passes through a contact lens and reaches the cornea. The measurement takes into account not only the lens material but also the thickness and design of the lens.

erysipelas acute infection of the skin and subcutaneous tissues.

esodeviation the deviation inward of the line of sight of the nonfixing eye from the point of fixation of the fixating eye.

esophoria tendency of the eye to turn inward.

esotropia manifest turning inward of the eye (convergent strabismus, or crossed eye).

evisceration surgical removal of the contents of the globe.

excentric fixation a monocular condition in which a parafoveal point is used for fixation. Usually the vision is very poor and the projection of that eye to a target is erroneous.

excimer a form of laser for ablation of the cornea. The word is a contraction of "excited" and "dimer."

exenteration surgical removal of the orbital region.

exodeviation the deviation outward of the line of sight of the nonfixing eye from the point of fixation of the fixating eye.

exophoria tendency of the eye to turn outward.

exophthalmos abnormal protrusion of the eyeball.

exotropia abnormal turning outward from the nose of one or both eyes (divergent strabismus).

extended wear contact lens wear in which the lenses may be worn continuously, day and night, without removal for up to 7 days.

extraocular muscles the six muscles that cause movement of the eye: medial and lateral recti, superior and inferior recti, and superior and inferior oblique.

extrinsic muscles external muscles of the eye that move the eyeball. Each eye has four recti and two oblique muscles.

eye grounds *see* fundus.

Farnsworth-Munsell 100-hue test a color-hue matching test to diagnose types and degrees of color blindness.

far-sightedness *see* hyperopia.

field of vision entire area that can be seen without shifting the eye.

fingerprint corneal dystrophy fine wavy lines resembling a fingerprint that appear on an otherwise normal cornea.

fissure elliptic space between the eyelids.

flare, aqueous the Tyndall effect, or the scattering of light in a beam directed into the anterior chamber, occurring as a result of increased protein content of the aqueous humor; a sign of severe inflammation of the iris and/or ciliary body.

flat cornea a cornea with a K value less than 41.00 diopters.

floaters small particles consisting of cells, pigment, or fibrin that move in the vitreous.

fluorescein an organic compound that is inert and used to stain the tear film for primarily rigid contact lens fitting and to assess the integrity of the cornea. It glows in the presence of ultraviolet light or cobalt blue light. It stains areas of epithelial damage yellowish green.

fluorescein angiography a procedure in which fluorescein dye is injected so that retinal choroidal circulation and iris circulation can be examined and photographed.

focal length the distance between the plane of a lens and the focal point of an object from infinity. The dioptric power is the reciprocal of this measurement in meters. All optical testing instruments and prescriptions use back focal lengths or back dioptric powers.

focal point the point at which distant light comes to a focus after being reflected or refracted.

focus point to which rays converge after passing through a lens.

fornix a loose fold of the conjunctiva, occurring where that part of the conjunctiva covering the eyeball meets the conjunctiva lining the eyelid.

fovea small depression in the retina at back of eye; the part of the macula adapted for most acute vision.

frequent replacement contact lens (also referred to as programmed or planned replacement contact lens) a hydrogel lens designed to be discarded and replaced at predetermined, regular intervals. The replacement cycle is usually 2 weeks, 1 month, or 3 months and cannot exceed 6 months.

Fuchs' dystrophy edema in the stroma associated with scarring on both the endothelium and the epithelium.

fundus inside of the eye, primarily the retina, the optic disc, and the retinal vessels that can be seen with an ophthalmoscope.

fusion power of coordination by which the images received by the two eyes become a single image.

gas-permeable lenses lenses that permit the passage of oxygen and carbon dioxide through the material.

ghost vessels empty vessels remaining after corneal invasion by blood vessels.

giant papillary conjunctivitis (GPC) also called giant papillary hypertrophy (GPH), a condition associated with contact lens wear, especially soft lens wear, marked by increasing lens awareness, itching, mucous discharge, formation of a coating on the contact lens, and papillae. The papillae form on the tarsal conjunctiva of the upper lid.

glare irregularly scattered light that interferes with the focused retinal picture and reduces visual acuity.

glaucoma an ocular disease having as its primary characteristic a sustained increase in intraocular pressure that the eye cannot withstand without damage to its structure or impairment of its function. This increased pressure can manifest in a variety of symptoms and signs, such as excavation of the optic disc, hardness of the eyeball, reduced visual acuity, seeing of colored halos around lights, visual field defects, and headaches. *Absolute glaucoma* is a final and hopeless stage of glaucoma in which the eye loses total light perception. *Acute glaucoma* is a sudden and painful type of glaucoma caused by a rapid rise in intraocular pressure. It is referred to as *angle-closure glaucoma*. *Congenital glaucoma* is caused by developmental anomalies in the region of the angle of the anterior chamber that present an obstruction to the drainage mechanism of the intraocular fluids. In *open-angle glaucoma*, the most common form, the angle of the anterior chamber is open. It usually is hereditary, is often symptomless, and produces slow erosion of the visual field.

glioma malignant tumor of the retina or optic nerve.

goniolens a contact lens designed to view the filtration angle of the anterior chamber.

gonioscope a magnifying device used in combination with strong illumination and a contact lens for examining the angle of the anterior chamber of the eye.

Gram staining the method of identifying bacteria and other microbes according to their reaction to a dye, that is, gram-positive or gram-negative.

granuloma a benign nodule that occurs as a result of a localized inflammation.

Gunn syndrome congenital ptosis associated with jaw winking.

guttata small whitish island deposits on Descemet's membrane that appear drop shaped.

hard lenses term sometimes used to refer to rigid lenses including polymethyl methacrylate (PMMA) and rigid gas permeable (RGP).

Hassali-Henie bodies drop-like particles of hyaline material seen in the periphery of Descemet's membrane.

hemangioma tumor arising from endothelial cells most frequently seen in the choroid.

hematoma swelling of the tissues caused by a large hemorrhage.

hemianopia blindness in one half of the visual field of one or both eyes. *Altitudinal hemianopia* is blindness of either the upper or the lower half of the visual field. *Bitemporal hemianopia* involves the temporal halves of the visual fields of both eyes. *Homonymous hemianopia* involves one-half of the visual field on the same side (right or left, nasal or temporal) in both eyes.

herpes simplex inflammatory condition of the conjunctiva, cornea, and iris caused by herpes simplex virus.

herpes zoster ophthalmicus inflammatory condition of the fifth cranial nerve, affecting the eyelid skin and eye structures.

herpetic keratitis recurring episodes of corneal epithelial inflammation caused by the herpes simplex virus.

heterochromia of iris a difference of color between the two irides.

heterophoria constant tendency of the eye to deviate from the normal position for binocular fixation, counterbalanced by simultaneous fixation prompted by the desire for singular binocular vision. Deviation is not usually apparent.

heterotropia an obvious or manifest deviation of visual axis of an eye out of alignment with the other eye. Synonyms are *crosseye* and *strabismus*.

high-order aberrations physical visual defects of multiple varieties, such as coma, trefoil, spherical aberrations, corneal scarring, and cataracts.

hippus marked variation in the size of the pupil. Could be spasmodic, rhythmic dilation, and constriction of the pupil (independent of illumination, fixation, or psychic stimuli).

HIV (human immunodeficiency virus) a virus causing a deficiency of the immune system, making the individual susceptible to a variety of infections.

homonymous *see* hemianopia.

hordeolum *see* stye.

hyalitis (asteroid) calcium-containing opacities in the vitreous.

hydrogel lens a soft lens that has an affinity to absorb and bind water into its molecular structure.

hydrophilic refers to the property of a material that has an affinity for water.

hyperopia (hypermetropia) a refractive error in which, because the eyeball is short or the refractive power of the lens is weak, the point of focus for rays of light from distant objects falls behind the retina; thus accommodation to increase the refractive power of the lens is necessary for distance vision, as well as near vision.

hyperphoria tendency of one eye to deviate upward, controllable by fixational efforts.

hypertropia deviation upward of one eye; not controllable by fixational efforts.

hyphema hemorrhage in the anterior chamber of the eye.

hypopyon cells pooled in the lower part of anterior chamber of the eye.

incipient pertaining to early changes.

injection a term sometimes used to mean congestion of ciliary or conjunctival blood vessels; redness of the eye.

interpupillary distance (or pupillary distance [PD]) is the distance in millimeters between the centers of the two pupils of both eyes.

interstitial keratitis inflammation of the middle layer of the cornea; found chiefly in children and young adults, and usually caused by transmission of syphilis from the mother to the unborn child.

intracorneal ring a ring of tissue inserted into the peripheral cornea to reduce myopic refractive errors.

intraocular pressure the pressure of the fluid within the eye measured in millimeters of mercury.

IOL intraocular lens.

iridectomy operation to remove iris tissue. In peripheral iridectomy, tissue is removed from the base of the iris; in full iridectomy, tissue is removed from the base to the pupillary margin.

iridocyclitis inflammation of the iris and ciliary body.

iris colored circular membrane suspended behind the cornea and immediately in front of the lens. The iris regulates the amount of light entering the eye by changing the size of the pupil.

iris bombé bulging forward of the midpart of the iris, thus severely narrowing the angle of the anterior chamber.

iritis inflammation of the iris; the condition is marked by pain, inflammation, discomfort from light, contraction of the pupil, and disorientation of the iris. It may be caused by injury, syphilis, rheumatism, gonorrhea, tuberculosis, or other systemic disease.

ischemia localized anemia of the retina caused by arterial constriction and subsequent visual grayout or blackout.

Ishihara's test a test for detecting defects in recognizing colors, based on the tracing of numbers or patterns in a series of multicolored charts or plates.

isopter a line connecting points that are of equal sensitivity to light.

jack-in-the-box phenomenon objects that appear to jump to view from the peripheral visual field when one wears strong plus lenses; occurs after cataract surgery.

Jackson cross cylinder a single lens composed of a plus cylinder and a minus cylinder of equal power located perpendicular to each other; used to refine the cylinder, axis, and power during refraction.

Jaeger's test types a test for near vision, in which lines of reading matter are printed in a series of type sizes.

K the keratometer reading of the corneal meridians.

Kayser-Fleischer ring pigmented ring encircling the cornea.

keratectomy removal of a portion of the cornea.

keratitis inflammation of the cornea; frequently classified as to type of inflammation and layer of cornea affected; for example, interstitial keratitis and phlyctenular keratitis.

keratitis sicca dryness of the cornea.

keratoconus (conical cornea) cone-shaped deformity of the cornea.

keratometer (ophthalmometer) an instrument that measures the central 3.3 mm of the anterior curvature of the cornea in its two meridians. The readings are called K readings. The measurement is in diopters, with the average cornea having a power of 42.00 to 48.00 diopters.

keratomileusis refractive surgery in which a portion of the cornea is removed, reshaped, and replaced.

keratopathy a noninflammatory disease of the cornea.

keratoplasty corneal transplant operation.

Kestenbaum rule a formula used to estimate the power of low-vision aid that is needed.

Krimsky method an assessment of eye deviation with the use of prisms to equalize the position of the corneal light reflex in each eye.

lacrimal apparatus the tear-producing and tear-disposal system of the eye.

lacrimal gland a gland that secretes tears; it lies in the upper outer angle of the orbit.

lacrimal sac the dilated upper end of the lacrimal duct.

lacrimation production of tears.

lagophthalmos a condition in which the lids cannot completely close.

lamellar keratoplasty operation in which only the diseased outer layers of the cornea are removed and the healthy donor cornea is sutured as a replacement.

laser an instrument that transforms an intense beam of light into energy that affects tissue; acronym for *l*ight *a*mplification by *s*timulated *e*mission of *r*adiation.

laser-assisted in situ keratomileusis (LASIK) a surgical laser vision correction procedure in which a thin flap of corneal tissue with a hinge is created, the flap is then retracted, the excimer laser is used to ablated the tissue beneath the flap and the flap is repositioned.

laser trabeculoplasty a treatment by laser light that shrinks the trabecular meshwork; used for the relief of glaucoma.

lens a piece of glass or other transparent substance shaped so that rays of light converge or scatter. Also the transparent biconvex body of the eye. An *aphakic lens* is a convex spectacle lens of high dioptric power, so named because its principal use is in the correction of vision in aphakia. In a *biconvex lens*, both surfaces are convex. It is used for the treatment of hyperopia ("far-sightedness"). In a *biconcave lens* both surfaces are concave. It is used in myopia ("near-sightedness"). A *bifocal lens* is constructed of two separate lenses, each having a different power. The upper portion is used for distance vision and the lower portion for near vision. A *cross cylinder* is a compound lens in which the dioptric powers in the principal meridians are equal but opposite in sign; it is usually mounted with the handle midway between the principal meridians. It is used to determine the axis and power needed for correcting astigmatism. A *luxated lens* is a crystalline lens of the eye that is completely displaced from the pupillary aperture. A *subluxated lens* is a crystalline lens of the eye that is partially displaced but remains in the pupillary aperture.

lensectomy a procedure to remove the clear crystalline lens to reduce high myopic errors.

leukokoria any pathologic condition, such as retrolental fibroplasia, that produces a white reflex in the pupillary area.

leukoma a very dense opacity of the cornea.

light adaptation power of the eye to adjust itself to variations in the amount of light.

light perception (LP) ability to distinguish light from dark.

light projection ability to determine the quadrantal direction of light.

limbus boundary between the cornea and the sclera.

low-order aberrations physical visual defects that consist of myopia, hyperopia, and astigmatism.

lupus erythematosus organic disease of collagen origin.

macrophthalmia abnormally large eyeball, resulting chiefly from infantile glaucoma.

macula lutea retinae small area of the retina that surrounds the fovea and that with the fovea comprises the area of the retina that gives distinct vision. Also referred to as the *yellow spot*.

magnification increase in size achieved by a lens system; the ratio of image size to object size.

malingering decreased vision to avoid something unpleasant.

Marfan syndrome disease of connective tissue, with eye involvement consisting of luxated lens and tremulous iris.

megalocornea an abnormally large cornea.

megalophthalmos *see* buphthalmos.

meibomian glands sebaceous glands of the eyelid.

meibomianitis inflammation of the meibomian glands.

melanoma pigmented tumor of the eye.

melanosis a condition characterized by abnormal deposits of melanin or pigment.

microcornea small cornea of 10 mm or less.

microphthalmia an abnormally small eyeball.

microscopic glasses magnifying lenses arranged on the principle of a microscope; occasionally prescribed for people with very poor vision.

miotic a drug that causes the pupil to contract.

mires the targets of the ophthalmometer that are reflected back from the cornea.

mirror writing inverting words while writing and a slowing of reading speed.

Mittendorf's dot a remnant of an embryonic hyaloid artery seen as a small dense floating opacity behind the posterior lens capsule.

monocular pertaining to or affecting one eye.

mucocele a pathologic swelling of a cavity caused by an accumulation of the mucoid material.

muscae volitantes small floating spots entoptically observed on viewing a bright uniform field; caused by minute embryonic remnants in the vitreous humor.

mydriasis enlargement of the pupil by the iris dilator muscle as occurs in darkness or in response to dilating drops.

mydriatic agent a drug that dilates the pupil.

myokymia twitching of individual muscle bundles of the eyelid.

myopia (near-sightedness) a refractive error in which the eyeball is too long in relation to its focusing power; thus the point of focus for rays of light from distant objects (parallel light rays) is in front of the retina.

myopic conus myopic crescent.

myotomy surgical division of muscle fibers.

nasal step depression of the nasal peripheral portion of the field. A sign of glaucoma.

near point of accommodation nearest point at which the eye can perceive an object distinctly. It varies according to the power of accommodation.

near point of convergence nearest single point at which the two eyes can direct their visual lines.

near vision the ability to perceive objects distinctly at normal reading distance or about 14 inches (35 cm) from the eyes.

nebula a faint or slightly misty corneal opacity.

needling surgical operation for opening a membrane following cataract surgery or in congenital cataracts in which the cataract or anterior capsule is pierced by a needle-like knife.

neovascularization recent formation of new blood vessels in a part, such as the cornea or retina.

neuritis inflammation of a nerve or nerves.

neuroblastoma a malignant tumor of the nervous system, one type of which is the retinoblastoma or tumor of the retina.

neuroophthalmology branch of ophthalmology that deals with the part of the nervous system associated with the eye.

neutralization the combining of two lenses of opposite powers to produce a resultant power of zero (one lens neutralizes the other).

night blindness a condition in which the sight is good by day but deficient at night or in faint light; seen in retinitis pigmentosa.

nystagmus an involuntary oscillating, rapid movement of the eyeball; it may be lateral, vertical, rotary, or mixed.

occluder an opaque or translucent device placed before an eye to obscure or block vision.

oculus dexter (OD) right eye.

oculus sinister (OS) left eye.

oculus uterque (OU) each eye.

ophthalmia inflammation of the eye or of the conjunctiva.

ophthalmia neonatorum an acute, purulent conjunctivitis of the newborn (sometimes defined as an inflamed or discharging eye in a newborn baby <2 weeks of age).

ophthalmic medical technician the separate occupational classification established by the U.S. Bureau of Labor's Standard Occupational Classification Committee in 2010 to encompass all three levels of the International Joint Commission on Allied Health Personnel in Ophthalmology (IJCAHPO) certification, Certified Ophthalmic Assistants (COA®), Certified Ophthalmic Technician (COT®), and Certified Ophthalmic Medical Technologist (COMT®) and to differentiate the ophthalmic medical assisting profession from "medical assisting."

ophthalmodynamometry measurement of the blood pressure in the retinal vessels of the eye.

ophthalmoplegia paralysis of one or more ocular muscles.

ophthalmoscope an instrument used in examining the interior of the eye.

optic atrophy degeneration of the nerve tissue that carries impulses from the retina to the brain.

optic chiasm crossing of the fibers of the optic nerves on the lower surface of the brain.

optic disc head of the optic nerve in the eyeball.

optic nerve special nerve of the sense of sight that carries impulses from the retina to the brain.

optic neuritis inflammation of the optic nerve.

optical center the point on a lens in which light rays are not bent. It corresponds to the thinnest portion of a minus lens and the thickest portion of a plus lens.

optical coherence tomography (OCT) a noninvasive diagnostic modality that provides high-resolution, cross-sectional imaging of ocular tissue in vivo. It is predominantly used to assess retinal and macular tissue and to study and monitor posterior ocular disease and glaucoma. The technique is similar to ultrasound except that it uses light of wavelength 843 nm rather than sound waves.

optotype a standardized symbol found on vision testing charts. It can consist of specially shaped letters, numbers, or geometric symbols.

ora serrata retinae anterior border of the retina.

orbit the bony cavity containing the eye, which is formed by the frontal, sphenoid, ethmoid, nasal, lacrimal, and maxillary bones.

orthokeratology the technique of flattening the cornea and thus correcting refractive errors by the use of a series of progressively flatter contact lenses.

orthoptic training series of scientifically planned exercises for developing or restoring normal teamwork of the eyes.

overrefraction determination of final lens power by performing a refraction over a contact lens.

pachometer a device used to measure the thickness of the cornea and the depth of the anterior chamber.

palpebral pertaining to the eyelid.

palpebral fissure opening between the eyelids.

pannus invasion of the cornea by infiltration and formation of new blood vessels.

panophthalmitis inflammation of the whole eyeball.

pantoscopic angle the angle of spectacle lenses when rotated on the X-axis to set the lens normal to the fixation axis below the horizon. Commonly measured as the angle between spectacle temple and the plane of the eyewear as angulated back from the perpendicular.

papilledema (papilloedema) edema of the optic nerve head; termed *choked disc* when caused by increased intracranial pressure.

papilloma a benign epithelial new growth.

Parinaud oculoglandular syndrome a group of clinical findings in which there is a unilateral granulomatous conjunctivitis often associated with an enlarged preauricular or submandibular lymph node.

pars planitis exudative edema on posterior portion of the retina.

partially sighted child for educational purposes, a child who has a visual acuity of 20/70 or less in the better eye after the best possible correction and who cannot use vision as the chief channel of learning.

perimeter an instrument for measuring the field of vision peripherally.

periorbita the loose connective tissue within the orbit.

peripheral vision ability to perceive the presence, motion, or color of objects outside the direct line of vision.

phacoanaphylaxis hypersensitivity to the protein of the crystalline lens.

phacoemulsification emulsification of a cataractous lens by ultrasound, permitting the material to be removed by aspiration.

phakic refers to an eye that still possesses its natural crystalline lens.

phlyctenular keratoconjunctivitis a variety of keratitis characterized by the formation of an inflammatory elevation on the cornea or conjunctiva. It usually occurs in young children and may be caused by poor nutrition, allergy, or tuberculosis.

-phoria a root word denoting a latent deviation in which the eyes have a constant tendency to turn from the normal position for binocular vision; used with a prefix to indicate the direction of such deviation (e.g., hyperphoria, esophoria, exophoria).

phoropter an instrument for determining the refractive state of the eye, phorias, and so on, consisting of a housing containing rotating disc with lenses, occluders, prisms, and pinholes.

photocoagulation procedure in which there is intentional burning by strong light. Vascular disease, tumors, and degenerative areas in the retina or the choroid may be treated by this means.

photophobia abnormal sensitivity to and discomfort from light.

photopic vision pertaining to vision in light-adapted conditions, mainly a cone function.

photorefractive keratotomy (PRK) a surgical procedure to correct vision by permanently changing the shape of the anterior central cornea using the excimer laser to remove, by vaporization, a small amount of the anterior corneal stroma just below the area of the corneal epithelium which is removed prior to the ablation. Post surgery the epithelium regenerates to cover the corneal defect.

phthisis bulbi a shrinking of the eyeball.

pinguecula yellowish, triangular thickening of bulbar conjunctiva, nasal or temporal to cornea.

pinhole disc a black disc with one or multiple openings that allow only central rays to pass through. Vision that is improved with a pinhole disc can be aided by spectacle lenses.

pleoptics a method of treating amblyopia ex anopsia by intense stimulation of light of the nonfoveal area to render the foveal area more receptive to fixational stimuli.

polycoria multiple pupils.

posterior chamber space between the back of the iris and the front of the lens; filled with aqueous.

posterior chamber (PC) lens an intraocular lens that is placed in the posterior chamber where a natural crystalline lens was previously located.

posterior pole of eye the center of the posterior curvature of the eyeball.

Prentice's rule formula for calculating prismatic effect induced at any point in the lens; the prism diopters equal the decentration (in centimeters) times the lens power (in diopters).

presbyopia a gradual lessening of the power of accommodation caused by a physiologic change that becomes noticeable about the age of 40 years.

Prince's rule a measuring scale used for determining a patient's near point of accommodation.

prism an optical system that deviates the path of light.

proptosis protrusion of the eye.

prosthesis replacement of a human eye by an artificial one.

pseudoisochromatic charts charts with colored dots of various hues and shades indicating numbers, letters, or patterns; used for testing color discrimination.

pseudophakia a condition in which an intraocular lens implant has replaced the crystalline lens.

pterygium a triangular fold of growing membrane that may extend over the cornea from the white of the eye. It occurs most frequently in people exposed to dust or wind.

ptosis (blepharoptosis) a drooping of the upper eyelid.

quadrantanopia blindness or loss of vision in a quarter sector of the visual field of one or both eyes.

recession operation to sever the eye muscle from its original insertion and reattach it more posteriorly on the sclera.

refraction deviation in the course of rays of light in passing from one transparent medium into another of different density; the sum of steps performed in arriving at a decision as to what lens or lenses (if any) will most benefit the patient.

refractive error a defect in the eye that prevents light rays from being brought to a single focus exactly on the retina.

refractive index the refractive power of a substance in comparison with that of air.

refractive media transparent parts of the eye having refractive power; cornea and lens. The aqueous and vitreous are transparent but contribute very little refractive power.

refractometry the measurement of refractive error.

resection operation to remove a portion of a muscle and tendon to shorten it; operation to remove a portion of the sclera to shorten it.

residual astigmatism the astigmatism present after the corneal astigmatism has been nullified by a contact lens. It is the astigmatism created by the crystalline lens of the eye.

retina innermost coat of the eye, formed of sensitive nerve elements and connected with the optic nerve.

retinal detachment a separation of the inner layer of the retina from the outer layer and the choroid.

retinitis inflammation of the retina.

retinitis pigmentosa a hereditary degeneration and atrophy of the retina; usually migration of pigment occurs.

retinoblastoma a malignant tumor of the retina.

retinopexy surgical reattachment of a detached retina.

retinoscope an instrument for determining the refractive state of the eye.

retinoscopy objective method of determining the refractive error of the eye by observing the movements of light reflected from the back of the eye.

retrobulbar behind the eyeball.

retrolental fibroplasia a disease of the retina in the premature infant in which the retina is partially or completely detached and pulled forward against the posterior surface of the lens.

rods and cones *see* cones and rods.

rose bengal a dye used to detect cells that are damaged or unprotected by native mucoproteins.

S, SC (sine correction) without correction; that is, not wearing prescribed lenses.

sac a bag-like structure.

safety glasses impact-resistant spectacles; available with or without visual correction for workshop or street-wear protection; used by adults and children.

Schirmer's test filter paper test for tear flow.

Schlemm's canal circular channel located deep in the limbus. The channel collects aqueous fluid from the anterior chamber to the episcleral veins. A circular canal situated at the junction of the sclera and cornea through which the aqueous is eliminated after it has circulated between the lens and the iris and between the iris and the cornea.

sclera white part of the eye; a tough covering that, with the cornea, forms the external protective coat of the eye.

scleritis inflammation of the sclera.

scotoma an area of reduced or lost vision in the visual field (relative or absolute scotomas).

scotopic vision vision in low light levels that involves rod photoreceptors.

second(s) of arc a second of arc is a tiny angle. A full circle consists of 360 degrees. One degree is divided into 60 minutes of arc. Each minute of arc contains 60 seconds of arc, so a second of arc is an angle that is 1/3600 of a degree. For instance, 20/20 vision in humans is the ability to resolve a spatial pattern separated by a visual angle of 1 minute of arc. A 20/20 letter subtends 5 minutes of arc total.

secretagogue an agent, such as a hormone or pharmaceutical that stimulates secretion.

siderosis bulbi deposit of iron pigment in the eyeball.

slit lamp lamp that provides a narrow beam of strong light; often used with a corneal biomicroscope for examination of the front portions of the eye.

small-incision intrastromal lenticular extraction (SMILE) a method of intrastromal keratomileusis in which a femtosecond laser is used to create 2 cuts within the cornea and 1 small superficial cut. A lenticule is produced of a specific shape and thickness, and is pulled mechanically true a 2-3 mm diameter corneal incision.

Snellen's chart chart used for testing central visual acuity, consisting of lines of letters, numbers or symbols in graded sizes drawn to Snellen's measurements. Each size is labeled with the distance at which it can be read by the normal eye. It is most often used for testing vision at a distance of 20 feet (6 m), but charts may be drawn for testing at reading distance (14 inches [35 cm]) or intermediate distances.

soft lens a contact lens composed either of *hydrogel* material, a watery gel-like material that contains more than 10% water, or of silicone.

spastic entropion turning in of lid margin.

spectacle blur blurred vision that lasts for 15 minutes or longer after a contact lens is removed and spectacles are used.

specular microscopy a noninvasive photographic technique using a reflected-light microscope that allows visualization and analysis of the corneal endothelial cell size, shape, and density.

spherical equivalent the equivalent of spectacle refraction expressed only as a sphere. To obtain it, take half of the cylinder and algebraically add it to the sphere.

spherical lens segment of a sphere, refracting rays of light equally in all meridians.

sterilization the complete death of all forms of bacteria, fungi, and spores.

stereocampimeter instrument used to measure the visual fields and determine central scotomas.

stereoscopic vision *see* depth perception.

staphyloma a bulging, or protrusion, of the cornea or the sclera.

strabismus squint; failure of the two eyes simultaneously to direct their gaze at the same object because of muscle imbalance. It may be convergent, divergent, alternating, or vertical.

stroma corneal layer underlying Bowman's membrane composed of dense strata of collagen fiber laid down in a regular manner. The stroma comprises about 90% of the cornea's thickness.

stye (hordeolum) acute inflammation of a sebaceous gland in the margin of the eyelid.

subluxation of lens incomplete dislocation of the crystalline lens.

symblepharon adhesion of conjunctiva of the eyelid to conjunctiva of the globe.

sympathetic ophthalmia inflammation of one eye caused by an inflammation of the other eye, without infection. May follow surgery or trauma.

synechia adhesion, usually of the iris to the cornea or angle structures (anterior) or the lens (posterior).

taco test a test to determine that a soft contact lens is not inside out by grasping the lens near its apex and folding it so the edge will roll in like a taco if it is not everted.

tangent screen a large, usually black curtain 1 or 2 meters in diameter, supported by a framework on which the central field of vision and the blind spot may be outlined; used for measuring the central field of vision.

tarsorrhaphy the stitching together of the upper and lower eyelids partially or completely to provide protection to the cornea.

tarsus framework of connective tissue that gives shape to the eyelid.

tear film breakup time (BUT) an evaluation of tear quality; the tear film will normally break up in 10 to 30 seconds and show dry spots. Any dry spot that appears in less than 10 seconds is pathologic.

tears a composite of secretions from lacrimal glands, accessory glands of Kraus and Wolfring, mucin-secreting goblet cells of the conjunctiva, meibomian-secreting tarsal glands, and oil-secreting glands of Teis.

telescopic glasses magnifying spectacles founded on the principles of a telescope; occasionally prescribed for improving very poor vision that cannot be helped by ordinary glasses.

temporal pallor loss of color (bleaching) of the temporal portion of the optic disc.

Tenon's capsule membranous tissue that envelops the whole eyeball except the cornea.

tension, intraocular pressure or tension of the contents of the eyeball.

thermokeratoplasty a form of heat that is used to shrink the collagen of the cornea and cause corneal steepening and reduction of hyperopic refractive error.

tonic pupil pupil that does not move with accommodation or direct light reflex.

tonography determination of the flow of aqueous humor into the eye and from the eye under the continuous pressure exerted by the weight of a tonometer over a 4- or 5-minute period.

tonometer instrument for measuring the pressure of the eye.

topography-guided photorefractive keratotomy (PRK) surgical technique that uses the excimer laser guided by corneal imaging to reduce irregular astigmatism by flattening steep areas and steepening flat areas; main indications are for keratoconus, pellucid marginal degeneration, and ectasia after laser vision correction

toxoplasmosis protozoal disease leading to inflammatory uveitis, strabismus, and nystagmus.

trabecular meshwork the drainage network in the iridocorneal angle through which aqueous humor leaves the eye.

trabeculectomy surgical removal of a portion of the trabeculum for improved outflow of aqueous in glaucoma patients.

trachoma a form of infection of the conjunctiva and cornea caused by a specific virus that, in the chronic form, produces severe scarring of the eyelids and cornea.

transposition the process of changing a spectacle prescription from a plus to a minus cylinder or vice versa without changing its refractive value. A + 2.00 + 1.00 × 90 lens is equivalent to a + 3.00 − 1.00 × 180 lens. The rule is to add the cylinder to the sphere, change the sign of the cylinder and rotate the axis by 90 degrees.

trephining removing of a circular button, or disc, of tissue.

trichiasis inversion of the eyelashes, resulting in impingement on the eyeball and subsequent irritation.

trochlea a ring-like structure of fibrocartilage attached to the frontal bone through which passes the tendon of the superior oblique muscle of the eyeball.

-tropia a root word denoting an obvious deviation from normal of the axis of the eyes (strabismus); used with a prefix to denote the type of strabismus (e.g., heterotropia, esotropia, exotropia).

tunnel vision contraction of the visual field to such an extent that only a small area of central visual acuity remains, thus giving the affected individual the sensation of looking through a tunnel.

ulcer, corneal pathologic loss of substance of the surface of the cornea caused by progressive erosion and necrosis of the tissue.

uvea entire vascular coat of the eyeball, consisting of the iris, ciliary body, and choroid.

uveitis inflammation of the vascular coat of the eye.

VA abbreviation for visual acuity.

vaccinia autoinoculation of smallpox vaccine causing corneal or lid lesions.

vascularization increased blood vessels occurring in a cornea.

verruca solid lesion on lid margin.

version referring to a binocular eye movement.

vertex distance distance from the posterior surface of the lens to the anterior surface of the eye (for measuring purposes, the closed lid). Important in aphakic prescriptions, in high myopia, and in high hyperopia.

vertigo dizziness, normally caused by disturbance in the inner ear.

vesiculation the formation of vesicles or blisters.

virulence the disease-producing properties of a microorganism.

VISC vitreous infusion suction cutter; used to cut and remove portions of the vitreous.

vision act or faculty of seeing; sight.

visual purple a pigment in the outer layers of the retina, a photochemical substance mediating light into nerve impulses.

visuscope an instrument designed to determine the type of monocular fixation in amblyopia.

vitreous transparent, colorless mass of soft, gelatinous material filling the eyeball behind the lens.

vitreous opacities *see* floaters.

von Graefe's sign a delay in downward movement of the upper eyelid as it follows the eyeball to downward gaze; seen in thyroid disease.

Vossius' ring a ring of iris pigment granules that is deposited on the anterior lens capsule after blunt trauma to the eye.

wavefront aberration the deviation in an optical system from the desired perfect planar wavefront propagation.

wavefront analyzer an instrument used to measure the way light travels through an eye's optical pathway and compares it with the pathway of light traveling through an optically perfect eye.

wavelength a physical property of light apparent in its color. Violet has a short wavelength, red a long wavelength. Different tissues absorb different wavelengths preferentially, making the various lasers useful for specific purposes.

Wirt stereo test a depth perception test. For a child, three lines of animals are shown from which to make a selection. If all three lines are correctly selected, the child has stereopsis of approximately 100 seconds of arc. For adults there are nine frames of raised rings, the first being the most obvious, the last the most difficult. If all are read correctly, stereopsis of 40 seconds of arc is present.

Worth four-dot test a test to detect amblyopia. The patient wears spectacles with a green lens and a red lens and looks at a target of one white, one red, and two green discs. If four discs are seen, there is no suppression of either eye. If three discs are seen, there is suppression; if five discs are seen, fusion is absent.

xanthelasma (xanthoma) small yellowish tumor of the eyelids, usually occurring in older adults or those with a high level of blood cholesterol.

xanthopsia a condition in which objects appear to be tinted yellow.

xerophthalmia drying of the eye surface, with loss of the corneal and conjunctival luster.

xerosis conjunctivae condition of dryness of the conjunctiva caused by the failure of its own secretory activity, or lack of tears.

yoke muscles muscles in opposite eyes that act together.

zonules the supporting fibers of the lens attached at their other end to the ciliary body.

Appendix | 1 |

Ocular emergencies

I. Ocular complications of systemic disease	
Disease	**Possible ocular findings**
Diabetes mellitus	Background retinopathy: retinal hemorrhages, exudates, and microaneurysms
	Preproliferative retinopathy: cotton-wool spots, intraretinal microvascular abnormalities
	Proliferative retinopathy: neovascularization, preretinal hemorrhage, vitreous hemorrhage, retinal detachment
Graves disease	Lid retraction, lid lag, exposure keratopathy, chemosis and injection, restriction of eye movements, proptosis, compressive optic neuropathy
Hypertension	Sclerosis of vessels in long-standing disease; narrowing of vessels, retinal hemorrhages and/or exudates in severe hypertension
Rheumatoid arthritis and other collagen vascular diseases	Dry eye, episcleritis, scleritis, peripheral corneal ulceration and/or melting
Cancer	Metastatic disease to choroid may result in retinal detachment; disease in the orbit can result in proptosis and restriction of eye movements (e.g., breast, lung cancer)
Sarcoidosis	Dry eye, conjunctival granulomas, iritis, retinitis
AIDS	Kaposi sarcoma, cotton-wool spots of retina, cytomegalovirus retinitis

II. Life-threatening ocular signs	
Findings	**Clinical significance**
White pupil	In an infant, retinoblastoma must be ruled out
Aniridia (iris appears absent)	May be autosomal dominant ($^2/_3$ s) or sporadic inheritance; in sporadic cases where the short arm of chromosome 11 is deleted, there is a 90% risk of developing Wilms' tumor; the risk in other sporadic cases is approximately 20%
Thickened corneal nerves (slit lamp)	Part of the multiple endocrine neoplasia syndrome type IIB; must rule out medullary carcinoma of the thyroid; pheochromocytoma and parathyroid adenomas

Continued

II. Life-threatening ocular signs—cont'd

Findings	Clinical significance
Retinal angioma	May be part of von Hippel-Lindau syndrome; autosomal dominant inheritance with variable penetrance; must rule out hemangioblastomas of the central nervous system, renal cell carcinoma, and pheochromocytoma
Multiple pigmented patches of fundus	Lesions represent patches of congenital hypertrophy of the retinal pigment epithelium; may be part of Gardner's syndrome, characterized by multiple premalignant intestinal polyps together with benign soft tissue tumors (lipomas, fibromas, sebaceous cysts) and osteomas of the skull and jaw; a complete gastrointestinal investigation is indicated; if a diagnosis of Gardner's syndrome is made, prophylactic colectomy is indicated because of the potential for malignant degeneration of colonic polyps
Third-nerve palsy with a dilated pupil	Must rule out an intracranial aneurysm or neoplastic lesion; CT scan and/or MRI should be performed on an emergency basis
Papilledema	Must rule out an intracranial mass lesion; CT scan and/or MRI should be performed on an emergency basis
Pigmentary degeneration of the retina and motility disturbance	May represent the Kearns-Sayre syndrome; must rule out a cardiac condition disturbance with an annual electrocardiogram; may develop an intraventricular conduction defect, bundle block, bifascicular disease, or complete heart block; patient must be prepared for the possible need to implant a pacemaker

III. Ocular complications of systemic medications

Medication	Ocular complications
Amiodarone	Superficial whorl-like keratopathy
Chlorpromazine	Anterior subcapsular cataracts
Corticosteroids	Posterior subcapsular cataracts, glaucoma
Digitalis	Blurred vision, disturbed color vision
Ethambutol	Optic neuropathy
Hydroxychloroquine	Superficial keratopathy and bull's-eye maculopathy
Indometacin	Superficial keratopathy
Isoniazid	Optic neuropathy
Nalidixic acid	Papilledema
Sildenafil	Optic neuropathy
Tamsulosin	Cataract surgery complications secondary to floppy iris and intraoperative miosis
Tetracycline	Papilledema
Thioridazine	Pigmentary degeneration of the retina
Vitamin A	Papilledema

IV. Differential diagnosis of the nontraumatic red eye

Feature	Condition		
	Acute conjunctivitis	**Acute iritis**	**Acute glaucoma**
Symptoms	Redness, tearing ± discharge, itching	Redness, pain, photophobia	Redness, severe pain, nausea, vomiting
Appearance	Conjunctival injection	Ciliary injection	Diffuse injection
Vision	Normal; can be blurred secondary to discharge	Moderate reduction	Marked reduction, halo vision
Cornea	Clear	May see keratic precipitates	Hazy secondary to edema
Pupil	Normal	Small, sluggish to light	Semidilated, nonreactive
Secretions	Tearing to purulent	Tearing	Tearing
Test and comments	Smears may show etiology; bacterial infection = polycytes; viral infection = monocytes; allergy = eosinophils	Slit lamp will show cells and flare in the anterior chamber	Elevated intraocular pressure
Treatment	Antibiotic Vigamox*	Steroids, cycloplegics	Pilocarpine, Travatar Z*, Duotrav*, Azarga*, Diamox*, mannitol, laser surgery

*Trademark or registered product.

V. Differential diagnosis of viral, bacterial, and allergic conjunctivitis

Feature	Viral	Bacterial	Allergy
Discharge	Watery	Purulent	Watery
Itching	Minimal	Minimal	Marked
Preauricular lymph node	Common	Absent	Absent
Stain and smear	Monocytes	Bacteria	Eosinophils
	Lymphocytes	Polycytes	

VI. Differential diagnosis of red eye in contact lens wearers

Diagnosis	Findings	Mechanism	Treatment
Corneal abrasion	Epithelial defect; stains with fluorescein	Mechanical, hypoxia	Antibiotic drops (e.g., Vigamox*)
Superficial punctate keratitis	Punctate corneal staining	Mechanical, chemical toxicity	Artificial tears (e.g., Systane ULTRA*)
Giant papillary conjunctivitis	Papillary reaction of superior tarsal conjunctiva	Immunologic, mechanical	Mast cell stabilizer (e.g., Patanol* drops)

Continued

VI. Differential diagnosis of red eye in contact lens wearers—cont'd

Diagnosis	Findings	Mechanism	Treatment
Sterile infiltrates	Corneal infiltrate; epithelium usually intact	Immunologic	Antibiotic drops (assume infected)
Infected ulcer	Corneal infiltrate with ulceration; stains with fluorescein	Infection (e.g., *Pseudomonas, Staphylococcus aureus,* etc.)	Corneal scraping for Gram stain and culture. Fortified antibiotic drops, Vigamox*

AIDS, acquired immunodeficiency syndrome; *CT*, computed tomography; MRI, magnetic resonance imaging.

Reproduced with permission from Stein RM, Stein HA. *Ocular Emergencies*. 6th ed. Montreal: Medicopea; 2016.

Appendix | 2 |

Following universal precautions

The best way to reduce occupational risk of "bloodborne" infection is to follow universal precautions based on the concept that every patient should be treated with the same level of precautionary and preventive measures to ensure the safety of everyone involved, including healthcare personnel. The following list of universal precautions is extracted from the Occupational Safety and Health Administration (OSHA) regulation "Occupational exposure to bloodborne pathogens." Please refer to this publication for complete instructions and precautionary guidelines. Ophthalmic medical personnel should regularly review all universal precautions presented there, ensure that they understand them completely, and adhere to them at all times.

1. Wash hands before and after patient contact, and immediately if hands become contaminated with blood or other body fluids.
2. Wear gloves whenever there is a possibility of contact with body fluids.
3. Wear masks whenever there is a possibility of contact with body fluids via airborne route.
4. Wear gowns if exposed skin or clothing is likely to be soiled.
5. During resuscitation procedures, ensure that pocket masks or mechanical ventilation devices are readily available for use.
6. Clean spills of blood or blood-containing body fluids with a solution of household bleach (sodium hypochlorite) and water in a 1:100 solution for smooth surfaces and a 1:10 solution for porous surfaces.
7. Healthcare professionals who have open lesions, dermatitis, or other skin irritations should not participate in direct patient care activities or handle contaminated equipment.
8. Contaminated needles should never be bent, clipped, or recapped. Immediately after use, contaminated sharp objects should be discarded into a puncture-resistant "sharps" container designed for this purpose.

9. Contaminated equipment that is reusable should be cleaned of visible organic material, placed in an impervious container, and returned to central hospital supply or some other designated place for decontamination and reprocessing.
10. Instruments and other reusable equipment used in performing invasive procedures should be disinfected and sterilized as follows:
    • Equipment and devices that enter the patient's vascular system or other normally sterile areas of the body should be sterilized before being used for each patient
    • Equipment and devices that touch intact mucous membranes, but do not penetrate the patient's body surfaces, should be sterilized when possible, or undergo high-level disinfection if they cannot be sterilized before being used for each patient
    • Equipment and devices that do not touch the patient or that only touch intact skin need only be cleaned with a detergent or as indicated by the manufacturer
11. Body fluids to which universal precautions always apply are as follows: blood, serum/plasma, semen, vaginal secretions, cerebrospinal fluid, vitreous fluid, synovial fluid, pleural fluid, pericardial fluid, peritoneal fluid, amniotic fluid, and wound exudates.
12. Body fluids to which universal precautions apply only when blood is visible in them are as follows: sweat, tears, sputum, saliva, nasal secretions, feces, urine, vomitus, and breast milk.

Optimal infection control in the eye care setting is based on the assumption that all specified human body fluids are potentially infectious. Many transmissible diseases of the external eye, such as adenoviral conjunctivitis, cause redness that immediately indicates infection. Other infectious agents, however, can be present on the ocular surface without causing inflammation. Human immunodeficiency virus (HIV), hepatitis B virus, hepatitis C virus, rabies virus, and the agent of Creutzfeldt-Jakob disease are not immediately obvious without systemic clues or laboratory testing. Every patient must be approached as potentially contagious. Guidelines for routine ophthalmic examinations include the following:

- Wash hands between patient examinations. Use disposable gloves if an open sore, blood, or blood-contaminated fluid is present. Using cotton-tipped applicators to manipulate the eyelids can also minimize direct contact.
- Avoid unnecessary contact. Eyedropper bottles used in the office should not directly touch the eyelids, eyelashes, or ocular surface of any patient. Individual sterile strips impregnated with dye are preferred where available.

- Disinfect all contact instruments after each use. Tonometer tips and pachometer tips should be soaked in diluted bleach or hydrogen peroxide after every use. Trial contact lenses must be disinfected between patients.
- Handle sharp devices carefully. Needles must always be discarded into puncture-resistant (sharps) containers.

References

Reproduced with permission from O'Hara MA. *Ophthalmic Medical Assisting: An Independent Study Course.* 6th ed. San Francisco: American Academy of Ophthalmology; 2017.

Reproduced with permission and with modifications from Reidy JJ. *Basic and Clinical Science Course, Section 8: External Disease and Cornea.* San Francisco: American Academy of Ophthalmology; 2012–2013.

Appendix |3|

Principles of informed consent

Informed consent

Informed consent permits the patient to exercise self-determination. The law imposes a "duty of disclosure" on the part of the physician.

Contents of an informed consent document

- Risks of procedure, including loss of vision
- Benefits of procedure
- Complications
- Alternative treatments
- Explanation of procedure
- Advantages of one procedure over another
- Significant issues (e.g., bilateral vs. sequential)

Duty of disclosure

1. To frankly answer all specific questions about the risk.
2. Without being questioned, to disclose:
   - The nature of the proposed procedure
   - The gravity of it
   - All material risks
   - All special and unusual risks in the particular circumstances
   - Alternative procedures available and their risks, including the consequences of no treatment

Material risks

A risk is material if it would be considered a significant issue by a reasonable person weighing the decision to consent to the procedure. A one in 1000 chance is probably not a material risk. A one in 100 chance is probably a material risk. Risks of very serious or grave consequence should be disclosed no matter how remote.

Special and unusual risks

The patient's particular circumstances, such as occupational, familial, and social circumstances, make certain risks significant to that patient (e.g., a risk of visual loss should be disclosed to a commercial pilot even if it is remote).

Consent

Consent may be written, oral, or implied from the circumstances (e.g., the patient holds out an arm for an injection).

Regardless of the form of the consent, the physician must be able to prove that the duty of disclosure was met before the consent was obtained. Therefore a prudent physician will make a note on the chart of the risks disclosed and the patient's comments or questions.

Exceptions

In an emergency, the duty of disclosure and obtaining consent is waived.

When the patient plainly does not wish to hear about the risks, the duty of disclosure is waived, but consent should be obtained and circumstances noted on the chart.

In rare circumstances, if the physician can prove that disclosing the risks would create a state of mind in the patient that would seriously hinder successful treatment, the duty of disclosure is waived but consent should be obtained and the circumstances noted on the chart.

Failure to disclose

When an undisclosed risk occurs and the patient sues and the court determines the risk should have been disclosed because it was material or because of the patient's particular circumstances, the physician will be liable if the court is satisfied that another person in the patient's position would have refused the treatment had the risks been disclosed.

For cosmetic purposes and for treatments for which there is little medical justification or urgency, liability of the physician is more likely if an undisclosed risk materializes. Therefore it is prudent to outline all of the risks.

Experimental procedures, particularly involving healthy volunteers, warrant utmost disclosure of risks.

The duty of disclosure also embraces what the surgeon knows or should know that the patient deems relevant to the patient's decision whether to undergo the operation. If the patient asks specific questions about the operation, then the patient is entitled to be given reasonable answers to such questions.

A risk that is a mere possibility ordinarily does not have to be disclosed, but if its occurrence may result in serious consequences, such as paralysis, blindness, or even death, then it should be treated as a material risk and should be disclosed.

The patient is entitled to be given an explanation as to the nature of the operation and its gravity.

Appendix | 4 |

Abbreviations and symbols in clinical use

Symbol/Abbr.	Meaning	Symbol/Abbr.	Meaning
$\smile$	combine with	E^1	esophoria for near
$<^a$	less than	EOM	extraocular movements
$>^a$	greater than	EOM	extraocular muscle
$\circ$	degree	EOMB	extraocular muscle balance
∞	infinity	ET	esotropia
Δ	prism diopter	ET_1	esotropia for distance
+	convex lens	ET^1	esotropia for near
−	concave lens	g	gram
A	applanation tensions	gt	drop (gutta)
ac	before meals (ante cibum)	HM	hand movements
Acc	accommodation	hs	at bedtime (hora somni)
add	addition	IO	inferior oblique (muscle)
ARC	abnormal retinal correspondence	Ic	between meals (inter cibum)
ASC	anterior subcapsular cataract	IR	inferior rectus (muscle)
AT or Appl	applanation tension	J1, J2, J3, etc.	test types for reading vision
BD	base down	KP	keratic precipitates
bid or bd	twice daily (bis in die)	L&A	light and accommodation
BI	base in	LE	left eye
BO	base out	LH	left hyperphoria
BU	base up	IOP	intraocular pressure
C or cyl	cylinder lens	LP	light perception
CC or c	with correction	LR	lateral rectus (muscle)
C/D	cup/disk ratio	mcg	microgram
CF	counting fingers	mg	milligram
D	diopter	mL or ml^b	milliliters
dd	disc diameters	mm	millimeter
E(T)	intermittent esotropia	MR	Maddox rod
E_1	esophoria for distance	MR	medial rectus (muscle)

N5, N6, etc.	test types for near vision	RE	right eye
ne rep or non rep	do not repeat	RH	right hyperphoria
NLP	no light perception	Rx	prescription (recipe)
NPA	near point of accommodation	S or sph	spheric lens
NPC	near point of convergence	s	without correction
NRC	normal retinal correspondence	SC	without correction
NV	near vision	Sig	label (signa)
occulent	eye ointment	SO	superior oblique (muscle)
OD	right eye (oculus dexter)	Sol	solution
OS	left eye (oculus sinister)	SR	superior rectus (muscle)
OT	ocular tension	ST	Schiotz tension
OU	both eyes (oculus uterque)	stat	at once
pc	after meals (post cibum)	Susp	suspension
PD or IPD	interpupillary distance	T	tension
PERRLA	pupils equal, round, reactive to light and accommodation	tid or td	three times daily (ter in die)
		tsp	teaspoon
PH	pinhole	ung	ointment (unguentum)
po	orally, by mouth (per os)	V	vision or visual acuity
Pr	presbyop	VAc or VAcc	visual acuity with correction
prn	as necessary, as needed (pro re nata)		
PRRE	pupils round, regular, and equal	VAs or VAsc	visual acuity without correction
PSC	posterior subcapsular cataract	VF	visual field
qd[c]	every day (quaque die)	W	wearing
q4h	every 4 hours (quaque quarta hora)	X(T)	intermittent exotropia
qh	every hour (quaque hora)	X_1	exophoria for distance
qid	four times daily (quarter in die)	X^1	exophoria for near
ql	as much as wanted (quantum libert)	XP	exophoria
qs	quantity sufficient	XT	exotropia

[a]The Joint Commission recommends writing "less than" or "greater than" for the symbols < and >.
[b]The Joint Commission states mL is preferred over ml.
[c]Abbreviation on the official "Do Not Use" list of The Joint Commission.

Optical constants of the eye[a]

Optical constants of the eye are summarized as follows:

- The curvature of the anterior face of the cornea is 7.5 mm.
- The index of refraction of the corneal tissue, the aqueous humor, and the vitreous equals 1.332.
- The distance separating the anterior pole of the cornea from the posterior pole of the crystalline lens is 3.6 mm.
- The curvature of the anterior face of the crystalline lens measures 10 mm.
- The curvature of the posterior face of the crystalline lens is 6 mm.
- The distance separating the anterior pole of the crystalline lens from the posterior pole of the crystalline lens is 4 mm.
- The main refraction index of the crystalline lens equals 1.40.
- The dioptric power of the cornea equals 44.26 diopters.
- The dioptric power of the crystalline lens alone, when both of its surfaces are immersed in a medium having an index of 1.332, equals 17.82 diopters.
- The total power of the eye equals 58.53 diopters.
- The distance of the first principal plane of the crystalline lens back of the anterior pole of the crystalline lens is 2.4 mm.
- The distance of the second principal plane of the crystalline lens ahead of the posterior pole of the crystalline lens is 1.4 mm.
- The distance separating these two planes is 0.4 mm.
- The distance of the principal plane of the whole eye behind the anterior pole of the whole cornea is 1.370 mm.
- The distance of the second principal plane of the whole eye behind the anterior pole of the whole cornea is 1.664 mm.
- The distance separating these two planes is 0.294 mm.

[a]Reproduced with permission from Hartstein J. *Basics of Contact Lenses Manual*. San Francisco: American Academy of Ophthalmology; 1979.

Appendix | 6 |

Metric conversion (United States)

	When you know	Multiply by (approximation)	To find
Length	inches (in)	2.54	centimeters (cm)
	feet (ft)	30.48	centimeters (cm)
	miles (mi)	1.61	kilometers (km)
Area	square inches (sq in)	6.45	square centimeters (cm^2)
	square miles	2.60	square kilometers (km^2)
Weight	ounces (oz)	28.35	grams (g)
	pounds (lb)	0.45	kilograms (kg)
Volume and capacity	teaspoons (tsp)	4.93	milliliters (mL)
	tablespoons (tbsp)	14.78	milliliters (mL)
	fluid ounces (fl oz)	29.57	milliliters (mL)
	cups (c)	0.24	liters (L)
	pints (pt)	0.47	liters (L)
	quarts (qt)	0.95	liters (L)
	gallons (gal)	3.79	liters (L)
	cubic inches (cu in)	16.3871	cubic centimeters (cc)
Speed and velocity	miles per hour (mph)	1.61	kilometers per hour (km/h)
	feet per second (fps)	30.48	centimeters per second (cm/s)
Temperature	Fahrenheit temperature (°F)	($5/9$ after subtracting 32)	Celsius temperature (°C)

Mass
 1 lb = 0.45 kg
 1 kg = 2.21 lb
 $1/2$ oz = 15.55 g
 1 oz = 31.103 g

Length
 1 in = 2.540 cm
 1 ft = 0.3048 m
 1 mile = 1.61 km
 10 millimeters (mm) = 1 cm = 0.3937 in

100 cm = 1 m = 39.37 in
1000 m = 1 km = 0.62137 mile

Volume (United States)

1 q = 0.946 L
1 gal = 3.79 L
$^{1}/_{2}$ oz = 14.786 mL
1 oz = 25.573 mL
1 mL = 1 cc = 0.0338 fl oz

10 cl = 1 deciliter (dL) = 6.102 in^2
1 dL = 0.10 L = 0.211 liquid pt
10 dL = 1 L = 1.057 liquid qt
100 L = 1 hectoliter (hl) = 26.425 gal

Temperature

0° Celsius = 32° Fahrenheit
0° Fahrenheit = − 17.78° Celsius
100° Celsius = 212° Fahrenheit

Supplementary resources

Books, eBooks, downloadable PDFs, DVDs, CD-ROMs

American Academy of Ophthalmology. *Basic and Clinical Science Course* (13 sections). San Francisco: American Academy of Ophthalmology; 2022–2023 (Updated annually).

American Academy of Ophthalmology. *Care and Handling of Ophthalmic Microsurgical Instruments*. 4th ed. San Francisco: American Academy of Ophthalmology; 2017.

American Academy of Ophthalmology. *Focal Points® Modules* (Serial Publications, eBook, Print, Audio. Access to 100+ issues in digital archives). San Francisco: American Academy of Ophthalmology; 2010–2022 (Published and revised as appropriate).

American Academy of Ophthalmology. *Introducing Ophthalmology: A Primer for Office Staff*. 3rd ed (Online). San Francisco: American Academy of Ophthalmology; 2013.

American Academy of Ophthalmology. *Ophthalmic Coding Coach* (Print and Online). San Francisco: American Academy of Ophthalmology; 2021.

American Academy of Ophthalmology. *The Dispensing Ophthalmologist eBook*. San Francisco: American Academy of Ophthalmology; 2021.

American Academy of Ophthalmology. *Ultimate Documentation Compliance Training for Scribes and Technicians* (Online). San Francisco: American Academy of Ophthalmology; 2021.

American Association for Pediatric Ophthalmology and Strabismus. *AAPOS Vision Screening Kit*. San Francisco: American Association for Pediatric Ophthalmology and Strabismus; 2021.

American Heart Association. *Advanced Cardiovascular Life Support (ACLS): Provider Manual*. 16th ed. Dallas: American Heart Association; 2016.

American Heart Association. *American Heart Association 2015 Guidelines for CPR and ECC*. Dallas: American Heart Association; 2015.

American Heart Association. *2015 Handbook of Emergency Cardiovascular Care for Health Providers*. Dallas: American Heart Association; 2015.

Association of Technical Personnel in Ophthalmology. *ATPO Exam Review Flash Cards (COA®, COT®, COMT®, ROUB®, OSA)*. Association of Technical Personnel in Ophthalmology; 2010, 2013, 2015.

Blais BR. *AMA Guides to the Evaluation of Ophthalmic Impairment and Disability: Measure the Impact of Visual Impairment on Activities of Daily Life*. Chicago: American Medical Association; 2011.

Blomquist PH. *Practical Ophthalmology: A Manual for Beginning Residents*. 7th ed. San Francisco: American Academy of Ophthalmology; 2015.

Byrne SF, Green RL. *Ultrasound of the Eye and Orbit*. 2nd ed. New Delhi: Jaypee Brothers Medical Publishers; 2010.

Cassin B, Rubin ML. *Dictionary of Eye Terminology*. 6th ed. Gainesville, FL: Triad Publishing; 2011.

Corboy JM. *The Retinoscopy Book: An Introductory Manual for Eye Care Professionals*. 5th ed. Thorofare, NJ: Slack; 2003.

Dansby-Kelly A. *Ophthalmic Procedures in the Operating Room and Ambulatory Surgery Center*. 4th ed. San Francisco: American Society of Ophthalmic Registered Nurses; 2016.

Dean EC, Gomez JL, Welch RM, et al. *Essentials of Ophthalmic Nursing Books 1, 2, 3 & 4*. San Francisco: American Society of Ophthalmic Nurses; 2014–2015.

DuBois L. *Clinical Skills for the Ophthalmic Examination: Basic Procedures*. 2nd ed. Thorofare, NJ: Slack Inc.; 2005.

Erickson B, Modi Y. *The Yale Guide to Ophthalmic Surgery*. Philadelphia: Wolters Kluwer/Lippincott Williams & Wilkins; 2011.

Faye EE, Chan-O'Connell L, Fischer M, et al. *The Lighthouse Clinician's Guide to Low Vision Practice*. New York: Lighthouse International; 2011.

Fraunfelder FT, Fraunfelder FW, Chambers W. *Drug-Induced Ocular Side Effects: Clinical Ocular Toxicology*. 8th ed. Philadelphia: Elsevier; 2021.

Friedman NJ, Kaiser PK, Pineda R. *The Massachusetts Eye and Ear Infirmary Illustrated Manual of Ophthalmology*. 5th ed. Philadelphia: Elsevier; 2021.

Goldberg S, Tattler W. *Ophthalmology Made Ridiculously Simple with CD (Atlas)*. 5th ed. MedMaster: Miami; 2019.

Harper RA, editor. *Basic Ophthalmology: Essentials for Medical Students* (Print and eBook). 18th ed. San Francisco: American Academy of Ophthalmology; 2016.

Hoffer KJ. *IOL Power*. Thorofare, NJ: Slack Inc.; 2011.

Henderer JD. *Dictionary of Eye Terminology*. 7th ed. San Francisco: American Academy of Ophthalmology; 2019.

Hung D, Lumbroso B. *Optical Coherence Tomography Angiography of the Eye: OCT Angiography*. Thorofare, NJ: Slack Inc.; 2017.

International Joint Commission on Allied Health Personnel in Ophthalmology. *IJCAHPO CD Lecture Packets*. St. Paul, MN: International Joint Commission on Allied Health Personnel in Ophthalmology; Multiple dates.

International Joint Commission on Allied Health Personnel in Ophthalmology. *IJCAHPO's Clinic CE Subscription. More than 160 online courses*. St Paul, MN: International Joint Commission on Allied Health Personnel in Ophthalmology; Continuously updated.

International Joint Commission on Allied Health Personnel in Ophthalmology. *IJCAHPO Learning Systems—A Series of 6*

Simulated Courses: Keratometry, Lensometry, Ocular Motility, Retinoscopy/Refinement, Tonometry and Visual Fields (CD-ROM). St Paul, MN: International Joint Commission on Allied Health Personnel in Ophthalmology; Multiple dates.

International Joint Commission on Allied Health Personnel in Ophthalmology. *IJCAHPO Refinements Modules (Series of Clinical Topics for Ophthalmic Medical Personnel).* St Paul, MN: International Joint Commission on Allied Health Personnel in Ophthalmology; 1997–2022.

International Joint Commission on Allied Health Personnel in Ophthalmology. *IJCAHPO Simulation and Interactive Courses.* St. Paul, MN: International Joint Commission on Allied Health Personnel in Ophthalmology; Multiple dates.

International Joint Commission on Allied Health Personnel in Ophthalmology. *IJCAHPO Study Guides (COA®, COT®, COMT®).* St. Paul, MN: International Joint Commission on Allied Health Personnel in Ophthalmology; 2019.

International Joint Commission on Allied Health Personnel in Ophthalmology. *Ophthalmic Assisting 101. Online course.* St. Paul, MN: International Joint Commission on Allied Health Personnel in Ophthalmology; Multiple dates.

International Joint Commission on Allied Health Personnel in Ophthalmology. *Scribe Pocket Guide—The Role of the Ophthalmic Scribe.* St. Paul, MN: International Joint Commission on Allied Health Personnel in Ophthalmology; 2019.

International Joint Commission on Allied Health Personnel in Ophthalmology/Association of Technical Personnel in Ophthalmology. *IJCAHPO/ATPO Pocket Guide: A Clinical Skills and Reference Guide for the Ophthalmic Technician.* 2nd ed. St. Paul, MN: International Joint Commission on Allied Health Personnel in Ophthalmology; 2012.

Jogi R. *Basic Ophthalmology.* 5th ed. New Delhi: Jaypee Brothers Medical Publishers; 2016.

Jost A. *Train the Trainer—Ophthalmic Training Strategies that Work.* Lexington, KY: Association of Technical Personnel in Ophthalmology; 2019.

Kahook MY, Schuman JS. *Chandler and Grant's Glaucoma.* 5th ed. Thorofare, NJ: Slack Inc.; 2013.

Kanski JJ. *Signs in Ophthalmology: Causes and Differential Diagnosis* (Print and eBook). Elsevier/Mosby: St Louis; 2010.

Karlsson VC. *Systematic Approach to Strabismus.* 2nd ed. Thorofare, NJ: Slack Inc.; 2009.

Kolker RJ, Kolker AF. *Subjective Refraction and Prescribing Glasses: The Number One (or Number two) Guide to Practical Techniques and Principles.* 3rd ed. Thorofare, NJ: Slack, Inc.; 2018.

Ledford JK, Hoffman J. *Quick Reference of Eye Terminology.* 5th ed. Thorofare, NJ: Slack Inc.; 2008.

Ledford JK, Lens A. *Principles and Practice in Ophthalmic Assisting: A Comprehensive Textbook.* Thorofare, NJ: Slack Inc.; 2018.

Leitman MW. *Manual for Eye Examination and Diagnosis.* 9th ed. Oxford: Wiley-Blackwell; 2016.

Lens A. *Optics, Retinoscopy and Refractometry.* 2nd ed. Thorofare, NJ: Slack Inc.; 2005.

Levine LA, Nilsson SFE, Hoeve JV, et al. *Adler's Physiology of the Eye, Expert Consult.* 11th ed. St Louis: Elsevier/Mosby; 2011.

Machin H. *Ophthalmic Operating Theatre Practice: A Manual for Lower-Resource Setting* (Print and Downloadable PDF). 2nd ed. London: International Center for Eye Health, London School of Hygiene and Tropical Medicine; 2016.

Marmor MF, Ravin JG. *The Artist's Eyes: Vision and the History of Art.* New York: Abrams; 2009.

Martonyi CL, Charles F, Bahn CF, Meyer RF. *Slit Lamp: Examination and Photography.* 3rd ed. Sedona, AZ: Time One Ink; 2007.

Milder B, Rubin ML. *The Fine Art of Prescribing Glasses. Without Making a Spectacle of Yourself.* 3rd ed. Gainesville, FL: Triad Publishing; 2004.

Mukherjee PK. *Ophthalmic Assistant.* New Delhi: Jaypee Brothers Medical Publishers; 2013.

Nelson LB, Levin AV. *Wills Eye Strabismus Surgery Handbook.* Thorofare, NJ: Slack Inc.; 2015.

O'Hara MA. *Ophthalmic Medical Assisting: An Independent Study Course.* 6th ed. San Francisco: American Academy of Ophthalmology; 2017.

Phillips N, Hornacky A. *Berry & Kohn's Operating Room Technique.* 14th ed. Philadelphia: Elsevier; 2022.

Pacheco L. *Care and Handling of Ophthalmic Microsurgical Instruments.* 4th ed. San Francisco: American Society of Ophthalmic Registered Nurses; 2017.

Riordan-Eva P. *Vaughan & Asbury's General Ophthalmology.* 19th ed. New York: McGraw-Hill/Lange; 2017.

Rubin ML. *Optics for Clinicians,* 25th anniversary ed. Gainesville, FL: Triad Publishing; 1993.

Saine PJ, Tyler ME. *Ophthalmic Photography.* 2nd ed. Philadelphia: Elsevier/Butterworth-Heinemann; 2001.

Salmon J. *Kanski's Clinical Ophthalmology: A Systematic Approach.* 9th ed. Philadelphia: Elsevier/ Saunders; 2021.

Schwartz GS. *Around the Eye in 365 Days.* Thorofare, NJ: Slack Inc.; 2009.

Shukla AV. *Clinical Optics Primer for Ophthalmic Medical Personnel: A Guide to Laws, Formulae, Calculations and Clinical Applications.* Thorofare, NJ: Slack Inc.; 2009.

Singh AD, Hayden BC. Ophthalmic Ultrasonography. Philadelphia: Elsevier/Saunders; 2012.

Sisson C. *Ophthalmic Imaging: Posterior Segment Imaging, Anterior Eye Photography and Slit Lamp Biomicrography (Applications in Scientific Photography).* New York: Routledge; 2018.

Slack Inc. Publishers. *The Basic Bookshelf for Eye Care Professionals (Series of Clinical Topics for Ophthalmic Medical Personnel).* Thorofare, NJ: Slack Inc.; 1998–2016.

Stein HA, Stein RM, Freeman MI, et al. *Ophthalmic Dictionary and Vocabulary Builder–For Eye Care Professionals.* 4th ed. New Delhi: Jaypee-Highlights Medical Publishers; 2012.

Stein R, Stein H. *Management of Ocular Emergencies.* 6th ed. Montreal: Mediconcept; 2016.

Steinert RF. *Cataract Surgery.* 3rd ed. Philadelphia: Elsevier/ Saunders; 2010.

Tasman W, Jaegar EA. *Duane's Clinical Ophthalmology on DVD-ROM,* 2013 ed. Philadelphia: Lippincott Williams & Wilkins; 2013.

Tille P. *Bailey & Scott's Diagnostic Microbiology.* 14th ed. St. Louis: Elsevier/Mosby; 2018.

Tortora GJ, Funke BR, Case CL, et al. *Microbiology: An Introduction* (Print and eBook), 13th ed. London: Pearson; 2018.

Trob JD. *The Physician's Guide to Eye Care.* 4th ed. San Francisco: American Academy of Ophthalmology; 2012.

Wang M. *Corneal Topography: A Guide for Clinical Application in the Wavefront Era.* 2nd ed. Slack: Thorofare. NJ; 2012.

Welch RM, Waldo MN. *Ophthalmic Procedures in the Office and Clinic,* 4th ed. San Francisco: American Society of Ophthalmic Registered Nurses; 2017.

Index

Note: Page numbers followed by *b* indicate boxes *f* indicate figures, and *t* indicate tables.